The Oxford Handbook of
Intellectual Disability and Development

OXFORD LIBRARY OF PSYCHOLOGY

Editor-in-Chief PETER E. NATHAN

The Oxford Handbook of Intellectual Disability and Development

Edited by

Jacob A. Burack

Robert M. Hodapp

Grace Iarocci

Edward Zigler

OXFORD
UNIVERSITY PRESS

OXFORD
UNIVERSITY PRESS

Published in the United States of America by Oxford University Press, Inc.,
198 Madison Avenue, New York, NY, 10016
United States of America

Oxford University Press, Inc. publishes works that further
Oxford University's objective of excellence in research, scholarship, and education

Oxford is a registered trade mark of Oxford University Press in the UK and in certain other countries

This handbook is an update of the *Handbook of Mental Retardation and Development*
(1998, Cambridge University Press).

Library of Congress Cataloging-in-Publication Data

The Oxford handbook of intellectual disability and development / edited by
Jacob A. Burack ... [et al.].
    p. cm.
Includes index.
ISBN 978-0-19-530501-2
1. Mental retardation. 2. Developmental disabilities. 3. People with mental disabilities. I. Burack, Jacob A. II. Title:
Handbook of intellectual disability and development.
RC570.O96 2011
362.196'89—dc22   2010054102

978-0-19530501-2

1 3 5 7 9 10 8 6 4 2

Typeset in Adobe Garamond Pro
Printed on acid-free paper
Printed in the United States of America

SHORT CONTENTS

OXFORD LIBRARY OF PSYCHOLOGY

The *Oxford Library of Psychology*, a landmark series of handbooks, is published by Oxford University Press, one of the world's oldest and most highly respected publishers, with a tradition of publishing significant books in psychology. The ambitious goal of the *Oxford Library of Psychology* is nothing less than to span a vibrant, wide-ranging field and, in so doing, to fill a clear market need.

Encompassing a comprehensive set of handbooks, organized hierarchically, the *Library* incorporates volumes at different levels, each designed to meet a distinct need. At one level are a set of handbooks designed broadly to survey the major subfields of psychology; at another are numerous handbooks that cover important current focal research and scholarly areas of psychology in depth and detail. Planned as a reflection of the dynamism of psychology, the *Library* will grow and expand as psychology itself develops, thereby highlighting significant new research that will impact on the field. Adding to its accessibility and ease of use, the *Library* will be published in print and, later on, electronically.

The *Library* surveys psychology's principal subfields with a set of handbooks that capture the current status and future prospects of those major subdisciplines. This initial set includes handbooks of social and personality psychology, clinical psychology, counseling psychology, school psychology, educational psychology, industrial and organizational psychology, cognitive psychology, cognitive neuroscience, methods and measurements, history, neuropsychology, personality assessment, developmental psychology, and more. Each handbook undertakes to review one of psychology's major subdisciplines with breadth, comprehensiveness, and exemplary scholarship. In addition to these broadly conceived volumes, the *Library* also includes a large number of handbooks designed to explore in depth more specialized areas of scholarship and research, such as stress, health and coping, anxiety and related disorders, cognitive development, or child and adolescent assessment. In contrast to the broad coverage of the subfield handbooks, each of these latter volumes focuses on an especially productive, more highly focused line of scholarship and research. Whether at the broadest or most specific level, however, all of the *Library* handbooks offer synthetic coverage that reviews and evaluates the relevant past and present research and anticipates research in the future. Each handbook in the *Library* includes introductory and concluding chapters written by its editor to provide a roadmap to the handbook's table of contents and to offer informed anticipations of significant future developments in that field.

An undertaking of this scope calls for handbook editors and chapter authors who are established scholars in the areas about which they write. Many of the nation's and world's most productive and best-respected psychologists have agreed to edit *Library* handbooks or write authoritative chapters in their areas of expertise.

For whom has the *Oxford Library of Psychology* been written? Because of its breadth, depth, and accessibility, the *Library* serves a diverse audience, including graduate students in psychology and their faculty mentors, scholars, researchers, and practitioners in psychology and related fields. Each will find in the *Library* the information they seek on the subfield or focal area of psychology in which they work or are interested.

Befitting its commitment to accessibility, each handbook includes a comprehensive index, as well as extensive references to help guide research. And because the *Library* was designed from its inception as an online as well as a print resource, its structure and contents will be readily and rationally searchable online. Further, once the *Library* is released online, the handbooks will be regularly and thoroughly updated.

In summary, the *Oxford Library of Psychology* will grow organically to provide a thoroughly informed perspective on the field of psychology, one that reflects both psychology's dynamism and its increasing interdisciplinarity. Once published electronically, the *Library* is also destined to become a uniquely valuable interactive tool, with extended search and browsing capabilities. As you begin to consult this handbook, we sincerely hope you will share our enthusiasm for the more than 500-year tradition of Oxford University Press for excellence, innovation, and quality, as exemplified by the *Oxford Library of Psychology*.

Peter E. Nathan
Editor-in-Chief
Oxford Library of Psychology

ABOUT THE EDITORS

Jacob A. (Jake) Burack, Ph.D., is Professor of School/Applied Child Psychology and Human Development in the Department of Educational and Counselling Psychology at McGill University, Director of the McGill Youth Study Team (MYST), and a researcher at Hôpital Rivière-des-Prairies.

Robert M. Hodapp, Ph.D., is a Professor of Special Education in the Department of Special Education at Vanderbilt Peabody College and Director of Research at Vanderbilt University Center for Excellence in Developmental Disabilities.

Grace Iarocci, Ph.D., is Associate Professor of Developmental and Clinical Psychology in the Department of Psychology at Simon Fraser University, a Michael Smith Foundation for Health Research Scholar, and Director of the Autism and Developmental Disorders Lab at SFU.

Edward Zigler, Ph.D., is Sterling Professor of Psychology (Emeritus) at Yale University, founder and Director Emeritus of Yale's Edward Zigler Center in Child Development and Social Policy. He is a member of the Institute of Medicine and the American Academy of Arts and Sciences. In the 1970s, he was the founding Director of the U.S. Office of Child Development (now ACYF) and Chief of the U.S. Children's Bureau.

CONTRIBUTORS

Leonard Abbeduto
Waisman Center
University of Wisconsin-Madison
Madison, Wisconsin

Michal Al-Yagon
School of Education
Tel-Aviv University
Tel-Aviv, Israel

Armando Bertone
Neuroscience Laboratory for Research in
Education in Developmental Disorders
Department of Neurology and
Neurosurgery
McGill University
Montreal, Quebec, Canada

Anjali K. Bhatara
Laboratoire Psychologie de la Perception
Université Paris Descartes
CNRS UMR 8158
Paris, France

Nancy Brady
Schiefelbusch Institute for Life Span
Studies
University of Kansas
Lawrence, Kansas

Jon Brock
Macquarie Centre for Cognitive Science
Macquarie University
Sydney, Australia

Jacob A. Burack
Department of Educational &
Counselling Psychology
McGill University
Hôpital Rivières-des-Prairies
Montreal, Quebec, Canada

Robin S. Chapman
Emerita, Dept. of Communicative Disorders
University of Wisconsin
Madison, Wisconsin

Kim M. Cornish
Institute for Brain Development and
Repair and Centre for Developmental
Psychiatry & Psychology
Monash University, Australia

Tamara Dawkins
McGill University
Montreal, Quebec, Canada

Mayada Elsabbagh
Centre for Brain and Cognitive
Development
Birkbeck, University of London
London, United Kingdom

James T. Enns
Department of Psychology
University of British Columbia
Vancouver, British Columbia, Canada

Anna J. Esbensen
Waisman Center
University of Wisconsin
Madison, Wisconsin

Rinat Feniger-Schaal
Department of Psychology
University of Haifa
Haifa, Israel

Deborah J. Fidler
Department of Human Development and
Family Studies
Colorado State University
Ft. Collins, Colorado

Heidi Flores
Department of Educational and
Counselling Psychology
McGil University
Montreal, Quebec, Canada

Laraine Masters Glidden
Department of Psychology
St. Mary's College of Maryland
St. Mary's City, Maryland

Amanda Gulsrud
Semel Institute for Neuroscience and
Human Behavior
University of California
Los Angeles, California

Penny Hauser-Cram
Department of Applied Developmental
and Educational Psychology
Boston College
Chestnut Hill, Massachusetts

Robert M. Hodapp
Vanderbilt Kennedy Center &
Department of Special Education
Nashville, Tennessee

Patricia Howlin
Institute of Psychiatry
King's College London
London, United Kingdom

Mariëtte Huizinga
Department of Psychology
University of Amsterdam
The Netherlands

Grace Iarocci
Department of Psychology
Simon Fraser University
Burnaby, British Columbia, Canada

Laudan Jahromi
School of Social and Family Dynamics
Arizona State University
Tempe, Arizona

Christopher Jarrold
School of Experimental Psychology
University of Bristol
Bristol, United Kingdom

Connie Kasari
Graduate School of Education and
Information Studies
University of California, Los Angeles
Los Angeles, California

Annette Karmiloff-Smith
Centre for Brain and Cognitive
Development
Birkbeck, University of London
London, United Kingdom

Elizabeth Kay-Raining Bird
School of Human Communication
Disorders
Dalhousie University
Halifax, Nova Scotia, Canada

Alexandra P.F. Key
Vanderbilt Kennedy Center &
Department of Hearing and
Speech Sciences
Vanderbilt University
Nashville, Tennessee

Cary S. Kogan
Department of Educational
Psychology
McGill University
Montreal, Quebec, Canada

Nina Koren-Karie
School of Social Work
University of Haifa
Haifa, Israel

Sara T. Kover
Waisman Center
University of Wisconsin-Madison
Madison, Wisconsin

Marty Wyngaarden Krauss
Office of the Provost
Brandeis University
Waltham, Massachusetts

Barbara Landau
Department of Cognitive Science
Johns Hopkins University
Baltimore, Maryland

Daniel J. Levitin
Department of Psychology
Department of Educational
Counseling Psychology
McGill University
Montreal, Quebec, Canada

Malka Margalit
School of Education
Tel Aviv University
Tel Aviv, Israel

Andrea McDuffie
Waisman Center
University of Wisconsin-Madison
Madison, Wisconsin

Carolyn B. Mervis
Department of Psychological and
Brain Sciences
University of Louisville
Louisville, Kentucky

Joanna Moss
Cerebra Centre for
Neurodevelopmental Disorders
School of Psychology
University of Birmingham
Birmingham, United Kingdom

Alison Niccols
Department of Psychiatry &
Behavioural Neurosciences
Offord Centre for Child Studies
McMaster University
Hamilton, Ontario, Canada

Chris Oliver
Cerebra Centre for
Neurodevelopmental Disorders
School of Psychology
University of Birmingham
Birmingham, United Kingdom

David Oppenheim
Department of Psychology
University of Haifa
Haifa, Israel

Stephen A. Petrill
Department of Human Development and
Family Science
The Ohio State University
Columbus, Ohio

Mafalda Porporino
McGill University
Montreal, Quebec, Canada

Eve-Marie Quintin
Center for Interdisciplinary
Brain Sciences Research
Stanford University
Palo Alto, California

Natalie Russo
Department of Pediatrics
Albert Einstein College of Medicine
Bronx, New York

Department of Psychology
Syracuse University
Syracuse, New York

Gaia Scerif
Department of Experimental Psychology
University of Oxford
Oxford, United Kingdom

Louis A. Schmidt
Offord Centre for Child Studies
Department of Psychology,
Neuroscience & Behaviour
McMaster University
Hamilton, Ontario, Canada

Marsha Mailick Seltzer
Waisman Center
University of Wisconsin
Madison, Wisconsin

Karen Thomas
Department of Medicine
McMaster University
Hamilton, Ontario, Canada

Tricia A. Thornton-Wells
Department of Molecular Physiology
& Biophysics
Vanderbilt University
Nashville, Tennessee

Stefano Vicari
Department of Neuroscience
Institute of Research and
Clinical Care
Bambino Gesù Children's Hospital
Rome, Italy

Nurit Yirmiya
Department of Psychology
School of Education
Hebrew University of Jerusalem
Jerusalem, Israel

Edward Zigler
The Edward Zigler Center in Child
Development and Social Policy
Yale University
New Haven, Connecticut

PREFACE

Our goal with this volume was to update developments in the field of developmental theory and research as they apply to the study of persons with intellectual disability (ID). Although the volume is not entirely exhaustive on the topic, it reflects the excellence of the work in the field and the vast contributions of developmental researchers, their thinking, and their science. As noted in the opening and closing chapters of the volume, we clearly know considerably more about persons with ID than we did even a decade or two ago. And this knowledge provides us a map, or maybe many maps, to the direction(s) that we need to follow to continue to both better our science and to better the lives of persons with ID. With these goals in mind, we dedicate this volume to Eunice Shriver, who devoted so much of her life and used her position in the world to advance the well-being of persons with ID and their families.

As is the case with any edited volume, the success of this handbook was mostly contingent on folks other than those who have their name on the front cover. Accordingly, we are grateful to many. First and foremost, we are indebted to the authors of the various chapters who agreed to share the fruits of their hard work and scholarship, and uniformly provided excellent contributions. We thank Catharine Carlin, who enthusiastically recruited this volume and provided both friendship and sage advice throughout the long, but enjoyable, process. We thank Sarah Harrington who took over as the OUP editor of the volume near the beginning of the production phase and provided much support and insight about maximizing the contribution of the volume. We thank Chad Zimmerman, the Development Editor at OUP for his positive and upbeat work on the beginning stages of the transformation of the manuscript into a book. We thank Antonio Orrantia and Emily Perry, the Production Editors at OUP, and Aravind Raveendran, the Project Manager from Glyph International, for their thorough and thoughtful managing of the volume as it is being prepared for publication. We thank Phil Porter for allowing us to use his artwork on the cover, and Marsha Seltzer and Pat Mitchell of the Waisman Center at the University of Wisconsin for suggesting and arranging the use of Mr. Porter's artwork. We are grateful to the many members of the McGill Youth Study Team (MYST) who, under the guidance of Heidi Flores, formatted and edited the volume; they include Janice LaGiorgia, Stephanie Rishikof, Ariel Stee, Kira Barey, Kara Soerono, Colin Campbell, Elaina Zendegui, France Laine, Dana Hayward, Fallyn Leibovitch, Alexandra D'Arrisso, Cassandra Rodgers, Jenny Hoppenheim, and Megan McConnell. The work on the volume by the MYST members and by Jacob A. (Jake) Burack was supported by a research grant from the Social Sciences and Humanities Research Council of Canada to JAB.

We hope that this project is consistent with the legacy of Eunice Shriver, and that it contributes in meaningful ways to bettering the lives and the positions in life of persons with ID and of their families.

Jacob A. Burack, Robert M. Hodapp,
Grace Iarocci, and Edward Zigler

CONTENTS

PART 1

Introduction and Overview

CHAPTER 1

The More You Know the Less You Know, But That's OK: Developments in the Developmental Approach to Intellectual Disability

Jacob A. Burack, Natalie Russo, Heidi Flores, Grace Iarocci, *and* Edward Zigler

Abstract

The adage "the more you know, the less you know" may best describe the contributions of the developmental approach to the study of persons with intellectual disability. Based on this premise, we trace the development of the approach from its origins in the 19th century, and highlight both the advances and difficulties of an increasingly precise science that involves differentiating among etiological groups and fine-tuned developmental concepts. We also provide an overview of the five sections of the volume.

Keywords: Intellectual disability, intellectual development, developmental approach, cognition, defect approach

The adage that "the more you know, the less you know" might best describe the contributions of the developmental approach to the study of persons with intellectual disability (ID). The tremendous growth of developmentally oriented research in the two decades since our (Hodapp, Burack, & Zigler, 1990) first volume on *The Developmental Approach to Mental Retardation* led to remarkable advances in understanding the developmental pathways of persons with ID across all areas of functioning in relation to specific etiologies and ages (e.g., see Burack, Hodapp, & Zigler, 1998). The broadening of the scope involves the implementation of the framework of the whole person, in which personality, the social and emotional characteristics of the person, and familial and larger contextual factors are considered in addition to cognitive functioning. Yet, the original adage also serves to highlight the vast task of precisely charting functioning in all the areas, sub-areas, and sub-sub-areas of functioning for each of the many different etiologies of ID at different ages in relation to familial, community, and environmental factors. Accordingly, the adoption of a developmental framework entails more fine-grained

theory, more sophisticated experimental methodologies and, as a result, more knowledge about persons with ID at levels of both precision and breadth than could ever have been anticipated in prior conceptualizations.

The increased sophistication in science and specificity of knowledge highlight the futility of attempts to generalize findings across the heterogeneous group that we refer to as persons with ID and clearly renders meaningless the notion of a single grouping or field of research under the title of ID. Thus, the seemingly large advances in understanding only serve to set the stage for encounters with greater and increasingly fine-tuned, complex, and intertwined questions associated with etiology-specific conceptualizations within the context of developmental theory and considerations (for reviews, see Burack, Evans, Klaiman, & Iarocci, 2001; Burack, Root, & Shulman, 1996; Hodapp & Burack, 2006)—*the more we know, the more we know how little we know.*

Although facing the enormity of the developmental task may be daunting, it is preferable to the prior state of research on ID, in which the research contribution might have best been described as a variation of our adage, or, "the more we think we know, the less we really know." In that context of monolithic pronouncements of the origins of ID regardless of etiology, in which persons with ID were considered a homogenous group (for a discussion of predevelopmental conceptualizations of persons with intellectual disability, see Burack, 1990), big stories abounded, but none was scientifically sound and little was known about the nuances of each group or individual. Although each of more than 1,000 etiologies associated with ID differs from all the others in meaningful ways in virtually every aspect of functioning, persons with ID were grouped together as if they were a single entity, thereby obscuring important characteristics associated with the individual etiologies. Flawed research methodologies, including the obviously erroneous practice of matching persons with and without ID on chronological age (CA), led to false claims of defects among persons with ID in a variety of areas of functioning (for discussions of these shortcomings, see Burack et al., 2001; Iarocci & Burack, 1998). Thus, much was thought to be known about ID on a grand scale, but the reality was that the lack of theoretical and scientific precision left the field in the shambles of ignorance—*the more we knew, the less we knew.*

Yet, this is not a call of despair. The goal of the developmental approach was to promote the vision of theoretically sophisticated and methodologically precise research that can be cobbled together to provide a more precise understanding of persons with ID. This approach has its origins in 19th-century writings of Langdon Down and William Wetherspoon Ireland, who pioneered etiologically-specific research, and in the 20th-century writings by developmental theorists, including Heinz Werner, Edward Zigler, Dante Cicchetti, and their colleagues, who promoted the interface of developmental psychology and the study of ID. This approach finds fruition in the 21st-century sophistication of experimental technology and empirical methodology in the study of genetics, brain functioning, behavior, social and interpersonal functioning, and emotional well-being, as well as in the study of the relations among them. Through this synergy, the key to understanding the heterogeneous group of persons who fall under the diagnostic heading of ID is a bottom-up process, with small but fine-tuned and precise empirical "stories" of smaller homogeneous groupings, rather than a top-down process with bigger and more general, but

essentially flawed accounts. With the developmental approach, we know much more about persons with ID than we have in the past, but are also painfully aware of the extent to which we only tap the surface of all there is to know; thus, the more we know, the less we know, but that is OK, because— *the more we know the less we know, the more we (really) know.*

Theoretical Shift from a Singular Defect to a More Fine-tuned Understanding of Development

The study of cognitive and neurocognitive functions or abilities may best highlight the contributions of the developmental approach to ID. These types of functions were the primary focus of scientific research on ID during the second half of the 20th century, when most empirical work in the field was characterized by a race to identify "the deficit" that was the primary cause or marker of reduced intellectual functioning. Those who undertook this frantic search emphasized broad constructs of cognition that were considered essential across all domains of functioning, including cognitive rigidity, memory processes, discrimination learning, and attention–retention capabilities, among many others (for a review of these approaches, see Burack, 1990). With the use of experimental paradigms that were sophisticated for the time, researchers presented compelling evidence of deficient performance in virtually all of these areas of functioning, and each specific defect was touted as the central cause of ID. Unfortunately, the evidence was fatally flawed as the researchers failed to consider essential and seemingly obvious conceptual and methodological issues, such as the inherent differences in developmental levels of functioning between persons with and without ID of the same CA, the multiplicity of etiologies associated with ID, the uniqueness of each etiology with regard to phenotypic expression, and social factors related to the life experiences of persons with ID (for reviews, see Burack et al., 2001; Hodapp & Zigler, 1986).

In critiquing and debunking the various claims of the defect theorists, Zigler and colleagues (e.g., Hodapp, Burack, & Zigler, 1990b, 1998; Zigler, 1967, 1969; Zigler & Balla, 1982; Zigler & Hodapp, 1986;) highlighted these formerly ignored issues as the hallmarks of a nascent approach to ID that would be based on classic developmental theory. As the developmental approach evolved, the critiques led to the growth of more sophisticated conceptual and methodological frameworks that, in turn, resulted in more nuanced and precise understandings of persons with ID. For example, in his classic early articulation of this approach, Zigler (1967) proposed the "two group approach to mental retardation" and argued that persons for whom the cause of ID was familial should be differentiated from those for whom ID could be classified as organic. In this framework, persons with familial ID are simply those at the lower end of the normal distribution of intelligence whose development should, therefore, be typical in every way except that it occurs at a slower rate and reaches a lower asymptote. In contrast, persons with ID associated with organic causes could not be expected to show typical patterns of development because of the lack of integrity of their physiological systems. Differences between these groups were not expected in the developmental sequence of the acquisition of skills within any given domain of functioning as these sequences are considered to be universal (for a review, see Hodapp, 1990), but rather in the profile of functioning across domains (Burack, 1990; Weiss, Weisz, & Bromfield, 1986; Weisz & Yeates, 1981; Zigler & Hodapp, 1986). As the two-group approach was extended, each of the more than 1,000 etiologies and subetiologies (e.g., trisomy 21, mosaicism, and translocation forms of Down syndrome [DS]) was associated with a unique pattern of strengths and weaknesses, and in many occasions, with a specific profile of developmental trajectory (see Burack, Hodapp, & Zigler, 1988; Dykens & Hodapp, 1999).

The impact of Zigler's theory is reflected in several methodological considerations that are now considered fundamental to research on ID. The first methodological impact is reflected in the issue of developmental level and the use of mental age (MA) matching to compare the performance between groups of persons with ID in relation to other groups, most commonly typically developing persons, to determine whether specific aspects of functioning are commensurate with or impaired relative to the comparison group. When compared to typically developing persons, the use of MA matching provides an implicit measure of functioning in relation to the expected developmental level for that function.

The second advance in research is reflected in the study of profiles of cognition and social functioning that are etiology specific. As advances in the field of genetics led to the discovery of even more etiologies associated with ID, the need to further differentiate groups became apparent, and the quest to find the core deficit of ID was largely abandoned in favor of the characterization of strengths and weaknesses across etiologies.

Considering Developmental Level

The most obvious, and therefore the most troubling, of the essential flaws that were inherent to the defect approach is that the groups of persons with and without ID within a study were typically matched on CA (for a discussion of the implications of these problematic outcomes, see Burack et al., 2001). By definition, then, those persons with ID were lower functioning than those without ID and would be expected to perform worse on any task that was age-appropriate and sufficiently sensitive to differentiate between groups with considerably different levels of functioning. Yet, despite the inevitability of the findings of group differences, the defect theorists cited the impaired performance among the persons with ID as evidence of a core deficit.

In highlighting one example of the extent to which advocates of the defect approach misled the field, Burack et al. (2001) and Iarocci and Burack (1998) demonstrated that the notion of attention as the core (or at least a central) defect, which was perpetuated from the 1960s through the 1990s, was based on a series of articles in which matching was exclusively based on CA. Accordingly, Burack and colleagues argued that the findings of a deficit was inevitable for virtually every aspect of attention. In other words, the proponents of the attention defect theory had simply found that "lower functioning persons were functioning at lower levels than higher functioning persons." This, of course, is not at all surprising, and not at all informative. In contrast, Iarocci and Burack highlighted in a review of the literature that when matching was based on MA, attentional functioning was generally developmentally appropriate with some exceptions in certain aspects of functioning among persons with specific syndromes.

One common argument among the proponents of CA matching is that this approach allows for the identification of areas of "sparing of abilities." The idea is that if persons with IDs perform similarly to a CA-matched group of typically developing persons in a specific area of functioning, then that area could be considered to be uniquely "spared." Unfortunately, this reasoning is inconsistent with fundamental tenets of experimental research. The failure to find group differences can rarely be considered unqualified, or even strong, evidence that the groups perform similarly. Rather, this finding is more likely the consequence of one or more methodological problems. In the case of research on persons with ID, the failure to find group differences is often due to the use of participant groups that are not functioning at the developmental levels at which differences in the specific area of functioning might optimally be identified. For example, if an area of functioning emerges at age X, testing groups considerably prior to age X would not elicit group differences since the area of functioning would not have yet developed for even the typically developing persons, and both typically developing children and children with ID would display poor levels of performance. Conversely, differences would be less likely to be elicited at ages that are significantly older than age X as persons with ID would have had ample opportunity to attain the requisite skills, even if their development was slower as compared to typically developing persons. Even in the case in which the participants are all at the ideal age for finding group differences, the failure to find these differences might be attributable to the lack of sufficient sensitivity of the task to differentiate level of performance among groups. Thus, without more evidence, the failure to find group differences tells us little about the relative abilities of the groups, and the case for the "sparing of abilities" is more likely a consequent of problematic methodology than of any meaningful characteristic of the specific group.

The obvious, and simplest, solution to the matching problem of comparing groups with different levels of ability is to utilize groups with similar levels of ability. In the study of cognitive and cognitive-related tasks among persons with and without intellectual disabilities, the relevant aspect of developmental level is intellectual functioning, or MA, and the task is to include groups of persons with and without ID that are similar on these measures. In this way, findings of deficits among persons with IDs cannot simply be attributed to the generally lower levels of functioning. Rather, the case might be made that the deficit in the area of interest among the group of persons with ID is evident even when general functioning is equated. This is, of course, a much stronger argument than when the level of functioning differs between the groups. Thus, the original call to match by MA, or general developmental level (for a review, see Burack et al., 2001), was a meaningful improvement over the CA-matching strategies of yesteryear since the apparent deficits of persons with ID could not be simply attributed to a priori levels of development and functioning.

Despite these advantages of MA as the primary matching variable, the increased precision that is associated with MA only serves to highlight that the process of matching is inherently flawed. It is used to equate two groups that are essentially different, so that they can be compared on some variable-thereby allowing researchers to conclude that any discrepancies in performance or scores can be considered a consequence of some essential difference, rather than of any a priori differences between the groups. However, the inherent difficulty with this type of task is that groups that are essentially different are, in fact, essentially different. For example, a group of children with DS can be matched to typically developing children on MA, but many crucial differences between the groups can effect performance on the relevant tasks, including differences in developmental rate, CA, a life time of experiences, physical and motor abilities, and interaction styles, among many others.

Even in the imaginary scenario in which a person with ID and a typically developing person have the exact same MA for a moment in time, they would differ in many different ways. By definition, the typically developing child would have attained the given MA at a faster rate and at a younger age, whereas the person with ID would have lived longer and had more life experiences. And, the nature of those past life experiences would likely have varied considerably, as typically developing children are likely to have experienced considerably more successes and positive reinforcement than their peers with ID. Their futures would also diverge. In the case of an "ideal" test with perfect sensitivity and reliability, the moment after the MAs of the two children are perfectly commensurate, the typically developing child would surge ahead.

Despite some conceptual concerns about the trajectory of MA, basic MA matching is particularly useful in the study of persons whose ID is familial, who, like typically developing persons, are thought to show relatively flat profiles across cognitive domains. However, with the advent of primary interest in the different etiological groups and in the differences in profile among them, general scores of MA were no longer sufficient to mitigate against claims of a priori differences between the groups.

Among others, Burack et al. (2004) highlight the need to utilize matching measures that are even more precise than MA, so that the matching is not by some general construct of developmental level but rather is linked to the development of abilities that are pertinent to the specific function or task.

This strategy minimizes the chances that differences in performance between the groups might be an artifact of a specific relative strength or weakness displayed by one of the groups in the area of functioning related to the experimental task.

The advances in matching by specific aspects of developmental level allow for considerably more precise assessments of the implications of various findings but, as in many other examples of development, progress is also associated with some reorganization. For example, the intricacies and difficulties in optimizing matching strategies even led to some recent calls to forego matching in favor of the use of regression models that allow researchers to chart developmental changes (e.g., Jarrold & Brock, 2004). Thus, the discussions are less about "the way" or even "best way" to match, but rather, more humbly, the "least bad way" for the specific study. These types of discussions both highlight the essential contribution of the consideration of developmental level and matching strategies to understanding the performance in specific aspects of functioning among persons with ID and point the way to the need for continued development of the thinking and research in this field.

The Developmental Approach as Represented in This Volume

This volume differs from many Handbooks as the contributors were not simply assigned specific topics to review, but rather were asked to provide original conceptual contributions in their general areas of research. Thus, they were able to uniquely frame their chapters in ways that could maximize their contribution to both the volume and the general literature. As a result, the chapters differ considerably in their orientation. In some chapters, specific topics are discussed in relation to different etiological groups, whereas the focus in others is on a specific etiological group in relation to a given topic. We imposed a structure of five general sections, with each focused on a domain of functioning or aspect of life that is inherent to an integrated, transactional perspective of development within the context of the unique manifestations evident across the specific etiological groups associated with ID. The focus of the first section is genetics, with examples of the expression of genes in various etiological groups. The next two sections are focused on the development of cognition and of language. The focus of the fourth section is socioemotional development and the fifth on the relationships among persons with ID, the members of their families, and

the broader environment. In all cases, the emphasis is on delineating a more fine-tuned understanding of ID by focusing on developmental processes for one or more well-defined etiological groups.

In the opening section on genetics, intelligence, and behavior, Iarocci and Petrill focus on ID that is not associated with a specific disorder or condition, but rather is thought to be due to natural genetic variation. They review the history of the two-group approach and the need to differentiate between organic and nonpathological forms of ID, and highlight the concept of "polygenic inheritance" to discuss extreme variations in IQ, and in particular, the low IQ that is found in the nonorganic type of ID. In the next two chapters, the focus is the relationship of specific genetic syndromes in relation to behavioral phenotypes. Elsabbagh and Karmiloff-Smith discuss genetic, developmental, neuroanatomical, and behavioral characteristics of persons with Williams syndrome (WS) and depict how these characteristics are incorporated into theoretical models of gene–environment interactions. Cornish, Bertone, Kogan and Scerif focus specifically on fragile X syndrome (FXS), a particularly striking case of gene–behavior interaction, as the level of intellectual impairment of a person with FXS is inextricably linked to the number of repeats of a particular DNA sequence. With the greater the number of the repeats, the greater the severity of the disorder and the intellectual impairments associated with it.

The second section is on cognitive development. In the opening chapter, Landau highlights the manner in which a fine-tuned understanding of a specific etiological group can inform about general developmental processes—in this case, the organization and development of spatial representation are examined through the unique example of WS. Landau proposes that development involves the specialization of function, factors that constrain each specialized system, and the importance of timing in the emergence of brain and cognitive systems, and she applies these principles to the development of spatial representation among both persons with WS and typically developing persons. The focus of the next several chapters in this section is a specific aspect of cognitive development and the extent to which relevant performance is impaired in different etiological groups. Iarocci, Porporino, Enns, and Burack update the review of literature on attention from the first edition of the Handbook as they examine the finding on disparate aspects of attention among persons with various etiologies, including

DS, WS, and FXS. They apply a framework for understanding developmental change and stability in selective attention that is based on the fundamental dimensions of attentional selection. Specifically, they explore whether attentional selection occurs with or without awareness and whether the origin of the selective process is exogenous, and does not require learning, or is endogenous, and involves learning and prior experience. Vicari reports on specific profiles of memory capacities among persons with IDs of different etiologies, especially individuals with DS and WS. Consistent with a neuropsychological approach, distinct memory profiles among persons with genetic syndromes can be traced to the characteristics of brain development and architecture. Jarrold and Brock refer to Baddeley's (1986) model, in which working memory involves the combined functioning of a central control system (the central executive) and two peripheral short-term memory systems (the phonological loop and the visuo-spatial sketch pad) that are specialized for the maintenance of verbal and visuo–spatial information, respectively. Jarrold and Brock highlight the range of working memory impairments found across the genetic syndromes associated ID. Russo, Dawkins, Huizinga, and Burack examine various aspects of executive functioning among person with DS, FXS, Prader-Willi syndrome, and phenylketonuria. They structure their interpretation of findings to fit within the context of a developmental framework and consider the methodological issues inherently related to the study of executive function among persons with IDs. Bhatara, Quintin, and Levitin address the link between intelligence and musical ability among individuals with WS, DS, FXS, tuberous sclerosis complex, and Rett syndrome. Key and Thornton-Wells end the section with an introduction to event-related potential and magnetic resonance imaging technology for studying cognition among persons with ID, and they illustrate how these methods are used with persons with DS, Prader-Willi syndrome, WS, and FXS. Across the chapters in this section, the need to differentiate by specific etiology is highlighted as the groups are unique in so many ways, even as they share the common criterion for ID of a significantly lowered intellectual functioning.

In the section on language development, the focus is on the development of language within specific etiological groups, with two chapters on DS and one each on FXS and WS. Chapman and Kay-Raining Bird summarize the strengths and weaknesses of the emerging language profile among children, adolescents, and young adults with DS. Kay-Raining Bird and Chapman focus on literacy, and highlight the evidence that interventions can improve emergent literacy, word recognition and decoding skills, orthographic knowledge, and phonological awareness among persons with DS. Abbeduto, McDuffie, Brady, and Kover provide a comprehensive characterization of language problems typically associated with FXS. They describe the extent and profile of delays and impairments, the syndrome-specific features and within-syndrome variation of the linguistic profile, and how both are influenced by genetic and environmental factors. Mervis considers research on early language acquisition, and on the language abilities of school-aged children and adolescents with WS. She argues that, rather than providing evidence for the independence of language from cognition, the evidence from WS is consistent with their interdependence throughout development. As in the case of cognitive development, the chapters on language highlight the unique patterns of development seen across different etiologies, and highlight the need for a more fine-tuned understanding of the relevant developmental trajectories.

The fourth section is on social-emotional development, and the chapters are organized so that each addresses a different aspect of study, with one on general social-emotional development, one on social-emotional development in relation to brain activity, and one in relation to the diagnosis of autism and dual diagnoses. Kasari, Jahromi, and Gulsrud highlight essential developmental milestones in social-emotional development for typical child development and use this model as a framework for considering the extent to which children with developmental disabilities are delayed or different in their emotional development. They address several areas of emotional development, including emotion recognition and understanding, emotional expressions, emotion responsiveness, and emotion regulation among children with autism, DS, and FXS. Niccols, Thomas, and Schmidt synthesize the current state of research on the relationship among brain, behavior, and social-emotional development in children with the six most common genetic syndromes associated with an ID, including DS, FXS, 22q11.2, Williams, Prader-Willi, and Angelman syndromes. They conclude that the increased prevalence of some socioemotional difficulties in children with genetic syndromes may be partially explained by neurodevelopmental differences. Moss, Howlin, and Oliver provide an extensive review of the assessment and presentation of autism spectrum disorder and related behaviors among individuals with severe ID associated with several genetic syndromes, including tuberous sclerosis complex, FXS, DS, WS, and Angelman, Coffin-Lowry, Cohen, Rett, and Cornelia de Lange syndromes. The relatively frequent comorbidity between certain syndromes and autism spectrum disorder suggests possible links that might inform about the syndrome, autism spectrum disorders, and the relationship between them. The unique patterns of social-emotional development and prevalence of autism spectrum disorders across different etiologies highlights that etiological differences extend beyond the domains of functioning, cognition, and language most associated with ID to affect every aspect of individuals' lives.

The final section of this volume is on relationships between persons with ID and the various members of their family across the lifespan. In delineating the issues faced by family members, especially mothers, some of the contributions include first-person accounts. Glidden focuses on the reactions of parents to raising a child with an ID. She addresses reports of both positive and negative reactions, as well as the intensity and duration of the reaction to having children with DS, FXS, and Smith Magenis, Prader-Willi, and other forms of ID. Hauser-Cram, Howell-Moneta, and Young discuss the physical and behavioral characteristics of children with DS and WS that influence their social interactions, and conclude that similarities and contrasts between profiles of children with each syndrome are informative for those who seek possible avenues of intervention for promoting optimal mother–child interactions when the child has a genetic etiology. Feninger-Schaal et al. provide a review of attachment theory, with an emphasis on factors relating to the parents' representation of their children, as reflected both in their insightfulness into the experiences of their child and their reactions to their child's diagnosis. Both factors impact caregiving behavior and the attachment that children form to their parents. Al-Yagon and Margalit examine parents' perspectives on having children with DS in an attempt to characterize family sources of stress and coping. Fidler contrasts two frameworks used for understanding the effect on families of children with different etiologies including DS, FXS, WS, Smith Magenis syndrome, Prader-Willi syndrome, and Angelman syndrome. One is an etiology-specific framework rooted in Hodapp's (1997) notion of direct and indirect effects in families of children with ID of different

etiologies, and the other is a bioanthropological framework that provides a more distal account of child eliciting factors in children with disabilities and takes into account evolutionary influences on parent–child relationships. Esbensen, Seltzer, and Krauss present a life course perspective on research on families of persons with specific genetic syndromes. They focus on patterns of individual developmental trajectories, with an emphasis on the effect of context on outcome. The editors conclude the volume with some reflections on its contributions to the theory, research, and understanding of persons with intellectual disability from a developmental perspective, and outline directions for future work in the field.

As developmental approaches to understanding persons with ID continue to emerge, the contributions to this volume provide conceptual foundations for examining the developmental trajectories across persons with any of the many different etiologies. More than 40 years after Zigler's (1967) initial call to arms for a developmental approach to ID, and 20 years after our initial volume (Hodapp, Burack, & Zigler, 1990)—*the more we know, the more we know we need to know (even) more.*

Acknowledgments

Work on this chapter was supported by funding from the Social Sciences and Humanities Research Council of Canada to Jacob A. (Jake) Burack.

References

Burack, J. A. (1990). Differentiating mental retardation: The two-group approach and beyond. In R. M. Hodapp, J. A. Burack, & E. Zigler (Eds.), *Issues in the developmental approach to mental retardation* (pp. 27–48). New York: Cambridge University Press.

Burack, J. A., Evans, D. W., Klaiman, C., & Iarocci, G. (2001). The mysterious myth of attention deficit and other defect stories: Contemporary issues in the developmental approach to mental retardation. *International Review of Research in Mental Retardation, 24,* 299–320.

Burack, J. A., Hodapp, R., & Zigler, E. (1988). Issues in the classification of mental retardation: Differentiating among organic etiologies. *Journal of Child Psychology and Psychiatry, 29,* 765–769.

Burack, J. A., Hodapp, R. M., & Zigler, E. (1998). *Handbook of mental retardation and development.* New York: Cambridge University Press.

Burack, J. A., Iarocci, G., Flanagan, T. D., & Bowler, D. M. (2004). On mosaics and melting pots: Conceptual considerations of comparison and matching strategies. *Journal of Autism and Developmental Disorders, 34,* 65–73.

Burack, J. A., Root, R. R., & Shulman, C. (1996). The developmental approach to mental retardation. *Child and Adolescent Psychiatric Clinics of North America, 5,* 781–796.

Dykens, E. M., & Hodapp, R. M. (1999). Behavioural phenotypes towards new understandings of people with developmental disabilities. In N. Bouras (Ed.), *Psychiatric and behavioural disorders in developmental disabilities and mental retardation* (pp. 96–108). Cambridge: Cambridge University Press.

Dykens, E. M., & Hodapp, R. M. (2001). Research in mental retardation: Toward an etiologic approach. *The Journal of Child Psychology and Psychiatry and Allied Disciplines, 42*, 49–71.

Hodapp, R. M. (1990). One road too many? Issues in the similar-sequence hypothesis. In R. M. Hodapp, J. A. Burack, & E. Zigler (Eds.), *Issues in the developmental approach to mental retardation* (pp. 49–70). New York: Cambridge University Press.

Hodapp, R. M. (1997). Direct and indirect behavioral effects of different genetic disorders of mental retardation. *American Journal on Mental Retardation, 102*, 67–79.

Hodapp R. M., & Burack, J. A. (2006). Developmental approaches to children with mental retardation: A second generation? In D. J. Cohen & D. Cicchetti (Eds.), *Developmental psychopathology: Risk, disorder, and adaptation* (2nd ed., pp. 235–267) Hoboken, NJ: John Wiley & Sons.

Hodapp, R. M., Burack, J. A., & Zigler, E. (1990). The developmental perspective in the field of mental retardation. In R. M. Hodapp, J. A. Burack, & E. Zigler (Eds.), *Issues in the developmental approach to mental retardation.* New York: Cambridge University Press.

Hodapp, R. M., Burack, J. A., & Zigler, E. (1998). Developmental approaches to mental retardation: A short introduction. In J. A. Burack, R. M. Hodapp, & E. Zigler (Eds.), *Handbook of mental retardation and development.* New York: Cambridge University Press.

Iarocci, G., & Burack, J. A. (1998). Understanding the development of attention in persons with mental retardation: Challenging the myths. In J. A. Burack, R. M. Hodapp, & E. Zigler (Eds.), *Handbook of mental retardation and development* (pp. 349–381). New York: Cambridge University Press.

Jarrold, C., & Brock, J. (2004). To match or not to match? Methodological issues in autism-related research. *Journal of Autism and Developmental Disorders, 34*, 81–86.

Weisz, B., Weisz, J. R., & Bromfield, R. (1986). Performance of retarded and nonretarded persons on information-processing tasks: Further tests of the similar structure hypothesis. *Psychological Bulletin, 100*, 157–175.

Weisz, J. R., & Yeates, K. O. (1981). Cognitive development in retarded and nonretarded persons: Piagetian tests of the similar structure hypothesis. *Psychological Bulletin, 90*, 153–178.

Zigler, E. (1967). Familial mental retardation: A continuing dilemma. *Science, 20*(3760), 292–298

Zigler, E. (1969). Developmental versus difference theories of mental retardation and the problem of motivation. *American Journal of Mental Deficiency, 73*, 536–556.

Zigler, E., & Balla, D. (1982).Introduction: The developmental approach to mental retardation. In E. Zigler & D. Balla (Eds.), *Mental retardation: The developmental-difference controversy.* Hillsdale, NJ: Erlbaum.

Zigler, E. & Hodapp, R. (1986). *Understanding mental retardation.* New York: Cambridge University Press.

PART 2

Genes and Behavior

Behavioral Genetics, Genomics, Intelligence, and Mental Retardation

Grace Iarocci *and* Stephen A. Petrill

Abstract

This chapter provides an overview of the current evidence on the behavioral genetic etiology of mental retardation. It begins with a history of the two-group approach and the need to differentiate between organic and nonpathological forms of mental retardation. Then, it presents evidence that genetic and environmental factors that contribute to variation in IQ in the general population may also lead to low IQ in persons with familial mental retardation. The chapter continues with a review of the new behavioral genetic work to identify DNA markers for intelligence. It outlines methodological challenges, with particular emphasis on how these issues pertain to the search for an etiological link between familial mental retardation and normal variation in general cognitive ability. It concludes with a discussion of familial mental retardation within the broader scope of the reciprocal relation between genetic and environmental influences.

Keywords: Familial mental retardation, behavioral genetic etiology, IQ, DNA markers, intelligence, cognitive ability

Within the last decade, the fields of molecular and behavioral genetics experienced remarkable technological and methodological innovation. These advances brought about significant progress in the identification of the causes of mental retardation associated with major chromosomal anomalies or single-gene disorders such as fragile X and Williams syndromes. Recent reviews list over 200 genetic mutations associated with mental retardation (e.g., Zechner et al., 2001) and, as of 2007, over 800 polymorphisms were associated with the term "mental retardation" in the Online Mendelian Inheritance in Man (OMIM) database that account for mental retardation in two-thirds of the individuals in the moderate to profound range of mental retardation (Stromme & Hagberg, 2000). However, for persons with a mild range of mental retardation (e.g., IQ from 50 to 70), the causes for their low IQ are still largely unknown (Hodapp & Dykens, 1996). Persons in this IQ range constitute an estimated 2.28% of the 3.04% of cases of mental retardation in the general population (Zigler & Hodapp,

1986). Thus, the majority of cases of mental retardation have not benefited from behavioral genetic advances (Raynham, Gibbons, Flint, & Higgs, 1996).

It is estimated that over 50% of individuals diagnosed with mild mental retardation show no known pre-, peri-, or postnatal cause for their lowered IQ (Zigler & Hodapp, 1986) and, although delayed, cognitive development is as orderly and organized as that of their typically developing peers (Hodapp & Zigler, 1990, 1995). Mental retardation in these cases may be familial and nonpathological, constituting the lower end of the normal distribution of cognitive ability (Zigler, 1967, 1969). Most individuals with familial mental retardation are capable of living independently and maintaining a job; however, as we enter the technologically sophisticated and competitive society of the 21st century, their plight becomes increasingly notable (Brown, 2000; Plomin, 1999a; Zetlin & Morrison, 1998).

In this chapter, we provide an overview of the current evidence on the behavioral genetic etiology of mental retardation. The chapter begins with a history of the two-group approach and the need to differentiate between organic and nonpathological forms of mental retardation. *Familial mental retardation* is defined as a nonpathological form of mental retardation using the behavioral genetic concept of polygenic inheritance. Then, evidence is presented that genetic and environmental factors that contribute to variation in IQ in the general population may also lead to low IQ in persons with familial mental retardation. The chapter continues with a review of the new behavioral genetic work to identify DNA markers for intelligence. Methodological challenges are outlined, with a particular emphasis on how these issues pertain to the search for an etiological link between familial mental retardation and normal variation in general cognitive ability. The discovery of polygenes that, working together, may account for the approximately 50% of intellectual variation due to genetic factors has implications for understanding both genetic and environmental contributions to the development of children with familial mental retardation. Thus, the chapter concludes with a discussion of familial mental retardation within the broader scope of the reciprocal relation between genetic and environmental influences.

The Two-group Approach to Mental Retardation

The differentiation between organic and nonpathological forms of mental retardation has a long history and was initially impelled by the notion that identifiable differences in physical, medical, or behavioral symptoms reflected particular underlying etiologies (Burack, 1990; Dykens, 1995; Lewis, 1933; Werner & Strauss, 1939; Zigler, 1967). The classification of mental retardation according to etiology dates back to the 17th century, when Felix Platter, a physician, grouped persons with mental retardation into two subtypes. One subtype included persons who displayed "simple-minded" behavior beginning in early infancy, whereas a second subtype included persons who, in addition to exhibiting "simple-minded" behavior, were born with physical deformities and were presumed to suffer from an underlying organic defect.

Down (1887) introduced the notion of developmental causes of mental retardation. Tredgold (1908) further articulated the notion of developmental delay and noted that mental retardation of the "primary type" was due to genetic factors, whereas the "secondary type" was due to environmentally based delay in the development of a potentially

normal brain. Even these rudimentary classifications in type of mental retardation instilled some order to the study of mental retardation and generated several subsequent theories and empirical study on the distinction between organic and familial (nonorganic) etiologies of mental retardation.

Parallel to these events, Galton (1869, 1883, 1889), a geneticist concerned with the study of mental ability and the inheritance of genius, grouped people on the basis of social class or influence. This was his best estimate of mental capacity, as standardized intelligence tests were not available at that time. Galton proposed that the distribution of people in the various classes was Gaussian and symmetrical. He estimated that the number of "eminent" men would be matched by the number of "imbeciles" and suggested that intelligence has a normal distribution pattern in the general population. Although considered unsophisticated by today's standards, Galton's work on quantifying the variation in human intelligence was pioneering. However, Galton's idea that intelligence had a normal distribution needed to be refined, as the actual distribution of intelligence in the population was not symmetrical (Lewis, 1933).

With the development of standardized tests of intelligence, his successors were able to show that, contrary to the theoretical predictions from the normal curve on which IQ scores are based, the frequency of persons with mental retardation that fall within 2 or 3 standard deviations (SD) below the mean is consistent with the 2.3% expected in a normal distribution, but that the number that fall below 3 SD below the mean was significantly greater than the expected .3% (Pearson & Jaederholm, 1914; Roberts, Norman, & Griffiths, 1938; Penrose, 1970). To explain these findings, two distributions of intelligence were proposed; one reflecting the normal population and another, smaller population whose performance was influenced by processes (possibly pathological) that were different from those that determine normal variation in intelligence (see Figure 2.1).

The empirical evidence supported earlier clinical observations and suggested that the population of persons with mental retardation was not homogenous; at least two distinct etiological groups existed (Dingman & Tarjan, 1960). One group was thought to comprise persons with mild mental retardation who suffered from poor but nonpathological genetic factors. This group was thought to represent the low end of the normal distribution of IQ (Lewis, 1933; Penrose, 1963; Zigler, 1967). In contrast, another group consisted of persons with more severe

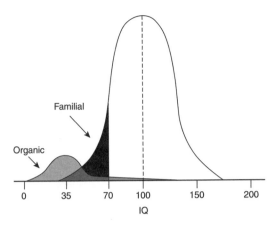

Fig. 2.1 Distributions of IQ among persons with familial or intergenerational mental retardation and those with organic mental retardation. From Zigler, E., & Hodapp, R.M. [1986]. *Understanding mental retardation* (p. 73). New York: Cambridge University Press; reprinted with permission.

mental retardation that was associated with pathological processes (e.g., genetic defect, organic insult) that interfered in specific ways with cognitive development (Burack, 1990).

Although this work represents a significant contribution to the two-group approach, the problem of confounding etiology with severity of mental retardation remained a limitation. For example, the region at the lower negative tail of the normal distribution, where the two distributions overlap, is likely to consist of both people with known causes of mental retardation and those without an identifiable pathology (see Figure 2.1). Moreover, even persons with identified genetic forms of mental retardation, such as Down syndrome (DS), vary in severity of mental retardation and may function in the range of mild mental retardation (Rutter et al., 1996; Simonoff, Bolton, & Rutter, 1996, 1998). Thus, classification based solely on IQ did not adequately account for the heterogeneity of mental retardation. The two-group distinction needed a legitimate basis for differentiating etiology. The developmental perspective was particularly useful in conceptualizing nonpathological mental retardation because it was grounded in empirical work on typical development.

Developmental Contributions to the Two-group Approach

A major milestone was achieved in research on mental retardation when leading developmental theorists, such as Werner and Straus (1939) and later Zigler (1967), used the knowledge and principles of typical development to inform their study of persons with mental retardation. Werner and Strauss

emphasized the difference between endogenous and exogenous mental retardation. The former referred to mental retardation that was associated with a family history of mental retardation, no organic damage, and positive response to modifications in the environment. The latter was commonly associated with pathological damage, no family history of mental retardation, and little benefits from environmental changes (Kephart & Strauss, 1940) (see Table 2.1).

Although the distinction in taxonomy was not new, the developmental approach emphasized the underlying developmental processes that are integrally associated with the etiology of mental retardation, as opposed to the external, behavioral indices of mental retardation (e.g., IQ level). In 1967, Zigler integrated the work of Werner and Strauss (1939) with that of others (Kounin, 1941; Lewis, 1933) and advanced the two-group theory of mental retardation, marking the most prolific period in the field of mental retardation. The developmental perspective provided a framework for generating and testing hypotheses about the etiology of mental retardation in relation to differences in rate of development.

The theoretical premise of Zigler's two-group approach was that mental retardation could be classified into two broad categories on the basis of organic and nonorganic etiology and that markedly different patterns of development across and within domains of functioning could be predicted on the basis of these different etiologies. He argued that the nonorganic group consisted of persons with familial mental retardation due to the nonpathological transmission of poor cognitive endowment from their parent(s) with similarly low cognitive ability. Conversely, the organic group included persons with more severe mental retardation that was due to a specific prenatal, perinatal, or postnatal organic affliction with etiology-specific consequences on development.

Over the next several years, Zigler and his colleagues examined persons with no known cause for their retardation and compared this group with those persons whose retardation was due to an identifiable organic cause. The most compelling evidence for the link between familial mental retardation and nonpathological cognitive delay is based on a series of studies that showed that, although the rate of development was slower among persons with familial mental retardation, they followed the same sequences of development and showed similar patterns of cognitive development across domains

Table 2.1 The definition, diagnosis, causes, and characteristics of organic and familial mental retardation

	Organic	Familial
Definition	Individual shows a clear organic cause of mental retardation	Individual shows no obvious cause of retardation Family member may have mental retardation
Diagnosis	Typically at birth or infancy	School-age
	Frequent comorbidity	No comorbidity
	No change in mental retardation (MR) status	Likely, upon leaving school
Causes	Prenatal (genetic disorders, accidents in utero)	Polygenic (i.e., parents of low IQ)
	Perinatal (prematurity, anoxia)	Environmentally deprived
	Postnatal (head trauma, meningitis)	Undetected organic conditions
Characteristics	More prevalent in moderate, severe, and profound mental retardation	More prevalent in mild mental retardation
	Equal or near-equal rates across all ethnic and socioeconomic status (SES)	Higher rates within minority groups and low-SES groups
	More often associated with other physical disabilities (e.g., epilepsy, cerebral palsy)	Few associated physical disabilities
	Often accompanied by severe health problems	Health within normal range
	IQ most often below 50	IQ rarely below 50
	Siblings usually of normal intelligence	Siblings often at lower levels of intelligence
	Appearance often marred by physical stigmata	Normal appearance
	Mortality rate higher (more likely to die at a younger age than the general population)	Normal mortality rate
	Often dependent on care of others throughout life	With some support can lead an independent existence as adults
	Unlikely to mate and often infertile	Likely to marry and produce children of low intelligence
	Unlikely to experience neglect in home	More likely to experience neglect in their homes

Compiled from Hodapp & Dykens, 1996; MacMillan, Siperstein, & Gresham, 1996; and Zigler, Balla, & Hodapp, 1984.

when compared to typically developing peers of the same mental age (MA) (Weisz & Yeates, 1981; Hodapp & Zigler, 1997). With few exceptions (e.g., Weiss, Weisz, & Bromfield, 1986), Zigler's application of developmental principles to persons with familial mental retardation was supported (Iarocci & Burack, 1998). Despite several refinements and extensions to the original two-group formulation (Cicchetti & Sroufe, 1976; Cicchetti & Pogge-Hesse, 1982; Hodapp & Zigler, 1990) and disputes over its functional significance (Goodman, 1990), it remains the most influential theory on the etiology of familial mental retardation (Burack, 1990).

An area of concern, however, is the lack of recent growth in research on nonpathological mental retardation. The future of mental retardation research depends largely on continued nurturance of both branches of the two-group taxonomy. Yet, current trends indicate a widening gap between our knowledge of organic syndromes and non-pathological mental retardation (King, State, Shah, Davanzo, & Dykens, 1997; Plomin, 1999a; Rutter, Simonoff, & Plomin, 1996; Simonoff, Bolton, & Rutter, 1996; State, King, & Dykens, 1997). There is both substantial breadth and depth of knowledge concerning the genetic conditions that cause organic mental retardation. Conversely, there is a paucity of information regarding the nonpathological genetic pathways that contribute to familial mental retardation.

The organic branch of the two-group theory flourished largely as a result of the introduction of new molecular genetic technologies that contributed to the identification of genetic defects that cause mental retardation. Further, the differentiation of organic forms of mental retardation according to genetic etiology allowed researchers to more thoroughly study specific behavioral phenotypes and chart developmental profiles of persons with specific syndromes. In particular, a proliferation of psychiatric genetic studies of mental retardation has occurred over the past 20 years. The specific genetic mechanisms are described in greater detail elsewhere (see Butler & Meaney, 2005) and fall into several categories of noninherited (occurring at the time of meiosis or conception) and inherited (passed down from parents to offspring) mutations. For example, cri du chat syndrome is characterized by small head size, a broad nasal ridge, and most importantly, in infancy and early childhood, a cry resembling a cat's meow. Cri du chat has been linked with a constellation of genes located on the short arm of chromosome 5 (Overhauser et al., 1994; Gersh et al., 1995; Mainardi et al., 2001). Rett syndrome, on the other hand, is a disorder associated with a period of 6–18 months of normal development, followed by a slowing and then a loss of acquired cognitive and motor skills, resulting in a loss of speech, autistic features, and mental retardation. Rett syndrome has been localized to a set of mutations in the MECP2 gene located in the long arm of the X-chromosome (Amir et al., 1999).

In comparison, the search for identifiable genetic and environmental markers for nonpathological familial mental retardation has proven more difficult (Plomin, 1999a; Zigler & Hodapp, 1986). However, the conditions for growth in this area are currently favorable (Nokelainen & Flint, 2002). Substantive knowledge is available on the genetics of general cognitive ability. In addition, quantitative behavioral genetic techniques have been developed to study individuals with IQs in the extreme range. Thus, early speculations that familial mental retardation involved familial transmission of multiple genes that additively contribute to cognitive disability (Lewis, 1933; Zigler, 1967) may now be reformulated into testable hypotheses. The primary goal is to identify the polygenes that additively accumulate genetic risk and, that in tandem with environmental risk factors, increase an individual's susceptibility to familial mental retardation.

The Two-group Approach: Current Developments
Mild Mental Retardation Shows a Familial Link

Early epidemiological studies compared persons with mental retardation and consistently showed a link between the individual's level of severity of retardation (mild or severe) and their family pedigree. For example, if one parent had mild mental retardation, the risk of retardation in their children was about 20%, and if both parents were afflicted, the risk was nearly 50%. However, severe mental retardation occurred independently of familial and sociocultural risk factors (Johnson, Ahern & Johnson, 1976; Reed & Reed, 1965; Roberts, 1952). These findings also hold up in the context of current prospective analyses of the broader population of children with and without mental retardation.

Broman and colleagues (1975) conducted an extensive longitudinal study relating prenatal and perinatal events to adverse outcomes from birth to 8 years. The study included a sample of 17,432 Caucasian and 19,419 African American children. At 7 years of age, children were tested with the Wechsler Intelligence Scale for Children (WISC-R). For the 7-year-old lower functioning children, the Stanford-Binet Intelligence Scale, Vineland Social Maturity Scale, Catell Infant Intelligence Scale, or the Bayley Scale of Infant Mental Development (BSID) were administered. IQs were estimated for those children who were considered untestable or were institutionalized at age 7.

Children who scored less than 50 on the IQ tests were classified with severe mental retardation, and those with IQs between 50 and 69 were classified with mild mental retardation. There was a 0.5% rate of severe mental retardation and 1.2% rate of mild mental retardation among the Caucasian children. Among the African American children, 0.7% scored in the severe range and 4.6% in the mild range. In both samples, substantially more children with severe retardation than mild retardation manifested organic pathologies such as DS, post-traumatic deficits, central nervous system (CNS) malformations, cerebral palsy, epilepsy, and sensory deficits.

In the Caucasian population, higher rates of retardation were found among the relatives of children with mild mental retardation, whereas among the relatives of children with severe retardation a familial link was not evident. In the African American population, familial patterns did not show a clear distinction between relatives of children with severe and mild mental retardation (Nichols, 1984). However, Nichols (1984) noted that if he shifted the IQ distribution for the African American population downward, it appeared more consistent with the two-group theory. Nichols (1984) suggested that the downward shift in the IQ distribution in the African American population has an environmental basis. Alternatively, the discrepancies in IQ scores may be due to limitations in the measurement tools. This account is consistent with evidence that certain standardized tests used to assess IQ may be culturally biased and may be particularly problematic when used to assess African American children (Grados-Johnson & Russo-Garcia, 1999).

Another study based on the same sample found a 12-fold increase in the frequency of retardation among full siblings of children with mild retardation and significantly more affected relatives than found among the children with severe retardation (Broman, Nichols, Shaughnessy, & Kennedy, 1987). The average IQ of siblings of the group with severe mental retardation was normal (IQ = 103), whereas the mean IQ of siblings of the children with mild mental retardation was below average (IQ = 84.8). Twenty-one percent of the siblings of the children with mild mental retardation were also found to function in the mentally retarded range. The authors concluded that mild but not severe mental retardation shows a familial link with normal variation in general intelligence (Broman et al., 1987). For African American children, familial patterns did not indicate a clear distinction between relatives of children with severe and mild mental retardation, as most mental retardation appeared to be of the familial type.

Mild Mental Retardation Is More Prevalent in Low Socioeconomic Environments

In addition to familial links, epidemiological studies consistently point to an association between mild mental retardation and low socioeconomic status (SES) (Birch et al., 1970; Broman, Nichols, Shaughnessy, & Kennedy, 1987; Hagberg, Hagberg, Lewerth, & Lindberg, 1981a,b; Rao, 1990; Richardson & Koller, 1996). For example, Broman et al. (1987) classified children according to SES and found that the child's SES level was associated with mental retardation as measured at 7 years. In the lowest SES group (bottom 25%), 3.34% scored in the mental retardation range, whereas only 1.31% and .3% of children from middle (50%) and high (top 25%) SES groups scored in that range. For the African American groups, the relationship between SES and

IQ was even stronger. In the lowest SES group, 7.75% scored in the mental retardation range and 3.59% and 1.19% scored in the mental retardation range in the middle and highest SES groups, respectively. The findings establish a clear link between low SES and mild mental retardation. However, in interpreting these findings, it is important to note that social class status is often confounded with racial or ethnic background, and their independent effects on cognitive ability have not been established (Helms, 1992).

Richardson and Koller (1996) used social class as an indirect marker of psychosocial adversity and found that, for children with moderate to severe mental retardation (IQ<50), the prevalence was generally evenly distributed among five levels of social class (measured as a function of type of employment). A marked increase in the prevalence of mild mental retardation (IQ 60–69) was noted at the lower end of the class scale. To determine overrepresentation or underrepresentation of mental retardation in a particular class, the researchers calculated the expected number of children with mental retardation within a social class and divided by the actual number in the social class. Children with IQs between 60 and 69 were underrepresented in the highest social classes but overrepresented (three times greater than expected) in the lowest social classes (Richardson & Koller, 1996).

Although mild mental retardation appears to be concentrated in socially disadvantaged segments of the population, there is little evidence that psychosocial deprivation alone could cause mental retardation (Clarke, 1985). For example, most children who experience psychosocial adversity do not develop mental retardation, suggesting that other, possibly genetically driven processes may also play a significant role (Richardson & Koller, 1996). Suboptimal or disadvantaged environments hold a variety of factors that together may moderate the genetic influences on intelligence.

Mild Mental Retardation Is Associated with Subtle Organic Anomalies

The population of children with mild mental retardation is also at risk for inherited abnormalities, prenatal and perinatal adversities, postnatal malnutrition and toxicity, illnesses, and other vulnerabilities that may affect the developing brain (McGue, 1997). In some cases of unknown etiology, undetected genetic and organic anomalies may account for the mental retardation (Akesson, 1984, 1986; Hagberg et al., 1981a, b). Akesson (1986) reviewed Swedish population studies conducted in the mid 1980s and concluded that persons with mild mental retardation had a higher than expected (by the normal curve) rate and range of organic pathologies. For example, in one study of a rural, northern community in Sweden, a significant proportion (25%) of persons with mild mental retardation had a major genetic disorder, chromosomal defect, or organic handicap (e.g., hypothyroidism, viral disease, hydrocephalus, epilepsy, cerebral palsy) (Blomquist, 1981). In another study of a large Swedish city, persons with mild mental retardation showed increased rates (4%–19%) of mild chromosomal abnormalities. Heavy maternal alcohol consumption during pregnancy was confirmed in 8%–9% of cases with mild mental retardation and suspected in other cases (Hagberg et al., 1981a,b). In the central region of Sweden, additional physical impairments (e.g., visual defects, hearing problems, movement difficulties) were found in 75% of cases with mild mental retardation (Gostason, 1985). More recent findings also revealed subtle chromosomal abnormalities in children with unexplained mental retardation (Knight et al., 1999) and an association between mild mental retardation and pre-, peri-, and postnatal risk factors (McGue, 1997).

Based on a review of the literature on organic etiology among persons with mild mental retardation, Zigler and Hodapp (1986) acknowledged that the incidence of organic anomalies within this group may be greater than previously estimated. According to the authors, this is not surprising, as persons with mild mental retardation do not constitute a homogeneous group, and finer differentiations within this group are required to better identify the subgroup of persons with nonpathological, familial mental retardation.

Familial Genes and Environment Interactively Contribute to Mild Mental Retardation

There is a prevailing view in the field of mental retardation that the interplay between nature (genetics) and nurture (environments) is a consequence of the additive effects of independent and separate influences despite considerable empirical evidence that the process is best characterized as dynamic, synergistic, and interdependent (Plomin, 1994; Plomin & Rutter, 1998; Rutter et al., 1996).

Richardson and Koller (1996) demonstrated the powerful interactive impact of familial genetic and environmental influences on low cognitive ability. They examined the frequency of biomedical factors, family pedigree, and psychosocial adversity among children with mild mental retardation. Biomedical factors included major genetic disorders or X-linked disorders, cerebral palsy, micro- and macrocephaly, autism, cerebral malformation, epilepsy, dysmorphic syndrome, teratogen, and small for gestational age. The family pedigree factor was measured on the basis of the proportion of the child's relatives who had received mental retardation services. A five-point scale, ranging from stable to markedly unstable, was used to measure family stability and infer the degree of psychosocial adversity (Richardson, Koller, & Katz, 1985).

Among the children with mild mental retardation, psychosocial adversity as a single factor was present in only 21% of cases and, in combination with other biomedical factors, it was present in less than 34% of cases (Richardson & Koller, 1996). However, in combination with family pedigree, psychosocial adversity had a greater impact on IQ. Jointly, these factors were present in 85% of persons with mild mental retardation (Richardson & Koller, 1996). The implication is that persons with mild mental retardation are vulnerable to a host of genetic, organic, and environmental risk factors, the effects of which may be, in some cases, subtle and difficult to detect. Attributing primacy to either genetic or environmental causes of mental retardation is not warranted.

Zigler and colleagues challenge overly simplistic accounts of the etiology of mental retardation, whether based predominantly on a nature or nurture theme, since these are unlikely to lead to a better conceptualization of the complex interrelationship between genes and environments (Scarr & Weinberg, 1978; Zigler & Hodapp, 1986). As an alternative, they championed an interactionist perspective that emphasizes the dynamic interplay among genetic and environmental factors. Specifically, interactionists believe that intelligence emerges through the coalescence of inherited developmental structures and the organism's ongoing and active engagement with the environment (Fischer & Bullock, 1984; Thelen & Smith, 1998). Thus, interactionists favor the concept of reaction range, viewing intelligence as both structured and malleable, with different potential phenotypes as probable outcomes from the same genotype in response to varying environmental supports (Scarr-Salapatek, 1973; Fischer, Bullock, Rotenberg, & Raya, 1993). Within this framework, intelligence is likened to an elastic band, whereby environmental conditions may broaden or constrain inherent potential, but only within the limits of the structure (i.e., inherited familial polygenes) that maintains its integrity.

The availability of new behavioral genetic techniques (e.g., the identification of microdeletions of chromosomes [Flint et al., 1995] and DF extremes analysis [named for its developers, DeFries & Fulker, 1985, 1988]) may lead to discoveries of both subtle, previously undetected pathological etiologies of mild mental retardation and polygenes that account for normal variation in cognitive ability. Differentiations based on genetic etiology, in turn, will facilitate research on the specific role of environments on the development of both pathological and nonpathological mental retardation.

Polygenic Inheritance of Familial Mental Retardation

Epidemiological family and twin studies are used extensively to assess the extent to which familial resemblance is due to genetic and environmental sources of variance in relation to the phenotypic variance on measured IQ (Broman, Nichols, & Kennedy, 1975; Nichols, 1984; Plomin, 1994). Reviews conducted over the past 40 years have yielded consistent findings (Erlenmeyer-Kimling & Jarvik, 1963; Bouchard & McGue, 1981; Chipuer, Rovine, & Plomin, 1990; Plomin & Spinath, 2004). Collapsing across the dozens of available twin and adoption studies involving tens of thousands of participants across the entire lifespan, about 50% of the differences in intelligence can be attributable to genetic variance, with the remaining 50% due to nongenetic variance. This finding is largely stable, irrespective of the geographical location of the sample, and is also consistent across group factors such as verbal ability, spatial ability, and perceptual speed (Plomin, DeFries, McClearn, & McGuffin, 2001). However, differences emerge when the data are grouped by sample age. The heritability of intelligence increases, rising from 20% in infancy to 40% in young childhood to 80% in adulthood (Boomsma, 1993; McCartney, Harris, & Bernieri, 1990; McGue, Bouchard, Iacono, & Lykken, 1993; Plomin, 1986; Plomin, Fulker, Corley, & DeFries, 1997), remaining substantial even into old age (McClearn et al., 1997). At the same time, shared environmental influences decline to zero by adolescence. Nonshared environment (including error) remains significant throughout the lifespan.

Quantitative genetic researchers have also employed multivariate approaches to examine the relationship among cognitive skills, both measured at the same point in time as well as across measurement occasions. In general, genetic influences account largely for the relationship among different aspects of cognitive performance when assessed at the same point in time (Petrill, 2002; Plomin & Kovas, 2005). Similarly, genetic influences account largely for the stability in cognitive performance across measurement occasions (see Petrill et al., 2004). Genetic influences are increasingly important throughout the lifespan and tend to promote stability across different aspects of cognitive performance, both concurrently and longitudinally. Shared environmental influences are important in early childhood but dissipate by adolescence. The nonshared environment (and error), and some age-specific genetic effects promote discontinuity between aspects of cognitive performance both concurrently and longitudinally.

These genetic approaches are important because they have done much to move the field beyond nature versus nurture arguments. Most now agree that both genes and environments are important to understanding individual differences in intelligence. This is a useful starting point for thinking about disability. However, the univariate genetic results described above examine genetic and environmental influences across the range of ability, but do not specifically examine the etiology of developmental disabilities. One approach is to examine the concordance among family members for mental impairment. In this case, twins, called *probands*, are selected based on a particular cutoff for mental ability and then compared to their co-twins. If the monozygotic (MZ) co-twins are more likely to be impaired than dizygotic (DZ) twins, then genetic influences are implicated. If MZ and DZ co-twins are equally likely to be impaired, then shared environmental influences are assumed. Finally, nonshared environment (and error) is implied to the extent that there is no concordance between probands and co-twin.

Although a useful first step, probandwise concordance rates suffer from two limitations. First, concordance rates are categorical, in that twins are selected into disabled and nondisabled groups. Thus, concordances do not provide quantitative estimates of genetic and environmental influences that can be tested for statistical significance. A second problem is that probandwise concordance rates are blind to the base rates of the disorder in the population. A twin concordance of .80 from a population in which the disorder has a prevalence rate of .08 means that being from the same family leads to markedly increased risk. In contrast, a twin concordance of .80 does not indicate any increased risk in a population with a prevalence rate of .80.

Therefore, behavioral genetic researchers examining mental disability have employed a more powerful analytic approach, called DF extremes analysis (DeFries & Fulker, 1986, 1988). The general idea is that, because intelligence is distributed quantitatively, co-twins will be more similar to their probands even if they do not necessarily cross the threshold into disability. As shown in Figure 2.2, MZ and DZ probands are selected for mental disability. The MZ and DZ co-twin means are then examined. Some of these co-twins are also disabled but some of the co-twins are also within the normal range. If the co-twin mean is the same as the unselected population, then the correlation among family members is zero. If the co-twin mean is the same as the proband mean, then the correlation among family members is 1.0. If MZ co-twins are more similar to probands than were DZ twins, then genetic influences are inferred. The statistic that measures this effect is called *group heritability* (h_g^2), which estimates the extent to which the mean difference between the disabled group and the unselected population is due to genetic factors. To the extent that MZ and DZ co-twins are similar, then shared environmental influences are assumed (called c_g^2).

Additionally, the DF approach can also be used to examine whether the genetic and environmental influences in developmental disability are different from those found in the unselected population. In the case of mental impairment versus unselected mental ability, h_g^2 in the disability group can be similar to or different from h^2 in unselected general cognitive ability. If disability is different from ability,

then we can conclude that there is discontinuity in how genes and environments impact disability versus ability. In contrast, if disabled and unselected groups are similar, then there are two possible interpretations. First, it is possible that the genetic environmental influences and processes underlying developmental disability are continuous with those in the unselected population. In this case, disability would be the tail of the normal range of ability. Another possible interpretation is that different genes and environments are operating, but their relative importance is similar for disability and ability.

With these approaches, evidence is found both for and against continuity between disability and ability. In early childhood, Spinath et al. (2004) suggested that h_g^2 is higher in mild mentally impaired children assessed at 2, 3, and 4 years of age ($h_g^2 = .49$) versus unselected children ($h^2 = .24$). In contrast, Petrill et al. (1997) suggested that genetic and environmental influences on mild mental impairment in 24-, 36-, and 48-month-old children were not significantly different from the unselected population. There are some important differences between these two studies. First, Spinath et al. examined the Twins Early Development Study (TEDS), a population-based sample of 3,886 twins, whereas the study by Petrill et al. was based on a more modest sample derived from the MacArthur Longitudinal Twin Study (MALTS). Second, the TEDS data utilized parent report whereas the MALTS was based on psychometric tests.

In older twins, Petrill et al. (2001) examined low cognitive ability in nondemented twin pairs drawn

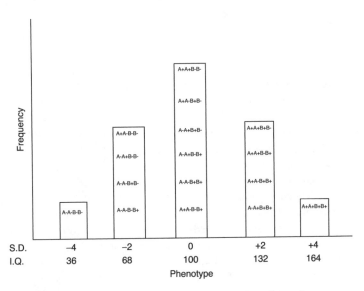

Fig. 2.2 Gottesman's five-gene model of the Normal distribution of IQ. The hypothetical case of two genes contributing to IQ, each including a maternal and a paternal allele that is either enhancing or nonenhancing with regard to IQ.

from the OctoTwin Study, a sample of 351 pairs of 80-year-old and older Swedish twin pairs (McClearn et al., 1997). Petrill et al. (2001) found that h_g^2 was zero in nondemented elderly adults selected for low general cognitive ability.

Despite the possible exceptions in very early life (Spinath et al., 2004) and very late life (Petrill et al., 2001), previous studies examining cognitive ability and disability at other ages have almost universally suggested that h^2 is similar in magnitude to h_g^2 (Petrill et al., 1997, 1998; Plomin et al., 2001; Plomin & Thompson, 1993; Saudino et al., 1994) irrespective of sample differences. This pattern extends beyond general cognitive ability to reading-related outcomes (Fisher & DeFries, 2002) as well as mathematics (Haworth et al., 2007; Kovas, Haworth, Petrill, & Plomin, in press). Although these findings cannot rule out the possibility that different genes and environments are operating at the extremes, the data suggest that continuity between the normal range and extremes is a working hypothesis. Thus, in most cases, "abnormal" is the quantitative extreme of "normal," as suggested by the two-group theory. Another important related question is whether the same genes and environments operate across different kinds of disability. As noted above, genetic influences at the extremes appear to be largely the same as those in the normal range of ability. Furthermore, when examining unselected samples, there is substantial evidence for genetic covariance across cognitive abilities. Thus, a reasonable working hypothesis is that genes related to one disability will be associated with other disabilities. Preliminary evidence indicates that genetic influences are largely stable across reading, mathematics, and language disability (see Plomin & Kovas, 2005).

Molecular Genetics

Given the quantitative genetic evidence, the goal in molecular genetic studies using the quantitative trait locus (QTL) perspective has been to identify those genes that predict a portion of the variance in intelligence, not to find "the" gene that determines whether children will develop mental retardation. To date, these studies have largely employed a "candidate gene" approach, in which candidate DNA markers are selected for analysis based on some a priori criterion. Although no consistent replicated results have been obtained, there is some evidence for associations across three basic classes of candidate genes (see Payton, 2005; Plomin, 2006, for a fuller discussion). The first category of markers is related to *synaptic transmission*. These include

glutamate receptor-modulating synaptic glutamate (GRM3; Egan et al., 2004), serotonin transporter (SLC6A4, Payton et al., 2004), nicastrin (NCSTN, Deary et al., 2005), adrenergic α2A receptor (ADRA2A; Comings et al., 2000), brain-derived neurotrophic factor (BDNF; Egan et al., 2003; Hariri et al., 2003; Tsai, Hong, Yu, & Chen, 2004), cholinergic muscarinic 2 receptor (CHRM2; Comings et al., 2003; Gosso et al., 2006), and dopamine receptor D_2 (DRD2; Bartres-Fair et al., 2002; Tsai et al., 2002, Ball et al., 1998; Moises et al., 2001). The largest number of reports for a synaptic transmission marker has emerged for catechol-O-methyltransferase (COMT) across numerous studies with diverse samples and methods of assessment. In the original report, Egan et al. (2001) found an association between COMT and the Wisconsin Card Sort Test. This finding was replicated by three independent studies with the same measure (Joober et al., 2002; Malhotra et al., 2002; Rose et al., 2004) as well as in four other studies with different measures (Bilder et al., 2002; Diamond et al,. 2004; Goldberg et al., 2003; Nolan et al., 2004). However, this finding was not replicated in three studies (Tsai et al., 2003; Bachner-Melman et al., 2005; Plomin et al., 1995). Additionally, a more recent analysis by Kennedy et al. (in press) found no effect with a sample (n >5,000) larger than all the other studies combined.

A second category involves candidate genes related to brain development. Associations are reported between intelligence and cathepsin D (CTSD; Payton et al., 2003), muscle segment homeobox 1 (MSX1; Fisher et al., 1999; Hill et al., 2002), succinate-semialdehyde dehydrogenase (SSADH, Plomin et al., 2004), and β-synthase (CBS, Barbaux et al., 2000). A third category involves the influence of inflammatory mechanisms on cognitive dysfunction. These include insulin-like growth factor II receptor (Chorney et al., 1998, not replicated in the same group by Hill et al., 2002), insulin-like growth factor II (Bachner-Melman et al., 2005), and histocompatability complex, class II, DRβ1 (HLA-DRB1; Payton et al., 2005; Shepherd et al., 2004).

Finally, a number of studies have found both evidence for (Deary et al., 2002, 2004; Jonker et al., 1998; Small et al., 2000; Staehelin et al., 2999) and against (Mayeaux et al., 2001; Pendelton et al., 2002; Puttonen et al., 2003; Smith et al., 1998; Turic, Fisher, Plomin, & Owen, 2001) the association between allele e-4 of the apolipoprotein gene (APOE-4) and intelligence.

In sum, the literature has led to several key findings. It is clearly possible and useful to identify genes that contribute to DS, Rett syndrome, and other organic forms of mental retardation. However, this "major gene" approach does not appear to be an appropriate model for understanding the majority of cases of low cognitive performance, emanating from the quantitative distribution of cognitive ability. Quantitative genetic evidence suggests strongly that theories of mental retardation must account for the substantial heritability and genetic stability of psychometric intelligence. That said, attempts to identify and replicate the DNA polymorphisms underlying the quantitative genetic literature have remained elusive.

This state of affairs may lead some to pessimistic conclusions that it is simply not possible to find DNA polymorphisms related to familial intelligence. However, it is important to keep in mind that the advent of new molecular genetic techniques is spurring a field-wide transformation in the understanding of genetic influence on complex disease (Glazer, Nadeua, & Aitman, 2002; Botstein & Risch, 2003). Advances in the ability to scan the genome, coupled with advances in statistical genetics, have opened up new ideas concerning genetic models for complex diseases. Typically, genes have been dichotomized into two categories: those major genetic effects that are not only rare, but also large in effect as to be both necessary and sufficient to cause a disease (such as Rett syndrome); or those common variants that act as risk factors across the range of ability and are genes "for" cognitive disability in the sense that individuals with a certain set of polymorphisms are more likely to also fall below the threshold of mental impairment (see Plomin, Owen, & McGuffin, 1994). More recently, there has been discussion in the genetic literature about a possible third genetic mechanism relevant to complex diseases like mental retardation. In particular, more recent research has suggested that the aggregation of mildly deleterious mutations in the human population is an important possible third mechanism for the genetics of complex diseases (Prichard et al., 2001). These mutations are similar to the major gene hypothesis in the sense that they are relatively rare but different in that these mutations are small in effect. Conversely, mildly deleterious markers are similar to the common variant hypothesis in the sense that they are small in effect but different in that they are rare as opposed to common and one-tailed—they act to increase risk. Recent analyses using publicly available genome banks suggest around 53% of mutations in the human genome may be rare, but mildly deleterious (Kryukov, Pennachio, & Sunyaev, 2007). Most molecular genetic studies of intelligence have explicitly looked for common as opposed to rare polymorphisms.

Moreover, all molecular genetic studies of intelligence to date have examined differences in DNA structure—whether the presence or absence of a particular pattern of polymorphisms is correlated with cognitive functioning. These structural differences are only the beginning point in understanding how genes impact behavior. Continually emerging evidence points to the importance of gene–environment processes in the genetics of complex outcomes like intelligence and mental retardation. Consider the classic example of phenylketonuria. (PKU). This disorder, discovered in the 1930s, is caused by a mutation in the phenylalanine hydroxylase gene (*PAH*; Woo et al., 1983). Left untreated, this mutation leads to severe mental retardation but can be prevented by dietary changes. Moreover, quantitative genetics has also highlighted the importance of gene–environment processes. Gene–environment processes are important because they provide additional possible mechanisms to explain the high heritability of intelligence and associated mental disability described earlier in this chapter. In particular, heritability is based on the difference between MZ and DZ twins. Monozygotic twins may be more similar due to direct genetic effects (genes have a direct impact on the biological processes related to intelligence) but may also be more similar due to indirect genetic effects. The increased genetic similarity for MZ twins leads to twins experiencing more similar environments relative to DZ twins, which increases MZ twin similarity. In the case of *reactive/evocative* G × E correlation, environments are provided to an individual by others as a reaction to his or her genetically influenced behavior. *Active* G × E correlation occurs when a child seeks out environments based upon his or her genetically influenced characteristics (Plomin, DeFries, & Loehlin, 1977). Scarr and McCartney (1983) proposed that these effects become increasingly salient over the course of development as children gain more control over situations and experiences that are more likely to be compatible with their genetically influenced characteristics. Quantitative genetic studies have also shown the importance of gene × environment interaction, or the nonlinear association between genetic and environmental influences. For example, Rowe, Jacobson, and Van den Oord (1999) found that parental education moderated the heritability of verbal IQ in a sample of adolescents. The heritability of IQ was lower in low SES families, a finding replicated by Turkheimer et al. (2002).

Conclusion

Clearly, the emerging molecular genetic and gene–environment literatures suggest that further study is needed to bridge the gap between estimating genetic effects versus identifying the genetic processes in nonpathological mental retardation. It has only been 50 years since Crick and Watson first characterized the structure of DNA. In that time, enormous progress has been made in the fields of molecular biology and statistics that have allowed for large-scale studies examining the etiology of complex behaviors and diseases like mental retardation. Most have moved beyond examining *whether* genes or environments are important to intelligence and mental retardation, but there is a great deal of work ahead to understand not only *how* genes and environments affect cognitive ability and disability, but how these findings impact the ways in which we conceptualize, diagnose, and treat mental handicaps. These efforts will involve study at multiple levels of analysis. For example, Plomin and Crabbe (2000) have referred to "bottom-up" approaches that start at genes and work up through cells to behavior, and "top-down" approaches that start at complex behavior then look for genes. Others have postulated that endophenotypes, such as neuroanatomical correlates offer the best hope for finding genes because they are "in between" genes and complex behavior (see Dick et al., 2006). It is clearly far too early to dismiss any of these approaches.

In closing, an important limiting factor in the search for genes for intelligence and mental retardation is that, despite over 100 years of study, the neuroanatomical and biological underpinnings of intelligence are still poorly understood. Genes are operationally defined constructs. They are stretches of DNA that produce amino acids. Their effect on complex outcomes is based on how the outcome is defined. Greater precision in the definition of intelligence, its biological underpinnings, and the numerous subtypes of mental retardation are necessary.

Glossary

Allele: One member of a pair or series of genes that occupy a specific position on a specific chromosome.

Allelic Association = association= linkage disequilibrium: Refers to covariation between allelic variation in a marker and phenotypic variation in the population. Occurs when the restriction fragment length polymorphism (RFLP) is located very close to the trait gene, and therefore is almost never separated during meiotic crossing over of chromosomes. The advantages of association are that it is equally appropriate for a continuous dimension and a dichotomous disorder, and it allows the use of large samples of unrelated individuals, which can be used to provide sufficient power to detect associations that account for a small amount of variance. It can also be thought of as the presence of specific alleles at marker loci contiguous to QTLs at higher frequencies than expected by chance. Considered this way, it is clear that the power of association to detect a QTL depends not only on the magnitude of the effect of the QTL on the trait but also on the magnitude of linkage disequilibrium between the QTL and a marker. Research suggesting that levels of linkage disequilibrium differ in different populations (e.g., different ethnic populations) complicates this matter.

Behavioral Genetics: A branch of genetics that investigates possible connections between a genetic predisposition and observed behavior. Research in behavioral genetics examines the effects of genotype and environment on a range of phenotypic traits such as anxiety, intelligence, sexual orientation and antisocial behavior.

Central Nervous System (CNS) Malformation: Abnormal or anomalous formation or structure, of the portion of the vertebrate nervous system consisting of the brain and spinal cord.

Cerebral Palsy: A disorder usually caused by brain damage occurring at or before birth and marked by muscular impairment. Often accompanied by poor coordination, it sometimes involves speech and learning difficulties.

Chromosome: A threadlike body in the cell nucleus that carries the genes in a linear order.

Comorbidity: The overlapping of two or more disorders at a rate that is greater than would be expected by chance alone.

Concordance Rate: The presence of a rate of a given trait in both members of a pair of twins.

Congenital: Of or relating to a condition that is present at birth, as a result of either heredity or environmental influences: a congenital heart defect; congenital syphilis.

Cretinism: A congenital condition caused by a deficiency of thyroid hormone during prenatal development and characterized in childhood by dwarfed stature, mental retardation, dystrophy of the bones, and a low basal metabolism. Also called congenital myxedema.

DF extremes analysis: Uses quantitative data for continuous traits rather than artificially dichotomizing the traits. It measures differential regression to the mean, and thereby yields "group" statistics that address the etiology of the average difference on a quantitative trait between the selected group and the rest of the population. It assumes that if a particular disorder, such as mental retardation, is linked genetically with a measured quantitative trait, such as IQ, then the probands will be more similar for identical than for fraternal twins (there will be less regression to the mean).

Deoxyribonucleic acid (DNA): A nucleic acid that carries the genetic information in the cell and is capable of self-replication and synthesis of RNA. DNA consists of two long chains of nucleotides twisted into a double helix and joined by hydrogen bonds between the complementary bases adenine and thymine or cytosine and guanine. The sequence of nucleotides determines individual hereditary characteristics.

Dizygotic (DZ) twins: Nonidentical or DZ twins, like other siblings, share, on average, 50% of their genes.

DNA pooling: Pools DNA from cases and controls and compares the two pooled results for DNA markers. It is conceptually similar to genotyping two individuals (one pooled group of cases and one pooled group of controls) for each DNA marker rather than genotyping each individual (although individual genotyping can be used to confirm the results of DNA pooling).

Dysmorphic syndrome: Related to dysmorphism, abnormality of shape.

Eclampsia: Related to eclampsia, coma and convulsions during or immediately after pregnancy, characterized by edema, hypertension, and proteinuria.

Environment: An individual's environment is to be understood very broadly. It includes everything that influences an individual's phenotype, apart from his or her genotype. Environmental factors include where a person lives and how many siblings he or she has, but also biological factors such as to which chemicals a person might have been exposed to before and after birth.

Etiology: The study of the causes of disorders. With respect to childhood disorders, etiology considers how biological, psychological, and environmental processes interact.

Family Pedigree: An individual's ancestors, used in human genetics to analyze Mendelian inheritance of certain traits, especially of familial diseases.

Family Studies: Studies of genetically related individuals that explore familial aggregation and inherited risk of a disease or disorder.

Fragile X syndrome: An inherited disorder caused by a defective gene on the X chromosome and causing mental retardation, enlarged testes, and facial abnormalities in males and mild or no effects in heterozygous females. It is the most common inherited cause of mental retardation.

Gamete: A mature sexual reproductive cell having a single set of unpaired chromosomes.

Gestational: Of or relating to gestation. Gestation is the period of development in the uterus from conception until birth; pregnancy.

Genotype: The genetic makeup, as distinguished from the physical appearance, of an organism or a group of organisms. The combination of alleles located on homologous chromosomes that determines a specific characteristic or trait.

Group heritability (GH): The extent to which the mean difference between the extreme group and the unselected population is due to heritable factors.

Group Common Environment (GCE): The extent to which the mean difference between the extreme group and the unselected population is due to shared family environmental factors. GF, GH and GCE are all elements of DF analysis.

Group familiality (GF): The regression to the mean of the quantitative trait score of the sibling on a proband selected for an extreme quantitative trait score. The more that the siblings regress to the population mean the lower the familiality. When MZ twins > DZ twin group familiality implies group heritability.

Heritability: Describes the proportion of the variance of a trait that is attributable to genetic influences in the population

Hippocampus: A complex neural structure (shaped like a sea horse) consisting of gray matter and located on the floor of each lateral ventricle; intimately involved in motivation and emotion as part of the limbic system; has a central role in the formation of memories.

Hydrocephalic: Related to hydrocephalus, a usually congenital condition in which an abnormal accumulation of fluid in the cerebral ventricles causes enlargement of the skull and compression of the brain, destroying much of the neural tissue.

Hypothyroidism: Insufficient production of thyroid hormones. A pathological condition resulting from severe thyroid insufficiency, which may lead to cretinism or myxedema.

Linkage analysis: Attempts to determine whether a DNA marker and a trait gene are within millions of nucleotide base pairs on the same chromosome. Detects deviations from independent assortment for a marker and a disease locus within families. Linkage is not powerful in detecting QTLs of small effect size; however, it is possible to scan the entire genome with just a few hundred markers. Sib-pair QTL linkage is more powerful than traditional linkage because it assumes a quantitative distribution, but it cannot detect QTLs that account for less than 10% of the variance.

Macrocephaly: Abnormal largeness of the head. Also called megacephaly, megalocephaly.

Marker genes: Genes with a known function related to the trait being investigated (e.g., intelligence). Targeted in allelic association.

Meiosis: The process of cell division in sexually reproducing organisms that reduces the number of chromosomes in reproductive cells from diploid to haploid, leading to the production of gametes in animals and spores in plants.

Microcephaly: Abnormal smallness of the head.

Microdeletions: Extremely small loss, as through mutation, of one or more nucleotides from a chromosome.

Mitochondrial: Related to mitochondrion, a spherical or elongated organelle in the cytoplasm of nearly all eukaryotic cells, containing genetic material and many enzymes important for cell metabolism, including those responsible for the conversion of food to usable energy. Also called chondriosome.

Molecular Genetics: The branch of genetics that deals with the expression of genes by studying the DNA sequences of chromosomes.

Monozygotic (MZ) twins: MZ twins come from the same fertilized egg and are genetically identical; that is, they have 100% of their genes in common.

Morphology: The branch of biology that deals with the form and structure of organisms without consideration of function.

Neurotransmitter: A chemical substance, such as acetylcholine or dopamine, that transmits nerve impulses across a synapse.

Nomenclature: The procedure of assigning names to the kinds and groups of organisms listed in a taxonomic classification: *the rules of nomenclature in botany.*

Nonadditive Genetic Variance: Genetic factors that contribute to variance in a nonadditive way. Important because they do not contribute much to resemblance between relatives, except in the case of identical twins. Implied when the phenotypic correlation for first-degree relatives is less than half the correlation for identical twins; e.g., in the case of dominance and epistasis.

Nonshared Environment: Environmental influences not shared by children growing up in the same family (e.g., peer relationship).

Normal Distribution: A theoretical frequency distribution for a set of variable data, usually represented by a bell-shaped curve symmetrical about the mean. Also called *Gaussian distribution.*

Nucleotide: Any of various compounds consisting of a nucleoside combined with a phosphate group and forming the basic constituent of DNA and RNA.

Paralytic: A person affected with paralysis.

Perinatal: Of, relating to, or being the period around childbirth, especially the 5 months before and 1 month after birth: *perinatal mortality; perinatal care.*

Phenotype: The constitution of an organism as determined by the interaction of its genetic constitution and the environment. An individual's phenotype consists of all his or her measurable or observable properties and characteristics aside from his or her genes. These could include characteristics such as hair color, height, and IQ score. Researchers in behavioral genetics often include such diverse traits as marital status, taste in music, and religious beliefs as part of the phenotype.

Polygenes: Any of a group of nonallelic genes, each having a small quantitative effect, that together produce a wide range of phenotypic variation. Also called *multiple factor, quantitative gene.*

Polygenic Inheritance: The sum of characteristics genetically transmitted through polygenes from parents to offspring.

Postnatal: Of or occurring after birth, especially during the period immediately after birth.

Post-traumatic Deficits: Physical or cognitive difficulties following injury or resulting from it: *posttraumatic amnesia.*

Prenatal: Existing or occurring before birth.

Profound Mental Retardation: An IQ level below 20 or 25.

Reaction range: The phenotype or behavioral expression of the genotype will vary with the potential range of environmental conditions. Environments that are favorable for a particular trait will broaden the potential range of outcomes, whereas unfavorable conditions will narrow the range.

Shared Environment: Environmental influences shared by children growing up in the same family (e.g., socioeconomic status).

Teratogen: An agent, such as a virus, a drug, or radiation, that causes malformation of an embryo or fetus.

Twin Studies: Studies of MZ and DZ twins allow researchers to examine what proportion of the total phenotypic variance is explained by genetic fac-tors, shared environmental factors, and nonshared environmental factors. Greater similarity or correlation between MZ twins than DZ twins indicates a genetic influence.

Quantitative Trait Loci (QLT): "Susceptibility" genes. QTLs are genes of a relatively small effect size that contribute interchangeably and additively, like probabilistic risk factors. Each QTL can be seen as one gene in a multigene system.

References

Akesson, H. O. (1984). Intelligence and polygenic inheritance. A dogma to re-examine. *Acta Paediatrica Scandinavica, 73*(1), 13–17.

Akesson, H. O. (1986). The biological origin of mild mental retardation. A critical review. *Acta Psychiatrica Scandinavica, 74*(1), 3–7.

Bilder, R. M., Volavka, J., Czobor, P., Malhotra, A. K., Kennedy, J. L., Ni, X., et al. (2002). Neurocognitive correlates of the COMT Val[158] met polymorphism in chronic schizophrenia. *Neuropsychopharmacology, 29*(11), 1943–1961.

Birch, H. G., Richardson, S. A., Baird, D., Horobin, G., & Illsley, R. (1970). *Mental subnormality in the community: A clinical and epidemiological study.* Baltimore: Williams & Williams.

Blomquist, H. K. S., Gustavson, K. H., & Holmgren, G. (1981). Mild mental-retardation in children in a northern Swedish county. *Journal of Mental Deficiency Research, 25,* 169–186.

Botstein, D., & Risch, N. (2003). Discovering genotypes underlying human phenotypes: Past successes for Mendelian disease, future approaches for complex disease. *Nature Genetics, 33*, 228–237.

Broman, S., Nichols, P. L., & Kennedy, W. (1975). *Preschool IQ: Prenatal and early developmental correlates.* Oxford, UK: Lawrence Erlbaum.

Broman, S., Nichols, P. L., Shaughnessy, P., & Kennedy, W. (1987). *Retardation in young children: A developmental study of cognitive deficit.* Hillsdale, NJ: Erlbaum.

Brown, R. I. (2000). Quality of life: Challenges and confrontation. In K. D. Keith, & R. L. Schalock (Eds.), *Cross-cultural perspectives on quality of life* (pp. 347–361). Washington, DC: American Association on Mental Retardation.

Burack, J. A. (1990). Differentiating mental retardation: The two group approach and beyond. In J. A. Burack, R. M. Hodapp, & E. Zigler (Eds.), *Issues in the developmental approach to mental retardation* (pp. 27–48). New York: Cambridge University Press.

Butler, M. G., & Meaney F. J. (Eds.).(2005). *Genetics of developmental disabilities.* Boca Raton: Taylor & Francis Group.

Chipuer, H. M., Rovin, M., & Plomin, R. (1990). LISREL modeling: Genetic and environmental influences on IQ revisited. *Intelligence, 14*, 11–29.

Chorney, M. J., Chorney, K., Seese, N., Owen, M. J., Daniels, J., McGuffin, P., et al. (1998). A quantitative trait locus (QTL) associated with cognitive ability in children. *Psychological Science, 9*, 1–8.

Cicchetti, D., & Sroufe, L. A. (1976). The relationship between affective and cognitive development in Down's syndrome infants. *Child Development, 47*(4), 920–929.

Cicchetti, D., & Pogge-Hesse, P. (1982). Possible contributions of organically retarded persons to developmental theory. In E. Zigler, & D. Balla (Eds.), *Mental retardation: The developmental-difference controversy.* Hillsdale, NJ: Erlbaum Associates.

Clarke, A. D. B. (1985). Mental-retardation: A life-cycle approach (Drew, C. J., Logan, D. R., & Hardman, M. L., Eds.). *British Journal of Mental Subnormality, 32*, 117.

Deary, I. J., Whiteman, M. C., Pattie A., Starr, J. M., Hayward, C., Wright, A. F., et al. (2002). Cognitive change and the APOE epsilon 4 allele. *Nature, 418*, 932.

Deary, I. J., Hamilton, G., Hayward, C., Whalley, L. J., Starr, J. M., & Lovestone, S. (2005) Nicastrin gene polymorphisms, cognitive ability level and cognitive ageing. *Neurosci Lett, 373*, 110–114.

Defries, J. C., & Fulker, D. W. (1985). Multiple-regression analysis of twin data. *Behavior Genetics, 15*, 467–473.

Defries, J. C., & Fulker, D. W. (1988). Multiple regression analysis of twin data: Etiology of deviant scores versus individual differences. *Acta Geneticae Medicae et Gemellologiae, 37*(3–4), 205–216.

Diamond, A., Briand, L., Fossella, J., & Gehlbach, L. (2004). Genetic and neurochemical modulation of prefrontal cognitive functions in children. *American Journal of Psychiatry, 161*(1), 125–132.

Dick, D. M., Jones, K., Saccone, N., Hinrichs, A., Wang, J. C., Goate, A. et al. (2006). Endophenotypes successfully lead to gene identification: Results from the collaboration study on genetics of alcoholism. *Behavior genetics, 36*(1), 112–126.

Dingman, H. F., & Tarjan, G. (1960). Mental retardation and the normal distribution curve. *American Journal of Mental Deficiency, 64*, 991–994.

Down, J. L. (1887). *Mental affections of children and youth.* London: J. & A. Churchill.

Dykens, E. M. (1995). Measuring behavioral phenotypes: Provocations from the new genetics. *American Journal on Mental Retardation, 99*, 522–532.

Dykens, E. M., Hodapp, R. M., Ort, S. I., & Leckman, J. F. (1993). Trajectory of adaptive-behavior in males with fragile x-syndrome. *Journal of Autism and Developmental Disorders, 23*, 135–145.

Erlenmeyer-Kimling, L., & Jarvik, L. (1963). Genetics and intelligence: A review. *Science, 142*, 1477–1479.

Fischer, K. W., & Bullock, D. (1984). *Cognitive development in school-age children: Conclusions and new directions. Development during middle childhood* (pp. 70–146). Washington, DC: National Academy Press.

Fischer, K. W., Bullock, D. H., Rotenberg, E. J., & Raya, P. (1993). *The dynamics of competence: How context contributes directly to skill. Development in context* (pp. 93–117). Hillsdale, NJ: Erlbaum.

Fisher, S. E., & DeFries, J. C. (2002). Developmental dyslexia: Genetic dissection of a complex cognitive trait. *Nature Review Neuroscience, 3*, 767–780.

Fisher, P. J., Turic, D., Williams, N. M., McGuffin, P., Asherson, P., Ball, D., et al. (1999). DNA pooling identifies QTLs on chromosome 4 for general cognitive ability in children. *Human Molecular Genetics, 8*(5), 915–922.

Flint, J., Corley, R., DeFries, J. C., Fulker, D. W., Gray, J. A., Miller, S., & Collins, A. C. (1995). A simple genetic basis for a complex psychological trait in laboratory mice. *Science, 269*(5229), 1432–1435.

Galton, F. (1869). *Hereditary genius: An inquiry into its laws and consequences.* London: Watts and Co.

Galton, F. (1883). *Inquiries into human faculty and its development.* London: MacMillan.

Galton, F. (1889). *Natural inheritance.* London: MacMillan.

Goldberg, T. E., Egan, M. F., Gscheidle, T., Coppola, R., Weickert, T., Kolachana, B. S., et al. (2003). Executive subprocesses in working memory: Relationship to catechol-O-methyltransferase Val158Met genotype and schizophrenia. *Archives of General Psychiatry, 60*(9), 889–896.

Goodman, J. F. (1990). Problems in etiological classifications of mental retardation. *Journal of Child Psychology & Psychiatry & Allied Disciplines, 31*(3), 465–469.

Gosso, M. F., van Belzen, M. J., de Geus, E. J. C., Polderman, J. C., Heutink, P., Boomsma, D. I., et al. (2006). Association between the CHRM2 gene and intelligence in a sample of 304 Dutch families. *Gene, Brain and Behavior, 5*(8), 577–584.

Gostason, R. (1985). Psychiatric illness among the mentally retarded. A Swedish population study. *Acta Psychiatrica Scandinavica. Supplementum, 318*, 1–117.

Grados-Johnson, J., & Russo-Garcia, K. A. (1999). Comparison of the Kaufman Brief Intelligence Test and the Wechsler Intelligence Scale for Children-Third Edition in economically disadvantaged African American youth. *Journal of Clinical Psychology, 55*(9), 1063–1071.

Hagberg, B., Hagberg, G., Lewerth, A., & Lindberg, U. (1981a). Mild mental retardation in Swedish school children. I. Prevalence. *Acta Paediatrica Scandinavica, 70*(4), 441–444.

Hagberg, B., Hagberg, G., Lewerth, A., & Lindberg, U. (1981b). Mild mental retardation in Swedish school children. II. Etiologic and pathogenetic aspects. *Acta Paediatrica Scandinavica, 70*(4), 445–452.

Hariri, A. R., Goldberg, T. E., Mattay, V. S., Kolachana, B. S., Callicott, J. H., Egan, M. F., et al. (2003). Brain-Derived neurotrophic factor val 66 met polymorphism affects human memory-related hippocampal activity and predicts memory performance. *The Journal of Neuroscience. 23*(17), 6690–6694.

Haworth, C. M. A., Kovas, Y., Petrill, S. A., & Plomin, R. (2007). Developmental origins of low mathematics performance and normal variation in twins from 7 to 9 years. *Twin Research and Human Genetics, 10,* 106–117.

Helms, J. E. (1992). Why is there no study of cultural equivalence in standardized cognitive-ability testing. *American Psychologist, 47,* 1083–1101.

Hill, L., Chorney, M. J., Lubinski, D., Thompson, L. A., & Plomin, R. (2002). A quantitative trait locus not associated with cognitive ability in children: A failure to replicate. *Psychological Science: a Journal of the American Psychological Society, 13*(6), 561–562.

Hodapp, R. M., & Dyckens, E. M. (1996). Mental retardation. In E. J. Mash, & R. A. Barkley (Eds.), *Child psychopathology* (pp. 362–389). New York: Guildford.

Hodapp, R. M., & Zigler, E. (1990). Applying the developmental perspective to individuals with Down syndrome. In D. Cicchetti, & M. Beeghly (Eds.), *Children with Down syndrome: A developmental perspective* (pp. 1–28). New York: Cambridge Univ. Press.

Hodapp, R., & Zigler, E. (1997). New issues in the developmental approach to mental retardation. In W. E. MacLean (Ed.), *Ellis' handbook of mental deficiency, psychological theory and research* (3rd ed.). Mahwah: NJ: Lawrence Earlbaum Associates, Inc.

Iarocci, G., & Burack, J. A. (1998). Understanding the development of persons with mental retardation: Challenging the myths. In J. A. Burack, R.M. Hodapp, & E. Zigler (Eds.), *Handbook of mental retardation and development* (pp. 349–381). New York: Cambridge University Press.

Johnson, C. A., Ahern, F. M., & Johnson, R. C. (1976). Level of functioning of siblings and parents of probands of varying degrees of retardation. *Behavior Genetics, 64*(4), 473–477.

Jonker, C., Schmand, B., Lindeboom, J., Havekes, L. M., & Launer, L. J. (1998). Association between apolipoprotein E epsilon4 and the rate of cognitive decline in community-dwelling elderly individuals with and without dementia. *Archives of Neurology, 55,* 1065–1069.

Joober, R., Gauthier, J., Lal, S., Bloom, D., Lalonde, P., Rouleau, G., et al. (2002). Catechol-O-methyltransferase Val-108/158-Met gene variants associated with performance on the Wisconsin Card Sorting Test. *Archives of General Psychiatry, 59,* 622–663.

Kephart, N. C., & Strauss, A. A. (1940). A clinical factor influencing variations in IQ. *American Journal of Orthopsychiatry, 10,* 343–351.

King, B. H., State, M. W., Shah, B., Davanzo, P., & Dykens, E. (1997). Mental retardation: A review of the past 10 years. *Child and Adolescent Psychiatry, 36*(Part I), 1656–1663.

Knight, S. J., Regan, R., Nicod, A., Horsley, S. W., Kearney, L., Homfray, T., et al. (1999). Subtle chromosomal rearrangements in children with unexplained mental retardation. *Lancet, 354*(9191), 1676–1681.

Kounin, J. S. (1941). Experimental studies of rigidity. II. The explanatory power of the concept of rigidity as applied to feeble-mindedness. *Character & Personality; A Quarterly for Psychodiagnostic & Allied Studies, 9,* 273–282.

Kryukov, G. V., Pennacchio, L. A., & Sunyaev, S. R. (2007). Most rare missense alleles are deleterious in humans: Implications for complex disease and association studies. *The American Journal of Human Genetics, 80,* 727–739.

Lewis, A. (1993). Inheritance of mental disorders. *Eugenics Review, 25,* 79–84.

Mainardi, P. C., Perfumo, C., Cali, A., Coucourde, G., Pastore, G., Cavani, S., et al. (2001). Clinical and molecular characterisation of 80 patients with 5p deletion: Genotype-phenotype correlation. *Journal of Medical Genetics. 38,* 151–158.

MacMillan, D. L., Siperstein, G. N., & Gresham, F. M. (1996). A Challenge to the viability of mild mental retardation as a diagnostic category. *Exceptional Children, 62,* 356–371.

Malhotra, A. K., Kestler, L. J., Mazzanti, C., Bates, J. A., Goldberg, T., & Goldman, D. (2002). A functional polymorphism in the COMT gene and performance on a test pf prefrontal cognition. *The American Journal of Psychiatry, 159,* 652–654.

Mayeux, R., Small, S. A., Tang, M., Tycko, B., & Stern, Y. (2001). Memory performance in healthy elderly without Alzheimer's disease: Effects of time and Apolipoprotein-E. *Neurobiology of Aging, 22(4),* 683–689.

McCartney, K., Harris, M. J., & Bernieri, F. (1990). Growing up and growing apart: A developmental meta-analysis of twin studies. *Psychological Bulletin, 107,* 226–237.

McClearn, G. E., Johansson, B., Berg, S., Pedersen, N. L., Ahern, F., Petrill, S. A., & Plomin, R. (1997). Substantial genetic influence on cognitive abilities in twins 80 or more years old. *Science, 276*(5318), 1560–1563.

McGue, M. (1997). The democracy of the genes. *Nature, 388*(6641), 417–418.

McGue, M., Bouchard, T. J., Iacono, W. G., & Lykken, D. T. (1993). Behavioral genetics of cognitive ability: A life span perspective. In R. Plomin, & G. E. McClearn (Eds.), *Nature, nurture and psychology* (pp. 59–76). Washington, D.C.: American Psychological Association.

Nichols, P. L. (1984). Familial mental retardation. *Behavior Genetics, 14*(3), 161–170.

Nokelainen, P., & Flint, J. (2002). Genetic effects on human cognition: Lessons from the study of mental retardation syndromes. *Journal of Neurology, Neurosurgery & Psychiatry, 72,* 287–296.

Nolan, K. A., Bilder, R. M., Lachman, H. M., & Volavka, J. (2004). Catechol O-methyltransferase Val158Met polymorphism in schizophrenia: Differential effects of Val and Met alleles on cognitive stability and flexibility. *The American Journal of Psychiatry, 161,* 359–361.

Pearson, K., & Jaederholm, G. A. (1914). *On the continuity of mental defect.* London: Dalau & Co.

Pendleton, N., Payton, A., van den Boogerd, E. H., Holland, F., Diggle, P., Rabbitt, P. M., et al. (2002). Apolipoprotein E genotype does not predict decline in intelligence in healthy older adults. *Neuroscience Letters, 10,* 74–76.

Penrose, L. S. (1963). Measurements of likeness in relatives of trisomics. *Annals of Human Genetics, 27*(2), 183–187.

Penrose, L. S. (1970). Measurement in mental deficiency. *British Journal of Psychiatry, 116*(533), 369–375.

Petrill, S. A. (2002). The case of general intelligence: A behavioral genetic perspective. In R. J. Sternberg, & E. L. Grigorenko (Eds.), *The General Factor of Intelligence: How General is it?* (pp. 281–298) Mahwah: Lawrence Erlbaum Associates.

Petrill, S. A., Ball, D. M., Eley, T. C., Hill, L., Plomin, R., McClearn, G. E., et al. (1998). Failure to replicate a QTL association between a DNA marker identified by EST00083 and IQ. *Intelligence, 25,* 179–184.

Petrill, S. A., Johansson, B., Pedersen, N. L., Berg, S., Plomin, R., Ahern, F., & McClearn, G. E. (2001). Low cognitive functioning in nondemented 80+ year old twins is not heritable. *Intelligence, 29*, 31–43.

Petrill, S. A., Lipton, P. A., Hewitt, J. K., Plomin, R., Cherny, S. S., Corley, R., et al (2004). Genetic and environmental contributions to general cognitive ability through the first 16 years of life. *Developmental Psychology, 40*, 805–812.

Petrill, S. A., Saudino, K., Cherny, S. S., Emde, R. N., Hewitt, J. K., Fulker, D. W., & Plomin, R. (1997). Exploring the genetic etiology of low general cognitive ability from 14 to 36 months. *Developmental Psychology, 33*(3), 544–548.

Plomin, R. (1994). Genetic research and identification of environmental influences. *Journal of Child Psychology and Psychiatry, 35*, 817–834.

Plomin, R. (1997). Identifying genes for cognitive abilities and disabilities. In R. J. Sternberg, & E. L. Grigorenko (Eds.), *Intelligence, heredity, and environment.* New York: Cambridge University Press.

Plomin, R. (1999). Genetic research on general cognitive ability as a model for mild mental retardation. *International Review of Psychiatry, 11*, 34–36.

Plomin, R. (2001). Genetic factors contributing to learning and language delays and disabilities. *Genetic Contributions to Learning and Language Delays and Disabilities, 10*(2), 259–277.

Plomin, R., DeFries, J. C., & Loehin, J. C. (1977). Genotype-environment interaction and correlation in the analysis of human behavior. *Psychological Bulletin, 84*(2), 309–322.

Plomin, R., McClearn, G. E., Smith, D. L., Skuder, P., Vignetti, S., Chorney, M. J., et al. (1995). Allelic associations between 100 DNA markers and high versus low IQ. *Intelligence, 21*, 31–48.

Plomin, R., & Crabbe, J. C. (2000). DNA. *Psych Bull, 126*, 806–828.

Plomin, R., & Kovas, Y. (2005). Generalist genes and learning disabilities. *Psychological Bulletin, 131*, 562–617.

Plomin, R., & Rutter, M. (1998). Child development, molecular genetics, and what to do with genes once they are found. *Child Development, 69*(4), 1223–1242.

Plomin, R., & Spinath, F. M. (2004). Intelligence: Genetics, genes, and genomics. *Journal of Personality and Social Psychology, 186*, 112–129.

Plomin, R., & Thompson, L. A. (1993). Genetics and high cognitive ability. In G. R. Bock & K. Ackrill (Eds.), *The origin and development of high ability* (pp. 67–84). London: Ciba Foundation Symposium 178.

Plomin, R., Turic, D. M., Hill, L., Hill, L., Turic, D, E., Stephens, M., Williams, J., et al. (2004). A functional polymorphism in the succinate-semialdehyde dehydrogenase (aldehyde dehydrogenase 5 family, member A1) gene is associated with cognitive ability. *Molecular Psychiatry, 9*(6), 582–586.

Rao, J. M. (1990). A population-based study of mild mental handicap in children: Preliminary analysis of obstetric associations. *Journal of Mental Deficiency Research, 34*, 59–65.

Raynham, H., Gibbons, R., Flint, J., & Higgs, D. (1996). The genetic basis for mental retardation. *QJM: monthly journal of the Association of Physicians, 89*(3), 169–175.

Reed, E. W., & Reed, S. C. (1965). *Mental retardation: A family study.* Philadelphia: Saunders.

Richardson, S. A., & Koller, H. (1996). *Twenty-two years: Causes and consequences of mental retardation.* Cambridge, MA: Harvard University Press.

Richardson, S. A., Koller, H., & Katz, M. (1985). Relationship of upbringing to later behavior disturbance of mildly mentally retarded young people. *American Journal of Mental Deficiency, 90*(1), 1–8.

Roberts, J. A. (1952). The genetics of mental deficiency. *Fraser; Eugenics Review, 44*, 71–83.

Roberts, J. A., Norman, R. M., & Griffiths, R. (1938). Studies on a child population. IV. The form of the lower end of the frequency distribution of Stanford-Binet intelligence quotients with advancing age. *Annals of Eugenics, 8*, 319.

Rosa, A., Peralta, V., Cuesta, M. J., Zarzuela, A., Serrano, F., Martinez-Larrea, A., et al. (2004). New evidence of association between COMT gene and prefrontal neurocognitive function in healthy individuals from sibling pairs discordant for psychosis. *The American Journal of Psychiatry, 161*(6), 1110–1112.

Rutter, M., Simonoff, E., & Plomin, R. (1996). Genetic influences on mild mental retardation: Concepts, findings and research implications. *Journal of Biosocial Science, 28*(4), 509–526.

Saudino, K. J., Plomin, R., & Pederson, N. L. (1994). The etiology of high and low cognitive ability during the second half of the life span. *Intelligence, 19*(3), 359–371.

Scarr, S., & Weinberg, R. A. (1978). The influence of "family background" on intellectual attainment. *American Sociological Review, 43*, 674–692.

Scarr-Salapetek, S. (1973). Unknowns in the IQ equation. In F. Rebelsky, & L. Dorman (Eds.), *Child development and behavior* (2nd ed.). Oxford, UK: Alfred A. Knopf.

Simonoff, E., Bolton, P., & Rutter, M. (1996). Mental retardation: Genetic findings, clinical implications and research agenda. *Journal of Child Psychology and Psychiatry, 37*(3), 259–280.

State, M. W., King, B. H., & Dykens, E. (1997). Mental retardation: A review of the past 10 years. Part II. *Journal of the American Academy of Child Adolescent Psychiatry, 36*, 1664–1671.

Stromme, P., & Hagberg, G. (2000). Aetiology in severe and mild mental retardation: A population-based study of Norwegian children. *Developmental Medicine and Child Neurology, 42*, 76–86.

Thelen, E., & Smith, L. B. (1998). Dynamic systems theories. In R. M. Lerner, & W. Damon (Eds.), *Handbook of child psychology.* (5th ed., Vol. 1, pp. 563–633). New York: Wiley.

Turic, D., Fisher, P. J., Plomin, R., & Owen, M. J. (2001). No association between apolipoprotein E polymorphisms and general cognitive ability in children. *Neuroscience Letters, 299*, 97–100.

Tredgold, A. F. (1908). *Mental deficiency: Amentia.* (pp. 410). Oxford, UK: Balliere.

Weiss, B., Weisz, J. R., & Bromfield, R. (1986). Performance of retarded and nonretarded persons on information-processing tasks: Further tests of the similar structure hypothesis. *Psychological Bulletin, 100*(2), 157–175.

Weisz, J. R., & Yeates, K. O. (1981). Cognitive development in retarded and nonretarded persons: Piagetian tests of the similar structure hypothesis. *Psychological Bulletin, 90*(1), 153–178.

Werner, H., & Strauss, A. (1939). Problems and methods of functional analysis in mentally deficient children. *Abnormal & Social Psychology, 34*, 37–62.

Zetlin, A. G., & Morrison, G. M. (1998). Adaptation through the life span. In J. A. Burack, & R. M. Hodapp (Eds.), *Handbook of mental retardation and development.* (pp. 481–503). New York: Cambridge University Press.

Zigler, E. (1967). Familial mental retardation: A continuing dilemma. *Science, 155*, 292–298.

Zigler, E., & Hodapp, R. M. (1986). *Understanding mental retardation.* New York: Cambridge University Press.

The Contribution of Developmental Models Toward Understanding Gene-to-Behavior Mapping: The Case of Williams Syndrome

Mayada Elsabbagh *and* Annette Karmiloff-Smith

Abstract

This chapter discusses the ways in which research findings about the genetic, developmental, neuroanatomical, and behavioral characteristics of persons with Williams syndrome (WS) are incorporated into theoretical models of gene–environment interactions, and it critically evaluates the rationale and assumptions of each approach. It demonstrates that, despite the wealth of findings from research into WS, developmental questions concerning the link of genes to behavioral outcomes are yet to be resolved. The chapter discusses three approaches to the neurocognitive study of WS, including neuropsychological approaches; bridging gene, brain, and cognition; and developmental approaches. Differences in objectives, assumptions, hypotheses, and consequently, the in methodology of these approaches are addressed. The analysis will focus on how these approaches apply to WS as an illustration of their broader applicability to special populations in general.

Keywords: Williams syndrome, neuropsychological approaches, bridging approach, cognition, gene-to-behavior mapping

Among the fundamental questions in the study of cognitive neuroscience is the differential contribution of genes and environment to behavior. Two broad theoretical orientations make different claims about the nature of interactions between genes and environment. According to neuroconstructivist approaches, the genetic influence is constraining, but the environment plays an active role in shaping behavioral outcomes (Elman et al., 1996; Karmiloff-Smith, 1998). Conversely, according to some neuropsychological theories, certain behavioral outcomes are genetically predetermined, and the environment acts only as a trigger (Chomsky, 1975; Pinker, 1994).

The question of how much genes contribute to behavioral outcomes has largely been framed within the issue of the independence of behavioral domains and the brain systems that mediate them (i.e., the extent to which these systems can be regarded as *modular*). Broadly speaking, the concept of modularity concerns the degree to which perceptual and cognitive systems develop and function independently of one another. Exactly what constitutes a module varies widely across disciplines and theoretical approaches. Fodor (1983) provides the most explicit definition of modularity. In his view, a module is a perceptual input system that meets several criteria, including that they are domain specific, operating exclusively on certain types of input, and localized in particular brain areas. Although this strict definition of modularity has been challenged, other forms in the adult human mind/brain are generally accepted. For example, there is little controversy that highly specialized areas of the visual cortex selectively process specific dimensions of the visual experience, such as color and orientation. However, for higher-level cognition, the extent to which a specific brain region can be thought of as the "language module" or the "face module" is more controversial. The study of special populations provides an illustration of the modularity debates and provides a rich source of evidence. The assumption is that developmental disorders provide unique opportunities to understand the link between genes and behavioral outcomes. For example, Williams syndrome (WS) traditionally gained considerable attention from researchers in the field of cognitive neuroscience because of the apparent independence of language from the rest of cognition, supporting a genetically prespecified language faculty (Pinker, 1999; Gopnik, 1990). *why match on language?*

Developmentalists have addressed the implications of cross-domain relations and disassociations within the context of developmental theory (Burack, Hodapp, & Zigler 1998). For instance, those who favor the notion of progressive modularization (Karmiloff-Smith, 1992) challenge the view that developmental disorders, including WS, support genetically prespecified modules. According to this neuroconstructivist view, explanations of the behavioral profile observed in this population, and more generally in typical and atypical development, must extend beyond descriptions of inter- or intradomain dissociations. Rather, they must be done through examinations of behavior over the course of developmental time and investigations of more basic processes that underlie performance in cognitive domains (Elman et al., 1996; Karmiloff-Smith, 1998).

The goal of this chapter is to discuss the ways in which research findings about the genetic, developmental, neuroanatomical, and behavioral characteristics of persons with WS are incorporated into theoretical models of gene–environment interactions, and to critically evaluate the rationale and assumptions of each approach. Our review will demonstrate that, despite the wealth of findings from research into WS, developmental questions concerning the link of genes to behavioral outcomes are yet to be resolved.

We will discuss three approaches to the neurocognitive study of WS, including neuropsychological approaches; bridging gene, brain, and cognition; and developmental approaches. Differences in objectives, assumptions, hypotheses, and consequently, in the methodology of these approaches are addressed next. Our analysis will focus on how these approaches apply to WS as an illustration of their broader applicability to special populations in general.

Neuropsychological Approaches

The main objective of the adult neuropsychological approach is to use patterns of impairment in the adult to arrive at a theory of typical cognitive processes and brain structure. The theoretical construct of modularity (Fodor, 1983) is a central concept for the neuropsychological approach, and can be thought of as one of its axioms. Seeking evidence for the functional components of cognition, modular analysis extensively involves demonstrating double dissociations (DD). Different versions of modular analysis share a similar logic. The adult brain damage version of DD is typically described using the following scenario: After a brain injury, Patient A loses the capacity to perform task X but can still perform task Y. Another Patient, B, shows the opposite pattern: He can perform Y but not X. In this case, researchers infer that functions X and Y are doubly dissociated, in that they function independently of one another. A further inference is that the sites of lesion in Patients A and B are causal for functions X and Y, respectively. These inferences are used to construct a model of which areas of the brain are responsible for which functions.

In the more recent field of developmental, rather than adult neuropsychology, the objective is mainly to arrive at a model of the normal child state from patterns of developmental impairment and developmental disorders, including WS. The extension of the adult DD logic to development is questionable since WS, like most conditions of developmental disorders, is not associated with frank neurological lesions. Thus, the logic is modified in the developmental case. Child A has learned skill X but not skill Y. Another Child, B, has learned Y but not X. On those bases, the developmental dissociation between X and Y is inferred. However, the application of modular analysis to adult and child acquired disorders does not necessarily imply genetic specification of a modular architecture, and this is even accepted by those who are proponents of the applicability of the adult neuropsychological approach to the child (e.g., Temple, 1997). Yet another stronger version of DD is used to support a particular claim, namely, genetic modularity: Due to genetic impairment, Child A fails to learn skill X but learns skill Y. Another Child, B, shows the opposite pattern: He learns Y but not X. In this case, researchers infer that skills X and Y map onto the mutated gene or the specific set of genes in each case. The child is deemed to be missing the necessary module to develop the skill in question.

What are the assumptions embedded in the logic of DD in relation to genetic disorders? The most critical assumptions are (a) that specific brain substrates underlie dissociable functional components—the *dissociability assumption*; and (b) that lesions or disorders cause the subtraction of the affected module, reflected in functional impairment on tasks relevant to that module, while all other functions operate normally—the *subtractivity or* residual normality assumption.

Evidence for genetic modularity has come from the study of developmental disorders like WS. Initial excitement about WS was motivated by the inference that the uneven behavioral profile in this syndrome demonstrated the independence of language from general cognition (Bellugi, Lichtenberger, Mills, Galaburda, & Korenberg, 1999). Although more recently a more complex picture of strengths and deficits within each domain has begun to emerge, WS is still described as a disorder in which we find "striking preservation" of language, and face processing alongside severe visuospatial deficit (Bellugi, Lichtenberger, Jones, Lai, & St. George, 2000). Individuals with WS do not exhibit the expected performance levels based on their chronological age (CA) on standardized tests assessing a wide range of visuospatial and visuoconstructive skills, which include pattern construction (e.g., block design), visual–motor integration, visuospatial memory, and orientation judgment (Bellugi, Bihrle, Jernigan, Trauner, & Doherty, 1990; Bellugi, Sabo, & Vaid, 1988; Mervis, Morris, Bertrand, & Robinson, 1999; Wang, Doherty, Rourke, & Bellugi, 1995). Individuals with WS do not even exhibit expected performance levels based on their overall mental age (MA) on some of these tasks, including tests of visual reception, closure, and memory (Crisco, Dobbs, & Mulhern, 1988). Furthermore, individuals with WS score below MA-matched individuals with Down syndrome (DS) on a subset of these standardized spatial measures (Bellugi et al., 1999). These difficulties cannot be attributed to visual neglect (Bellugi et al., 1988; Wang et al., 1995) nor do they strictly result from motor impairment, since individuals with WS perform well on some motor tasks like tracing complex figures (Bellugi et al., 1988).

In contrast to their performance on visuospatial and visuoconstructive tests, most adolescents and adults with WS perform within the normal range expected for their CA on standardized tests of face and object discrimination and recognition (Bellugi et al., 1988, 1990; Udwin & Yule, 1991; Wang et al., 1995). However, in experimental studies of face perception in WS, subtle abnormalities are frequently reported depending on the task. When asked to match faces on a number of dimensions

including emotional expression, identity, and lip-reading, individuals with WS performed at the level of MA-matched controls but below the level of the CA-matched comparison group (Deruelle, Mancini, Livet, Casse-Perrot, & de Schonen, 1999). Recognition of basic facial emotions was found to be worse in individuals with WS relative to CA-matched controls, but their performance on this task did not differ from MA-matched controls (Gagliardi et al., 2003).

In a stricter application of modular analysis, WS and another developmental condition, namely, specific language impairment (SLI), have been taken as a doubly dissociated pair of the rule-based versus associative memory language systems, implying genetically specified modules for these two domains (Pinker, 1999). Evidence for this claim comes from investigations of English past-tense formation. Children with SLI have difficulties in past-tense formation and crucially do not exhibit an advantage for regular over irregular past-tense formation (Ulman & Gopnik, 1999). Conversely, WS children are claimed to display a particular difficulty in generating irregular past-tense forms, whereas the regular past-tense forms are unproblematic (Clahsen & Almazan, 1998). This led to the conclusion that behavioral components in developmental disorders are dissociable (*dissociability*) and that development and performance in the unaffected domains is normal (*residual normality*).

Nevertheless, claims of dissociability and residual normality have been challenged based on findings from WS. Once fine-grained methods are used to assess participants, clear-cut selective patterns of impairment and sparing are no longer found, invalidating the assumption of residual normality. Subtle abnormalities are found in virtually all domains, including ones generally described as areas of strength, such as language and face processing (e.g., Grant, Karmiloff-Smith, Berthoud, & Christophe, 1996; Karmiloff-Smith et al., 2004; Thomas et al., 2001). Although patters of strength and weakness are found in WS, performance within individuals across various domains is highly correlated (Mervis et al., 1999), contradicting the assumption of dissociability.

In addition to these findings, other patterns of performance in WS are difficult to fit within a modular framework. For instance, equivalent levels of performance found in areas of strength in WS may be driven by atypical processing strategies. For example, in face processing tasks, individuals with WS seem to be driven by a predominantly featural processing strategy, unlike typically developing individuals, who reply more on a configural strategy (Deruelle et al., 1999; Karmiloff-Smith, 1997; Karmiloff-Smith et al., 2004). Similarly, it is suggested that proficiency in language and music in WS is mediated by atypical auditory strategies (Elsabbagh, Cohen, & Karmiloff-Smith, 2010; Elsabbagh, Cohen, Cohen, Rosen, & Karmiloff-Smith, in press). Consistent with these behavioral differences, different brain structures from those found in typical circumstances are involved in language and face processing in WS (Grice et al., 2001; Mills et al., 2000). These atypical patterns of brain specialization are difficult to explain in terms of preserved or impaired modules.

Generally, the utility of applying a strictly modular approach to investigating developmental disorders has been challenged (Karmiloff-Smith, 1998). Modular analysis lends itself to unconstrained flexibility in the face of inconsistent data; a modular framework can, without fail, carve existing modules into increasingly smaller components or keep adding new modules to accommodate a given behavioral pattern. This infinite decomposition is exemplified by the modular analysis of the cognitive profile observed in WS, as linguistic knowledge is claimed to be separated from general cognition (Pinker, 1999; Gopnik, 1990). Language in WS was subsequently carved into components for rule-based versus memory-based systems for syntax (Clahsen & Almazan, 1998) and separated face processing and object processing from the rest of visuospatial skills (Bellugi et al., 1990; Udwin & Yule, 1991; Wang et al., 1995). This seemingly infinite refinement of cognitive architecture raises the possibility that it is simply the task itself that can account for what is deemed to be a module, shedding doubt on the falsifiability of modular theories.

Does WS present a case for "intact" and "impaired" modules across various cognitive domains? If so, does this pattern support genetically prespecified modular architecture? This view fails to capture the complexities of the behavioral profile in WS and indicates that the use of developmental disorders as evidence for genetic modularity is theoretically and empirically flawed.

Bridging the Gene, the Brain, and Cognition

The rationale of the bridging approach is that understanding developmental disorders must be done through specifying the unique profile presented by each condition and elucidating the key aspects that differentiate these profiles (Bellugi et al., 1999, 2000; Mervis et al., 2000). Researchers aim to provide a multifaceted view of the molecular genetics on the one hand, and the neuroanatomical and cognitive phenotype on the other, to enhance our understanding of the neurobiological bases of WS. This would allow us to match cognitive abnormalities with their probable bases in genetic and neuroanatomical abnormalities (Bellugi et al., 2000).

In mapping the cognitive profile of WS, researchers focus on higher-level domains, such as language and visuospatial processing, seeking selective patterns of impairment and sparing, mostly in late childhood and adulthood. Other syndromes, such as DS, have been used as comparison groups against which these selective patterns seem to clearly emerge. The picture of striking language abilities in the face of serious visuospatial impairment in WS is primarily based on comparing profiles of individuals with WS and DS who are matched on MA. For instance, relative to individuals with DS, individuals with WS are worse on several standardized spatial measures, but reveal more proficiency on many receptive and expressive language skills (Bellugi et al., 1999).

Since the goal of the research is to map impaired genes to impaired behavior alongside an otherwise normal brain, it is no surprise that the hallmark of this mapping is the search for dissociations, both between as well as within domains (Bellugi et al., 2000). Similar to the neuropsychological approach, assumptions of *dissociability* and *residual normality* resonate here too. Therefore, the bridging approach can be thought of as a special application of the neuropsychological model to WS.

We have already addressed why applying adult neuropsychological models to developmental cases has been seriously challenged. Here, we illustrate, with examples from the research on WS, how the bridging approach is useful in mapping genetic and neuroanatomical patterns to behavioral profiles. These examples, particularly the link between neuroanatomy and behavior, are abundant in the literature and have covered almost all major physical, behavioral, and social characteristics of the WS phenotype.

Gene-to-Behavior Mapping

The WS critical region contains some 28 genes, all of which are missing in 98% of cases. Variable deletion cases are found among a few individuals with full-blown WS, but mainly among individuals who exhibit cardiovascular impairments (supravalvular aortic stenosis; SVAS) but do not usually share other major characteristics of WS. These cases may provide clues regarding the relationship between specific missing genes and specific phenotypic outcomes (Frangiskakis et al., 1996; Tassabehji et al., 1996). For instance, the Elastin deletion usually causes heart and pulmonary defects (Bellugi et al., 1999; Tassabehji et al., 1999), but what about other characteristics of WS? Can researchers use the same logic to infer a link between specific gene deletions and cognitive-level deficits? Using a simple subtraction procedure, the bridging approach has linked genes to cognitive outcomes based on variable deletion cases (Bellugi et al., 1999).

At first blush, this bridging model is appealing, and a few of its predictions have gained some empirical support. For instance, the deletion of the LIMK1 gene has been linked to visuospatial deficit (Frangiskakis et al., 1996). However, this was not replicated in another study of two individuals who had identical deletions and who scored within the normal range of intellectual abilities in general, and in all the visuospatial tasks in particular (Gray, Karmiloff-Smith, Funnell, & Tassabehji, 2006). Furthermore, graded effects of LIMK1 expression on visuospatial skills were not found in a group of individuals with variable partial deletions (i.e., smaller than the WS critical region). The visuospatial abilities of individuals with deletion of only Elastin and LIMK1 did not differ from individuals with larger partial deletions. The entire group of variable deletion cases performed within the normal range indicates that LIMK1 deletion does not, in isolation, cause visuospatial deficit (Tassabehji et al., 1999).

How can these findings be reconciled? The inconsistency can be attributed to at least two sources. One is that the differences in findings demonstrate that direct linking between the two levels cannot be achieved without taking into account the developmental process that mediates the effects of genes on behavior (Elman et al., 1996). If gene expression were probabilistic, one would expect the group of individuals with LIMK1 deletions as a whole to have a higher incidence of visuospatial deficits, but not all individuals in the group may show this pattern. Another possibility is that, although not behaviorally apparent, the deletion has subtle effects on the domain. Gray et al. (2006) do not favor this claim, since they have conducted detailed testing of their deletion patients and still did not find subtle impairments in the spatial domain. However, they did not investigate subtle

differences in strategies of processing, which are thought to be an important aspect of gene expression (Scerif & Karmiloff-Smith, 2005). A combination of these two possibilities could then explain the variability in gene expression across individuals.

Neuroanatomy-to-Behavior Mapping

In a manner not so different from gene-to-behavior mapping in WS, researchers also juxtapose patterns of structural "intactness" or "impairment" in the brain onto their functional counterparts, relying on adult models of which areas preserve which functions. Various neuroanatomical abnormalities in WS have been mapped to function in this manner. For example, the basis of visuospatial deficits is claimed to be the reduction in size of the cortical and subcortical extrastriate visual pathways (Reiss et al., 2004), coupled with higher cell packing density in some of these regions (Galaburda, Holinger, Bellugi, & Sherman, 2002). Conversely, the relative preservation of auditory processing, language, face, and emotion functions is thought to be due to the enlargement of the size of the amygdala, orbital and medial prefrontal cortices, superior temporal gyrus, and the fusiform gyrus, coupled with increased gray matter density in these areas (Reiss et al., 2000, 2004). It is also proposed in other models that impairment in dorsal pathways underlies deficits in visuospatial functions, whereas intact ventral pathways mediate strengths in face processing (Atkinson et al., 1997; Reiss et al., 2004), as well as in language, music, and other auditory functions (Holinger et al., 2005).

Although precise and comprehensive, certain details of the above claims are problematic, given our limited understanding of the correspondence between structural brain differences and functional abilities. In WS, the analysis drawing direct links between the two has lent itself to unconstrained flexibility in the face of inconsistent data. For example, in explaining the hypersociability and proficiency in face processing in WS, Reiss and colleagues (2004) report an "increase of up to 30% in emotion–face areas relative to overall reduction in brain volume." A different study of the same "emotion–face areas" provided a contradictory result, in which dramatic reduction in the size of the amygdala (almost half of the normal size) was found postmortem in one patient with WS (Galaburda & Bellugi, 2000). Although the authors of the latter study acknowledged the difficulty of generalization based on a single case, they nonetheless interpret their finding regarding the relationship between neuroanatomy and function in the opposite direction, in which the reduction in amygdala size was taken as the basis for the lack of stranger anxiety, and hence hypersociability in WS.

Generally speaking, are bigger, thicker, or denser brains necessarily better? How do volumetric and cellular differences translate to function? Can such bridging approaches provide any answers that are not circular (e.g., individuals with WS have good face processing because they have an enlarged fusiform area, then better face processing is associated with an enlarged fusiform area)? Some appreciation of these issues has very recently begun to emerge in research on WS. Drawing functional implications of the abnormal cortical thickness and complexity in the WS brain, Thompson and colleagues (2005) note that differences in cortical structures in either direction (thickening or thinning) may reflect deficits, but may also reflect compensatory mechanisms varying among individuals.

These issues are not uncommon in the field of developmental disorders. In a comprehensive review, Scerif and Karmiloff-Smith (2005) critically evaluate further applications of "cognitive genetics" to various genetic neurodevelopmental disorders including SLI, fragile X, and DS. The crucial limitation of these applications is not simply that they ignore the developmental process by which genes give rise to cognitive outcomes, but that they also ignore the complexities of the relationship between neural processes and behavioral outcomes in the original models on which these claims are based. Hence, drawing on these divisions in explaining the entirety of the behavioral profile in WS is obviously overly simplistic.

For decades, much of neuropsychology has focused on where functions/behaviors are localized. Rarely challenged, this focus has been carried into research on developmental disorders. Indeed, far more emphasis has been given to the *where* question at the expense of the *why* question. Beyond claims of genetic specification, very little is understood about why, in default circumstances, a region takes on certain functions and not others.

Despite the wealth of data that the bridging approach has generated, many shortcomings are associated with direct linking of genotypic and phenotypic outcomes. Although genes obviously contribute to behavioral outcomes, it is more likely that the mapping between these is indirect and highly experience-dependant. Gene-to-behavior mapping is rarely one-to-one but comes about in interaction within the genetic level, and between the genetic level and the organism's internal and external environment (Elman et al., 1996; Karmiloff-Smith, 1998). Deviant neuroanatomical or neurophysiological characteristics observed in WS may be a result rather than the cause of the behavioral patterns observed.

Developmental Approaches

Although the crucial role of biological constraints in shaping behavioral outcomes is acknowledged in developmental theories, the contribution of the developmental process and environmental interaction is equally emphasized (Elman et al., 1996). According to this view, domain-specific outcomes are achieved through a process of progressive modularization (Karmiloff-Smith, 1992), thus challenging the claim that a static model can be used to explain development in both the typical and atypical case. Genetic abnormalities result in differential selection and processing of input eventually giving rise to alternative forms of brain organization. Hence, it is essential to understand the developmental process itself, including atypical interactions over development. Instead of seeking specific patterns of impairment, researchers seek to identify subtle effects across all domains, including ones in which behavior is proficient. The latter would highlight any processes that differ from the default ones seen in typical development.

Although capturing these developmental changes is essential, it is no simple task. Traditionally, development in atypical circumstances has been viewed as falling into one of two categories: delay or deviance. The goal of most studies has been to assess how the experimental group differs from a norm; that is, whether differences in performance between groups can be attributed to the disorder itself. Different comparison or "matching" procedures are used to assess questions regarding delay or deviance in the behavior of the experimental group relative to the comparison group. These groups can be comprised of typical individuals who are matched on a number of factors such as CA, MA, or performance level in a specific domain (e.g., linguistic ability), as well as on other potentially relevant characteristics such as gender. They can also be individuals with other specific or nonspecific developmental disorders matched on similar criteria.

These traditional categories of delay and deviance do not capture additional possibilities of the nature of differences between experimental and comparison groups. The target population can (a) be delayed in the onset of a given ability, but then catch up to age-appropriate performance; (b) develop slower than average from beginning to mastery; or (c) reach a plateau without attaining mastery (Burack, Iarocci, Bowler, & Mottron, 2002). Alternatively, the target population may (d) exhibit an uneven profile, in which a given ability has a different developmental progression relative to age or language level for example (Leonard, 1999). Hence, these different comparison procedures can be criticized for failing to capture several aspects of development itself. For example, the futility of CA matching and the complexities of choosing the appropriate MA matching strategy in developmental disorders have been extensively discussed (see for e.g., Burack et al., 2002; Jarrold & Brock, 2004; Mervis & Klein-Tasman, 2004).

In studies on WS, patterns of proficiency and impairment are based on comparisons of the WS group to a CA-matched group, an MA-matched group, or to a group of individuals with a different developmental disorder, such as DS. By contrast, many researchers acknowledge that large-scale longitudinal studies in developmental disorders can be powerful in enriching our understanding of these conditions. However, in view of the practical limitations associated with these types of studies, researchers frequently make inferences on the basis of snapshots of development. This is particularly problematic, given that a developmental framework is essential in understanding these conditions (Burack et al., 1998; Cicchetti & Cannon 1999; Karmiloff-Smith, 1998; Rutter & Sroufe, 2000). In the same way that examining a stationary vehicle tells us very little about its velocity, researchers who study children are not necessarily conducting developmental research. Issues of developmental change are not only theoretically important, but they are also significant on empirical grounds. Findings among individuals with WS indicate that certain characteristics of the behavioral profiles observed in adults with the syndrome may differ from those observed in infants or in children with WS (Paterson, Brown, Gsodl, Johnson, & Karmiloff-Smith, 1999; Vicari et al., 2004).

Some researchers stress the importance of building task-specific *developmental trajectories* (Karmiloff-Smith, 1998; Karmiloff-Smith et al., 2004); rather than matching on the basis of CA or MA, performance of the target group can be compared against a trajectory of typical comparison groups, in which patterns of developmental change and developmental stability emerge more clearly. The idea is that assessing change in performance level over developmental time, even if cross-sectional, is more useful in elucidating

atypical trajectories than are snapshots captured at different moments in time and averaged over the group. However, some of the problems frequently encountered in building developmental trajectories are the disparity in age ranges if the sample size is small, and the difficulty in devising tasks that are usable for a wide range of ages. Nevertheless, tracing developmental trajectories in WS has been done with a fair degree of success for a variety of skills, including visual attention, language, face processing, and numerical skills (Ansari & Karmiloff-Smith, 2002; Karmiloff-Smith et al., 2004; Scerif, Cornish, Wilding, Driver, & Karmiloff-Smith, 2004; Thomas et al., 2001).

When building developmental trajectories, an important source of evidence for developmental approaches is research on infancy. This provides insights into precursors to different atypical pathways by indicating whether outcomes observed in older children and adults are already apparent at the outset or are a result of subsequent development. For instance, infants with WS do not initially present with the same pattern of behavioral strengths and weaknesses usually described among adults with WS (Paterson et al., 1999). Generally, infants with WS exhibit delays in several milestones. including language, fine motor coordination, and gross motor skill (Nicholson & Hockey, 1993; Plissart & Fryns, 1999). Furthermore, examining the developmental process of domains, such as language, highlights qualitative differences between infants with WS and typically developing infants. For instance, infants with WS are late in acquiring language (Laing et al., 2002; Singer-Harris, Bellugi, Bates, Jones, & Rossen, 1997). Infants' segmentation of the speech stream is seriously delayed in toddlers with WS relative to typically developing toddlers (Nazzi, Paterson, & Karmiloff-Smith, 2003).

A further goal of developmental approaches is not only to understand differences in the timing of developmental milestones, but also the qualitative nature of the process across various domains in these clinical populations, even for those domains in which behavioral performance is at a proficient level, as in the case of language and face processing in WS. Some atypical patterns observed early on in most infants with WS include an unusual sensitivity to noise, which persists into adulthood but improves for most individuals (Klein, Armstrong, Greer, & Brown, 1990; Van Borsel, Curfs, & Fryns, 1997). Infants with WS exhibit extended and intense looking behavior toward adult faces (Mervis et al., 2003). Other patterns of deviance from the typical milestones observed in infants with WS include differences in pointing and the onset of the vocabulary spurt (Laing et al., 2002; Mervis & Bertrand, 1997).

Despite the late emergence of most abilities, performance on certain language measures tends to improve over time in children with WS well into their teens (Bellugi et al., 1999). However, this can hardly be described as "typical." If there were a single feature that could be described as "striking" about this syndrome, it would be the verbal fluency found in many older children and adults. Some researchers hypothesize that the basis of this fluency is good articulatory capacities and a well-developed phonological system (Grant et al., 1996; Thomas & Karmiloff-Smith, 2003; Volterra, Capiric, Pezzini, & Sabbadini, 1996). Such developed capacities might mask the difficulties people with WS have in other domains of language. For instance, relative to MA-matched comparisons, individuals with WS exhibit more difficulties in phonological awareness tasks, such as rhyme detection and phoneme deletion (Laing, Hulme, Grant, & Karmiloff-Smith, 2001), as well as in nonword repetition tasks (Grant et al., 1996).

A number of findings also support qualitatively different mechanisms in online processing in several domains. For instance, individuals with WS are better local than global processors, as shown by paradigms of visuospatial processing of hierarchical stimuli (Bihrle, Bellugi, Delis, & Marks, 1989; Deruelle et al., 1999). They rely more on featural properties than configural properties when processing faces (Deruelle et al., 1999; Karmiloff-Smith et al., 2004). Moreover, when processing unfamiliar melodies, individuals do not benefit from the same cues that typically developing individuals use. They are able to use pitch cues, which rely on tracking the absolute value of individual notes but not contour cues, which rely on tracking the pattern of rise and fall of the notes (Deruelle, Schon, Rondan, & Mancini, 2005; Elsabbagh et al., in press).

Studying the neural correlates of areas of proficiency in WS also supports atypical patterns of specialization at the brain level. Face processing in WS appears to be atypical when investigated with event-related potentials (ERPs). Although there are marked differences in neural responses to upright versus inverted faces in typically developing persons, these are less differentiated in individuals with WS (Grice et al., 2001; Mills et al., 2000). In the language domain, atypical neural correlates of syntactic and semantic processing have been reported in ERP studies. Individuals with WS do not show the same left anterior asymmetry to grammatical function words found in typically developing children (Mills et al., 2000). They also do not exhibit the same N400 found in normal controls in response to semantic anomaly; instead, they show an uncharacteristic positivity at 200 ms (Mills et al., 2000).

To delineate atypical brain and behavioral organization, cross-syndrome comparisons of associated skills that modulate development of higher-level domains is an area of growing focus in developmental models (Brown et al., 2003; Grice et al., 2003; Scerif et al., 2004). For instance, visuospatial and constructive skills, the areas of greatest deficit for individuals with WS, have benefited from cross-syndrome comparisons. Difficulties in these domains are apparent early on in infancy and childhood in WS. Toddlers with WS show impairment in planning visual saccades (Brown et al., 2003) and in visual search for targets among distractors (Scerif, et al., 2004). In late childhood and adulthood, low-level visual deficits in WS are also present in attentional shifting (Lincoln, Lai, & Jones, 2002) and in low-level perceptual grouping (Grice et al., 2001; Farran, 2005). Infant studies of visual attention in toddlers with WS and fragile X syndrome revealed that, although both populations exhibit overall impairment in searching for targets among distractors, each group showed a qualitatively different pattern of errors (Scerif et al., 2004), implying diverging paths of development in these two clinical groups. Researchers adopting a developmental approach are also particularly interested in cross-domain comparisons of different syndromes. Rather than seeking patterns of impairment and sparing, developmentalists investigate the cognitive processes underlying differences in developmental pathways in different disorders (Scerif & Karmiloff-Smith, 2005).

Genes, the Brain, and Development

Studies of gross neural anatomy, morphology, and cytoarchitectonics reveal widespread abnormalities in the WS brain at multiple levels. Compared to normal individuals, the overall brain volume in WS is reduced to about 80% (Reiss et al., 2000). The reduction is not, however, even across all brain areas. Cerebral volume is close to that found among typically developing persons (around 90%) and is proportionally enlarged in the WS brain, whereas brainstem volume is reduced (around 80%) (Reiss et al., 2000). Additionally, gray matter volume is close to that found in typical comparison groups, whereas white matter volume is

(Reiss et al., 2000). In addition to these gross volumetric abnormalities, cortical thickness and complexity (i.e., cortical folding and sulcal patterning) differ in individuals with WS relative to typically developing persons. Overall, surface complexity is significantly increased in WS, particularly in right perisylvian and inferior temporal areas, with cortical thickness being most marked in the perisylvian cortex (Thompson et al., 2005). Furthermore, increased gyrification is present in the right parietal and occipital, as well as left frontal areas (Schmitt et al., 2002).

Abnormalities in the WS brain also encompass neuronal organization in the cortex. Postmortem studies of WS indicate that the average size of neurons in the visual cortex (area 17) is larger in individuals with WS compared to controls. This increase in neuronal size, coupled with normal or sometimes decreased cell packing density in these areas, is taken to suggest increased subcortical connectivity in the WS brain (Galaburda & Bellugi, 2000). Other cytoarchitectonic differences found in the WS brain include exaggerated horizontal neuronal orientation found across cortical regions (Galaburda et al., 2002). Studies of brain biochemistry are limited, but there is some evidence indicating abnormal levels of the compounds regulating brain metabolism, particularly in the cerebellum (Rae et al., 1998). Yet, these studies are mostly restricted to adults. We therefore have sparse understanding of the developmental mechanisms giving rise to these brain abnormalities.

The findings presented here clearly illustrate that the genetic mutations in WS have widespread effects on brain architecture. Such genetic and neuroanatomical abnormalities are likely to contribute to the complex pattern of behavioral and cognitive strengths and weaknesses in this neurodevelopmental disorder. However, our understanding of how variation in genetic and neuroanatomical characteristics in WS relate to behavioral outcomes is very limited. Further understanding of how these two levels are related would help in evaluating their influence on behavioral tasks such as language. To delineate the relationship between brain and behavior, developmentalists argue that certain brain areas take on the functions they do, not because these ~~ specifically designed for that function, but ~~rea with the computational ~~ particularly well suited to ~~ents of that domain (Elman ~~ords, a *domain-relevant* region ~~cific over time (Karmiloff-~~ntermediate view is that the

typical patterns of cortical specialization for social stimuli emerge during development as a result of interactions and competition between regions that begin with only broadly tuned biases (Johnson, 2001). According to the latter view, some skills may be present at birth, whereas others become increasingly specialized over time, showing gradual developmental changes leading to adult-like processing patterns. In support of this, infants as young as 2 months of age show activation in areas similar to those found in adults in response to faces. However, the activated network in infants is broader, encompassing areas such as the prefrontal cortex (de Haan et al., 2003; Johnson et al., 2005; Tzourio-Mazoyer, De Schonen, Crivello, Reutter, Aujard, & Mazoyer., 2002). Thus, many regions may initially compete for the processing of given inputs, with the special computational properties of one region ultimately winning out. However, a full specification of what those computational properties are is as yet largely unknown. Recent studies have begun to search for the principles, which apply to both typical and atypical development, governing the relationship between neural and functional architecture. For instance, a link has been established between overall brain size and hemispheric connectivity over time (Lewis & Elman, 2008). Variations in brain size over the course of development appear to have an impact on the development and specialization of various functional circuits and their cross-hemispheric relations. This principle has been used in explaining individual differences among normal individuals (e.g., differences in brain connectivity in men and women), as well as in contributing to the explanation of various developmental disorders such as autism. Elucidating further principles of brain neuroanatomy and function is essential in future theorizing.

In sum, converging evidence from the various methodologies reviewed above suggests that modules are the final outcomes of the developmental process, as opposed to prerequisites to it. Furthermore, the progressive development of modules, both in infancy and adulthood, is tightly bound to experience. Developmental disorders are cases in which development takes alternative, atypical pathways.

Yet, how far can we take arguments for brain reorganization and atypical developmental pathways in special populations? Although experience-dependent plasticity appears to be a hallmark of our species' brains, if the brain were infinitely plastic, and alternative modes of organization were always possible, then we would not find behavioral manifestations of developmental disorders. However, in the same

Age range

way that plasticity is not infinite, alternative forms of organization are also limited, and not all give rise to optimal outcomes. After two decades of productive research, there is growing acceptance in the field of a general influential principle: "development itself is the key to understanding developmental disorders" (Karmiloff-Smith, 1998, p. 389). However, developmental approaches still have far to go in delimiting the developmental principles relating genes and behavior and specifying how these are altered in atypical development.

Conclusion

The aims and assumptions of different theoretical approaches shape the questions and conclusions drawn regarding what cases of genetic developmental disorders like WS can reveal about the architecture of the mind/brain, and in turn what research in cognitive neuroscience has to offer by way of explanation and possible remediation of these disorders. Classically, WS has been used to demonstrate the dissociation of cognitive skills, and some theories have gone even further to map the behavioral characteristics in these disorders to specific genetic and neuroanatomical underpinnings. On the other hand, developmentalists who favor the idea of progressive specialization forcefully challenge this approach, emphasizing that the study of developmental disorders must extend beyond simply describing such inter- or intradomain dissociations to include changes in behavior over time and the study of more basic, domain-relevant processes that gradually lead to the patterns observed later in development (Karmiloff-Smith, 1998).

References

Ansari, D., & Karmiloff-Smith, A. (2002). Atypical trajectories of number development: a neuroconstructivist perspective. *Trends in Cognitive Science, 6,* 511–516.

Atkinson, J., King, J., Braddick, O., Nokes, L., Anker, S., & Braddick, F. (1997). A specific deficit of dorsal stream function in Williams syndrome. *Neuroreport, 27,* 1919–1922.

Bellugi, U., Bihrle, A., Jernigan, T., Trauner, D., & Doherty, S. (1990). Neuropsychological, neurological, and neuroanatomical profile of Williams syndrome. *American Journal of Medical Genetics, 6,* 115–125.

Bellugi, U., Lichtenberger, L., Jones, W., Lai, Z., & St. George, M. (2000). The neurocognitive profile of Williams syndrome: A complex pattern of strengths and weaknesses. *Journal of Cognitive Neuroscience, 12 supplement,* 7–29.

Bellugi, U., Lichtenberger, L., Mills, D., Galaburda, A., & Korenberg, J. (1999). Bridging cognition, the brain and molecular genetics: Evidence from Williams syndrome. *Trends in Neurosciences, 22,* 197–207.

Bellugi, U., Sabo, H., & Vaid, J. (1988). Spatial deficits in children with Williams Syndrome. In J. Stiles-Davis, &

M. Kritchevsky (Eds.), *Spatial cognition: Brain bases and development* (pp. 273–298). Hillsdale, NJ: Lawrence Erlbaum Associates.

Bihrle, A., Bellugi, U., Delis, D., & Marks, S. (1989). Seeing either the forest or the trees: Dissociation in visuospatial processing. *Brain and Cognition, 11,* 37–49.

Brown, J., Johnson, M. H., Paterson, S., Gilmore, R., Gsödl, M., Longhi, E., & Karmiloff-Smith, A. (2003). Spatial representation and attention in toddlers with Williams syndrome and Down syndrome. *Neuropsychologia, 41,* 1037–1046.

Burack, J. A., Hodapp, R. M., & Zigler, E. (1998). *Handbook of mental retardation and development.* New York: Cambridge University Press.

Burack, J. A., Iarocci, G., Bowler, D. M., & Mottron, L. (2002). Benefits and pitfalls in the merging of disciplines: The example of developmental psychopathology and the study of persons with autism. *Development and Psychopathology, 14,* 225–237.

Chomsky, N. (1975). *Reflections on language.* New York: Columbia University Press.

Cicchetti, D., & Cannon, T. D. (1999). Neurodevelopmental processes in the ontogenesis and epigenesis of psychopathology. *Development and Psychopathology, 11,* 375–393.

Clahsen, H., & Almazan, M. (1998). Syntax and morphology in Williams syndrome. *Cognition, 68,* 167–198.

Crisco, J., Dobbs, J., & Mulhern, R. (1988). Cognitive processing of children with William syndrome. *Developmental Medicine and Child Neurology, 30,* 650–656.

De Haan, M., Johnson, M. H. & Halit, H. (2003). Development of face-sensitive event-related potentials during infancy: A review. *International Journal of Psychophysiology, 51,* 45–58.

Deruelle, C., Mancini, J., Livet, M. O., Casse-Perrot, C., & de Schonen, S. (1999). Configural and local processing of faces in children with Williams syndrome. *Brain & Cognition, 41,* 276–298.

Deruelle, C., Schon, D., Rondan, C., & Mancini, J. (2005). Global and local music perception in children with Williams syndrome. *Neuroreport, 25,* 631–634.

Elman, J. L., Bates, E., Johnson, M. H., Karmiloff-Smith, A., Parisi, D., & Plunkett, K. (1996). *Rethinking innateness: A connectionist perspective on development.* Cambridge, MA: MIT Press.

Elsabbagh, M., Cohen, H., & Karmiloff-Smith, A. (2010). Discovering structure in auditory input: Evidence from Williams syndrome. *American Journal on Intellectual and Developmental Disabilities, 115,* 128–139.

Elsabbagh, M., Cohen, H., Cohen, M., Rosen, S. & Karmiloff-Smith, A. (in press). Severity of Hyperacusis predicts individual differences in speech perception in Williams Syndrome. *Journal of Intellectual Disability Research.*

Farran, E. (2005). Perceptual grouping ability in Williams syndrome: Evidence for deviant patterns of performance. *Neuropsychologia, 43,* 815–822.

Fodor, J. (1983). *Modularity of mind.* Cambridge, MA: MIT Press.

Frangiskakis, J., Ewart, A., Morris, C., Mervis, C., Bertrand, J., Robinson, B., et al. (1996). LIM-Kinase 1 hemizygosity implicated in impaired visuospatial constructive cognition. *Cell, 86,* 59–69.

Gagliardi, C., Frigerio, E., Burt, D. M., Cazzaniga, I., Perrett, D. I., & Borgatti, R. (2003). Facial expression recognition in Williams syndrome. *Neuropsychologia, 41,* 733–738.

Galaburda A. M., & Bellugi, U. (2000). V. Multi-level analysis of cortical neuroanatomy in Williams syndrome. *Journal of Cognitive Neuroscience, 12 supplement,* 74–88.

Galaburda, A. M., Holinger, D. P., Bellugi, U., & Sherman, G. F. (2002). Williams syndrome: Neuronal size and neuronal-packing density in primary visual cortex. *Archives of Neurology, 59*, 1461–1467.

Gopnik, M. (1990). Genetic basis of grammar defect. *Nature, 347*, 26.

Grant, J., Karmiloff-Smith, A., Berthoud, I., & Christophe, A. (1996). Is the language of people with Williams syndrome mere mimicry? Verbal short-term memory in a foreign language. *Cahiers de Psychologie Cognitive, 15*, 615–628.

Gray, V., Karmiloff-Smith, A., Funnell, E., & Tassabehji, M. (2006). In-depth analysis of spatial cognition in Williams syndrome: A critical assessment of the role of the LIMK1 gene. *Neuropsychologia, 44*, 679–685.

Grice, S. J., de Haan, M., Halit, H., Johnson, M. H., Csibra, G. & Karmiloff-Smith, A. (2003). ERP abnormalities of Illusory contour perception in Williams Syndrome. *NeuroReport, 14*, 1773–1777.

Grice, S., Spratling, M. W., Karmiloff-Smith, A., Halit, H., Csibra, G., de Haan, M., & Johnson, M. H. (2001). Disordered visual processing and oscillatory brain activity in autism and Williams syndrome. *Neuroreport, 12*, 2697–2700.

Holinger, D. P., Bellugi, U., Korenberg, J. R., Mills, D. L., Reiss, A. L., Sherman, G. F., & Galaburda, A. M. (2005). Relative sparing of primary auditory cortex in Williams syndrome. *Brain Research, 1037*, 35–42.

Jarrold, C., & Brock, J. (2004). To match or not to match? Methodological issues in autism-related research. *Journal of Autism and Developmental Disorders, 34*, 81–86.

Johnson, M. H. (2001). Functional brain development in humans. *Nature Reviews Neuroscience, 2*, 475–483.

Johnson, M. H., Griffin, R., Csibra, G., Halit, H., Farroni, T., de Haan, M., Tucker, L. A., et al. (2005). The emergence of the social brain network: evidence from typical and atypical development. *Development and Psychopathology, 17*, 599–619.

Karmiloff-Smith, A. (1992). *Beyond modularity: A developmental perspective on cognitive science.* Cambridge, MA: MIT Press.

Karmiloff-Smith, A. (1997). Crucial differences between developmental cognitive neuroscience and adult neuropsychology. *Developmental Neuropsychology, 13*, 513–524.

Karmiloff-Smith, A. (1998). Development itself is the key to understanding developmental disorders. *Trends in Cognitive Sciences, 2*, 389–398.

Karmiloff-Smith, A., Thomas, M., Annaz, D., Humphreys, K., Ewing, S., Brace, N., et al. (2004). Exploring the Williams syndrome face processing debate: The importance of building developmental trajectories. *Journal of Child Psychology and Psychiatry, 45*, 1258–1274.

Klein, A. J., Armstrong, B. L., Greer, M. K., & Brown, F. R. (1990). Hyperacusis and otitis media in people with WS. *Journal of Speech and Hearing Disorders, 55*, 339–3444.

Laing, E., Butterworth, G., Ansari, D., Gsödl, M., Longhi, E., Panagiotaki, G., et al. (2002). Atypical development of language and social communication in toddlers with Williams syndrome. *Developmental Science, 5*, 233–246.

Laing, E., Hulme, C., Grant, J., & Karmiloff-Smith, A. (2001). Learning to read in Williams syndrome: Looking beneath the surface of atypical reading development. *Journal of Child Psychology and Psychiatry, 42*, 729–739.

Leonard, L. (1999). *Children With Specific Language Impairment.* Cambridge, MA: MIT Press.

Lewis, J. D., & Elman, J. L. (2008). Growth-related neural reorganization and the autism phenotype: A test of the hypothesis that altered brain growth leads to altered connectivity. *Developmental Science, 11*, 135–155.

Lincoln, A., Lai, Z., & Jones, W. (2002). Shifting attention and joint attention dissociation in Williams syndrome: Implications for the cerebellum and social deficits in autism. *Neurocase, 8*, 226–232.

Mervis, C. B., & Bertrand, J. (1997). Developmental relations between cognition and language: Evidence from Williams syndrome. In L. Adamson, & M. Romski (Eds.), *Research on communication and language disorders: Contributions of to theories of language development* (pp.75–106). New York: Brooks.

Mervis, C. B., & Klein-Tasman, B. P. (2004). Methodological issues in group-matching designs: Alpha levels for control variable comparisons and measurement characteristics of control and target variables. *Journal of Autism and Developmental Disorders, 34*, 7–17.

Mervis, C. B., Morris, C. A., Bertrand, J., & Robinson, B. F. (1999). Williams syndrome: Findings from an integrated program of research. In H. Tager-Flusberg (Ed.), *Neurodevelopmental disorders: Contributions to a new framework from the cognitive neurosciences* (pp. 65–110). Cambridge, MA: MIT Press.

Mervis, C. B., Morris, C. A., Klein-Tasman, B. P., Bertrand, J., Kwitny, S., Appelbaum, L. G., & Rice, C. E. (2003). Attentional characteristics of infants and toddlers with Williams syndrome during triadic interactions. *Developmental Neuropsychology, 23*, 243–268.

Mervis, C. B., Robinson, B. F., Bertrand, J., Morris, C. A., Klein-Tasman, B. P., & Armstrong, S. C. (2000). The Williams syndrome cognitive profile. *Brain and Cognition, 44*, 604–628.

Mills, D. L., Alvarez, T. D., St. George, M., Appelbaum, L. G., Bellugi, U., & Neville, H. (2000). III. Electrophysiological studies of face processing in Williams syndrome. *Journal of Cognitive Neuroscience, 12 supplement*, 47–64.

Nazzi, T., Paterson, S., & Karmiloff-Smith, A. (2003). Early word segmentation by infants and toddlers with Williams syndrome. *Infancy, 4*, 251–271.

Nicholson, W., & Hockey, K. (1993). Williams syndrome: A clinical study of children and adults. *Journal of Pediatrics, 29*, 468–472.

Paterson, S. J., Brown, J. H., Gsodl, M. K., Johnson, M. H., & Karmiloff-Smith, A. (1999). Cognitive modularity and genetic disorders. *Science, 286*, 2355–2358.

Pinker, S. (1994). *The language instinct.* New York: William Morrow and Company.

Pinker, S. (1999). *Words and rules.* London: Weidenfeld & Nicolson.

Plissart, L., & Fryns, J. P. (1999). Early development (5–48 months) in Williams syndrome: A study of 14 children. *Genetic Counseling, 10*, 151–156.

Rae, C., Karmiloff-Smith, A., Lee, M. A., Dixon, R. M., Grant, J., Blamire, A. M., et al. (1998). Brain biochemistry in Williams syndrome: Evidence for a role of the cerebellum in cognition? *Neurology, 51*, 33–40.

Reiss, A. L., Eckert, M. A., Rose, F. E., Karchemskiy, A., Kesler, S., Chang, M., et al. (2004). An experiment of nature: Brain anatomy parallels cognition and behavior in Williams syndrome. *Journal of Neuroscience, 26*, 5009–5015.

Reiss, A. L., Eliez, S., Schmitt, J. E., Straus, E., Lai, Z., Jones, W., & Bellugi, U. (2000). IV. Neuroanatomy of Williams syndrome: A high-resolution MRI study. *Journal of Cognitive Neuroscience, 12 supplement*, 65–73.

Rutter, M., & Sroufe, L. A. (2000). Developmental psychopathology: Concepts and challenges. *Development and Psychopathology, 12*, 265–296.

Scerif, G., Cornish, K., Wilding, J., Driver, J., & Karmiloff-Smith, A. (2004). Visual selective attention in typically developing toddlers and toddlers with fragile X and Williams syndrome. *Developmental Science, 7,* 116–130.

Scerif, G., & Karmiloff-Smith, A. (2005). The dawn of cognitive genetics? Crucial developmental caveats. *Trends in Cognitive Sciences, 9*, 126–135.

Schmitt, J. E., Watts, K., Eliez, S., Bellugi, U., Galaburda, A. M., & Reiss, A. L. (2002). Increased gyrification in Williams syndrome: Evidence using 3D MRI methods. *Developmental Medicine & Child Neurology, 44*, 292–295.

Singer-Harris, N., Bellugi, U., Bates, E., Jones, W., & Rossen, M. (1997). Contrasting profiles of language development in children with Williams and Down syndromes. *Developmental Neuropsychology, 13*, 345–370.

Tassabehji, M., Metcalfe, K., Fergusson, W. D., Carette, M. J., Dore, J. K., Donnai, D., et al. (1996). LIM-kinase deleted in Williams syndrome. *Nature Genetics, 13*, 272–273.

Tassabehji, M., Metcalfe, K., Karmiloff-Smith, A., Carette, M. J., Grant, J., Dennis, N., et al. (1999). Williams syndrome: Use of chromosomal microdeletions as a tool to dissect cognitive and physical phenotypes. *American Journal of Human Genetics, 64*, 118–125.

Temple, C. (1997). *Developmental cognitive neuropsychology.* London: Psychology Press.

Thomas, M., Grant, J., Barham, Z., Gsödl, M., Laing, E., Lakusta, L., et al. (2001). Past tense formation in Williams syndrome. *Language and Cognitive Processes, 2*, 143–176.

Thomas, M., & Karmiloff-Smith, A. (2003). Modeling language acquisition in atypical phenotypes. *Psychological Review, 110*, 647–682.

Thompson, P. M., Lee, A. D., Dutton, R. A., Geaga, J. A., Hayashi, K., Eckert, M. A., et al. (2005). Abnormal cortical complexity and thickness profiles mapped in Williams syndrome. *Journal Neuroscience, 25*, 4146–4158.

Tzourio-Mazoyer, N., De Schonen, S., Crivello, F., Reutter, B., Aujard, Y., & Mazoyer, B. (2002). Neural correlates of woman face processing by 2-month-old infants. *Neuroimage, 15*, 454–461.

Udwin, O., & Yule, W. (1991). A cognitive and behavioural phenotype in Williams syndrome. *Journal of Clinical and Experimental Neuropsychology, 13*, 233–244.

Ulman, M. T., & Gopnik, M. (1999). Inflectional morphology in a family with inherited specific language impairment. *Applied Psycholinguistics, 20*, 51–117.

Van Borsel, J., Curfs, L. M., & Fryns, J. P. (1997). Hyperacusis in Williams syndrome: A sample survey study. *Genetic Counseling, 8*, 121–126.

Vicari, S., Bates, E., Caselli, M. C., Pasqualetti, P., Gagliardi, C., Tonucci, F., & Volterra, V. (2004). Neuropsycho-logical profile of Italians with Williams syndrome: An example of a dissociation between language and cognition? *Journal of the International Neuropsychological Society, 10*, 862–876.

Volterra, V., Capirci, O., Pezzini, G., & Sabbadini, L. (1996). Linguistic abilities in Italian children with Williams syndrome. *Cortex, 32*, 663–677.

Linking Genes to Cognition: The Case of Fragile X Syndrome

Kim M. Cornish, Armando Bertone, Cary S. Kogan, *and* Gaia Scerif

Abstract

This chapter draws together the plethora of findings from a decade of research on fragile X syndrome (FXS) in order to demonstrate how disruption to a single gene can impact across multiple levels (brain, cognitive, behavioral levels) and across developmental time. It begins by describing how some of the major advances in genetic, cognitive, and brain technologies have facilitated a decade of exploration of the gene–brain–behavior relationship in developmental disorders. It then illustrates the fruitfulness of this approach using the case of FXS. It focuses on the current knowledge of the fragile X cognitive phenotype and highlights the importance of using a cross-syndrome perspective to further delineate "signature" profiles. The chapter concludes with future research directions that specifically focus on comparisons of cross-syndrome performance over developmental time and the use of the cross-cultural context to delineate the contributions of similar genes within the context of different cultural environments to the developmental outcomes of different disorders.

Keywords: Fragile X syndrome, genetic disorders, signature profiles, developmental disorders, developmental cognitive neuroscience

Through advances over the past decade, the seemingly disparate fields of molecular genetics, developmental neuropsychology, and brain imaging provide scientists and clinicians with a unique window on the cognitive phenotypic outcomes of disorders with differing genetic etiologies. Previous research in the 1960s and 1970s had tended to ignore the role of etiology in explaining cognitive and behavioral deficits in disorders of mental retardation and instead had proposed that a common cognitive deficit accounted for mental retardation across different disorders (for exceptions, see Burack, 1992; Burack, Hodapp, & Zigler, 1988, 1990; and the introductory chapter of this Handbook; these provide extensive reviews of the broader literature on the importance of cross-syndrome comparisons in understanding developmental disorders).

One of the major strengths of this new multidisciplinary approach to understanding developmental disorders is that it clarifies which behaviors are more dependent on the overall degree of cognitive impairment (i.e., syndrome-general deficits, no matter what the specific cause; for example, processing speed differences or low IQ); and which behaviors reflect impairment unique to a particular disorder (syndrome-specific) and/or cognitive domain (i.e., domain-specific deficits, such as inhibitory control difficulties or difficulties in face processing). Although understanding the impact of a gene(s) on phenotypic outcomes accrues more targeted information for syndrome-specific early intervention programs, the relationship between genetic etiology and phenotypic outcome is always complex and rarely linear. Research must therefore be guided by the most current knowledge of how genes can impact across multiple levels, from the cellular level to early brain development and all the way through to the cognitive and behavioral end states.

Against this background, we propose to demonstrate the need to recognize the unique "signature" profiles that distinguish one genetic disorder from another and from the typically developing trajectory. Using the example of fragile X syndrome (FXS), we aim to demonstrate the impact of disruption to a single gene on the developing brain and the resulting cognitive pathways across the lifespan. A further aim of this chapter is to illustrate the importance of cross-syndrome analyses, especially for disorders that, at first glance, appear to share commonalities in phenotypic outcomes. The question guiding this research is to what extent symptom overlap implies common developmental pathways or etiologies.

To put this research into context, we will focus first on describing how some of the major advances in genetic, cognitive, and brain technologies have facilitated a decade of exploration of the gene–brain–behavior relationship in developmental disorders. We will then proceed to illustrate the fruitfulness of this approach using the case of FXS. We will focus on the current knowledge of the fragile X cognitive phenotype and highlight the importance of using a cross-syndrome perspective to further delineate signature profiles. We conclude with future research directions that specifically focus on comparisons of cross-syndrome performance over developmental time and the use of the cross-cultural context to delineate the contributions of similar genes within the context of different cultural environments to the developmental outcomes of different disorders.

The Emerging Discipline of Developmental Cognitive Neuroscience

The term *developmental cognitive neuroscience* was introduced in the past few years to encapsulate an exciting innovation that merges previously disparate disciplines including cognitive science, neurobiology, neuroscience and psychology into the study of typical and atypical cognitive development. The quest to understand the neurobiological basis in the developing organism across multiple cognitive domains, such as perception, attention, memory, learning, language, and executive functions, culminated in a wealth of multidisciplinary research initiatives in which the trajectories of early brain development and their impact across the lifespan were examined (for a review see Munakata, Casey, & Diamond, 2004). More recently, an emphasis was placed on understanding the mechanisms that drive atypical brain development in disorders with a specific genetic etiology (e.g., FXS, Williams syndrome). This surge in interest in linking genes to brain development to atypical behavior was brought about by two

important advances: a move away from the prevailing assumption that brain development follows a pre-specified genetic "map" of brain structure (see de Haan, Johnson, Halitf, 2003, for a historical perspective), and that development plays only a minimal role, if any, in shaping subsequent cognitive changes. Instead, an increasing focus is now placed on defining two distinct fundamental levels of description: the developmental changes leading to atypical brain development, and their underlying developmental mechanisms at the *molecular, genetic, and network levels*; and the changes at the *cognitive level* that result from atypical brain development. The second advance is the development of new methods in elucidating brain–behavior relations in the context of cognitive development.

Following recent evidence against genetic pre-specification, significant advances at the *neurobiological level* reveal the interplay between predisposing genetic anomalies associated with forms of mental retardation and experience-dependent neuronal processes. These mechanisms of neuroplasticity (for example, synaptic pruning) occur preferentially during development and include synaptogenesis, synaptic remodeling and elimination, dendritic spine formation, myelination, and pre- and postnatal neurogenesis. A particularly powerful method for elucidating these processes is the evaluation of long-term potentiation (LTP) and depression (LTD) in the hippocampus of transgenic mouse models of various forms of mental retardation (Bear, Huber, & Warren, 2004; Costa & Grybko, 2005; Hou et al., 2006; Li, Pelletier, Perez Velazquez, & Carlen, 2002; Meng, et al., 2002; Moretti et al., 2006; Siarey, Villar, Epstein, & Galdzicki, 2005). Long-term potentiation and depression are thought to be mechanisms of synaptic strengthening and weakening, respectively, and therefore allow measuring distinct aspects of neuroplasticity directly. Although disruptions of LTP or LTD are common in all murine models of developmental disorders, and presumably in affected humans as well, each condition demonstrates its own unique pattern of functional impairment. For example, in FXS, the fragile X mental retardation protein (FMRP) is not expressed. A consequence of this is the dysregulation of translation of downstream proteins normally involved in glutamate-mediated synaptic remodeling (Bear et al., 2004). Without FMRP, dendritic spines, rich sites of synapses, do not develop normally. A comprehensive study of spine abnormalities in cortical pyramidal neurons of developing *Fmr1* knock-out mice suggests that the pathology is most evident during cortical synaptogenesis (1 week postnatally). This implicates FMRP as necessary for normal synaptogenesis during a critical period for cortical development (Nimchinsky, Oberlander, & Svoboda, 2001).

The dendritic spine abnormalities that appear to be a neuronal phenotype associated with FXS suggests that FMRP is an important factor in synapse formation. In support of this idea, FMRP levels are found to increase in response to behavioural conditions that are known to induce synaptic plasticity in brain areas associated with particular behavioural tasks (Irwin et al., 2000b). For example, exposing rats to a complex visual environment resulted in increases in FMRP expression in the visual cortices of these animals as compared to cortices of inactive controls. Similarly, exposure to unilateral whisker stimulation selectively increases FMRP levels in the barrel cortex. This process is mediated by activation of a specific type of glutamate receptors, metabotropic glutamate receptors (mGluR, for a full review of the mGluR theory of FXS, see Bear et al., 2004). Evidence has also been found for enhanced LTD in hippocampal preparations from *fmr1* knock-out mice, a process also triggered by mGluR activation. These results further support the idea that FMRP is an important mediator of synaptic plasticity (Antar & Bassell, 2003).

Emerging evidence further suggests that the various disparate molecules affected in various disorders may belong to one or several key molecular pathways involved in neuroplasticity (Bardoni & Mandel, 2002). One such pathway linking a variety of molecules, including FMRP, appears to affect neuroplasticity through mechanisms responsible for synaptic remodeling (Yang et al., 1998). Without normal functioning of key molecules such as FMRP, environmental signals that occur during development cannot shape the development of brain areas such as the hippocampus. The result is the variety of cognitive and behavioural phenotypes associated with specific disorders.

Cognitive Level

At the *cognitive level*, the neuroconstructivist approach, pioneered by Karmiloff-Smith (1997, 1998, Scerif & Karmiloff-Smith, 2005; Karmiloff-Smith, Ansari, Campbell, Scerif, & Thomas, 2006) was critical in demonstrating the dynamic role of development itself in defining many developmental disorders. By applying a neuroconstructivist approach to understanding atypical development, most notably with regard to her work on Williams syndrome (see Morris,

Lenhoff, & Wang, 2006, for a comprehensive recent review), Karmiloff-Smith argued that phenotypic outcomes in developmental disorders cannot simply result from a juxtaposition of impaired and intact cognitive modules that are innately specified from infancy. Instead, the cognitive phenotype results from a dynamic interplay of factors from the biological and brain levels, such as the impact of the gene on pre- and postnatal brain development, to the cognitive level, such as hemisphere specialization, progressive selection, and processing of different types of input, and then to the behavioral and environmental levels, such as behavioral rigidity, impulsivity, and hyperactivity. One possibility is that any subtle differences at these levels during early development act as determinants to the range of phenotypic outcomes that some disorders can display. The multiple interactions between levels also allows for alternative developmental pathways that will interact all the way from the genetic origin through to the behavioral end state (Karmiloff-Smith, 1997, 1998). In essence, one cannot make the a priori assumption that the effects of genetic dysfunctions through development are replicas of outcomes in adulthood: Starting states in early childhood may be different and thus need to be empirically tested. Most recently, this approach has been adopted by Cornish, Scerif, and colleagues to explain the developing phenotype in FXS (a syndrome that results from the silencing of a single gene on the X chromosome) (Cornish, Scerif, & Karmiloff-Smith, 2007a; Cornish, Levitas, & Sudhalter, 2007; Scerif et al., 2004, 2005; Scerif, Cornish, Wilding, Driver, & Karmiloff-Smith, 2007).

Complementing the first advance in developmental cognitive neuroscience as a move toward understanding gene–environment interactions, the second advance comes from the development of new methods that have proved so important in elucidating brain–behavior relations in the context of cognitive development. These methods include novel experimental cognitive paradigms and brain imaging techniques. In terms of *cognitive methodology*, the development of novel experimental paradigms that attempt to tease apart subtle features of performance within and between cognitive domains facilitated a greater understanding of syndrome-specific strengths and difficulties. Early studies in the 1980s reported findings that began to explore cognitive functioning using traditional IQ tests to examine potential discrepancies between verbal and nonverbal performance for FXS. These early findings set the scene for research programs beginning in the 1990s and continuing to the present, in which researchers began to unravel more finely tuned profiles of cognitive dysfunction—more skill-specific rather than global in nature (see Cornish et al., 2004a; Cornish, Sudhalter, & Turk, 2004b, for a review of these changes in perspectives). More specifically, by using novel experimental measures that are specifically designed for individuals with differing levels of intellectual ability, and with a focus on delineating performance across a single cognitive domain, such as visuospatial cognition, findings revealed unique profiles that differentiate developmental disorders from each other and from typically developing children. For example, in the visual–spatial domain, children with Williams syndrome display greatest impairment in processing global rather than local information (Bellugi, Lichtenberger, Jones, Lai, & St. George, 2000) compared to children with Down syndrome (DS), who show the reverse pattern, and those with FXS, who present with delay in processing both global and local information (Cornish, Munir, & Cross, 1998, 1999). Just as in the visual–spatial domain, differing profiles characterize the language domain: For example, FXS is characterized by impairments in pragmatics and speech fluency (Belser & Sudhalter, 2001; Benneto & Pennington, 2002; Cornish et al., 2004b), which contrasts with the language profile of Williams syndrome, which is characterized by a relative proficiency in language overall, but with subtle impairments across all language subdomains (Grant, Valian, & Karmiloff-Smith, 2002; Laing et al., 2002; Thomas et al., 2001; for reviews see Karmiloff-Smith & Thomas, 2003; Thomas & Karmiloff-Smith, 2003). This in turn contrasts with the profile of DS, which is characterized by general delay but with vocabulary skills better than syntax skills (Fowler, 1990, 1995; Chapman, 1997). Although using tasks of generalized intelligence may provide a first assessment of relative strengths and weaknesses, these initial findings need to be followed by detailed analyses, to avoid masking subtle differences at the processing level.

Brain Level

Neuroimaging (NI) techniques are instrumental in assessing the consequence of abnormal brain morphology and neurofunctional changes during atypical development. Applications of neuroimaging to special populations are indeed evolving. In addition to neuropathological studies, findings from NI studies of atypical development demonstrate both cortical and subcortical structural abnormalities using either computed tomography (CT) or structural magnetic resonance imaging (MRI) (see Gothelf, Furfaro, Penniman, Glover, & Reiss, 2005, for review). However, abnormal structures form part of widely distributed networks, and deficits may be observed across a broad range of activities. Therefore, although structural abnormalities can be associated with differing cognitive profiles, such data cannot alone forward syndrome-specific hypotheses regarding etiology-driven cognitive function.

A number of caveats need further consideration in originating syndrome-specific hypotheses. First, structural brain abnormality in individuals with severe mental retardation is quite common and therefore not diagnostic of specific syndromes (between 34% and 98%, Curry et al., 1997; between 35% and 40%, Schaefer and Bodensteiner, 1998), and second, abnormalities affect a wide range of brain structures (from 9% to 60%, Curry et al., 1997), with no clear consensus on syndrome-specific structures. However, with the advent of functional NI techniques, the research direction in this field has evolved, albeit gradually. Unlike structural techniques, functional NI techniques have the advantage of measuring the activation of a specific brain area in performance on a specific task, possibly leading to more syndrome-specific findings concerning functionally relevant changes in neuronal network development and information processing capabilities. Thus, as part of the emerging discipline of developmental cognitive neuroscience, functional NI is emerging as an important experimental tool (Reiss & Dant, 2003) in understanding the gene–brain–behavior relationship in developmental disorders.

Brief descriptions of three different types of NI measures currently employed to investigate brain functioning in developmental disorders are presented below.

Event-related potentials (ERPs) are measured using electroencephalogram (EEG), a noninvasive procedure that measures electrical brain activity patterns. These are series of characteristic negative "N" and positive "P" peak amplitude changes measured over time via electrodes placed on standard scalp locations that occur in preparation for, or in response to, perceptual, cognitive, and/or motor events; deviations of these negative or positive peaks (in terms of latency or amplitude) are interpreted as atypical functioning (see Picton et al., 2000, for a review of the basic technique). Due to their high temporal resolution and characteristic responses to early perceptual and attentional functioning, ERPs are used in the study of a variety of developmental disorders, including FXS (Cornish et al., 2004c) to assess information processing capabilities (usually visual and auditory) and how they are associated to higher-level, cognitive functioning.

Functional (fMRI) complements structural techniques, in that it provides high-resolution, noninvasive measures of neural activity during certain cognitive-behavioral-affective tasks relative to a predetermined baseline. Locally activated brain regions are defined by brain hemodynamics; increased blood flow/volume/velocity is revealed using the blood oxygen level dependent (BOLD) measures. Functional MRI has been used to study a range of developmental disorders including FXS (for example, see review by Hessl, Rivera, & Reiss, 2004).

Diffusion tensor imaging (DTI; Basser, Mattiello, & LeBihan, 1994; for an application to FXS see Barnea-Goraly et al., 2003) is a new MRI technique that measures water diffusion in the brain, which can be used to estimate the regularity of white matter, as an indirect measure of myelination and neural connectivity. It therefore provides unique information on how connections across cortical and subcortical areas may vary across developmental disorders. This technique will be instrumental in assessing how a single gene mutation like FXS disrupts neural networks, rather than simply specific areas of cortex, and will highlight their role in mediating different aspect of cognition and behavior.

Defining the Gene–Brain–Behavior Correlates in Developmental Disorders: The Case of Fragile X Syndrome

Fragile X syndrome is central to fulfilling the unifying aspirations of the developmental cognitive neuroscience approach. The reason for this is two-fold. First, the prevalence of fragile X makes it the world's most common hereditary cause of mental retardation, affecting 1 in 4,000 males and 1 in 8,000 females (Kooy, Willesden, & Oostra, 2000; Turner, Webb, Wake, & Robinson, 1996). Second, compared to multigenic disorders, such as Williams syndrome, FXS allows for clear relationships to be drawn between the loss of expression of a single gene and the phenotypes observed at various levels of description (i.e., genetic, cellular, and brain level, and cognitive and behavioral level). In the following section, we describe the major advances in the field of developmental cognitive neuroscience facilitating a deeper understanding of the cognitive signature and trajectories of individuals with different developmental disorders. Here, we focus specifically on FXS.

The Genetic and Cellular Level

Fragile X syndrome is caused by a defect in the fragile X mental retardation 1 gene (*FMR1*), located near the end of the long arm of the X chromosome. *FMR1* carries a CGG trinucleotide repeat region in the 5′ untranslated region that becomes expanded in fragile X. In males, it is almost always associated with mental retardation. In unaffected individuals, between 7 and 60 repeats occur, with 30 repeats found on the most common allele. In clinically affected individuals, the CGG repeat region expands to over 200 repeats, resulting in gene silencing and, as described above, this leads to the loss of the encoded protein FMRP in all cells including neurons. Individuals possessing alleles with between 55 and 200 repeats are considered *premutation carriers*, and their cells do express a fraction of normal FMRP levels. The frequency of the fragile X premutation in the general population is estimated to be 1 in 250 females (Rousseau, Rouillard, Morel, Khandijian, & Morgan, 1995), 1 in 813 males (Dombrowski et al., 2002), and has generally been associated with intellectual and cognitive functioning in the average range (but see recent studies by Aziz et al. (2003), Cornish et al. (2005a), and Cornish et al. (2008). Premutations are unstable when transmitted from carrier mother to offspring, with the associated risk of giving rise to the fragile X phenotype should further expansion of the premutation to the full mutation range (i.e., >200 repeats) occur (O'Donnell & Warren, 2002). In the full mutation condition, absent FMRP likely affects the functioning of other genes, potentially giving rise to abnormal expression of other proteins that it regulates (Brown et al., 2001). The extent of effects of *FMR1* silencing on other genes with which it interacts is not fully understood. Nonetheless, at the genetic level it is now well established that *FMR1* is the only gene involved in the pathogenesis of fragile X and that the loss of FMRP has a detrimental impact on subsequent brain development. In this regard, a key question has been to identify how the absence of FMRP results in the fragile X phenotype. A model of how the lack of FMRP might lead to the cognitive and behavioral phenotype of FXS has been proposed, and there is mounting evidence that FMRP acts to transport mRNAs from the nucleus to locations within the cytoplasm and to the dendrites (Jin & Warren, 2000). Taken together with findings that FMRP regulates protein synthesis locally through its association with polyribosomes, Jin and Warren (2000) proposed that the protein is critical for normal neuronal development and function. This idea is supported by findings that suggest that FMRP is involved in dendritic spine formation, a process that is known to be important for synaptic development and plasticity. Abnormal dendritic spine formation is observed in human autopsy material of fragile X patients as well as in the brains of *fmr1* knock-out mice, an animal model of FXS that also lack expression of FMRP (Comery et al., 1997; Hinton, Brown, Wisniewski, & Rudelli, 1991). This hypothesis is strengthened by recent evidence that FMRP expression can be altered by activation of mGluRs (Bear et al., 2004). Activation of these receptors is necessary for normal synapse formation (Cho & Bashir, 2002). Researchers have speculated that the dendritic spine abnormalities might occur due to the absence of FMRP because those mRNAs normally bound to and regulated by the protein are freely unbound in the cytoplasm and therefore might offset the balance of cellular translation, competing for ribosomes that would normally be used to translate other transcripts (see review by O'Donnell & Warren, 2002). The normal function of FMRP is inferred from the consequences of the lack of the protein in neurons of individuals who are affected by FXS or in those from the *fmr1* knock-out mouse model of the syndrome. Abnormal dendritic spine morphogenesis of cortical neurons is consistently found in the brains of both fragile X individuals and *fmr1* knock-out mice (e.g., Comery et al., 1997; Irwin, Galvez, & Greenough, 2000; Irwin et al., 2001). In particular, dendritic spines are found in higher density, with a greater proportion that appear immature. This suggests dendritic elimination and pruning deficits due to the lack of FMRP. In contrast to earlier reports, the pathology of dendritic spines in cortical neurons in mice was found to be most severe during the first 2–4 weeks of life and largely absent upon maturation (Nimchinsky et al., 2001). This finding emphasizes the potential critical interaction between developmental processes and *FMR1* expression and highlights the possibility that FMRP may play a different role during development than during adulthood. In addition to abnormalities in spine formation, there are reported alterations in FMRP levels in response to sensory stimulation, behavioral conditions, or direct infusion with agonists for the mGluR (Antar, Afroz, Dictenberg, Carroll, & Bassell, 2004; Irwin et al., 2000b; Todd & Mack, 2000; Weiler et al., 1997). Furthermore, blockade of both N-methyl-D-aspartate (NMDA) and mGluR in the somatosensory cortex of rats was shown to have the effect of blocking increased production of FMRP in the barrel cortex (Todd, Malter,

& Mack, 2003). Taken together, findings of dendritic spine dysmorphogenesis and activity-dependent expression of FMRP implicate the protein as an important factor in synaptic plasticity and function.

The Brain Level

Findings from both structural and functional neuroimaging studies highlight a vulnerability of specific brain regions in full mutation males and females. For example, there is a decreased size of the posterior vermis of the cerebellum (Mostofsky et al., 1998; Reiss, Alyward, Freund, Joshi, & Bryan, 1991). Other brain areas whose function is affected by *FMR1* status include the caudate nucleus (Eliez, Blasey, Freund, Hastie, & Reiss, 2001) and the hippocampus (Kates, Abrams, Kaufmann, Breiter, & Reiss, 1997; Reiss, Lee, & Freund, 1994). Findings of several studies established a correlation between identified structural abnormalities and the degree of cognitive impairment in the full mutation. For example, posterior vermis volumes were found to be positively correlated with performance on specific measures of intelligence, visual–spatial ability, and executive function, thus suggesting a role of this structure in determining performance on these tasks (Mostofsky et al., 1998). As mentioned earlier, the use of ERP is a feasible tool to examine brain activity in individuals with FXS is emerging. For example, Castrén et al. (2003) have demonstrated abnormal processing in the auditory afferent pathways or in the corresponding cortical receiving areas, reflected by increased amplitude of the N1 component to standard tones in their study, possibly underlying hypersensitivity to sound in fragile X. Moreover, other studies also reported unusual posterior and frontal activations among fragile X adults in comparison to healthy adult participants, suggestive of abnormal cortical dendritic pruning and inhibition (Cornish et al., 2004c).

Alongside structural MRI and ERP measures, fMRI has been the neuroimaging technique of choice for investigating brain structure–function associations in both typical and atypical development. However, studies employing fMRI to investigate FXS are to date limited to female participants with the full mutation (e.g., Kwon et al., 2001). Nevertheless, findings have already demonstrated potential in defining the underlying neural etiology of atypical cognitive functioning associated with the disorder, and in some instances as a function of FMRP expression. For example, both Rivera et al. (2002) and Kwon et al. (2001) demonstrated that reduced parietal activation recorded in adults with fragile X was related to FMR1 protein expression, with possible implications for the visual–spatial and control difficulties reported at the cognitive level. In addition, Tamm and colleagues (2002) used fMRI to demonstrate that deficits in cognitive interference during a counting Stroop task may by the result of atypical recruitment of frontoparietal brain regions.

Most recently, DTI MRI, as described previously, has been employed with the fragile X population by Barnea-Goraly et al. (2003), who found white matter alterations in females with FXS in several brain regions, including frontal-caudate circuits, as well as in sensory–motor areas, bilaterally. These findings indicate that such abnormal white matter connectivity in these neural networks may underlie some of the abnormal integrative information processing deficits reported in FXS.

In summary, ERP, fMRI, and DTI technologies will undoubtedly become increasingly integral tools for linking structural and functional abnormalities in the many disorders associated with mental retardation. Critically, neural changes associated with disorders like FXS will need to be tracked over developmental time, as this is a key dimension in understanding the trajectories that characterize cross-syndrome similarities and differences at the cognitive level.

The Cognitive Level

Mental retardation is seen as the most defining cognitive feature of boys with FXS, with almost all affected males presenting with IQs within the moderate-severe range of impairment and with profiles emerging as young as 3 years of age (Skinner et al., 2005). In females, the phenotypic variation is such that some females show subclinical learning disabilities (Bennetto & Pennington, 2002), whereas approximately 50% display more moderate to severe mental retardation, similar in profile to males with fragile X. The X inactivation status of the fragile X female is seen as the major contributor to the heterogeneity of intellectual disability and the broad range of neurocognitive deficits. However, FXS is not defined by mental retardation alone, and there is strong evidence for a syndrome-specific "signature" of strengths and challenges that serve to differentiate individuals with FXS from individuals with other genetic forms of mental retardation (see Cornish, Turk, & Hagerman, 2008, for a review).

To date, two major recent research efforts have helped to define fragile X at the cognitive level. The first has been a series of in-depth studies of the correlation between the fragile X genetic mutation and the cognitive profiles. The second has been to elucidate the correct mapping between behavioral symptomatology and cognitive mechanisms, which may differ across syndromes. This research is useful for breaking down cognitive domains into their component parts, to fully capture the subtleties of cross-syndrome similarities and differences.

Studies examining the relationship between measures of molecular and cognitive severity have contributed to our understanding of the impact of the lack of *FMR1* expression. Research has included boys and men with the full mutation, girls and women, and men who carry the premutation allele. Some studies have reported small but significant correlations. For example, both Kaufmann et al. (1999) and Bailey et al. (2001) report significant relationships between FMRP expression levels and measures of general intelligence as well as motor, social, adaptive, and language development. However, Bailey et al. (2001) included participants with partial full mutations (i.e., with mosaicisms) and males with partial expression of *FMR1*. Similarly, when full mutation female carriers are tested, results of visual–motor processing, visual analysis–synthesis, visual–motor integration, and five of the seven subtests of the Test of Visual–Perceptual Skills reveal significant negative correlations with mutation size (Block et al., 2000). However, when data are restricted to males with fully methylated full mutations, the associations with measures of development are not found to be significant (Bailey et al., 2001). Therefore, relationships between molecular and cognitive variables may only be relevant to individuals who maintain some expression of FMRP. Unfortunately, the vast majority of individuals with FXS have fully methylated full mutations, thus casting some doubt on the generalizability of findings with partial mutations. Focusing specifically on school-age affected children, Sherman et al. (2002) found a marginally statistically significant relationship between cognitive abilities and CGG repeat length. Unlike previous studies examining molecular correlates however, they controlled for overall cognitive abilities and found a positive correlation with verbal ability and a negative correlation with nonverbal reasoning. Controlling for overall cognitive abilities and examining specific domains of neuropsychological functioning may therefore provide more meaningful results.

Cornish et al. (1999) also examined a specific cognitive domain, that of visual cognition. They conducted a study comparing fragile X males to age- and developmentally matched participants on a battery of visual–motor tasks, such as the Block Design and Object Assembly subtests of the Wechsler Intelligence Scale for Children-Revised (WISC-R), the Triangles subtest of the Kaufman-ABC test, the Annett pegboard, and the Draw a Person task. Evaluation of visual–perceptual abilities was accomplished using the Gestalt closure task. Fragile X affected males were contrasted with three different comparison groups: an unaffected age-matched group, an unaffected developmentally matched group (matched according to receptive vocabulary ability), and an age-matched DS affected group. Importantly, Cornish et al. (1999) explored correlations between CGG repeat lengths of the fragile X participants and scores on the various neuropsychological measures. Although the results of this study suggested a syndrome-specific fragile X phenotype, in which affected individuals perform relatively better in the visual–perceptual compared to the visual–motor domain, there was little evidence for a correlation between task performance and CGG repeat length. A parallel study was also conducted with affected females, permitting the additional analysis of activation ratio, which is an estimate of the amount of cells that are actively producing normal levels of FMRP (Cornish et al., 1998). Similarly, neither activation ration nor CGG repeat length correlated significantly with task performance. These findings are not surprising, given that the lack of FMRP is largely an all-or-nothing event once a threshold of 200 CGG repeats is achieved or surpassed.

Studies Looking at FMRP Level and Cognition

Another methodological approach to elucidating the cognitive phenotype of FXS has been to explore the relationship between molecular variables and neural activity during the performance a specific neuropsychological task. Menon et al. (2000) conducted the first imaging study correlating FMRP expression levels with regional brain activity measured by fMRI in adolescent girls and women harboring the full mutation. Both the prefrontal (inferior and middle frontal cortex) and parietal (superior parietal lobe and supramarginal gyrus) cortices were differentially activated in fragile X participants during performance of a visual–spatial working memory task. Significant positive correlations were also found between FMRP expression levels obtained from lymphocytes and brain activation in the right inferior frontal cortex, left middle

frontal cortex, right middle frontal cortex, left supramarginal gyrus, and right supramarginal gyrus. Kwon et al. (2001) reported similar results for a standard working memory task (one-back and two-back visual–spatial working memory). Unlike typically developing comparison females matched for chronological age, activity in the prefrontal and parietal cortex in fragile X affected females did not increase, despite increases in working memory load. This functional deficit was also found to be positively correlated with expression levels of FMRP in the affected participants, thus suggesting that the protein is necessary for proper development of the frontal lobe.

Abnormal brain activation in frontal areas has also been reported in fragile X affected females while they performed an arithmetic task. Participants had to determine whether an arithmetic equation composed of either two or three operands was correct (Rivera et al., 2002). This task was chosen because arithmetic ability is one domain that is clearly impaired in affected females (Bennetto, Pennington, Porter, Taylor, & Hagerman, 2001; Shalev, Auerbach, Manor, & Gross-Tsur, 2000). Fragile X affected females were found to have a performance deficit for the 3-operand but not the 2-operand equations. Unlike the age-matched comparison group, brain activity in the various regions of interest measured did not increase with task difficulty in the fragile X group. Furthermore, activation of the bilateral prefrontal cortex, the motor/premotor cortex, the left supramarginal gyrus, and the left angular gyrus was positively correlated with FMRP levels during performance of the more difficult 3-operand task. These results support the idea that fragile X affected females demonstrate deficits in executive functioning only when cognitive load is high.

Male or female carriers of the *FMR1* mutation possess between 55 and 200 CGG repeats and are therefore deemed premutation status because they do not present with the same severity of deficits that is observed in the full mutation condition. Initially, it was thought that individuals harboring the premutation were indistinguishable from those who were unaffected. Apparently, this is not the case and in fact, more recent data suggest that there are identifiable cognitive strengths and weaknesses in this population. Furthermore, female carriers are more prone to developing premature ovarian failure and a subset of male carriers (>65 years) are more prone in later life to developing a newly discovered condition known as *fragile X tremor and ataxia syndrome*

(FXTAS). Because of the variability in repeat length in this population, it is also possible to examine correlations between repeat length and cognitive performance to infer gene–behavior relationships. Several studies have begun to explore potential relationships between subthreshold repeat length and degree of cognitive impairment.

Allingham-Hawkins et al. (1996) examined cognitive performance in 14 female premutation carriers revealing full-scale IQs within the average range, thus suggesting normal general intelligence among these participants. Furthermore, analysis of the correlation between CGG repeat length and measures of cognitive ability indicated no significant relationship between these variables. However, results of the proportion of fibroblasts expressing the active form of *FMR1* were positively correlated with full-scale IQ, suggesting that increased molecular severity does affect cognitive ability. Johnston et al. (2001) replicated the Allingham-Hawkins et al. (1996) study with a larger sample of female premutation carriers. Consistent with the earlier study, there were no significant correlations between expansion size and IQ. Despite average performance on the cognitive measures, in the study, females with large repeat sizes reported higher degrees of interpersonal sensitivity and depression on the Symptom Checklist-90-R. Allen et al. (2005) conducted an extensive study of male and female premutation carriers by examining IQ scores in 66 males and 217 females harboring a range of CGG repeat expansion sizes. A nominal amount of the variance (4%) in verbal IQ scores could be explained by the CGG repeat length and only in female carriers. Taken together, these studies suggest that CGG repeat length variability explains only a very small proportion of general cognitive abilities in premutation individuals.

In other studies, specific cognitive domains known to be affected in individuals with the full mutation were assessed in premutation individuals. Cornish et al. (2005c) investigated aspects of social cognition in premutation male carriers and found no correlation between CGG repeat length and measures of theory of mind. Neuropsychological measures of inhibitory control, selective attention, working memory, and visual–spatial cognition have also been evaluated in a large sample of premutation male carriers, and only inhibitory control was found to be significantly correlated with CGG repeat length (Cornish et al., 2008).

Whereas there is little evidence to suggest that measures of molecular severity correlate with general IQ scores, when specific domains of cognition are evaluated, some are correlated and some are not. This highlights the importance of selecting specific measures that reflect discrete cognitive abilities when one is interested in studying genetic–neurocognitive relationships in fragile X. In fact, measures of general intelligence may conceal subtle cognitive deficits that would only be apparent by selecting finer grained measures.

Another approach employed with the aim of understanding the interaction between the genetic and cognitive levels in FXS has been to gather data about sensory system functioning using a combination of neurobiological and behavioural methods (Kogan et al., 2004). Kogan et al. (2004) assessed the functional integrity of early visual processing in males affected by fragile X using psychophysical methods. In a parallel experiment, the authors examined autopsied brains of fragile X individuals to determine if a neuropathology exists within the areas of the visual system subserving early visual processing. Kogan et al. (2004) chose to investigate visual processing, in particular visual–motor and visual–construction abilities, because impairments have been previously identified as a specific area of weakness in fragile X (Cornish et al., 1999). They conjectured that the previously described deficits might be related to abnormal early sensory processing within the visual pathway responsible for visual–motor control. Kogan et al. (2004) used specific psychophysical stimuli to probe the visual system at various levels and demonstrated a selective impairment in affected participant's ability to processes information necessary for normal visual–motor control but not for information necessary for visual–perceptual abilities. These functional deficits were confirmed with evidence from postmortem brains of affected individuals, which showed abnormally small-sized neurons in the dorsal lateral geniculate nucleus, a thalamic structure that relays information required for visual–motor control.

Comparing Commonalities and Differences in Atypical Cognition and Behavior

A cross-syndrome perspective is vital in investigating atypical cognitive functioning because it clarifies which behaviors are more dependent on the overall degree of intellectual impairment no matter the specific cause, and which behaviors reflect impairment unique to a particular developmental disorder. In the case of FXS, behavioral problems include symptoms that mirror those of attention deficit hyperactivity disorder (ADHD) and autism spectrum disorder (ASD), two of the most common childhood psychiatric disorders. In recent years, research has begun to detangle the distinct cognitive profiles that separate FXS from ADHD and ASD.

Fragile X Syndrome and Attention Deficits

Among the most distinctive and pervasive behavioral features of young boys with fragile X are attentional and hyperactivity problems (e.g., Wilding, Munir, & Cornish, 2001; Hatton et al., 2002; Turk, 1998), the severity of which often leads to a clinical diagnosis of ADHD. In a series of studies by Cornish and colleagues (Cornish, Munir, & Wilding, 2002; Munir, Cornish, & Wilding, 2000; Wilding, Cornish, & Munir, 2002), cognitive attention profiles of children with FXS were compared to children with DS, following on from their earlier behavioral observations of severe attentional impairments in both these syndrome groups (e.g., Cornish, Munir, & Wilding, 1997). By incorporating a cognitive neuroscience perspective, Cornish et al. developed a computerized battery of tasks that teased apart the different cognitive subdomains of attention processing (selective attention, sustained attention, divided attention, and attentional control; see Cornish et al., 2004a for a review; Cornish et al., 2007; Munir et al., 2000; Wilding & Cornish, 2004). This research represented one of the first attempts to deconstruct, at the cognitive level, the attention profiles of children with differing developmental disorders. Using well-defined tests of attention (selective attention, sustained attention, and inhibition), both children with FXS and children with DS showed a joint vulnerability across many aspects of performance, especially on tasks that tap selective attention. However, children with fragile X displayed additional problems, most notably a profound impairment in inhibitory control, particularly apparent for skills that require attentional switching and the inhibition of task-irrelevant responses

In an extension of these childhood studies, Scerif and colleagues assessed toddlers and infants with FXS and found similar difficulties in attentional control when assessed with a touch screen-based task that required searching for targets among a variable number of distractors that were more or less similar to the targets in size (see Figure 4.1), toddlers with fragile X repeatedly touching targets that they had already found (Scerif et al., 2004, 2007), thus suggesting difficulties in inhibiting previously successful responses, a pattern that mirrored errors by older children with fragile X. Deficits in inhibiting simple but inappropriate eye movements

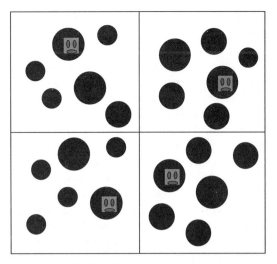

Fig. 4.1 Example of search displays presented on a computer touch-screen by Scerif, Cornish et al. (2004, in press). Children were asked (through verbal and non-verbal demonstration) to "find the king monster hiding under the large circles, but not the small ones" in displays that contained 10 target circles and up to 24 distractor circles. Touching a large circle displayed a marker face that remained in sight until the end of the search run (concluded by finding eight large circles in the display), whereas touching distractor small circles did not result in any reward. *Top-left*: Heterogeneous distractors (mainly dissimilar). *Top-right*: Heterogeneous distractors (mainly similar). *Bottom-left*: Homogeneous distractors (dissimilar). *Bottom-right*: Homogeneous distractors (similar).

were also demonstrated in infants with fragile X as young as 12 months old in an analogue of the antisaccade task (Scerif & Karmiloff-Smith, 2005). Furthermore, toddlers with William syndrome, when assessed using the touch screen task, confused targets and distractors much more than did toddlers with fragile X, who in turn produced more of these errors than typically developing participants, suggesting that, despite similarities in speed of search for all groups, and the fact that these children could accurately discriminate single target–distractor pairs, the two syndrome groups displayed strikingly different qualitative patterns of perceptual and attentional errors (Scerif et al., 2004).

Fragile X Syndrome and Autistic-like Features

Almost all children with fragile X display autistic-like characteristics that mirror typical autism, such as language delay, echolalia, and perseverative speech alongside poor eye contact, poor social interactions, and stereotypic movements (see Cornish, Turk, & Levitas, 2007a, for a review; Demark, Feldman, & Holden, 2003; Reiss & Freund, 1990). Recent estimates indicate a percentage of between 20% and 35%

of fragile X individuals will fulfil criteria for a clinical diagnosis of autism (see Hagerman, 2006; Rogers, Wehner, & Hagerman, 2001). At the cognitive level, a growing number of studies have begun to differentiate differing patterns of social cognitive performance in children with fragile X alone and children with autism alone, even though at first glance there are overlapping characteristics across a number of subdomains, notably reciprocal relationships (eye gaze avoidance, initiating social interactions) and in understanding the beliefs and intentions of others (theory of mind). However, closer inspection of performance reveals unique syndrome-specific signatures suggestive of differing atypical pathways. For example, eye gaze avoidance, although impaired in both fragile X and autism, is fundamentally different. Unlike children with autism who demonstrate a fundamental lack of interest in interacting with others, eye gaze behavior in fragile X does not appear to be the result of a lack of social awareness or communication. Instead, children with fragile X experience a unique pattern of hyperarousal and social anxiety that can cause them to avert their eyes in a social situation (to avoid the sensory stimulation of eye contact), although they may still wish to communicate socially (Wolff, Gardner, Paccla, & Lappen, 1989).

Likewise, a delay in theory of mind development has been well documented in children with autism (Baron-Cohen, 1999; Baron-Cohen, Leslie, & Frith, 1985) and in FXS (Cornish, Burack, Rahman, Munir, & Rossi, 2005b; Garner, Callias, & Turk, 1999). In their recent study, Cornish et al. (2005) reported that over 50% of children with fragile X were able to pass a first-order false-belief task (the Sally-Ann task), contrasting with 30% typically reported in children with autism. Subtle patterns in error profiles also differentiate FXS from autism when performance is compared on a task that requires a child to distinguish between his perception of an object (its *appearance*) and his actual knowledge of it (its *real identity*) (Baron-Cohen, 1989; Cornish et al., 2005). For example, a bottle of milk was shown to each child, who was asked to name the object and its color. An orange filter was then placed in front of the object and the child was asked the appearance question "Now, what color does the milk look?" and the reality question "What color is it really?" A correct response was that the milk looked orange but was really white. Two types of errors typically occur: one is a *phenomenist* error, in which the child states that the milk looked orange and really was orange, and the second is a *realist*

error when the child states that the milk looked white and really was white. Although children with fragile X and children with autism display considerable impairment on this task, their error patterns are qualitatively different from each other. Specifically, children with fragile X tended to make more realist errors, such that they ignored the appearance of an object and instead relied solely on real knowledge. In contrast, children with autism made more phenomenist errors, such that the perceptual information of an object, even if it contradicts the child's real knowledge of that object, overrides all other representations.

In sum, although at the behavioral level a range of characteristic appear to unite FXS and autism, at the cognitive level these same characteristics appear to serve very different purposes and are likely due to very different mechanisms and pathways underlying the two disorders.

Advancing Research Forward on Fragile X syndrome

Alongside the tremendous advances already made in our understanding of FXS, many avenues await further exploration. We have identified two core but currently unexplored avenues that warrant further research and investigation: the focus on developmental associations and dissociations across disorders and the impact of cross-cultural differences in the phenotypic outcomes of individuals with developmental disorders. These avenues will elucidate the diverging developmental dynamics of disorders otherwise summarily labeled as "mental retardation."

Avenue 1: Cross-syndrome Comparisons over Developmental Time

To explore how evolving cognitive functions diverge from normal development at different ages and across different disorders, it is necessary to study dissociations in cognitive performance across the lifespan rather than targeting a single age group. Tracing trajectories of cognitive functioning from infancy onward is critical, not only in individual neurodevelopmental disorders, but also through cross-syndrome comparisons, as has been advocated outside the domain of attention (see earlier references). We have only just begun to trace these from early infancy, by comparing infants, toddlers, children, and adults with fragile X to those with either Williams syndrome or DS, other developmental disorders characterized by inattention and hyperactivity (Cornish et al., 2008). Despite large overall delay and greater adult difficulties with selective attention, individuals with DS showed improvements by adulthood, whereas those with fragile X did not, especially for measures tapping inhibitory control. This divergence in syndrome-specific trajectories of performance also occurs in the field of numerical cognition, in which DS but not Williams syndrome shows improvement with age (Paterson, Girelli, Butterworth, & Karmiloff-Smith, 2006). Although in its infancy, this approach highlights unique insights emerging from cross-syndrome, multidomain comparisons charting developmental commonalities and syndrome-specific differences in developmental pathways.

Avenue 2: The Effects of Differing Sociocultural Contexts on the Developmental Trajectories of Atypical Children

To date, the majority of the research described in this chapter originates from research carried out in the West, and cross-cultural comparisons that specifically address cognitive phenotyping in atypical populations have yet to be explored in sufficient detail. However, in a recent China–West study, Karmiloff-Smith and colleagues have demonstrated the feasibility of this type of interdisciplinary research in terms of transferability of research methodologies across cultures, collection of large sample sizes from atypical populations, novel uses of recent biomedical and computer technologies (e.g., 3D photogrammetric scanning technology that provides 3D face images of Caucasian and now Chinese syndrome-specific dysmorphic faces), and large multisyndrome and cross-domain data sets (Cornish et al., 2005c). A specific goal of future research would be to use the cross-cultural context to delineate the contributions of similar genes within the context of different cultural environments to the developmental outcome of different syndromes. Developing unique cognitive experimental paradigms that can be used by Western and non-Western researchers, and that would be effective and applicable for typical and atypical children, would provide a first step in mapping trajectories of cognitive development (attention, perception, memory, number, language) in atypical populations across diverse cultures.

Conclusion

Our aim in this chapter has been to draw together the plethora of findings from a decade of research on FXS to demonstrate how disruption to a single gene can impact across multiple levels (brain, cognitive, behavioral levels) and across developmental time. This approach is directly inspired by a neuroconstructivist perspective on typical and atypical development, and finds its most novel contributions in first tracing process- and syndrome-specific developmental trajectories for FXS across levels of description. This focus was originally driven by neuroconstructivist perspectives on other developmental disorders with more complex genetic etiology and seemingly common behavioral profiles. Findings on FXS have further illustrated the key role of a developmental approach in understanding the cognitive processes that underlie relatively common behavioral phenotypes. Second, findings at the cognitive developmental level are now directly informed by a growing body of neuroscientific evidence. This extends earlier suggestions that similar cognitive profiles across developmental disorders such as FXS and autism may be better characterized by differences in the development of the neural circuitry supporting them. By situating research within the emerging field of developmental cognitive neuroscience, we have attempted to provide a framework for understanding the previous results from disparate levels of analysis and for inferring the design of future studies.

Acknowledgments

The research presented in this chapter was funded, in part, by grants from the Wellcome Trust, the National Institutes of Health, the Canadian Institutes of Health Research, and the Social Sciences and Humanities Research Council of Canada to Professor. Cornish; from the CIHR-Clinical Research Initiative Fellowship to Dr. Bertone; funding from the Faculty of Social Sciences at the University of Ottawa to Dr. Kogan; and from the Wellcome Trust and the Department of Experimental Psychology at the University of Oxford to Dr. Scerif.

References

Allen, E. G., Sherman, S., Abramowitz, A., Leslie, M., Novak, G., Rusin, M., et al. (2005). Examination of the effect of the polymorphic CGG repeat in the FMR1 gene on cognitive performance. *Behavior Genetics, 35*(4), 435–445.

Allingham-Hawkins, D. J., Brown, C. A., Babul, R., Chitayat, D., Krekewich, K., Humphries, T., et al. (1996). Tissue-specific methylation differences and cognitive function in fragile X premutation females. *American Journal of Medical Genetics, 64*(2), 329–333.

Antar, L. N., Afroz, R., Dictenberg, J. B., Carroll, R. C., & Bassell, G. J. (2004). Metabotropic glutamate receptor activation regulates fragile x mental retardation protein and FMR1 mRNA localization differentially in dendrites and at synapses. *Journal of Neuroscience, 24*(11), 2648–2655.

Antar, L. N., & Bassell, G. J. (2003). Sunrise at the synapse: The FMRP mRNP shaping the synaptic interface. *Neuron, 37*(4), 555–558.

Aziz, M., Stathopulu, E., Callias, M., Taylor, C., Turk, J., Oostra, B., Willemsen, R., & Patton, M. (2003). Clinical features of boys with fragile X premutations and intermediate alleles. *American Journal Medical Genetics Part B (Neuropsychiatric Genetics), 121B*, 119–127.

Bailey, D. B., Jr., Hatton, D. D., Tassone, F., Skinner, M., & Taylor, A. K. (2001). Variability in FMRP and early development in males with fragile X syndrome. *American Journal of Mental Retardation, 106*(1), 16–27.

Bardoni, B., & Mandel, J. L. (2002). Advances in understanding of fragile X pathogenesis and FMRP function, and in identification of X linked mental retardation genes. *Current Opinion in Genetics & Development, 12*(3), 284–293.

Barnea-Goraly, N., Eliez, S., Hedeus, M., Menon, V., White, C. D., Moseley, M., & Reiss, A. L. (2003). White matter tract alterations in fragile X syndrome: Preliminary evidence from diffusion tensor imaging. *American Journal of Medical Genetics Part B (Neuropsychiatric Genetics), 118B*, 81–88.

Baron-Cohen, S. (1989). Are autistic children behaviourists? An examination of their mental-physical and appearance-reality distinctions. *Journal of Autism and Developmental Disorders, 19*, 579–600.

Baron-Cohen, S. (1999). Theory of mind and autism: A 15-year review. In S. Baron-Cohen, D. Cohen, & H. Tager-Flusberg (Eds.), *Understanding other minds: Perspectives from autism and developmental cognitive neuroscience* (2nd ed., pp. 3–20). Oxford: Oxford University Press.

Baron-Cohen, S., Leslie, A. M., & Frith, U. (1985). Does the autistic child have a "theory of mind?" *Cognition, 21*, 37–46.

Basser, P. J., Mattiello, J., & LeBihan, D. (1994). MR diffusion tensor spectroscopy and imaging. *Biophysical Journal, 66*, 259–267.

Bear, M. F., Huber, K. M., & Warren, S. T. (2004). The mGluR theory of fragile X mental retardation. *Trends in Neuroscience, 27*(7), 370–377.

Bellugi, U., Lichtenberger, L., Jones, W., Lai, Z., & St. George, M. (2000). The neurocognitive profile of Williams syndrome: A complex pattern of strengths and weaknesses. *Journal of Cognitive Neuroscience, 12*, 7–29.

Belser, R. C., & Sudhalter, V. (2001). Conversational characteristics of children with fragile X syndrome: Repetitive speech. *American Journal on Mental Retardation, 106*, 28–38.

Bennetto, L., & Pennington, B. F. (2002). Neuropsychology. In R. J. Hagerman, & P. J. Hagerman (Eds.), *Fragile X syndrome: Diagnosis, treatment, and research* (3rd ed., pp 206–248). Baltimore: John Hopkins University Press.

Bennetto, L., Pennington, B. F., Porter, D., Taylor, A. K., & Hagerman, R. J. (2001). Profile of cognitive functioning in women with the fragile X mutation. *Neuropsychology, 15*(2), 290–299.

Block, S., Brusca-Vega, R., Pizzi, W. J., Berry-Kravis, E., Maino, D. M., & Treitman, T. M. (2000). Cognitive and visual processing skills and their relationship to mutation size in full and premutation female fragile X carriers. *Optometry and Vision Science: official publication of the American Academy of Optometry, 77*(11), 592–599.

Brown, V., Jin, P., Ceman, S., Darnell, J. C., O'Donnell, W. T., Tenenbaum, S. A., et al. (2001). Microarray identification of FMRP-associated brain mRNAs and altered mRNA translational profiles in fragile X syndrome. *Cell, 107*(4), 477–487.

Burack, J. A. (1992). Debate and argument: Clarifying developmental issues in the study of autism. *Journal of Child Psychology and Psychiatry and Allied Disciplines, 33*(3), 617–621.

Burack, J. A., Hodapp, R. M., & Zigler, E. (1988). Issues in the classification of mental retardation: Differentiating among organic etiologies. *Journal of Child Psychology and Psychiatry and Allied Disciplines, 29*(6), 765–779.

Burack, J. A., Hodapp, R. M., & Zigler, E. (1990). Toward a more precise understanding of mental retardation. *Journal of Child Psychology and Psychiatry and Allied Disciplines, 31*(3), 471–475.

Castrén, M., Pääkkönen, A., Tarkka, I. M., Ryynänen, M., & Partanen, J. (2003). Augmentation of auditory N1 in children with fragile X syndrome. *Brain Topography, 15*, 165–171.

Chapman, R. S. (1997). Language development in children and adolescents with Down syndrome. *Mental Retardation and Developmental Disabilities Research Reviews, 3*, 307–312.

Cho, K., & Bashir, Z. I. (2002). Cooperation between mGLU receptors: A depressing mechanism? *Trends in Neurosciences, 25*(8), 405–411.

Comery, T. A., Harris, J. B., Willems, P. J., Oostra, B. A., Irwin, S. A., Weiler, I. J., & Greenough, W. T. (1997). Abnormal dendritic spines in fragile X knockout mice: Maturation and pruning deficits. *Proceedings of the National Academy of Science, U S A, 94*(10), 5401–5404.

Cornish, K., Kogan, C., Turk, J., Manly, T., James, N., Mills, A., & Dalton, A. (2005a). The emerging fragile X premutation phenotype: Evidence from the domain of social cognition. *Brain and Cognition, 57*, 53–60.

Cornish, K., Sudhalter, V., & Turk, J. (2004b). Attention and language in fragile X. *Mental Retardation and Developmental Disabilities Research Reviews, 10*, 11–16.

Cornish, K., Swainson, R., Cunnington, R., Wilding, J., Morris, P. J., & Jackson, G. M. (2004c). Do women with fragile X syndrome have problems in switching attention: Preliminary findings from ERP and fMRI. *Brain and Cognition, 54*, 235–239.

Cornish, K. M., Burack, J., Rahman, A., Munir, F., & Rossi, N. (2005). Theory of mind in children with fragile X syndrome. *Journal of Intellectual Disability Research, 49*, 372–378.

Cornish, K. M., Levitas, A., & Sudhalter, V. (2007). Fragile X syndrome: The journey from genes to behaviour. In M. M. Mazzocco (Ed.), *Neurogenetic developmental disorders: Manifestation and identification in childhood* (pp.1–50). New York: MIT Press.

Cornish, K. M., Li, L., Kogan, C. S., Jacquemont, S., Turk, J., Dalton, A., et al. (2008). Age-dependent cognitive changes in carriers of the fragile X syndrome. *Cortex, 44*(6), 628–36.

Cornish, K. M., Munir, F., & Cross, G. (1998). The nature of the spatial deficit in young females with fragile-X syndrome: A neuropsychological and molecular perspective. *Neuropsychologia, 36*(11), 1239–1246.

Cornish, K. M., Munir, F., & Cross, G. (1999). Spatial cognition in males with fragile-X syndrome: Evidence for a neuropsychological phenotype. *Cortex, 35*(2), 263–271.

Cornish, K. M., Munir, F., & Cross, G. (2001). Differential impact of the FMR-1 full mutation on memory and attention functioning: A neuropsychological perspective. *Journal of Cognitive Neuroscience, 13*, 1–7.

Cornish, K. M., Munir, F., & Wilding, J. (1997). Is there a link between pattern of attention deficit and severity of behavioural problems in boys with fragile X syndrome? *Health and education professionals in attention deficit/hyperactivity disorder.* Hurstpierpoint, UK: International Psychology Services.

Cornish, K., Munir, F., & Wilding, J. (2002). A neuropsychological and behavioural profile of attention deficits in fragile X syndrome. *Revista de Neurologia, 33*(Suppl 1), S24–29.

Cornish, K. M., Scerif, G., & Karmiloff-Smith, A. (2007a). Tracing syndrome-specific trajectories of attention over the lifespan. *Cortex, 43*(6), 672–685.

Cornish, K., J. Turk, & Hagerman, R. (2008). The fragile X continuum: new advances and perspectives. *Journal of Intellectual Disability Research,* 52(Pt 6), 469–82.

Cornish, K., Turk., & Levitas, A. (2007a). Fragile X syndrome and autism: Common developmental pathways? *Current Pediatrics Reviews, 3*(1), 61–68.

Cornish, K. M., Turk, J., Wilding, J., Sudhalter, V., Kooy, F., Munir, F., et al. (2004a). Annotation: Deconstructing the attention deficit in fragile X syndrome. *Journal of Child Psychology and Psychiatry, 45,* 1042–1053.

Cornish, K. M., Zhao, Z., Fu, G., Shao, J., Hammond, P., Mill, D., et al. (2005c). Cognitive-brain phenotyping in Chinese children with genetic disorders. *Journal of Cognitive Neuroscience,* D85 Suppl. S.

Costa, A. C., & Grybko, M. J. (2005). Deficits in hippocampal CA1 LTP induced by TBS but not HFS in the Ts65Dn mouse: A model of Down syndrome. *Neuroscience Letters, 382*(3), 317–322.

Curry, C. J., Stevenson, R. E., Aughton, D., Byrne, J., Carey, J. C., Cassidy, S., et al. (1997). Evaluation of mental retardation: Recommendations of a consensus conference: American College of Medical Genetics. *American Journal of Medical Genetics, 72,* 468–477.

de Haan, M., Johnson, M. H., & Halit, H. (2003). Development of face-sensitive event-related potentials during infancy: A review. *International Journal of Psychophysiology: official journal of the International Organization of Psychophysiology, 51*(1), 45–58.

Demark, J. L., Feldman, M. A., & Holden, J. J. (2003). Behavioral relationship between autism and fragile x syndrome. *American Journal of Mental Retardation, 108*(5), 314–326.

Dombrowski, C., Levesque, S., Morel, M. L., Rouillard, P., Morgan, K., & Rousseau, F. (2002). Premutation and intermediate-size *FMR1* alleles in 10 572 males from the general population: Loss of an AGG interruption is a late event in the generation of fragile X syndrome alleles. *Human Molecular Genetics, 11,* 371–378.

Eliez, S., Blasey, C. M., Freund, L. S., Hastie, T., & Reiss, A. L. (2001). Brain anatomy, gender and IQ in children and adolescents with fragile X syndrome. *Brain, 24,* 1610–1618.

Fowler, A. (1990). Language abilities in children with Down syndrome: Evidence for a specific syntactic delay. In D. Cicchetti, and M. Beeghly (Eds.), *Children with Down syndrome: A developmental perspective* (pp. 302–328). Cambridge, UK: Cambridge University Press.

Fowler, A. (1995). Linguistic variability in persons with Down syndrome: Research and implications. In L. Nadel, and D. Rosenthal (Eds.), *Down syndrome: Living and learning in the community* (pp. 121–131). New York: Wiley-Liss.

Garner, C., Callias, M., & Turk, J. (1999). Executive function and theory of mind performance of boys with fragile-X syndrome. *Journal of Intellectual Disability and Research, 43*(Pt 6), 466–474.

Gothelf, D., Furfaro, J. A., Penniman, L. C., Glover, G. H., & Reiss, A. L. (2005). The contribution of novel brain imaging techniques to understanding the neurobiology of mental retardation and developmental disorders. *Mental Retardation and Developmental Disabilities Research Reviews, 11,* 331–339.

Grant, J., Valian, V., & Karmiloff-Smith, A. (2002). A study of relative clauses in Williams syndrome. *Journal of Child Language, 29,* 403–416.

Hagerman, R. (2006). Lessons from fragile X regarding neurobiology, autism, and neurodegeneration. *Journal of Developmental & Behavioral Pediatrics, 27*(1), 63–74.

Hatton, D. D., Hooper, S. R., Bailey, D. B., Skinner, M. L., Sullivan, K. M., & Wheeler, A. (2002). Problem behavior in boys with fragile X syndrome. *American Journal of Medical Genetics, 108,* 105–116.

Hessl, D., Rivera, S. M., & Reiss, A. L. (2004). The neuroanatomy and neuroendocrinology of fragile X syndrome. *Mental Retardation and Developmental Disabilities Research Reviews, 10*(1), 17–24.

Hinton, V. J., Brown, W. T., Wisniewski, K., & Rudelli, R. D. (1991). Analysis of neocortex in three males with the fragile X syndrome. *American Journal of Medical Genetics, 41*(3), 289–294.

Hou, L., Antion, M. D., Hu, D., Spencer, C. M., Paylor, R., & Klann, E. (2006). Dynamic translational and proteasomal regulation of fragile X mental retardation protein controls mGluR-dependent long-term depression. *Neuron, 51*(4), 441–454.

Irwin, S. A., Galvez, R., & Greenough, W. T. (2000). Dendritic spine structural anomalies in fragile-X mental retardation syndrome. *Cerebral Cortex, 10*(10), 1038–1044.

Irwin, S. A., Patel, B., Idupulapati, M., Harris, J. B., Crisostomo, R. A., Larsen, B. P., et al. (2001). Abnormal dendritic spine characteristics in the temporal and visual cortices of patients with fragile X syndrome: A quantitative examination. *American Journal of Medical Genetics, 98*(2), 161–167.

Irwin, S. A., Swain, R. A., Christmon, C. A., Chakravarti, A., Weiler, I. J., & Greenough, W. T. (2000b). Evidence for altered fragile-X mental retardation protein expression in response to behavioral stimulation. *Neurobiology of Learning and Memory, 74*(1), 87–93.

Jin, J., & Warren, S. T. (2000). Understanding the molecular basis of fragile X syndrome. *Human Molecular Genetics, 9*(6), 901–908.

Johnston, C., Eliez, S., Dyer-Friedman, J., Hessl, D., Glaser, B., Blasey, C., et al. (2001). Neurobehavioral phenotype in carriers of the fragile X premutation. *American Journal of Medical Genetics, 103*(4), 314–319.

Karmiloff-Smith, A. (1997). Crucial differences between developmental cognitive neuroscience and adult neuropsychology. *Developmental Neuropsychology, 13*(4), 513–524.

Karmiloff-Smith, A. (1998). Development itself is the key to understanding developmental disorders. *Trends in Cognitive Sciences, 2*(10), 389–339.

Karmiloff-Smith, A., Ansari, D., Campbell, L., Scerif, G., & Thomas, M. (2006). Theoretical implications of studying genetic disorders: The case of Williams syndrome. In C. A. Morris, H. M. Lenhoff, & P. P. Wang (Eds.), *Williams-Beuren syndrome: Research, evaluation and treatment* (pp. 254–273). Baltimore: The Johns Hopkins University Press.

Karmiloff-Smith, A., & Thomas, M. (2003). What can developmental disorders tell us about the neurocomputational constraints that shape development? The case of Williams syndrome. *Development and Psychopathology, 15,* 969–990.

Kates, W. R., Abrams, M. T., Kaufmann, W. E., Breiter, S. N., & Reiss, A. L. (1997). Reliability and validity of MRI measurement of the amygdala and hippocampus in children with fragile X syndrome. *Psychiatry Research, 75,* 31–48.

Kaufmann, W. E., Abrams, M. T., Chen, W., & Reiss, A. L. (1999). Genotype, molecular phenotype, and cognitive phenotype: Correlations in fragile X syndrome. *American Journal of Medical Genetics, 83*(4), 286–295.

Kogan, C. S., Boutet, I., Cornish, K., Zangenehpour, S., Mullen, K. T., Holden, J. J., et al. (2004). Differential impact of the FMR1 gene on visual processing in fragile X syndrome. *Brain, 127*(Pt 3), 591–601.

Kooy, R. F., Willesden, R., & Oostra, B. A. (2000). Fragile X syndrome at the turn of the century. *Molecular Medicine Today, 6,* 193–198.

Kwon, H., Menon, V., Eliez, S., Warsofsky, I. S., White, C. D., Dyer-Friedman, J., et al. (2001). Functional neuroanatomy of visuospatial working memory in fragile X syndrome: Relation to behavioral and molecular measures. *American Journal of Psychiatry, 158*(7), 1040–1051.

Laing, E., Butterworth, G., Ansari, D., Gsodl, M., Longhi, E., Panagiotaki, G., et al. (2002). Atypical development of language and social communication in toddlers with Williams syndrome. *Developmental Science, 5,* 233–246.

Li, J., Pelletier, M. R., Perez Velazquez, J. L., & Carlen, P. L. (2002). Reduced cortical synaptic plasticity and GluR1 expression associated with fragile X mental retardation protein deficiency. *Molecular and Cellular Neuroscience, 19*(2), 138–151.

Meng, Y., Zhang, Y., Tregoubov, V., Janus, C., Cruz, L., Jackson, M., et al. (2002). Abnormal spine morphology and enhanced LTP in LIMK-1 knockout mice. *Neuron, 35*(1), 121–133.

Menon, V., Kwon, H., Eliez, S., Taylor, A. K., & Reiss, A. L. (2000). Functional brain activation during cognition is related to FMR1 gene expression. *Brain Research, 877*(2), 367–370.

Moretti, P., Levenson, J. M., Battaglia, F., Atkinson, R., Teague, R., Antalffy, B., et al. (2006). Learning and memory and synaptic plasticity are impaired in a mouse model of Rett syndrome. *Journal of Neuroscience, 26*(1), 319–327.

Morris, C. A., Lenhoff, H. M., & Wang, P. P. (2006). (Eds.), *Williams-Beuren syndrome: Research, evaluation and treatment.* Baltimore: The Johns Hopkins University Press.

Mostofsky, S. H., Mazzocco, M. M., Aakalu, G., Warsofsky, I. S., Denckla, M. B., & Reiss, A. L. (1998). Decreased cerebellar posterior vermis size in fragile X syndrome: Correlation with neurocognitive performance. *Neurology, 50*(1), 121–130.

Munakata, Y., Casey, B. J., & Diamond, A. (2004). Developmental cognitive neuroscience: Progress and potential. *Trends in Cognitive Sciences, 8*(3), 122–128.

Munir, F., Cornish, K. M., & Wilding, J. (2000). A neuropsychological profile of attention deficits in young males with Fragile X syndrome. *Neuropsychologia, 38,* 1261–1270.

Nimchinsky, E. A., Oberlander, A. M., & Svoboda, K. (2001). Abnormal development of dendritic spines in FMR1 knockout mice. *The Journal of Neuroscience, 21*(14), 5139–5146.

O'Donnell, W. T., & Warren, S. T. (2002). A decade of molecular studies of fragile X syndrome. *Annual Review of Neuroscience, 25,* 315–338.

Paterson, S. J., Girelli, L., Butterworth, B., & Karmiloff-Smith, A. (2006). Are numerical impairments syndrome specific? Evidence from Williams syndrome and Down's syndrome. *Journal of Child Psychology and Psychiatry and Allied Disciplines, 47*(2), 190–204.

Picton, T. W., Bentin, S., Berg, P., Donchin, E., Hillyard, S. A., Johnson, R., et al. (2000). Guidelines for using human event-related potentials to study cognition: Recording standards and publication criteria. *Psychophysiology, 37*(2), 127–152.

Reiss, A., Alyward, E., Freund, L., Joshi, P. K., & Bryan, R. N. (1991). Neuroanatomy of fragile X syndrome: The posterior fossa. *Annals of Neurology, 29,* 26–32.

Reiss, A. L., & Dant, C. C. (2003). The behavioral neurogenetics of fragile X syndrome: Analyzing gene-brain-behavior relationships in child developmental psychopathologies. *Developmental Psychopathology, 15,* 927–968.

Reiss, A. L., & Freund, L. (1990). Fragile X syndrome, DSM-III-R, and autism. *Journal of the American Academy of Child and Adolescent Psychiatry, 29*(6), 885–891.

Reiss, A. L., Lee, J., & Freund, L. (1994). Neuroanatomy of fragile X syndrome: The temporal lobe. *Neurology, 44,* 1317–1324.

Rivera, S. M., Menon, V., White, C. D., Glaser, B., & Reiss, A. L. (2002). Functional brain activation during arithmetic processing in females with fragile X Syndrome is related to FMR1 protein expression. *Human Brain Mapping, 16*(4), 206–218.

Rogers, S. J., Wehner, D. E., & Hagerman, R. (2001). The behavioral phenotype in fragile X: Symptoms of autism in very young children with fragile X syndrome, idiopathic autism, and other developmental disorders. *Journal of Developmental and Behavioral Pediatrics, 22*(6), 409–417.

Rousseau, F., Rouillard, P., Morel, M. L., Khandjian, E. W., & Morgan, K. (1995). Prevalence of carriers of premutation-size alleles of the fmri gene—and implications for the population genetics of the fragile x syndrome. *American Journal of Human Genetics, 57,* 1006–1018.

Scerif, G., Cornish, K. M., Wilding, J., Driver, J., & Karmiloff-Smith, A. (2004). Visual search in typically developing toddlers and toddlers with fragile X or Williams syndrome. *Developmental Science, 7,* 118–130.

Scerif, G., Cornish, K., Wilding, J., Driver, J., & Karmiloff-Smith, A. (2007). Delineation of early attentional control difficulties in fragile X syndrome: Focus on neurocomputational mechanisms. *Neuropsychologia, 45*(8-4), 1889–1898.

Scerif, G., Cornish, K. M., Wilding, J., Driver, J., & Karmiloff-Smith, A. (2004). Visual search in typically developing toddlers and toddlers with fragile X or Williams syndrome. *Developmental Science, 7,* 118–130.

Scerif, G., & Karmiloff-Smith, A. (2005). The dawn of cognitive genetics? Crucial developmental caveats. *Trends in Cognitive Sciences, 3,* 126–135.

Scerif, G., Karmiloff-Smith, A., Campos, R., Elsabbagh, E., Driver, J., & Cornish, K. M. (2005). To look or not to look? Typical and atypical control of saccades. *Journal of Cognitive Neuroscience, 17,* 591–604.

Schaefer, G. B., & Bodensteiner, J. B. (1998). Radiological findings in developmental delay. *Seminars in Pediatric Neurology, 5*(1), 33–38.

Skinner, M., Hooper, S., Hatton, D. D., Robert, J., Mirrett, P., Schaaf, J., et al. (2005). Mapping nonverbal IQ in young boys with fragile X syndrome. *American Journal of Medical Genetics, 132A,* 25–32.

Shalev, R. S., Auerbach, J., Manor, O., & Gross-Tsur, V. (2000). Developmental dyscalculia: Prevalence and prognosis. *European Child and Adolescent Psychiatry, 9*(Suppl 2), II58–64.

Sherman, S. L., Marsteller, F., Abramowitz, A. J., Scott, E., Leslie, M., & Bregman, J. (2002). Cognitive and behavioral performance among FMR1 high-repeat allele carriers surveyed from special education classes. *American Journal of Medical Genetics, 114*(4), 458–465.

Siarey, R. J., Villar, A. J., Epstein, C. J., & Galdzicki, Z. (2005). Abnormal synaptic plasticity in the Ts1Cje segmental trisomy

16 mouse model of Down syndrome. *Neuropharmacology, 49*(1), 122–128.

Tamm, L., Menon, V., Johnston, C. K., Hessl, D. R., & Reiss, A. L. (2002). fMRI study of cognitive interference processing in females with fragile X syndrome. *Journal of Cognitive Neuroscience, 14*, 160–171.

Thomas, M. S. C., Grant, J., Barham, Z., Gsodl, M., Laing, E., Lakusta, L., et al. (2001). Past tense formation in Williams syndrome. *Language and Cognitive Processes, 16*, 143–176.

Thomas, M. S. C., & Karmiloff-Smith, A. (2003). Modeling language acquisition in atypical phenotypes. *Psychological Review, 110*, 647–682.

Turner, G., Webb, T., Wake, S., & Robinson, H. (1996). Prevalence of fragile X syndrome. *American Journal of Medical Genetics, 64*, 196–197.

Turk, J. (1998). Fragile X syndrome and attentional deficits. *Journal of Applied Research in Intellectual Disabilities, 11*, 175–191.

Wilding, J., Munir, F., & Cornish, K. M. (2001). The nature of attention differences between groups of children differentiated by teacher ratings of attention and hyperactivity. *British Journal of Psychology, 92*, 357–371.

Wolff, P. H., Gardner, J., Paccla, J., & Lappen, J. (1989). The greeting behavior of fragile X males. *American Journal of Mental Retardation, 93*, 406–411.

Yang, N., Higuchi, O., Ohashi, K., Nagata, K., Wada, A., Kangawa, K., et al. (1998). Cofilin phosphorylation by LIM-kinase 1 and its role in Rac-mediated actin reorganization. *Nature, 393*(6687), 809–812.

PART 3

Cognitive Development

The Organization and Development of Spatial Representation: Insights from Williams Syndrome

Barbara Landau

Abstract

This chapter uses the case of Williams syndrome (WS) to provide insight into the nature of human spatial representation and its development under normal circumstances. The chapter has four sections. The first starts with a discussion of the hallmark pattern of spatial breakdown observed in people with WS when they carry out visuoconstructive tasks, such as drawing and block construction. The second and third sections document aspects of the WS profile. The fourth section proposes a speculative hypothesis on how the cognitive profile in WS emerges, emphasizing the role of developmental time tables in the emergence of normal spatial cognitive profiles as well as the WS profile. This hypothesis provides a new way of thinking about the relationships among genes, brains, and minds in spatial cognitive development. It moves us away from a static and simplistic view of how genetic differences might cause cognitive differences, and toward a view that emphasizes the role of normal development and developmental timetables.

Keywords: Williams syndrome, human spatial representations, spatial breakdown, cognitive profile

Our experience of the spatial world is a unified one: We perceive objects and layouts with ease, act on objects and move through the world in a directed fashion, and we reflect on, recall, and talk about our spatial experience. Despite this impression of seamlessness, however, research over the past 30 years shows that the unified spatial world we consciously experience is the product of a highly specialized set of spatial representations, designed for different purposes. The coordination of these spatial systems results in our experience of a unified spatial world.

When part or parts of this system break down, either because of brain damage in adulthood or because of developmental disorder, scientists have the rare opportunity to probe the nature of the system. The study of people with Williams syndrome (WS)—a genetic disorder in which a small set of genes is deleted from chromosome 7—provides such an opportunity, as the syndrome is characterized by severe spatial impairment coupled with remarkable strength in language. The syndrome was first brought

to the attention of cognitive scientists by Ursula Bellugi and colleagues (Bellugi, Sabo, & Vaid, 1988), who suggested that it was an example of cognitive modularity, with one system emerging unimpaired (language) but another emerging profoundly impaired (space). The latter can be illustrated using examples from copying by children with WS (see Figure 5.1). The severe difficulty in visual–constructive tasks such as drawing occurs in both young children and adults with WS, with varying degrees of severity. It is considered a critical part of the clinical profile of people diagnosed with WS (Mervis et al., 2000).

The simplest inference from missing genes to a profile of severely imbalanced cognition is that a specific set of genes (deleted in the case of WS) is responsible for severe impairment in spatial representation; symmetrically, the strength of language in WS would reflect the insulation of language from the effects of the deleted genes. This could be viewed as evidence for cognitive modularity (e.g., Pinker, 1994),

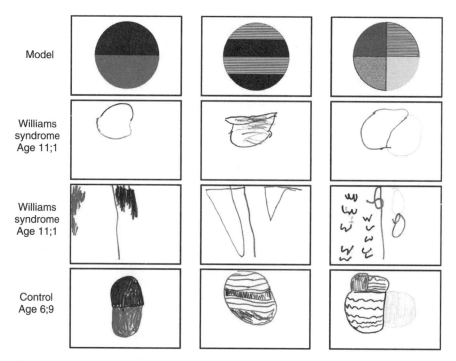

Fig. 5.1 Models (row 1) and sample copies by 11-year-old children with Williams syndrome (rows 2–3) and a normally developing 6-year-old child who is a MA match (row 4).

since genes would be viewed as directly responsible for the sparing or impairment of a particular cognitive system.

Although this strong interpretation of the cognitive profile is debatable, it is clear that the WS profile offers some surprising contrasts that shed unique light on the development of mind and brain in the context of genetic abnormalities. In this chapter, I will use the case of WS to drive our understanding of spatial representation in both people with WS and in normally developing children. I have two goals. The most important is to use the case of WS to provide insight into the nature of human spatial representation and its development under normal circumstances. This will require understanding the WS spatial breakdown; so, my second goal is to present a set of hypotheses about how the characteristic spatial–cognitive profile might result from a genetic deficit. The focus will be on understanding the *cognitive* level that emerges from this genetic deficit, in particular, how the WS spatial profile fits within the broader architecture of human spatial cognition.

Together, these two goals will lead to one of the main theses of this chapter: That understanding WS depends heavily on our understanding of normal spatial development, and its underlying principles. Using principles of normal development in this way can serve as a general model for thinking about developmental deficits. Briefly, I will consider three

principles of normal development: specialization of function, constraint within each specialized system, and the importance of timing in the emergence of brain and cognitive systems. Specialization of function is the idea that the spatial cognitive system is not a single monolithic system, but rather, is composed of different subsystems, specialized to carry out different spatial functions. Examples include vision for action (Milner & Goodale, 1995), navigation (Gallistel, 1990), face perception (Kanwisher, McDermott, & Chun, 1997), and object recognition (Palmieri & Gauthier, 2004). Constraint within each specialized system reflects the idea that each of these systems has different computational goals and mechanisms suited to solve its particular problem. For example, the computational goals of the object recognition system are quite different from those required for reaching for or acting on objects. The importance of timing reflects a rock-bottom assumption about human development; namely, that there are different timelines for development of both brain and cognitive functions. There is evidence for clear developmental time tables in brain development (Gogtay et al., 2004; Huttenlocher, 2002), and in selected aspects of spatial cognition (Newcombe & Huttenlocher, 2000), so timing will surely be a part of the story about how a person with WS comes to have a profile of spatial weakness in childhood and as an adult.

In addition to these three principles of normal spatial development, a fourth principle is required to understand how a genetic deficit can result in specific spatial impairments. This principle is: *Genes can target cognitive systems.* Although the action of genes can be understood at a molecular level, it follows from this principle that genes can also have effects on higher levels of organization, in this case, on spatial cognition. It does *not* follow from this principle that genes must have a one-to-one correspondence with cognitive systems, or with a particular cognitive component of a system. But it does follow that genes can have targeted effects on cognition. This effect is likely to be quite indirect in the case of cognition, but some possibilities (to be explored in this chapter) are that genes target cognitive systems either by altering developmental time tables or by altering the pattern of strengths in different brain functions. The characteristic cognitive profile of people with WS—and the difference between the WS profile and those with other syndromes such as Turner syndrome, Down syndrome, or autism spectrum disorders—shows that genes surely have targeted effects on cognitive systems. But what this statement does not tell us is exactly what these effects are, nor *how* they emerge. And, the story of how a small set of genes can have repercussions on a developing cognitive system is a very complex story indeed, to be explored in this chapter.

This chapter has four sections. The first will start with a discussion of the hallmark pattern of spatial breakdown observed in people with WS when they carry out visuoconstructive tasks such as drawing and block construction. These tasks are commonly used as straightforward clinical diagnostic tests, but—as will be shown—they are remarkably complex. Analysis of the task reveals components that tap into a range of spatial cognitive functions, and suggests a broad hypothesis about the nature of the spatial impairment: That the principal deficit in WS spatial organization occurs across functions guided by the dorsal and parietal areas of the brain, with relative sparing in spatial functions guided by the ventral stream. This hypothesis is given further credence by considering recent empirical evidence from the literature on spatial representation in monkeys, that, surprisingly, recruit many of the same processes when they copy figures and carry out block construction tasks. These processes are guided by dorsal and parietal areas of the monkey brain, and therefore provide a plausibility case for the same functions being disrupted by dorsal and parietal damage in people with WS.

In the second and third sections, I will use evidence from our lab and that of others to document aspects of the WS profile that are consistent with this broad hypothesis. The second section will cover functions of the ventral stream, and the third section will cover functions of the dorsal stream. In addition, these sections will reveal that the WS profile can be understood in terms of the principles of normal development discussed earlier. First, the evidence will show that the profile is consistent with specialization of function, because it is uneven across different kinds of spatial representation, with significant impairment in some areas of spatial representation but not in others. It will also show that the profile is consistent with specialization within subdomains of spatial cognition because performance is strongly constrained within each domain of knowledge, with detailed patterns of performance showing significant and highly specific internal structure. Finally, the evidence will show that the profile is consistent with the importance of timing, because the pattern of strengths and deficits show an unusual timing profile: People with WS perform like normal people of the same chronological age (CA) on some tasks, like normal people of the same mental age (MA) (but much younger CA) on other tasks, and like normal children who are much younger than MA matches on yet other tasks. I hope to convince the reader that this mixed profile maps neatly onto the first three principles of normal spatial organization and development, and provides an explanation within normal spatial development for why the WS profile is the way it is. In the fourth section, I will propose a speculative hypothesis on how the cognitive profile in WS emerges, emphasizing the role of developmental time tables in the emergence of normal spatial cognitive profiles, as well as in the WS profile. This hypothesis provides a new way of thinking about the relationships among genes, brains, and minds in spatial cognitive development. It moves us away from a static and simplistic view of how genetic differences might cause cognitive differences, and moves toward a view that emphasizes the role of normal development and developmental time tables.

The Issue of Comparison Groups

There is one more issue to discuss before turning to the review. This is the issue of how to understand performance levels; in particular, what makes an appropriate comparison group in the study of people with WS. Much research on WS is driven by the hypothesis of relative sparing and deficit across different cognitive domains. In its strongest form, the hypothesis of sparing would predict that people with WS should perform the same as normal individuals of the same CA matches (for whom overall IQ will surely be higher). This suggests that CA matches are the right comparison group. However, people with WS are mildly to moderately mentally retarded, so a prediction of performance equal to CA matches may be setting the bar inappropriately high. If people with WS perform more poorly than did their CA matches, this could be due to overall retardation, and not deficient cognitive representations or mechanisms specific to the syndrome (see Burack, 2011, Chapter 1, this volume, for additional reasons that CA matching is inappropriate).

For this reason, researchers have often tried to control for the effects of retardation by matching WS individuals on the basis of MA matches. Mental age matches are usually determined by equivalent performance on some presumably independent control variable (usually an IQ test). Typically, matches for retarded individuals will get the same raw score on some target test, but if they are normally developing people, they will often be chronologically younger than the WS individuals and have a higher overall IQ. The two strategies of matching for CA and separately matching for MA provide two different kinds of information, neither perfect. If the WS individuals are identical to CA matches, we might conclude there is no impairment, as has been shown for some aspects of face perception and object recognition (Landau, Hoffman, & Kurz, 2006; Tager-Flusberg, Plesa-Skwerer, Faja, & Joseph, 2003; although even this conclusion has been challenged, see Deruelle, Mancin, Livet, Casse-Perrot, & de Schonen, 1999). If they are no different from normally developing MA matches (who are typically younger, but are of the same "MA"), then we might once again conclude that there is no impairment specific to WS because performance is what one would expect given overall MA (i.e., the same as any other group that is retarded). Finally, if individuals with WS perform worse than their MA matches, then there is clearly some impairment, since performance is worse than one would expect even after equating for MA.

Although the most common approach is to match using either CA and/or MA control groups, there is a serious theoretical question of whether matching of either kind will provide exactly the right comparison. On the one hand, matching on the basis of CA assumes that one system can be completely intact, including its core representations and computations along with all of the more general cognitive mechanisms that must generally be engaged in carrying out any cognitive task— working memory, attention, vigilance, etc. This is a questionable assumption, especially since mental retardation surely reflects some general effects on mental processing. If our interest is in the structure of knowledge representations, we would want to factor out any consequences of poor working memory or general attention. On the other hand, matching on the basis of MA makes little sense, given that we know precious little about what either overall IQ or MA actually measures.

There are additional reasons to question the significance of either CA or MA matches. For example, Burack (2011, Chapter 1, this volume) points out that global MA matching may be less useful than matching on the basis of the targeted capacity; for example, a language match if one is testing some aspect of language, a visual–spatial match if one is testing some aspect of spatial processing. This approach is clearly more refined than the global matching approach, but still presents us with the problem that we do not necessarily know which of an infinite number of possible language tests is the "right" one; that is, the one that best reflects language capacity. Another serious problem is that different capacities develop at different rates, so it is very difficult to infer what should be the "equivalence" score on some target variable, even if we match carefully on the control variable (see Mervis & Klein-Tasman, 2004, for an excellent discussion of these and other problems in group matching designs.)

In our own research, we have used a different approach, one that is generally consistent with the developmental approach to mental retardation, first discussed by Zigler (1967). This view assumes that retardation represents the lower end of the normal curve; hence, the knowledge of a retarded individual should be similar to a normally developing individual, just "less," at any given point. Our approach is not to prejudge what the equivalence level should be—whether it should be the same as a person of the same CA, or same overall MA, or even the same MA on some particular task—but to determine equivalence by comparing performance among people with WS to the developmental curves generated by normally developing children on the tasks of interest. Some of these children will be CA matches, and some will be MA matches, and these can be useful for a first look at relative strengths and weaknesses. However, the more important comparison is to a range of normally developing children whose CAs span the MA and CA comparison groups, but also include children who are *younger* than MA matches. From this age range, we generate normal developmental curves for different aspects of spatial cognition, and then map the WS profile onto these normal developmental curves. From this, we can gain insight into the overall pattern of performance across different kinds of knowledge.

This approach is particularly important in the case of a broad investigation into spatial representations, because different spatial subsystems might normally develop at different rates, and therefore, might mature at different points in developmental time. Although there is evidence about brain development trajectories (Gogtay et al., 2004) and the development of selected aspects of spatial functioning (e.g., Newcombe & Huttenlocher, 2000), there is little to no evidence on the normal developmental time tables across a broad range of different kinds of spatial representations, including, for example, object representation, motion perception, action, imagery and mental transformations, spatial language, etc. Understanding the impairment in WS requires that we understand a broad range of spatial representational functions, and that we evaluate these against normal developmental trajectories. Without knowing whether different spatial capacities are normally acquired at different times, we cannot really evaluate the nature or meaning of an unusual pattern of performance.

Therefore, in what follows, I will describe findings in terms of comparisons to MA and CA matches, but I will also compare WS performance against a trajectory of normal development. In particular, I will ask whether the WS pattern of performance in some task(s) mirrors that of normally developing children *at some age*. Our evidence shows that, whereas WS people are severely impaired in aspects of spatial representation, they perform very much like normally developing children who are much younger than the relevant MA matches. Indeed, when they are impaired, they often perform like children who are around 4 years of age—the age equivalent that also best reflects their performance on the hallmark block construction task. This is no coincidence, as I will discuss in the last section of this chapter.

The Phenomenon: Copying Figures and Constructing Block Designs

The hallmark spatial deficit in people with WS is typically revealed by the fact that they have severe difficulty in carrying out "visuospatial constructive" tasks, which include copying figures (e.g., Test of Visual–Motor Integration or VMI; Beery & Buktenica, 1967) and constructing copies of designs from individual component blocks (e.g., the Differential Ability Scales or DAS; Elliott, 1990; the Wechsler Adult Intelligence Scale-Revised or WAIS-R; Wechsler, 1981). Figure 5.1 shows some examples of figures that have been copied by children with WS, in comparison to a child who is substantially younger, but has the same raw score on a standardized intelligence task (i.e., an MA match). The difference is obvious: The children with WS replicate the individual elements (and their colors, not shown in the panel), but do not put the elements together in a recognizable configuration. Remarkably, however, copying by children with WS—although abnormal for CA or even MA—is qualitatively quite similar to normally developing children who are 3–4 years of age and *younger* than the MA matches (Georgopoulos, Georgopoulos, Kurz, & Landau, 2004; Bertrand, Mervis, & Eisenberg, 1997). I return to this point later.

The same pattern of deficit—that is, inability to construct an accurate copy—is observed when WS individuals carry out a standardized block construction task. Although they can often (although not always) select the correct component blocks for a particular design, these blocks are not configured to accurately reproduce the overall design. A sample model and copy by a WS adult are shown in Figure 5.2.

An Early Hypothesis and Why It Is Wrong

The earliest observations of this deficit were made by Bellugi and colleagues (Bihrle, Bellugi, Delis, & Marks, 1989), who proposed that people with WS had a deficit in "global processing," with preserved ability to process the local features of a design, but impaired integration of these features; this could lead to failures in producing correct overall configurations. In principle, such a deficit could explain the great difficulty shown by people with WS in tasks such as copying and reconstructing designs, which require assembling individual parts into an overall form.

This proposed global processing deficit has, however, been ruled out by a number of findings. First, Pani, Mervis, and Robinson (1999) found that WS adults—like normal adults—can benefit from grouping cues during visual search. Both groups showed that their search was made easier when the target (such as a T) was presented in a group that

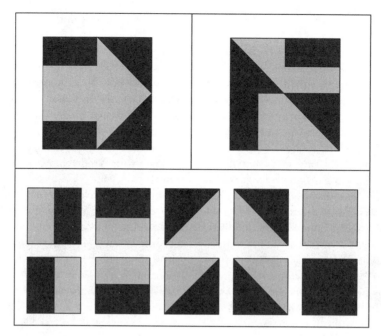

Fig. 5.2 Example of a block construction puzzle, including a model (*upper left*), the block choices (*bottom*), and an actual copy made by an adult with Williams syndrome (*upper right*).

was spatially separated from a group of confusable distracters (e.g., a group of Ls). Thus, WS adults can benefit from item groupings, showing that they can use global properties of an array (i.e., groups) to guide search. Second, Farran et al. (2003) found that although people with WS have great difficulty drawing configurations composed of individual local parts, they have no difficulty in perceptually matching these to identical global figures made up of the same parts. Thus, the observed deficit in constructing copies cannot be explained by a deficit in global perceptual processing.

A particularly compelling argument against the global processing deficit comes from recent work on the perception of visual illusions by people with WS. The perception of visual illusions provides strong evidence that the visual system takes into account global surrounding context. For example, when viewing a stimulus for the Muller-Lyer illusion (see Figure 5.3), typical adults judge the target elements (the two lines in the case of these illusions) as unequal in length, even though they are in fact equal. The illusion is produced by the surrounding contours (compare the control stimuli); hence, perceiving an illusion entails that the perceptual system has integrated information from the "global" visual context when evaluating the relative sizes of the target lines.

Palomares and colleagues showed that children and adults with WS are just as susceptible to visual illusions as typical adults (Palomares, Ogbonna,

Landau, & Egeth, 2009). We examined children and adults with WS (10–41 years old, mean age = 20 years, 9 months) on their tendency to perceive four classic illusions, including the Muller-Lyer, Ponzo, Kanisza, and Ebbinghaus illusions (see Figure 5.3 for examples of the first two). The processes of integration that produce the illusory effect are obligatory in normal adults—that is, we cannot help but see the lines as different in length even if we consciously *know* that they are equal. Palomares' findings show that this kind of obligatory integration occurs in both children and adults with WS, since they perceived the two lines as different in length when they were physically equal, and they do so to the same

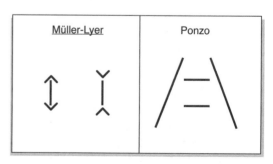

Fig. 5.3 Muller-Lyer and Ponzo illusions used by Palomares et al. (2009) to determine whether people with WS and normally developing children and adults perceive illusions to the same extent. People with WS judged the right hand line (Muller-Lyer) and the upper line (Ponzo) to be longer than its mate, consistent with perceiving the illusion.

extent as typical (non-WS) adults do. This rules out a deficit in at least some kinds of visual integration. One possibility is that the integration required for contextual effects, such as perception of illusions, represents a class of "implicit" spatial integration, which is unimpaired in WS, whereas visual–spatial construction tasks such as copying and block construction require "explicit" integration, which is severely impaired in WS (Palomares, 2006). Another interpretation is that perception of illusions is part of a modular, encapsulated system of visual processing (Pylyshyn, 2003), which is unimpaired in WS, whereas block construction tasks engage nonmodular central processes such as planning, voluntary shifts of attention, and memory.

In sum, findings cast doubt on the original global processing deficit as an explanation of the severe deficit among people with WS in copying and construction tasks. Indeed, as the next section reveals, tasks of copying and construction are quite complex, drawing on many different processes and mechanisms of spatial perception and cognition.

The Requirements of the Block Construction and Copying Tasks

The WS deficit in copying and block construction tasks is likely to occur at multiple levels beyond simple perception of the figures. This is because both of these tasks are remarkably complex, engaging many different component processes. Let's return to our example of the block task. To make a copy, the person is shown the model, provided blocks, and must use the blocks to assemble a copy (see example in Figure 5.2, after Hoffman, Landau, & Pagani, 2003). The model appears in one part of the screen, block choices in another, and the copy space in a third location, opposite the model. Hoffman et al. argued that this type of block construction task requires at least three steps, each of which engages a different set of cognitive processes:

1. *The model must be segmented into component parts–in this case, individual blocks.* In many block tasks, the emergent design is not coincident with the block-sized pieces that will ultimately form the pattern; so, people must use some voluntary selective attention processes to visually segment the model into the relevant block-sized pieces. Segmentation itself proves to be difficult for people with WS, and segmenting the model does result in better performance among WS individuals (Hoffman et al., 2003; Key, Pani, & Mervis, 1998).

2. *Individual blocks must be accurately selected from the available set.* Once a particular block-sized chunk is encoded, the observer must move his gaze to the area displaying individual blocks, and select the correct one. This step requires accurately representing the individual block, and holding it in working memory while the block choices are scanned for selection. In the version of the block task shown in Figure 5.2, accurately choosing the block entails representing the geometry of the target block (whether it is split vertically, horizontally, or diagonally) and the relative locations of the two colors in the halves of the block (in the figure, black and white).

3. The process of representing and retaining these block properties is also a problem for people with WS. Hoffman, Landau, and Pagani (2003) carried out an experiment similar to the full block construction task, except that people were only required to select a block that matched one that was specifically marked in the design (see Figure 5.4A). We found that children with WS (mean age 9;5, range 7–13;11) performed reliably more poorly than MA-matched children (mean age 5;9, range 5;1–6;4) and that their errors tended to preserve geometric structure, but violate the location of each color, resulting in mirror image errors. For example, if the marked block was vertically split, with black on the left and white on the right, children with WS would most often err by choosing a vertically split block whose colors were reversed. The same pattern held for typically developing children who were MA matches, but performance overall was much poorer among the children with WS, indicating that they experience significant problems in representing and holding in working memory the combination of color and direction (although not overall geometry) within a single block.

4. *Individual blocks must be corrected in the copy space.* The final step is placing individual blocks into the copy space in a location that is the *same* as in the copy. Here, *same location* is represented in an object-centered reference system, where the object is the model and the origin of the reference system is at the center of the model. Note that using other reference frames will not result in an accurate copy. For example, a person cannot use an egocentric frame of reference to accurately place the block in the copy space: Assuming that the model is to the person's left and the copy to his right, any location defined with respect to one's own body, head, or eye will result in erroneous placement of the block. A person cannot use a screen-based reference frame

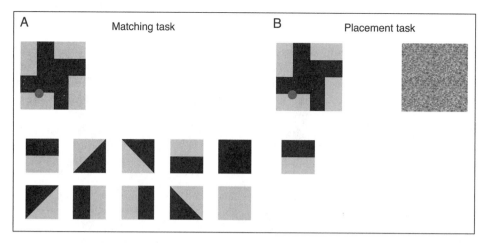

Fig. 5.4 Components of the block construction task. People were asked to either (A) select a single block that matched the target block in the model (Matching Task) or (B) move a single block to a location that matched that of the target block in the model (Placement Task). In both cases, a large dot indicated the target block in the model.

either, for similar reasons—the block's location in the model and its location in the copy will be in different locations relative to the screen. The only frame of reference that will work is the object-based system, and this must be converted into a parallel object-based system centered on the outline of the copy in the copy space. Thus, making an accurate copy requires coordinating several different frames of reference.

Children with WS have difficulty with this step as well. We carried out another experiment similar to the block task, except that children were shown the entire puzzle with one block marked, and a replica of the target block was positioned below the model. Children were asked to move this replica block into the correct location in the copy space (see Figure 5.4B). Again, children with WS performed more poorly than did typically developing children who were matched in MA, and their errors were often column (but not row) mislocations. For example, a block that was located to the left of the model's midline might now be placed to the right of the copy's midline.

These points highlight that the block construction task engages at least three crucial spatial–cognitive mechanisms. First, selective attention must be used to segment the design into block-sized chunks. Second, representation of the geometric structure of blocks and the relative locations of colors within this structure must be used to accurately select candidate blocks for the copy. Third, locations of the blocks in the model space (an object-based reference system) must be transformed into locations in the copy space (another object-based reference system), while ignoring both body- and screen-based reference systems.

What Is Wrong? Evidence From Monkeys That Draw and Carry Out Construction Tasks

The copying and construction deficits observed in people with WS are known more generally as *constructional apraxia*, which is a condition most commonly associated with damage to the parietal cortex of humans. Remarkable studies of construction abilities in monkeys provide us with a hint about the possible locus of damage in human constructional apraxia. In particular, these studies suggest that specific areas of the parietal cortex are responsible for the monkey's ability to represent locations of "missing elements" while they are carrying out tasks that are closely related to traditional block construction tasks (Chafee, Crowe, Averbeck, & Georgopoulos, 2005). By examining the neuronal activation that occurs as the monkey carries out these tasks, the studies provide us with information about which brain areas are likely to be involved in the hallmark block construction deficit of WS. Moreover, by doing so, they also suggest a broader hypothesis about the nature of the WS spatial deficit.

Chafee et al. begin by considering what component processes must be involved in a simple block construction task. Their analysis is consistent with the one proposed by Hoffman et al. (2003) in suggesting that attentional modulation, the intention to act, and the representation of spatial location must all play a role in copying a design. Focusing on the representation of a block's spatial location, Chafee et al. presented monkeys with simple block designs, all of which used a basic inverted T design plus one or two extra blocks, forming overall patterns

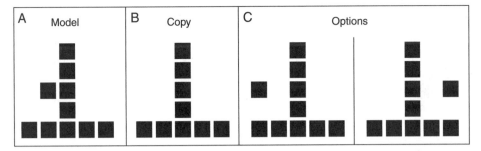

Fig. 5.5 Stimuli adapted from Chafee et al. (2005). A: Monkeys were shown a design composed of blocks arranged in an inverted T plus one additional block. B: They were then shown a copy with the single additional block missing. This was followed by (C) two options, each with a block that could complete the partial design. Patterns of neuronal activation were tuned to the location of the *missing* block, showing that the monkey encodes abstract locations. Adapted with permission of Oxford Journals.

slightly different from the basic T (see Figure 5.5A). After the monkey viewed one of these designs, it was removed from view and monkeys were now presented with the same block design, except that the one or two blocks that had been added to the T were no longer present (see Figure 5.5B). The monkey's task was to now select (by pressing a foot peddle) which of several blocks shown in various locations on the screen was the one needed to complete the design, rendering the overall design identical to the one originally seen. Monkeys learned to carry out this task quite well over a variety of block designs, with accuracy levels around 90%. To solve the task, the monkey would have had to represent the location of the *missing block* in the pattern. This is quite analogous to the problem that a person faces when he or she must construct a copy of an existing block pattern—by knowing where to place blocks in the (empty) copy space.

While the monkey was carrying out this task, neuronal recordings were made from a population of neurons in a small area of posterior parietal cortex (area 7a), near the intraparietal sulcus and the superior temporal sulcus. Analysis of these recordings showed that activation of a large subset of neurons in this area was tuned to the location of the missing block during the test trials. The patterns of activation occurred when the monkey observed the test stimuli; that is, the model with missing units (Figure 5.5B), and the particular patterns of activation were observed to correlate with the location of the *missing element*. These patterns were sustained whether the overall model and test forms were presented in the same location on the screen or in different locations, thus ruling out a purely retinotopic coding of the missing block's location and suggesting that the monkey had coded the missing block's location in an object-centered frame of reference (i.e., one centered on the model rather than the screen or the

monkey's body, head, retina, etc.). In control experiments, Chafee et al. showed these results could not be explained solely in terms of attentional modulation or intention to act.

The fact that the parietal cortex in monkey encodes such a representation suggests that a key brain area of the deficit in WS might be the homologous parietal areas in humans. These areas are known to also be important in regulating visual attention in both monkey and humans (Colby & Goldberg, 1999), and they are engaged during visual–manual action in both monkeys (Chafee et al., 2005) and humans (Milner & Goodale, 1995). According to Hoffman et al.'s (2003) analysis of the block construction task, each of these is an important component of the task, and each is required to accurately reproduce the copy. Recalling the earlier discussion, Hoffman et al. proposed that attentional processes are important in segmenting the overall design of the puzzle into block-sized chunks. Representing the object-based location of an individual block (and ignoring its egocentric or screen-based location) is crucial in placing the block into its correct space in the copy area. Clearly, the intention to act and the action itself are also important in placing each piece in the correct space. As I will describe later, each of these components is itself damaged in people with WS, thus providing strong convergence with the monkey work.

Deficient copying is another major hallmark of WS, and this too falls within the category of constructional apraxia. Averbeck et al. (2003) have shown that areas of the prefrontal cortex in monkeys are engaged during copying activity. Monkeys were trained to repeatedly copy simple geometric figures such as squares, triangles, and trapezoids, and neuronal recording revealed substantial activity in prefrontal cortex, which was specifically tuned to components of specific shapes during copying activity.

Not only was a majority of neurons specific to the shape being generated, the sequence of strokes composing each of the shapes—along with direction and length—was strongly related to the target shapes. The close proximity and anatomical connections between parietal and prefrontal cortex in monkey suggest that both of these areas are involved in representing abstract geometrical information required to carry out both copying and construction tasks (Averbeck, Chafee, Crowe, & Georgopoulos, 2003; Chafee et al., 2005).

A Hypothesis: Ventral Sparing, Dorsal/Parietal Weakness

The studies of monkeys' visual–spatial construction and drawing suggest a hypothesis about the hallmark deficit in WS: Areas of the parietal cortex, linked to prefrontal areas, may be damaged. If so, this would predict that other spatial cognitive functions that normally engage the parietal and frontal-parietal areas might also be impaired in people with WS.

The hypothesis that WS can be characterized as a deficit in dorsal stream functions—which engage parietal and prefrontal areas—has been suggested by others (Atkinson et al., 2003; Wang, Doherty, Rourke, & Bellugi, 1995), but supporting evidence has been somewhat limited. Several key questions must be answered before concluding that the deficit is indeed primarily one of the dorsal and parietal regions. First, if the parietal and prefrontal areas are selectively damaged, then is there sparing in areas of spatial representation that are known to engage different areas of the brain, such as those that are part of the ventral stream? Abundant evidence from neuroscience, neuropsychology, and psychophysiology suggests that the visual system is broadly divided into two streams—the dorsal stream, which generally is thought to process spatial information that is relevant to action, and the ventral stream, generally thought to process spatial information relevant to processing of objects and faces (see, e.g., Milner & Goodale, 1995). Evidence from the literature hints that, in WS, certain functions carried by the ventral stream may be relatively undamaged. For example, people with WS are known to perform very strongly in face recognition tasks (Bellugi et al., 1988; Wang et al., 1995), and recent evidence has shown that they are susceptible to the face inversion effect, performing like normal CA matches on tasks requiring face processing (Tager-Flusberg et al., 2003; but see Deruelle et al., 1999, for a different view).

Second, if the dorsal stream is damaged, is this quite general within the stream (including both parietal and prefrontal regions), resulting in impairment to a wide range of functions known to engage these areas? Or, is the impairment restricted to just certain functions?

Along with colleagues, I have been carrying out a program of research that has sought answers to both of these questions by examining a wide range of spatial functions known to engage the ventral and dorsal stream in humans. If the deficit in people with WS is specific to the dorsal stream, then we should observe sparing of ventral stream functions; if the deficit encompasses the dorsal stream as a whole, then we should observe quite general impairment across dorsal stream functions. In the next two sections, I will review our findings on functions that typically engage the ventral stream and those that typically engage the dorsal stream (see next two sections). Using evidence from both of these sets of functions, we will be able to determine whether the unusual profile of spatial sparing and breakdown in people with WS is consistent with sparing in ventral stream functions and impairment in dorsal stream functions, especially those engaging the parietal areas.

Spatial Functions That Typically Engage the Ventral Stream

In attempting to characterize the spatial impairment in WS, a central issue is whether the severe impairment observed in tasks such as block construction and drawing is generally observed across a wide variety of spatial representational functions. If so, then the spatial system of people with WS would look essentially "flat," with roughly equal impairment across a host of different tasks. For example, they might show a pattern of performance that is no different across a range of tasks relative to MA-matched children, or they might show a pattern of performance that is systematically and equally worse than that of MA matches. If we use normal developmental trajectories as the comparison, a flat pattern would mean performance that is no different across a range of tasks relative to a particular CA, say 6-year-olds. An alternative possibility is that the system is selectively impaired, with an uneven pattern of performance; for example, people with WS might perform no differently from MA matches for one class of tasks, but might show performance that is worse (or better) than MA matches for another class of tasks. Comparing to a normal developmental curve, people with WS might be different from

6-year-olds for one class of tasks, but no different from 4-year-olds for another class of tasks.

As a first attempt to evaluate this, our research group has examined a range of spatial functions, some of which might be relatively spared, with a pattern of performance better than MA matches or possibly no different from CA matches. Several functions that engage spatial representations—but do not directly appear to engage the parietal areas of the brain—include object representation, biological motion perception, and spatial language. In this section, I review evidence from our lab on these functions. Another obvious function is face perception, which is thought to engage a specific area of the ventral stream, and was initially suggested as a candidate for sparing in WS. Indeed, Tager-Flusberg et al. (2003) have shown that WS people show the face inversion effect, a signature of holistic processing shown in normal individuals. These findings are especially significant since they disconfirm the hypothesis that people with WS suffer from impairment in the ability to integrate elements into a unified whole. If they were impaired in this ability, people with WS would fail to process faces holistically, and would likely fail to show the inversion effect. The presence of a face inversion effect is consistent with other evidence (reviewed earlier and in the present section) showing that people with WS do not generally suffer from failure to perceptually integrate elements into a whole. For example, the perception of illusions requires integration from context, yet people with WS perceive illusions to the same extent as typically developing children and adults.

Object Representation

Although object recognition can sometimes be achieved on the basis of color or surface texture (bananas are yellow; artifacts often have smooth surfaces), one spatial property—object shape—is arguably the most important property used by the visual system for recognition. The computational solution to recognizing objects is complex because objects need to be identified regardless of changes in viewpoint, size, lighting, and so on (see Palmieri & Gauthier, 2004, for a review). In addition, many objects such as bears, trees, and people are nonrigid and therefore can change shape from one occasion to another. Object recognition processes must somehow pick out the invariant characteristics of object shape and discard the results of these irrelevant transformations. These processes of object recognition appear to be obligatory and can occur

extremely rapidly in adults. For example, Grill-Spector and Kanwisher (2005) found that people identify objects at about the same time as we realize that we have seen them.

In a series of experiments, we asked whether children with WS could accurately recognize (and identify) common objects when presented quite briefly (500 msec each), and under a variety of challenging conditions (Landau et al., 2006). In one condition, we presented full-color objects either in canonical or unusual orientations. Canonical orientations exposed many large and diagnostic parts of objects, whereas unusual orientations showed highly atypical views with few diagnostic parts (see Figure 5.6A and B for examples). Overall, children with WS (mean age 11;0, range 7;4–15;3) were comparable to MA-matched controls (MA, mean age 5;8, range 4;1–7;1) and only slightly worse than normally developing children of the same CA (CA controls, mean age 11;11, range 10;6–4;3), primarily in the unusual views condition. To make sure that the good performance of WS children was not based on nonshape features, such as color or texture, we also tested them on line drawings of the same objects (see Figure 5.6C and D for examples). The results were similar, with comparable performance for WS and MA-matched children and a small advantage for the CA group, mainly for objects shown in unusual views.

The performance of WS children—no different from MA children who are on average 6 years old—stands in marked contrast to their difficulty in block construction and drawing tasks. On the latter tasks, even adults with WS perform more like 4-year-olds. This indicates that the WS spatial profile is not flat, but rather, has at least one peak (object recognition) relative to visual–spatial construction tasks. In addition, there are other reasons to conclude that the mechanisms underlying object recognition are largely spared (see Landau et al., 2006, for full discussion).

Biological Motion and Other Motion Processing

Motion processing in people with WS has also been of interest, for two reasons. First, the literature suggests that processing of motion coherence (the ability to see elements moving together) engages the dorsal stream of the brain. As Atkinson and Braddick (2003) reasoned, if people with WS show significant deficits in processing of motion coherence, this would provide evidence for dorsal stream impairment. However, motion processing is also interesting because at least three different types of motion

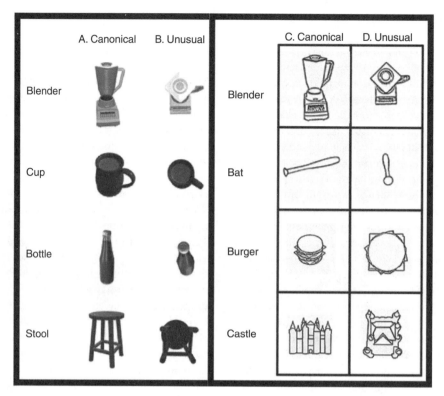

Fig. 5.6 Stimuli from object recognition experiments (Landau, Hoffman, & Kurz, 2006). Objects were presented with full color and surface texture, either in (A) canonical orientations or (B) unusual orientations. In a follow-up experiment, objects were presented as line drawings, again either in (C) canonical or (D) unusual orientations. Adapted with permission from Elsevier.

processing exist: Biological motion processing, motion coherence, and form-from-motion appear to be dissociable from each other (for evidence from single-cell recording in monkeys, see Maunsell & Van Essen, 1983; for evidence in human patients, see Cowey & Vaina, 2000; Vaina, Lemay, Bienfang, Choi, & Nakayama, 1990). Biological motion processing appears to engage an area of the brain that is more ventral than does motion coherence processing. Therefore, people with WS might show a pattern of peaks and valleys *within* the system of motion processing; and if so, the pattern could further shed light on the selectivity of the spatial impairment in WS. Our research group therefore studied the ability of people with WS to process three types of motion: biological motion, motion coherence, and form-from-motion.

A particularly compelling example of seeing shapes based on motion is biological motion perception, in which observers are able to quickly perceive a walking person based only on the motion of lights attached to the major joints (Johansson, 1973). This kind of motion perception involves the *global integration* of the local motion paths traced out by each of the joints. Taken singly, these local motion paths do not lead to a perception of biological motion. Thus, people with WS, who have sometimes been characterized as having deficits in the ability to see global shapes, might be expected to have difficulty with this task. However, we found that children with WS (mean age 11; 7: range 9;9–15;7) were comparable to and, in some cases, better than MA controls (mean age 6;5, range 4;3–7;3) in accurately judging the direction of locomotion of a point-light-walker (PLW) embedded in dynamic noise (Jordan, Reiss, Hoffman, & Landau, 2002).

The robustness of biological motion perception is consistent with the idea of specialization within spatial systems. To further probe robust representation in other systems of motion perception, we examined the performance of children and adults with WS (mean ages 14.3; 25;3, respectively) in three different motion perception tasks, including motion coherence, biological motion, and two-dimensional (2D) form-from-motion (Reiss, Hoffman, & Landau, 2005). Consistent with evidence from Nakamura et al. (2002), motion coherence thresholds were comparable to those of normal adults. Thresholds for biological motion were comparable or better than those of MA matches (mean age 6;1; range 4;11–7;7), consistent with our previous work (Jordan et al., 2002). People with WS were impaired (relative to MA matches) only in the 2D form-from-motion task. The relative difficulty with the form-from-motion task persisted into adulthood for people with WS, with adults failing to perform at levels beyond that of a normal 6-year-old child. This suggests developmental arrest in this type of motion processing.

The 2D form-from-motion task that was used by Reiss et al. was similar to one used by Atkinson et al. (1997), who also reported a motion processing deficit (although they characterized their task as one of motion coherence processing). It is also related to a task used by Mendes et al. (2005), who found that people with WS were deficient in processing three-dimensional (3D) structure from motion, although not 2D motion coherence. Mendes et al. explicitly linked the deficit in 3D structure from motion to a deficit in the magnocellular stream of the visual system, which feeds into the dorsal stream, suggesting that this type of motion perception might be compromised in WS due to a more general impairment in the dorsal stream.

These findings show that biological motion is not the only motion task preserved in people with WS; motion coherence is preserved as well. The selective impairment within the motion processing system suggests that people with WS do not have a "generalized" dorsal stream deficit. Evidence from animal studies suggests that motion coherence is processed in dorsal stream region V5/MT, and the relative sparing of this function in WS is inconsistent with the idea that all dorsal stream functions are impaired.

The underlying cause of difficulty in our 2D form-from-motion task remains to be determined, but one possibility is that this task relies strongly on the ability to segment a noisy signal from its background. People with WS seem to have difficulty with segmentation of parts from a surrounding whole. For example, Hoffman et al. (2003) found that performance in the block construction task by both normally developing and WS children improved when the blocks making up the model were separated from each other. Even when the blocks were separated, however, WS children continued to show a deleterious effect of the surrounding blocks, reflecting an inability to effectively separate individual blocks from their surrounding context. An alternative, suggested by Mendes et al. (2005), is that impairment may be specific to those motion tasks that selectively tap the magnocellular stream, such as the 3D form-from-motion explored in their paper.

Spatial Language: Motion Events

Mapping spatial experience into language engages a distinctly different kind of system from either object recognition or motion perception. We must, of course, perceive objects and their motions in order to say what has occurred in any motion event. But talking about what we see further requires that we map these percepts into a linguistic structure that obeys syntactic and semantic constraints on the expression of motion events (Jackendoff, 1983; Talmy, 1978, 1983).

In two series of experiments, we probed the spatial–linguistic knowledge of children with WS (mean age 9;7), testing whether they obeyed the constraints of English in describing simple motion events. In the first series, we showed children a series of brief, animated motion events, for example, a doll hopping into a small ring or a toy cow falling off the back of a wagon. After people viewed each event, they were asked to tell us "what happened" (Landau & Zukowski, 2003). Descriptions were analyzed in terms of both semantic and syntactic content, emphasizing the encoding of three key elements of the motion events that are encoded in languages of the world: The *figure* (a noun phrase in English, e.g., "a girl"), the *motion* (usually a verb, e.g., "hopped"), and the *path expression*, a combination of a *path-function* (usually a preposition, e.g., "into") and a *reference object* (a noun phrase, e.g., "a small ring").

The path expressions in English and other languages have significant internal structure. For example, paths are differentiated into three types: Goal paths represent the paths of figures moving toward a reference object, as in "The bunny hopped *to the hole*." Source paths represent the paths of figures moving away from a reference object, as in "The bunny hopped *away from the hole*." Via paths represent paths of figures moving past the reference object, as in "The bunny hopped *past the hole*." As shown by these examples, different terms are appropriate for different path types (e.g., *to* or *into* for goal paths, *off of* or *away from* for source paths). Moreover, the choice of a path word is conditioned by the type of reference object: Words like *onto* or *off of* are used when the surface of a reference object is pertinent; words like *into* or *out of* are used when containment is pertinent.

Landau and Zukowski (2003) found that children with WS performed no differently from normally developing MA-matched children (mean age 5;0), who both performed like normal adults in their choice of terms for the figure, motion, or path expressions. The only difference between children with WS and MA-matched children was in the frequency of expression of "source paths." When describing events in which the figure moved *away from* the reference object (source path expressions), WS children again produced well-formed expressions, but they omitted the entire path expression reliably more often than the MA-matched children. Both groups produced goal path expressions with the same frequency; the difference was only observed for source paths, which were omitted more often. These omissions are not grammatical failures, because sentences produced without source path expressions are perfectly grammatical. For example, a child with WS might tend to describe an event as "The girl fell," rather than "The girl fell off the swing." Both sentences are grammatical, and differ only in how much information about the path is encoded in the linguistic description.

These findings strongly suggest that there is sparing of the internal semantic and syntactic structure of spatial language among WS children. Lakusta and Landau (2005) provided further supporting evidence for this conclusion in a series of experiments examining the structure of path expressions for different event types, including manner of motion events, change of state events, transfer events, and attachment/detachment events, each encoded by a different sets of verbs. Children with WS (mean age 13;7) were no different from MA-matched controls (mean age 5;9), and both groups showed significant and appropriate modulation of both syntax and semantics, varying with event type. Moreover, Lakusta and Landau found that the pattern of dropping source paths is common across all event types, and occurs frequently in young, normally developing children down to age 3, which was the youngest group tested. Dropping source paths does not result in an ungrammatical utterance, nor a pragmatically odd one; it is a perfectly grammatical option to omit the source path in the contexts tested. The fact that young children and people with WS tend to omit source paths may be the result of a bias to represent and remember events in terms of their goal structure (see discussion in Lakusta & Landau, 2005; Lakusta, Wagner, O'Hearn, & Landau, 2007), which could then naturally result in a bias to encode goal paths at the expense of source paths. Note that such a bias to omit source paths does not represent a *linguistic*

deficit of any kind. Thus, I conclude that the control of linguistic structures required for the language of motion events—as well as language for other event types—is not impaired in children with WS.

These findings of normal internal structure in the linguistic system are echoed by findings from other investigators and in other areas of syntax and semantics. For example, although people with WS perform rather poorly on standardized tests of some syntactic structures, such as relative clauses (Grant, Valian, & Karmiloff-Smith, 2002), children and adults with WS can accurately produce complex subject and object-relative clauses when the pragmatic context is felicitous (Zukowski, 2001). In addition, recent studies of the semantics and syntax of logical terms such as *not* and *or* show that people with WS—who have clear deficits in some areas of cognition—nevertheless engage complex rules of syntax and semantics when producing and interpreting sentences involving interactions between these logical terms (Musolino, Chunyo, & Landau, 2010).

Weakness in Parietal Functions and More Generally, the Dorsal Stream

I have already discussed the hypothesis that the spatial profile of people with WS might be characterized as general strength in spatial functions engaging the ventral stream, but marked weakness in spatial functions engaging the dorsal stream. This hypothesis has been suggested by a number of other scientists, including Wang et al. (1995) and Atkinson and Braddick (2003). The evidence I reviewed in second section suggests strength in ventral stream functions, consistent with this hypothesis. What about dorsal stream functions?

The hallmark visual–constructive deficit is consistent with the idea that functions engaging the parietal regions of the brain are damaged. As suggested by the analysis of Hoffman et al. (2003) and discussed earlier in this chapter, analysis of the block construction task suggests that the task might heavily engage dorsal stream processes and representations. If this account is correct, then we should predict that people with WS should perform especially poorly (i.e., reliably worse than MA-matched children) on a broad range of tasks that also engage the dorsal stream. Using our analysis of the block construction task as an analytic tool, my colleagues and I have examined several spatial functions that are known—on independent grounds—to engage parietal areas, testing the hypothesis that these functions may generally be impaired in people with WS.

Visual–Manual Action

Much research on spatial function in the mind and brain has distinguished between the dorsal and ventral streams of processing in the visual system. Ungerleider and Mishkin (1982) suggested that these two streams have different processing characteristics, with the dorsal stream processing information about object locations ("where") and the ventral stream processing information about object identification ("what"). A more recent formulation by Milner and Goodale (1995) revised the original distinction to emphasize the functional consequences of visual processing in the two streams. Milner and Goodale's work centered on a patient who had sustained cortical damage due to carbon monoxide poisoning. She was severely impaired in a task requiring her to judge the orientation of a slot in a box, but was able to act, posting a letter into the same slot. This and other cases led Milner and Goodale to propose two separate functions of the visual system, carried by two different streams of visual processing in the brain. The "what" system is thought to engage the ventral stream of the brain, supporting tasks such as perception and object recognition. The "how" system is thought to engage the dorsal stream of the brain, supporting tasks such as grasping, posting, and other visual–manual actions that require online, continuous updating of the effectors relative to a stable target as the action is carried out.

In our lab, we have tested the what/how hypothesis as an explanation of the spatial deficit in people with WS. We adapted Milner and Goodale's tasks for use with children and adults with WS (mean ages 12, and 23;9, respectively), as well as MA-matched children (mean age 6;3) and other normal children who were younger than these MA matches (mean age 3;8) (Dilks, Hoffman, & Landau, 2008; see also Atkinson et al., 2003 for a similar task). Under the hypothesis that the dorsal stream is damaged in WS, we expected to find especially poor performance on a task requiring visually guided action, but markedly better performance on an analogous task requiring a perceptual judgment, but no directed action. If people with WS have damage to spatial systems engaging the dorsal stream, but less or none to areas engaging more ventral areas of the brain, they should exhibit marked deficits in the action task—even relative to MA matches—but they should not show such deficits in the analogous perceptual matching task.

In the action task, we asked people to pick up a dollar bill and insert it into a piggy bank whose slot could be set at any of four different angles of orientation.

In the perceptual matching task, we asked people to judge whether a manikin hand holding the dollar bill was ready to put the dollar into the slot, using the same test angles of orientation.

In the perceptual matching task, all people were highly accurate; children and adults with WS did not perform reliably worse than MA-matched children (who were on average 6 years old). Even normally developing 3- and 4-year-olds performed very accurately in this task, and there was little development between 3 and 6 among these normal children. This indicates that the task of perceptual matching tapped into a function that develops rapidly and is close to mature by age 4 (under these test conditions). The ability of people with WS to perform accurately in this task, and at roughly the same levels as normal 6-year-olds, suggests that this function is at worst only slightly impaired in people with WS.

In contrast, the action task showed large absolute differences across groups, and these differences were consistent with the hypothesis of dorsal stream damage in WS. Children and adults with WS performed reliably worse than normally developing MA matches (who were on average 6 years old). This suggests a large deficit among WS people even compared to MA-matched children who are much younger. However, the performance of WS people was indistinguishable from normally developing 3- to 4-year-old children, who also performed reliably worse than normally developing 6-year-olds.

These results reveal several things. First, there is considerable developmental change among normal children between ages 3 and 6 in the ability to carry out an accurate action (here, posting). The change over age among normal children was much more substantial in the action task than in the perceptual matching task, suggesting the possibility that normal development entails prolonged development of the dorsal stream relative to the ventral stream. Second, the results showed that the WS participants—both children and adults—were significantly impaired in the action task (even compared to MA matches), basically performing at the level of 3- to 4-year-old, normally developing children. This pattern among people with WS suggests developmental arrest at the level of a normal 3- to 4-year-old.

This is a strong hypothesis. However, it is supported by several facts. First, the children and adults with WS performed the same as normally developing 4-year-olds in the action task; that is, there was no developmental improvement beyond childhood in people with WS. Second, analyses of the qualitative pattern of performance across the different groups revealed that children and adults with WS had error patterns highly similar to those of normally developing 4-year-olds. They were also similar to normal 6-year-olds, factoring out overall accuracy. For example, all participant groups were very accurate on trials showing vertical and horizontal target orientations, and much less accurate on trials showing oblique orientations. All groups showed error patterns of nonrandom spread around the target orientations, with the magnitude of spread larger for people with WS and normal 4-year-olds relative to the normal 6-year-olds. The similarity in the qualitative nature of the spread suggests a common, underlying representation of orientation across the different groups, with differences occurring in the magnitude of the spread around the target orientation.

The overall pattern in the action and perception tasks suggests fragility in the visual–manual action system among people with WS, with disproportionate error around targets in the action task relative to the perceptual matching task (which requires no visual–manual action). The 3- to 4-year-old age equivalence for WS individuals was the same in both the perception and action tasks, but importantly, performance in the perception task was close to ceiling in normal children by age 3–4, whereas performance in the action task showed significant improvement among normal children between 4 and 6. Individuals with WS appear to perform about like 4-year-olds in both tasks, consistent with the idea of arrest at this developmental level.

Using and Coordinating Reference Frames

As noted in my discussion of the block construction task, one plausible reason for failure in these tasks is impairment in the ability to convert the representation of location of a single block (in the model) into its parallel location in a different space (i.e., the space that will be occupied by the copy). To understand more about this element of the task, we need to introduce the notion of a location within a single reference frame and the conversion of this representation into location in a second reference frame.

A frame of reference is a mental structure that specifies the location of a point relative to an origin and (for simplicity of discussion) two orthogonal axes (vertical and horizontal). Different reference frames have different origins, for example, the origin could be the center of the retina (retinocentric frame), the center of the body (egocentric frame), the center of an object (object-centered frame), etc.

In the block task, the goal is to place a block in the copy area in a location that is "the same" as the location of an identical block in the model area. But how is the "same location" defined? Starting with the encoding of a target block's location in the model (perhaps in a head-centered frame of reference), this location—in this reference frame—must be coordinated with the block's location in a body-centered frame of reference, which is needed to guide action. But the location in a body-based frame of reference will not suffice to reproduce location from the model to the copy area. This requires representing the block's location in a *model*-based frame of reference, and then converting this into a second object-based frame of reference, which is centered on the copy area. This successive conversion of location across frames of reference can ultimately result in an accurate block placement in the copy area.

Neuroscientists have shown that the coordination of frames of reference of various types occurs in frontal and parietal areas of the brain (Andersen & Zipser, 1988; Colby & Goldberg, 1999). For example, the ability to update eye movements requires transforming location from retinocentric to egocentric frames of reference, and the mechanism underlying this updating engages these areas. Toddlers with WS may be impaired in the updating of eye movements (Brown et al., 2003). Furthermore, the clear difficulties that WS people experience when they try to place individual blocks into parallel locations in a copy space suggests that they have difficulty in converting a location in a model's reference system to the same location in the copy area (Hoffman et al., 2003).

To directly examine difficulties in coordinating the reference systems for two separate and adjacent spaces, we have carried out two lines of research. In one, we found that children with WS (mean age 10;4) do represent location in terms of object-centered reference frames, but that the reference systems (and their component axes) are fragile and possibly truncated, with accurate representation of location confined to smaller regions than those shown by normally developing MA matches (mean age 5;5) (Landau & Hoffman, 2005). We asked children to match a sample array (a square with a dot nearby) to its identical copy. The sample was always shown in the center of one sheet of paper, and the test items (same, different) were shown on a sheet of paper placed below the sample sheet (see Figure 5.7). "Same" items were always identical to the sample, and the "different" items portrayed the dot moved by a small amount. The test items

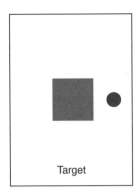

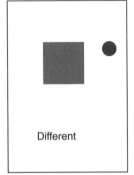

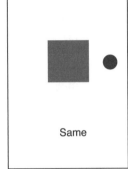

Fig. 5.7 Stimuli from reference-frame experiments (from Landau & Hoffman, 2005). People were shown a model displaying a target dot and a square and were instructed to match the array to one of the two below (that showed the dot "in the same place to the square"). Target dot locations sampled the space around the square, including locations that fell at varying distances on the extensions of the square's vertical, horizontal, and oblique axes.

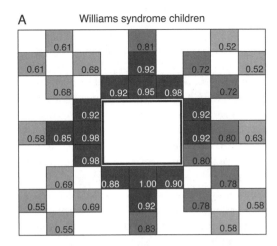

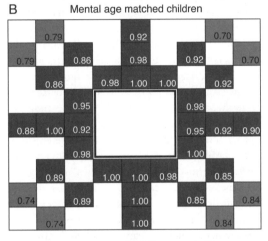

Fig. 5.8 Proportions correct for different sampled locations; (A) children with Williams syndrome children and (B) mental age-matched, normally developing children. Darker shades correspond to higher accuracy.

sampled a wide range of locations relative to the square, including locations that fell at varying distances on the extension of the square's vertical, horizontal, or oblique axes.

The results showed that children with WS could identify the "same location" as well as typically developing MA-matched children, but only for certain locations (see Figure 5.8). For example, all target locations in which the dot contacted the square were accurate at ceiling levels. In addition, targets with locations close to the square, but along the extension of the vertical or horizontal axes were also matched at very high levels of accuracy. Two important differences between the children with WS and typically developing MA controls did emerge, however. First, children with WS were reliably worse than MA matches for dots located at larger distances from the square, suggesting that representing locations in a single reference frame and/or converting one location to another reference frame is quite fragile, breaking down with any substantial distance from the reference object.

Second, although both normally developing children and those with WS performed worse for locations along the horizontal axis relative to the vertical axis, children with WS suffered more, again suggesting a fragile reference system.

In a second line of research, my colleagues and I are currently examining whether additional transformations across reference systems also show impairment. The task described earlier requires transformation from an object-based frame of reference centered on the upper panel to object-based frames centered on each test panel, to the left and right and below the upper panel. The task also requires only matching, which—although it clearly reveals some deficit—may not reflect the additional complexity inherent in the block construction task of actually *placing* a block in its new location. Therefore, we designed a new task that required placement of a target dot into a copy area, based on examining its location in a model on the person's left, and transferring it to the analogous location on the person's right (Landau, Hoffman, & Street, in progress).

In this task, children and adults with WS (mean age 21;9) as well as normal children at ages 4 (mean age 4;6), 6 (mean age 6;6), and 9 (mean age 9;9) examined a display showing a square with a dot located in one of 16 locations around it. This model display was presented to the person's left. They were then shown a copy panel (to their right) that displayed only the square, and were asked to place a dot in the same location relative to the square as in the model panel. In a first study, the location of the square within the copy panel was varied, with half of the trials showing the square in the same location in the copy panel as in the model panel, and half showing the square in a different location in the copy panel relative to the model (see Figure 5.9). When the square is in the same location relative to the panel in both model and copy, a person can place the new dot accurately by using a frame of reference centered on either the panel itself or the square. But when the square is in a different location relative to the panel in model and copy, the correct solution of the task requires ignoring the panel-based reference frame, and placing the dot using only the square-based frame of reference. In this task, people with WS performed at high levels of accuracy in both cases, but they performed

reliably better in cases in which the squares in model and copy were in the same place relative to the panel. When the squares in the model and copy are in the same place relative to the panel, the "same location" for the dot relative to the square can be coded in terms of either the square itself or the panel—both will give the same answer. But when the squares are in different places relative to the panel, the "same location" for the dot *must* be coded relative to the square, and not the panel. Using the "same location" relative to the panel will result in an error. The difference in performance under these two conditions suggests that the first is easier because the two candidate reference frames (panel, square) coincide; the second is more difficult because the two reference frames result in different representations of what is the "same location."

The findings from a second experiment reinforced this conclusion, revealing severe difficulties in coordinating locations within different frames of reference. The same task was used, except that the model square was rotated relative to the copy square (which was always shown upright); both squares were displayed in the same place relative to the panel. In this case, because the person must place the dot in the same place relative to the *model square*, this requires using only the model square as a frame of reference; that it, an object-based reference frame with the origin at the center of the model square. It also requires transforming the rotated object-based

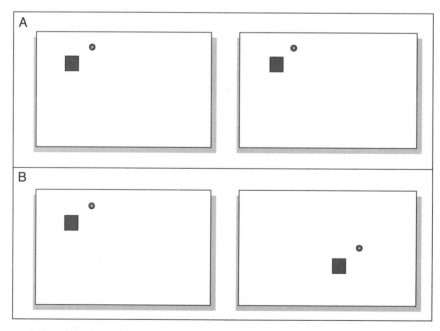

Fig. 5.9 Displays for "placing" task. People were shown the panel on the left, and must move the dot in the right hand panel to the "same place" relative to the square.

frame (in the model) into the upright one (in the copy). In this task, people with WS performed extremely poorly, showing errors that indicated great difficulty carrying out that transformation. Instead, they sometimes used the panel-based frame of reference, and sometimes adopted a kind of compromise solution, placing the dot in a location that was intermediate between the location required for the panel-based solution and the location required for the object-based solution.

Overall, the results of these experiments are consistent with the difficulty that children with WS have in putting blocks into the same location in a copy area after having inspected a model. Although they clearly can represent locations in terms of object-based reference systems that are organized by two primary orthogonal axes, the systems of people with WS are fragile. This fragility carries over into tasks requiring that one location be mapped onto another in a different reference system—a requirement for any copying task. Given the evidence for parietal involvement in the coordination of reference frames, these findings again suggest that dorsal and particularly parietal functions are impaired in WS.

Other Parietal Functions

The hypothesis of a dorsal stream deficit—especially involving parietal functions—suggests that many additional functions should be significantly impaired in people with WS. This is because the parietal areas are involved in many different cognitive functions, including modulation of visual attention (Colby & Goldberg, 1999), tracking of multiple objects (Culham et al., 1998), and even some processes involving the representation of number (Dehaene, Piazza, Pinel, & Cohen, 2003). My colleagues and I have tested the hypothesis of broader parietal involvement by examining a range of these functions. In several cases, we have found significant deficits among people with WS compared to MA-matched children. We have also found that the pattern of performance among people with WS is often quite similar to that of children who are younger than our MA matches—children who are on average 3–4 years old. This suggests a hypothesis of developmental arrest in certain parietal spatial functions, consistent with the suggestion I made earlier in the chapter.

One example that illustrates this pattern is found in the ability of people to keep track of multiple objects, when they are presented in stable locations and when they move around the screen on independent trajectories (O'Hearn, Landau, & Hoffman, 2005). Our experiments were patterned after those developed by Pylyshyn and colleagues using the *multiple object tracking* or MOT task (Pylyshyn & Storm, 1988; Scholl & Pylyshyn, 1999). These researchers showed that normal adults can—in this context—keep track of up to four different objects in a larger array as they moved over independent trajectories. These results have been interpreted as a visual capacity for representing and maintaining small sets of objects, up to a maximum of about four; there is recent discussion of whether these representations are the equivalent of an upper limit on the capacity of the visual attention or working memory system to maintain small sets of objects (see, e.g., Cowan, 2000).

In normal adults, the MOT task activates parietal and frontal cortex (Culham et al., 1998). If there is broad impairment in parietal areas in WS, then this cognitive function should show impairment. These areas of the brain are also known to undergo protracted development in normal children (Gogtay et al., 2004), hence the task could serve as a good litmus test to evaluate where people with WS fit on the normal developmental trajectory. Finally, the ability to mark and hold onto multiple objects could be crucial in a broad range of tasks, including the block construction task, since accurate performance likely involves keeping track of individual blocks in the model as one moves to select identical matching parts and assemble them in the copy space. Keeping track of this is crucial since the task requires continuous checking of the model and copy, looking back and forth between them to check the identity of target model blocks and their locations in the copy. The idea that object "pointers" or "indexes" are deployed via visual fixations to mark each block for later refixation suggests that multiple object tracking could be an important diagnostic of spatial breakdown in the block task (Ballard, Hayhoe, Pook, & Rao, 1997; Pylyshyn, 2000).

O'Hearn, Landau, and Hoffman (2005) asked whether such indexes are faulty in WS, possibly accounting in part for the deficit in the block task. Adapting the MOT task of Pylyshyn and Storm (1988), we presented children and adults with WS (mean age 18; range 10;5–38;11) and typically developing children ages 4, 5, and 6 with arrays of eight playing cards arranged randomly on a screen (see Figure 5.10). Between one and four of these were flipped over on cue to reveal a cat on the other side. These were then flipped back over, so that all

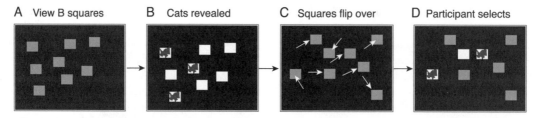

Fig. 5.10 Stimuli for the Multiple Object Tracking task (from O'Hearn et al., 2005). Observers view a panel with eight identical squares (A), some of which are flipped over to reveal cats (B). They are then flipped back (C), and all squares move along independent trajectories for several seconds. When the squares stop moving (D), people must select the squares that they think are hiding the cats. Panel (D) shows a (incorrect) response in which the person tracked two cats correctly, but not the third. Adapted with permission of Elsevier.

cards were identical, and then the cards either remained in their locations for several seconds (Static condition, a control) or moved about the screen on independent trajectories for the same amount of time (Moving condition). People were then asked to indicate where all the cats were "hiding" (i.e., which cards' reverse sides would reveal cats). The moving condition of this task can only be accomplished by continually tracking all target objects during the motion phase because targets and distractors (i.e., non-cat cards) are not otherwise distinguishable.

Children and adults with WS were impaired on the MOT task relative to MA matches (mean age 5;11), but they were not impaired relative to the MA children on the control task, which required that they remember the static locations of the hidden cats. Children and adults with WS tracked up to two objects, but normally developing MA matches tracked up to four. Comparing individuals with WS to normally developing children of different ages, we found that the people with WS (average age 18 years) performed at the level of 4-year-olds on the MOT task, but like 5-year-olds on the Static control task. We also found that there were large improvements in performance on the MOT task between the ages of 4 and 5 among normally developing children, suggesting that there is normally rapid development in the functions underlying this task during this age period. The pattern for people with WS again suggests arrested development around the age of a normally developing 4-year-old in the capacity to track multiple objects.

We are presently examining additional functions that normally engage parietal functions, and these show surprising convergence with the results of the MOT task, especially in the number of objects that can be visually represented at the same time. For example, we tested children and adults with WS in a subitizing task, briefly presenting from one to eight dots on a screen and asking people to report "how many" (O'Hearn, Landau, & Hoffman, 2011). Children and adults with WS could accurately report up to two or three dots, with a sharp drop in accuracy with larger numbers. Mental age matches (who were 5 and 6 years old) could accurately report up to four or five dots, whereas normally developing 4-year-olds reported either two or three dots, like the WS participants. The relative deficit in people with WS was not due to difficulty using number words. In a control condition, we presented the same displays for 5 seconds apiece, allowing explicit counting. In this condition, people with WS performed as well as MA-matched children (who were 5 and 6), and both groups could accurately count up to eight objects.

The apparent reduction in the number of objects that can be simultaneously tracked also emerged in a task modeled after Luck and Vogel (1997), who showed that normal adults could visually represent up to four objects (containing either one or multiple features) in short-term memory. Hoffman and Landau (2007) showed children and adults with WS (mean ages 11;8 and 24;0, respectively) briefly presented displays of one, three, or six objects (colored squares in the Color condition, and oriented lines in the Orientation condition). The first display appeared for 500 msec, followed 900 msec later by a second display shown for 500 msec, in which the entire display was identical to the first (Same condition) or changed just one object/feature combination—either the color of one of the squares or the orientation of one of the lines. Luck and Vogel had argued that detecting the identity or difference between such pairs of displays would require representing all of the objects in the display, and thus could provide a test of the number of objects one could represent in short-term memory at once. For normal adults, Luck and Vogel argued that this number is four—the same number as estimated by

Pylyshyn and colleagues for multiple object tracking, and the same number as most people report being the upper bound of the subitizing range (see Cowan, 2000, for review and theoretical discussion).

In our task, people with WS performed above chance on displays of one and three in the Color condition, but did so only for displays of one in the Orientation condition, suggesting a substantial difference between their capacity to detect color versus orientation changes. This is consistent with other difficulties observed in representing orientation (see, e.g., Dilks et al., 2008; also see Dilks, Reiss, Hoffman, & Landau, 2004). The crucial contrast, however, was between people with WS and MA matches (mean ages 15;4 and 6;8, respectively). In both conditions, normally developing children performed above chance for larger displays than did those with WS. In the Color condition, normal children performed above chance for one, three, or six squares; in the Orientation condition, they performed above chance for one or three lines. Thus, the people with WS again showed a deficit in the number of items they could accurately represent, relative to normally developing MA matches. The difference between color and orientation further suggests that some features are more difficult to represent, and suggests that the number of objects one can hold may depend to some extent on the objects' features.

The pattern of results across three very different types of tasks—multiple object tracking, subitizing, and detection of changes in an object set—is consistent in suggesting that people with WS have an unusually small capacity to process multiple objects. Although we are still far from a complete explanation, these results strongly suggest that a signature of the spatial deficit in WS is a range of abnormalities in spatial functions that engage parietal areas.

Spatial Representation, Brain Structure, and Developmental Timing: Review and a Speculative Hypothesis

The principal hypothesis discussed in this chapter is that the spatial profile of people with WS is uneven, with relative strength in functions that are normally carried by the ventral stream of the brain, and severe weakness or breakdown in functions that are normally carried by the dorsal stream of the brain, especially the parietal lobe. This division of labor—often described as "what" versus "where" or "how"—has been widely discussed within the literature on adult representation and brain function, and increasingly greater numbers of scientists are considering the

relative contributions to spatial cognition in early development. For example, several researchers have suggested that differences between the two streams of processing may be functionally important for development, and that the two streams may develop at different rates (Johnson, 2004; Neville & Bavelier, 2000). Given the uneven WS spatial profile, two questions naturally arise: First, is the uneven spatial profile in WS reflected in uneven activity of the different streams of the brain? Second, do differences in the relative time tables for normal development of the two streams play a role in producing the observed uneven profile in WS?

Studies of brain morphology and functioning are relatively recent and still incomplete; still, the profile is consistent with areas of relative sparing and other areas of abnormality (see Meyer-Lindenberg, Mervis, & Berman, 2006, for an excellent review). For example, several studies (some based on postmortem examination) report a range of structural abnormalities in the WS brain, including overall reduction in size, abnormalities of the corpus callosum, and abnormalities in cell size and packing in the primary visual cortex (Jernigan & Bellugi, 1990; Galaburda, Holinger, Bellugi, & Sherman, 2002; Mercuri et al., 1997). Evidence from structural magnetic resonance imagining (MRI) studies indicates reductions in both occipital and parietal areas (Eckert et al., 2005). Surface-based analyses of MRI data further indicate abnormalities in the depth of many sulci in the brains of people with WS (Van Essen et al., 2006). This set of structural abnormalities could play a role in functional abnormalities. But, to test such a link to cognition, we need studies in which people with WS are asked to carry out cognitive tasks while their brain activity is being observed.

Several such studies have revealed that the region of the intraparietal sulcus (IPS) may be crucially involved in the signature visual–construction deficit of people with WS. Meyer-Lindenberg et al. (2004) carried out a functional MRI (fMRI) study in which people with WS who had normal IQs passively viewed pictures such as houses and faces, identified such pictures, and matched relatively complex shapes to a standard. None of these tasks revealed different activation patterns compared to normal CA-matched controls. However, they did show abnormalities in two other types of tasks. One task required that people attend to the spatial location of house or face pictures (compared to a condition in which identity was attended). Another required that they determine whether the combination of two shapes could yield a third—an analogue of the block construction task. In these tasks, there was hypoactivation near the area of the IPS, compared to controls. Meyer-Lindenberg et al. suggested that the abnormalities in this area (the same location of decreased gray matter and sulcal depth found by others, e.g., Kippenhan et al., 2005) could create a "roadblock" in processing from earlier areas (inferior and posterior) to later areas (superior anterior). Other studies have shown normal retinotopic mapping (Olsen et al., 2009), consistent with the idea that earlier visual processing may be relatively normal. For example, people with WS perceive visual illusions to the same extent as do normal individuals (Palomares et al., 2006). And although people with WS have been reported to have higher than average levels of strabismus and difficulties with depth perception, these problems are not correlated with the signature visual–construction deficit (Atkinson et al., 2003). All this is consistent with the idea that the site of the primary deficit is in dorsal and parietal regions that are significantly involved in spatial representational mechanisms such as attentional modulation, coordination of frames of reference, and visual–motor control.

The mechanisms by which the WS brain arrives at these abnormalities is still unknown, but Meyer-Lindenberg et al. (2006) speculate that timing during early development may play a major role. They note that there are regional variations in volume and cortical thickness (Thompson et al., 2005), consistent with the hypothesis that developmental timing plays a role in cortical folding (Rakic, 2004). Meyer-Lindenberg suggests that the gray matter reductions in the area of the IPS could also lead to reductions in white matter, thus leading to abnormal connectivity.

Let us now turn to the idea that the normal developmental time table might also play a major role in the emergence of the signature spatial profile of people with WS. Inspection of timing profiles may provide an important framework for understanding unusual development—as is found in WS—as well as normal development. Indeed, Landau and Hoffman (2007) have argued that it is impossible to evaluate the timing profile for unusual populations without knowing what the typical developmental profile looks like. For example, different streams of processing may undergo different developmental time courses, *relative* to each other in *normal* development. It is possible, for example, that ventral stream functions become mature before dorsal stream functions (Neville & Bavelier, 2000).

If one stream of processing lags further behind the other in abnormal development, then we might see an uneven profile of spatial functions that exaggerates the profile seen in normal development. Indeed, Landau and Hoffman (2007) speculated that the profile of peaks and valleys in WS spatial representation may reflect an exaggeration of a *normal* asymmetry in the rate of development of the two streams, combined with early developmental arrest.

One of the most persistent puzzles about WS is the profile of peaks and valleys—both across aspects of spatial representation and across different knowledge domains. The earliest and most compelling description of WS still holds: People with WS have surprisingly strong language, both in an absolute and relative sense. In an absolute sense, people with WS can make accurate judgments about the grammaticality of complex sentences (Bellugi et al., 1988), and they can produce very complex sentences, such as those with both object and subject-relative clauses (Zukowski, 2001). These structures are very complex, and highly internally constrained; accurate production by people whose average overall IQ is 70 is surprising to even the strongest skeptic. Language is clearly a relative strength in WS.

But another sense of "relative" strength is also important. How does the language profile of people with WS compare to that of a normally developing child? Are complex structures such as object-relatives typically produced at age 4? At age 7? At age 18? Depending on the answer, we may have a very different picture of the developmental mechanisms at work.

The profile for spatial representations requires a similar analysis. There is no question that strengths and weaknesses are present. Block construction and other spatial tasks are clear weaknesses; even adults with WS perform like normal 4-year-old children. As I have discussed, they also perform like 4-year-olds in a range of other tasks, including multiple object tracking, visual–manual action, subitizing, and perhaps in other tasks that we are currently examining (e.g., coordination of reference frames, modulation of attention). These tasks—as a class—typically engage the dorsal stream and parietal areas of the brain, areas that are known to have significant structural and functional abnormalities. At the same time, there is significant strength in other sets of spatial tasks, including identifying objects in canonical perspectives, perceiving biological motion and motion coherence, and spatial language. Many of these fall into the general set of tasks that engage more ventral areas, consistent with the hypothesis that ventral stream functions tend to be strong.

But how does this profile of peaks and valleys look when it is compared to a normal developmental profile? We have speculated that the unusual spatial profile seen in WS is a consequence of two effects (Landau & Hoffman, 2007). First, as I've argued, the tasks we have used in our lab likely map onto two different systems or pathways in the brain, with the ventral stream developing early and the dorsal stream having a more protracted course of development. This predicts that younger normal children will show an imbalance in which cognitive functions that depend on the ventral stream may be stronger than those that depend on the dorsal stream. Older children will have a more balanced set of abilities as both systems approach maturity.

The second effect is particular to WS. We speculate that people with WS undergo very slow development of both streams, and that there is premature developmental arrest at the functional level of a normally developing 4-year-old child. This arrest could take place because of the early onset of puberty (Partsch et al., 1999), which might create changes in the efficiency of biological learning mechanisms. Such prolonged growth followed by functional arrest would result in the spatial imbalance characteristic of a 4-year-old: good performance in ventral stream tasks, with relative weakness in tasks that depend on the immature dorsal system. Of course, this pattern occurs for WS in a much older child, or an adult, and this will present as a seriously abnormal imbalance.

The basis for this speculation is the overall profile of strengths and fragility across the different aspects of spatial representation we have examined. People with WS perform *worse* than MA matches (roughly 6-year-olds) on tasks such as block construction and drawing (Georgopoulos et al., 2004; Hoffman et al., 2003), coordination of reference frames (Landau & Hoffman, 2005), multiple object tracking (O'Hearn et al., 2005), and visual–manual action ("posting," Dilks et al., 2008). At the same time, the overall performance and detailed internal structure of WS performance on these tasks is quite similar to that of 4-year-old, normally developing children. This suggests that the people with WS we have tested (usually age 10 and older) have reached the functional level of a normal 4-year-old for these tasks.

In contrast, people with WS perform at the same level or better than normally developing, MA-matched children in tasks tapping perception of biological motion and motion coherence (Reiss et al., 2005), object recognition under canonical or unusual views (Landau et al., 2006), and spatial language (Lakusta & Landau, 2005). Perceptual matching of orientation is almost equivalent to MA matches, even though visual–manual action using the same stimuli is much worse (Dilks et al., 2004; Dilks, Hoffman, & Landau, 2008). Our hypothesis predicts that those capacities that are relatively strong in WS should also emerge quite early in the normally developing child, whereas those that are severely impaired should develop later.

At present, the evidence is consistent with this story. For example, the crucial syntactic and semantic properties of spatial language for motion events are normally mastered by age 4, and shows strength in people with WS. Tasks requiring simple perceptual matching of two oriented lines elicit strong performance by normal 4-year-olds, and there is little development between ages 4 and 6. People with WS perform about like both 4- and 6-year-olds, showing strength, especially in comparison to parallel tasks requiring visual–manual action (Dilks et al., 2008).

These cases can be contrasted with spatial capacities that normally undergo more prolonged development. One example is object identification from unusual perspectives. Normal children show substantial development between ages 6 and 12, according to our data (Landau et al., 2006). People with WS show performance no different from 6-year-olds (also their MA matches), but worse performance than 12-year-olds. This ability clearly undergoes prolonged development in normal children, and WS individuals do not ever seem to reach the same level as normal 12-year-olds. Ongoing work in our lab suggests that there is little to no developmental change between age 4 and 6 in normally developing children's ability to identify objects presented from unusual perspectives. Therefore, the overall normal developmental profile suggests some capacity by age 4, which is roughly the same by age 6, and only develops to an adult level at age 12 or later. People with WS appear to hit the functional level of a 4- or 6-year-old normal child, but do not grow further.

Landau and Hoffman (2007) have idealized these different views of the unusual timing profile in two different ways, as illustrated in Figure 5.11. Both possibilities assume that there are normally different developmental trajectories—or rates of development—for each of the two streams of visual–spatial processing, dorsal and ventral (consistent with the view of Neville & Bavelier (2000). Figure 5.11A idealizes the situation in which relative shapes of the two trajectories (dorsal and ventral streams) are the same for WS people and normal children, but with an overall slower rate of development for

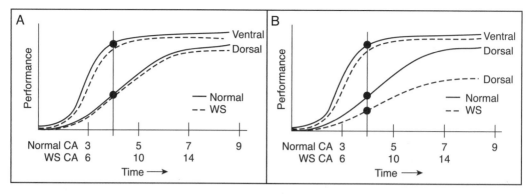

Fig. 5.11 Two hypothetical developmental trajectories for the dorsal and ventral streams in normal development and development of people with Williams syndrome (WS). Panel A shows the results of overall slowing of the dorsal stream in both groups, to an equivalent degree. Panel B shows different rates of development, with slower normal development of the dorsal stream, and exaggerated slowing of development in people with WS. In both panels, the vertical bar indicates the hypothetical result of developmental arrest.

WS people relative to normal children. In this scheme, the differences between the rates of development for the two streams are roughly equal, despite the overall slowing of development in the case of WS. For sake of argument, the WS rate is shown as half the rate (twice as slow) as normally developing children. This is shown by the difference in CAs for the two groups along the x-axis.[1] If we combine this profile with early arrest (due to puberty, perhaps), we would place the profile of the person with WS at roughly the level of a 4-year-old normally developing child (shown as the vertical line in the figure). Thus, people with WS might develop until they reach the functional level of a normal 4-year-old child, and then slow down or stop completely. Their profile would look like that of a normal 4-year-old but it would, of course, look very unusual in a 12- or 20-year-old person.

Figure 5.11B idealizes a different picture of timing, in which the relative shapes of the trajectories for the two streams are different for normally developing children than for people with WS. In this scheme, the dorsal stream in WS undergoes development that is even slower than that of the ventral stream, increasing the difference in early developmental profile between functions of the two streams. This situation would lead to an even greater lag in dorsal stream functions (relative to ventral functions) for people with WS, compared to normally developing people. Even if there were no arrest at the functional level of a 4-year-old, the dorsal stream functions would never reach normal levels, resulting in permanent developmental deficits in these functions.

These figures are obviously simplifications. For example, detection of coherent motion and perception

of biological motion are both, at least partly, dorsal stream functions but ones that develop early. Generally, early developing systems are ones that appear to be primarily "bottom-up" or automatic and consist of dedicated computational and neural machinery of great complexity, designed to carry out specific cognitive tasks given the right input (e.g., object recognition from canonical perspectives, language acquisition, etc.). People with WS perform at the level of MA matches or better on these tasks (we have yet to determine whether 4-year-old, normally developing children also perform at these levels). In contrast, tasks that are not likely to be carried out by such dedicated neural machinery, such as recognizing objects from unusual perspectives, appear to call on dorsal stream activation, particularly various areas of the parietal lobe. Landau and Hoffman (2007) speculated that tasks having a protracted course of development are those that require flexibility and control, and therefore require attention that can be flexibly modulated. This includes attentive multiple object tracking, visual–manual action requiring some precision (such as the posting task), and object recognition from unusual perspectives.

In this view, some apparent exceptions to the rule make sense. For example, despite overall strength in spatial language, people with WS have difficulty encoding direction in spatial terms (e.g., above–below, right–left). This is an area of spatial language that develops at around age 6 or 7 in normal children, and we have found that even WS adults still make systematic confusion errors between right and left (Landau & Hoffman, 2005). Although this is a language task (hence a putative ventral stream function), talking about left and right requires that a person accurately represent directional differences along an axis (the horizontal for left–right). Such differences are also involved in recognition of mirror-image differences. There is evidence that discrimination between mirror-image versions of objects depends on parietal areas. For example, damage to these areas in human adults leads to difficulties distinguishing mirror-image objects from each other (Priftis, Rusconi, Umilta, & Zorzi, 2003; Warrington & Taylor, 1973). Not surprisingly, people with WS are also impaired (relative to MA matches) at matching under brief delay in the context of mirror-image objects (Hoffman & Landau, 2006).

In sum, we speculate that normal differences in the time of emergence for different aspects of spatial representation can shed light on the WS spatial impairment. *Early emerging* spatial capacities seem to draw on primarily ventral functions, and these capacities would be important for tasks such as object recognition from canonical viewpoints, biological motion, and much of spatial language. Those capacities that appear to have a *more protracted developmental course* are likely to be the province of the dorsal stream, particularly parietal areas. These capacities underlie tasks such as multiple object tracking, visual–manual action, and object recognition from unusual perspectives.

Conclusion

Cases of genetic and developmental deficit have traditionally offered scientists the opportunity to understand how aspects of innate endowment and environmental experience can affect the development of cognitive capacity. In this chapter, I have used the case of WS to probe the nature of spatial representation, emphasizing the need to understand both strengths and deficits in this population, and to integrate this with an understanding of how normal development proceeds. The results of our studies have revealed that several major principles of normal development of spatial representations can help us understand the unusual developmental profile of people with WS and can also shed light on the processes of normal development, its structure and trajectories. These principles—specialization of function, constraint within spatial representational systems, and the importance of developmental timing—emphasize the remarkably resilient nature of human spatial representation and remind us that even in cases of genetic deficit, many aspects of normal spatial representation remain present. At the same time, the severe deficits observed in hallmark tasks—such as visual spatial construction and drawing—remind us that such tasks are a complex product of many different types of spatial representation, cobbled together for the unique purposes to which humans can apply their spatial knowledge. It appears to be these special products that are especially susceptible to impairment in people with WS, thus reminding us that genetic deficits are unlikely to have simple and direct effects on systems of human cognition, including those of space.

Note

1. By depicting development in terms of chronological age, I am assuming that we can draw meaningful conclusions by using normal developmental trajectories as a kind of measuring stick against which we can determine where people with WS lie along the developmental trajectory. Using this, we can also make predictions about where people with WS should fall relative to CA matches (compare the performance of a person with WS with that of a CA on the curve) or MA matches (take the chronological age of the MA match and find that person on the curve.) The point is that the WS profile can be meaningfully interpreted relative to a normal developmental curve, without using MA matching at all.

References

Andersen, R. A., & Zipser, D. (1988). The role of the posterior parietal cortex in coordinate transformations for visual-motor integration. *Canadian Journal of Physiology and Pharmacology, 66*, 488–501.

Atkinson, J., King, J., Braddick, O., Nokes, L., Anker, S., & Braddick, F. (1997). A specific deficit of dorsal stream function in William's syndrome. *Neuroreport: An International Journal for the Rapid Communication of Research in Neuroscience, 8*, 1919–1922.

Atkinson, J., Braddick, O., Anker, S., Curran, W., Andrew, R., Wattam-Bell, J., & Braddick, F. (2003). Neurobiological models of visuospatial cognition in children with Williams syndrome: Measures of dorsal-stream and frontal function. *Developmental Neuropsychology, 23*, 139–172.

Averbeck, B. B., Chafee, M. V., Crowe, D. A., & Georgopoulos, A. P. (2003). Neural activity in prefrontal cortex during copying geometrical shapes. *Experimental Brain Research, 150*, 142–153.

Ballard, D. H., Hayhoe, M. M., Pook, P. K., & Rao, R. P. N. (1997). Deictic codes for the embodiment of cognition. *Behavioral & Brain Sciences, 20*, 723–767.

Beery, K. E., & Bukrenica, N. A. (1967). *The Beery-Buktenica Developmental Test of Visual-Motor Integration.* Chicago: Follett Publishing.

Bellugi, U., Sabo, H., & Vaid, J. (1988). Spatial deficits in children with Williams syndrome. In J. Stiles-Davis, M. Kritchevsky, & U. Bellugi (Eds.), *Spatial cognition, brain bases, and development* (pp. 273–298). Hillsdale, NJ: Lawrence Erlbaum.

Bertrand, J., Mervis, C. B., & Eisenberg, J. D. (1997). Drawing by children with Williams syndrome: A developmental perspective. *Developmental Neuropsychology, 13*, 41–67.

Bihrle, A. M., Bellugi, U., Delis, D. C., & Marks, S. (1989). Seeing either the forest or the trees: Dissociation in visuospatial processing. *Brain & Cognition, 11*, 37–49.

Brown, J. H., Johnson, M. H., Paterson, S. J., Gilmore, R., Longhi, E., & Karmiloff-Smith, A. (2003). Spatial representation and attention in toddlers with Williams syndrome and Down syndrome. *Neuropsychologia, 41*, 1037–1046.

Burack, J. A., Russo, N., Flores, H., Iarocci, G., & Zigler, E. (2011). The more you know the less you know, but that's OK: Developments in the developmental approach to intellectual disability. In J. A. Burack, R. M. Hodapp, G. Iarocci, & E. Zigler (Eds.), *The Oxford handbook of intellectual disability and development*, 2nd ed. New York: Oxford University Press.

Chafee, M. V., Crowe, D. A., Averbeck, B. B., & Georgopoulos, A. P. (2005). Neural correlates of spatial judgment during object construction in parietal cortex. *Cerebral Cortex, 15*, 1393–1413.

Colby, C. L., & Goldberg, M. E. (1999). Space and attention in parietal cortex. *Annual Review of Neuroscience, 22*, 319–349.

Cowan, N. (2000). The magical number 4 in short-term memory: A reconsideration of mental storage capacity. *Behavioral and Brain Sciences, 24*, 87–185.

Cowey, A., & Vaina, L. M. (2000). Blindness to form from motion despite intact static form perception and motion detection. *Neuropsychologia, 38*, 566–578.

Culham, J. C., Brandt, S. A., Cavanagh, P., Kanwisher, N. G., Dale, A. M., & Tootell, R. B. H. (1998). Cortical fMRI activation produced by attentive tracking of moving targets. *Journal of Neurophysiology, 80*, 2657–2670.

Dehaene, S., Piazza, M., Pinel, P., & Cohen, L. (2003). Three parietal circuits for number processing. *Cognitive Neuropsychology, 20*, 487–506.

Deruelle, C., Mancini, J., Livet, M. O., Casse-Perrot, C., & de Schonen, S. (1999). Configural and local processing of faces in children with Williams syndrome. *Brain and Cognition, 41*, 276–298.

Dilks, D., Hoffman, J. E., & Landau, B. (2008) Vision for perception and vision for action: Normal and unusual development. *Developmental Science, 11*(4), 474–486.

Dilks, D., Reiss, J., Hoffman, J. E., & Landau, B. (2004, November). *Representation of orientation in Williams syndrome.* Paper presented at the Annual Meeting of the Psychonomics Society, Minneapolis, MN.

Eckert, M. A., Hu, D., Eliez, S., Bellugi, U., Galaburda, A., Korenberg, J., et al. (2005). Evidence for superior parietal impairment in Williams syndrome. *Neurology, 64*, 152–153.

Elliott, C. D. (1990). *Differential ability scales.* San Diego: Harcourt Brace Jovanovich.

Farran, E. K., Jarrold, C., & Gathercole, S. E. (2003). Divided attention, selective attention and drawing: Processing preferences in Williams syndrome are dependent on the task administered. *Neuropsychologia, 41*, 676–687.

Galaburda, A. M., Holinger, D. P., Bellugi, U., & Sherman, G. F. (2002). Williams syndrome: Neurological size and neuronal-packing density in primary visual cortex. *Archives of Neurology, 59*, 1461–1467.

Gallistel, C. R. (1990). *The organization of learning.* Cambridge, MA: MIT Press.

Georgopoulos, M. A., Georgopoulos, A. P., Kurz, N., & Landau, B. (2004). Figure copying in Williams syndrome and normal subjects. *Experimental Brain Research, 157*, 137–146.

Gogtay, N., Giedd, J. N., Lusk, L., Hayashi, K. M., Greenstein, D., Vaituzis, A. C., et al. (2004). Dynamic mapping of human cortical development during childhood through early adulthood. *Proceedings of the National Academy of Sciences of United States of America, 101*, 8174–8179.

Grant, J., Valian, V., & Karmiloff-Smith, A. (2002). A study of relative clauses in Williams syndrome. *Journal of Child Language, 29*, 403–416.

Grill-Spector, K., & Kanwisher, N. (2005). Visual recognition: As soon as you know it is there, you know what it is. *Psychological Science, 16*, 152–160.

Hoffman, J. E., Landau, B., & Pagani, B. (2003). Spatial breakdown in spatial construction: Evidence from eye fixations in children with Williams syndrome. *Cognitive Psychology, 46*, 260–301.

Hoffman, J. E., & Landau, B. (2006). *Can people with Williams syndrome perceive the spatial arrangement of visual parts?* Paper presented at the 3rd annual Williams syndrome workshop, Reading, England.

Hoffman, J. E., & Landau, B. (2007). *An unusually small limit on the number of objects that can be simultaneously represented: Evidence from people with Williams syndrome.* In preparation.

Huttenlocher, P. (2002). *Neural plasticity: The effects of environment on the development of the cerebral cortex.* Cambridge, MA: Harvard University Press.

Jackendoff, R. (1983). *Semantics and cognition.* Cambridge, MA: The MIT Press.

Jernigan, T. L., & Bellugi, U. (1990). Anomalous brain morphology on magnetic resonance images in Williams syndrome and Down syndrome. *Archives of Neurology, 47*, 529–533.

Johansson, G. (1973). Visual perception of biological motion and a model for its analysis. *Perception and Psychophysics, 14*, 201–211.

Johnson, M. (2004). *Developmental cognitive neuroscience.* London: Blackwell.

Jordan, H., Reiss, J. E., Hoffman, J. E., & Landau, B. (2002). Intact perception of biological motion in the face of profound spatial deficits: Williams syndrome. *Psychological Science, 13*, 162–167.

Kanwisher, N., McDermott, J., & Chun, M. M. (1997). The fusiform face area: A module in human extrastriate cortex specialized for face perception. *Journal of Neuroscience, 17*, 4302–4311.

Key, A. F., Pani, J. R., & Mervis, C. B. (1998). *Visuospatial constructive ability of people with Williams Syndrome.* Paper presented at the Sixth Annual Workshop on Object Perception and Memory, Dallas, TX.

Kippenhan, J. S., Olsen, R. K., Mervis, C. B., Morris, C. A., Kohn, P., Meyer-Lindenberg, A., & Berman, K. F. (2005). Genetic contributions to human gyrification: Sulcal morphometry in Williams syndrome. *Journal of Neuroscience, 25*, 7840–7846.

Lakusta, L., & Landau, B. (2005). Starting at the end: The importance of goals in spatial language. *Cognition, 96*, 1–33.

Lakusta, L., Wagner, L., O'Hearn, K., & Landau, B. (2007). Conceptual foundations of spatial language: Evidence for a goal bias in infants. *Language Learning and Development, 3*(3), 179–197.

Landau, B., & Hoffman, J. E. (2005). Parallels between spatial cognition and spatial language: Evidence from Williams syndrome. *Journal of Memory & Language, 53*, 163–185.

Landau, B., & Hoffman, J. E. (2007). Explaining selective spatial breakdown in Williams syndrome: Four principles of normal spatial development and why they matter. In J. Plumert, & J. Spencer (Eds.), *The emerging spatial mind.* Oxford: Oxford University Press.

Landau, B., Hoffman, J. E., & Kurz, N. (2006). Object recognition with severe spatial deficits in Williams syndrome: Sparing and breakdown. *Cognition, 100*, 483–510.

Landau, B., & Zukowski, A. (2003). Objects, motions, and paths: Spatial language in children with Williams syndrome. In C. Mervis (Ed.), *Developmental Neuropsychology: Special Issue on Williams Syndrome, 23*, 105–137.

Luck, S. J., & Vogel, E. K. (1997). The capacity of visual working memory for features and conjunctions. *Nature, 390*, 279–281.

Maunsell, J. H., & van Essen, D. C. (1983). The connections of the middle temporal visual area (MT) and their relationship to a cortical hierarchy in the macaque monkey. *Journal of Neuroscience, 3*, 2563–2586.

Mendes, M., Silva, F., Simoes, L., Jorge, M., Saraiva, J., & Castelo-Branco, M. (2005). Visual magnocellular and structure from motion perceptual deficits in a neurodevelopmental model of dorsal stream function. *Cognitive Brain Research, 25*, 788–798.

Mercuri, E., Atkinshon, J., Braddick, O., Rutherford, M., Cowan, F., Countrell, S., et al. (1997). Chiari I malformation and white matter changes in asymptomatic young children with Williams syndrome: Clinical and MRI study. *European Journal of Paediatric Neurology, 5*, 177–181.

Mervis, C. B., & Klein-Tasman, B. P. (2004). Methodological issues in group-matching designs: Alpha levels for control variable comparisons and measurement characteristics of control and target variables. *Journal of Autism and Developmental Disorders, 34*(1), 7–17.

Mervis, C. B., Robinson, B. F., Bertrand, J., Morris, C. A., Klein-Tasman, B. P., & Armstrong, S. C. (2000). The Williams syndrome cognitive profile. *Brain and Cognition, 44*, 604–628.

Meyer-Lindenberg, A., Kohn, P., Mervis, C., Kippenhan, J., Olsen, R., Morris, C., & Berman, K. (2004). Neural basis of genetically determined visuospatial construction deficit in Williams syndrome. *Neuron, 43*, 623–631.

Meyer-Lindenberg, A., Mervis, C. B., & Berman, K. F. (2006). Neural mechanisms in Williams syndrome: A unique window to genetic influences on cognition and behaviour. *Nature Reviews Neuroscience, 7*, 380–393.

Milner, A. D., & Goodale, M. A. (1995). *The visual brain in action*. New York: Oxford University Press.

Musolino, J., Chunyo, G., & Landau, B. (2010) Uncovering knowledge of core syntactic and semantic principles in individuals with Williams Syndrome. *Language learning and Development, 6*, 126–161.

Nakamura, M., Kaneoke, Y., Watanabe, K., & Kakigi, R. (2002). Visual information process in Williams syndrome: Intact motion detection accompanied by typical visuospatial dysfunctions. *European Journal of Neuroscience, 16*, 1810–1818.

Neville, H., & Bavelier, D. (2000). Specificity and plasticity in neurocognitive development in humans. In M. S. Gazzaniga (Ed.), *The cognitive neurosciences* (2nd ed., pp. 83–98). Cambridge, MA: MIT Press.

Newcombe, N., & Huttenlocher, J. (2000). *Making space: The development of spatial representation and reasoning*. Cambridge, MA: MIT Press.

O'Hearn, K., Landau, B., & Hoffman, J. E. (2005). Multiple object tracking in normally developing children and people with Williams syndrome. *Psychological Science, 16*, 905–9 PMCID: PMC2700022.

O'Hearn, K., Hoffman, J., & Landau, B. (2011) Small subitizing range in people with Williams syndrome. *Visual Cognition*, in press.

Olsen, R. K., Kippenhan, J. S., Japee, S., Kohn, P., Mervis, C. B., Saad, Z. S., Morris, C. A., Meyer-Lindenberg, A., & Berman,

K. F. (2009). Retinotopically defined primary visual cortex in Williams syndrome. *Brain, 132*(3), 635.

Palmieri, T. J., & Gauthier, I. (2004). Visual object understanding. *Nature Reviews: Neuroscience, 5*, 291–303.

Palomares, M., Ogbonna, C., Landau, B. & Egeth, H. (2009) Normal susceptibility to visual illusions in abnormal development: evidence from Williams Syndrome. *Perception, 38*(2), 186–199. PMCID: PMC2745710.

Palomares, M. (2006). *Normal and abnormal development of visuospatial integration: A perspective from Williams syndrome*. Ph.D. dissertation, Johns Hopkins University.

Pani, J. R., Mervis, C. B., & Robinson, B. F. (1999). Global spatial organization by individuals with Williams syndrome. *Psychological Science, 10*, 453–458.

Partsch, C. J., Dreyer, G., Goesch, A., Winter, M., Schneppenheim, R., Wessel, A., & Pankau, R. (1999). Longitudinal evaluation of growth, puberty, and bone maturation in children with Williams syndrome. *Journal of Pediatrics, 134*, 82–89.

Pinker, S. (1994). *The language instinct*. New York: William Morrow & Co.

Priftis, K., Rusconi, E., Umilta, C., & Zorzi, M. (2003). Pure agnosia for mirror stimuli after right inferior parietal lesion. *Brain, 126*, 908–919.

Pylyshyn, Z. W. (2000). Situating vision in the world. *Trends in Cognitive Science, 4*, 197–207.

Pylyshyn, Z. W. (2003). *Seeing and visualizing: It's not what you think*. Cambridge, MA: MIT Press.

Pylyshyn, Z. W., & Storm, R. W. (1988). Tracking multiple independent targets: Evidence for a parallel tracking mechanism. *Spatial Vision, 3*, 179–197.

Rakic, P. (2004). Genetic control of cortical convolutions. *Science, 303*, 1983–1984.

Reiss, J., Hoffman, J. E., & Landau, B. (2005). Motion processing specialization in Williams syndrome. *Vision Research, 45*, 3379–3390.

Scholl, B., & Pylyshyn, Z. (1999). Tracking multiple objects through occlusion: Clues to visual objecthood. *Cognitive Psychology, 38*, 259–290.

Talmy, L. (1978). Lexicalization patterns: Semantic structure in lexical forms. In T. Shopen, et al. (Eds.), *Language typology and syntactic description* (Vol. 3). New York: Cambridge University Press.

Talmy, L. (1983). How language structures space. In H. Pick, & L. Acredolo (Eds.), *Spatial orientation: Theory, research, and application*. New York: Plenum Press.

Tager-Flusberg, H., Plesa-Skwerer, D., Faja, S., & Joseph, R. M. (2003). People with Williams syndrome process faces holistically. *Cognition, 89*, 11–24.

Thompson, P. M., Lee, A. D., Dutton, R. A., Geaga, J. A., Hayashi, K. M., Eckert, M. A., et al. (2005). Abnormal cortical complexity and thickness profiles mapped in Williams syndrome. *The Journal of Neuroscience, 25*, 4146–4158.

Ungerleider, L. G., & Mishkin, M. (1982). Two cortical visual systems. In D. Ingle, M. Goodale, & R. Mansfield (Eds.), *Analysis of visual behavior*. Cambridge, MA: MIT Press.

Vaina, L. M., Lemay, M., Bienfang, D. C., Choi, A. Y., & Nakayama, K. (1990). Intact "biological motion" and "structure from motion" perception in a patient with impaired motion mechanisms: A case study. *Visual Neuroscience, 5*, 353–369.

Van Essen, D. C., Dierker, D., Snyder, A. Z., Raichle, M. E., Reiss, A. L., & Korenberg, J. (2006). Symmetry of cortical folding abnormalities in Williams syndrome revealed by surface-based analyses. *The Journal of Neuroscience, 26,* 5470–5483.

Wang, P. P., Doherty, S., Rourke, S. B., & Bellugi, U. (1995). Unique profile of visuo-perceptual skills in a genetic syndrome. *Brain & Cognition, 29,* 54–65.

Warrington, E. K., & Taylor, A. M. (1973). The contribution of the right parietal lobe to object recognition. *Cortex, 9,* 152–164.

Wechsler, D. (1981). *WAIS-R Manual: Wechsler Adult Intelligence Scale-Revised.* New York: Harcourt Brace Jovanovich, Inc. (The Psychological Corporation).

Zukowski, A. (2001). *Uncovering grammatical competence in children with Williams syndrome.* Dissertation thesis. Boston University, Boston, MA.

Zigler, E. (1967) Familial mental retardation: A continuing dilemma. *Science, 155,* 292–298.

Understanding the Development of Attention in Persons with Intellectual Disability: Challenging the Myths

Grace Iarocci, Mafalda Porporino, James T. Enns, *and* Jacob A. Burack

Abstract

This chapter focuses on the attentional abilities of the persons with specific etiologies. It begins with an extensive review of the literature on attention in persons with the most common organic forms of intellectual disability. It then summarizes the results of a survey of studies on attention in Down syndrome, fragile X, and Williams syndrome, and discusses the implications of these findings for future research in the area. The chapter proposes to apply a framework for understanding developmental change and stability in selective attention, a framework that initially emerged in the course of understanding the role of attention in automobile driving and was later applied to the development of attention over the typical human lifespan.

Keywords: Attention, attentional disability, intellectual disability, Down syndrome, fragile X syndrome, Williams syndrome

In the previous *Handbook of Mental Retardation and Development*, we challenged the "mysterious myth of attention deficit," and showed that the popular notion that persons with mental retardation (which we now refer to as intellectual disability, or ID) have a generalized attention deficit is not supported by the empirical evidence (Iarocci & Burack, 1998; also, see Burack, Evans, Klaiman, & Iarocci, 2001). Our conclusion was based on an assessment of the literature in terms of specific methodological variables related to the developmental approach to ID, including matching the various groups on meaningful measures of developmental functioning and differentiating among etiological subgroups of ID. Within these developmental guidelines, we highlighted two primary findings in the literature on attentional functioning among persons with ID. One, was that claims of deficits were most commonly found when the groups with and without ID were matched on chronological age (CA), and as persons with ID are by definition lower functioning than their CA-matched, typically developing peers, findings of impaired performance would be expected

on virtually every aspect of functioning, including attention. However, when groups were matched by mental age (MA), or some relevant measure of more general developmental level, the percentage of findings of impaired performance dropped considerably. The second finding was that the few examples of attentional deficit were found among persons with ID associated with a specific organic deficit, rather than among persons with familial ID, those apparently with no organic etiology who seem to simply reflect the lower end of the normal distribution of intellectual functioning. Thus, any attention deficits seem to be associated with organicity rather than low IQ, or ID, per se.

In this chapter, we extend our previous review and focus on the attentional abilities of those persons with specific etiologies, as studies of persons with specific types of organic forms of ID (e.g., Down syndrome [DS], Williams syndrome [WS], and fragile X syndrome [FXS]) may show deficits of attention relative to their general MA level. The attentional profiles of individuals with specific syndromes may be compared to provide insight into the underlying etiology and its impact on the cognitive development of these individuals. We begin with an extensive review of the literature on attention in persons with the most common organic forms of ID. We then summarize the results of a survey of studies on attention in DS, WS, and FXS, and discuss the implications of these findings for future research in the area. We propose to apply a framework for understanding developmental change and stability in selective attention, a framework that initially emerged in the course of understanding the role of attention in automobile driving (Trick, Enns, Mills, & Vavrik, 2004) and was later applied to the development of attention over the typical human lifespan (Enns & Trick, 2006). The main strength of this framework is that it differentiates the nature of the processes involved during a task (i.e., the level of effort needed to complete the task) from the origin of the underlying processes (i.e., whether the task involves innate or learned mechanisms). Attention, within this elaborated framework, is conceptualized as multifaceted, with some aspects remaining stable over the life course, while other aspects change with development. This is particularly useful in the study of different populations of persons with specific syndromes who may show atypical development of subcomponents of attention over time. Potentially unique attentional profiles may be identified with each of the specific syndromes.

A Conceptual Framework for Attention

The term *attention* has a popular connotation and is frequently used in common parlance to refer to a variety of activities. For example, a frequent directive to children in many situations is to "pay attention." However, when we consider the construct of attention from a scientific perspective, we begin to understand the complexity that underlies this colloquial statement. The construct of attention is thought to encompass a variety of functions, is used in a variety of contexts, and refers to several different processes. It includes the abilities to focus on relevant information while ignoring irrelevant sources, to search for new information, to compare and contrast dimensions of a visual image, to flexibly shift cognitive strategies to meet new task demands, to maintain focus on a task, and to physiologically facilitate the intake of information from the environment. Although each represents a different aspect of attention that requires the engagement of distinct mechanisms, the individual components commonly work together in a seamless and coordinated way to successfully contribute to the overall

processing of information from the environment (Enns, 1993).

Attention is critical to adaptive functioning throughout the lifespan. It helps the observer select a subset of stimuli for further processing from an infinite number of possible targets. The observer is then better able to manage and make sense of incoming input from his or her environment by prioritizing according to a particular goal or to the saliency of the input. Selective attention can best be understood in terms of a framework based on two fundamental dimensions (Trick et al., 2004; Enns & Trick, 2006). The first concerns whether selection occurs with or without awareness. Selection without awareness is automatic, effortless, and rapid. Selection with awareness is controlled, effortful, and often slow. The second dimension used to distinguish among the different aspects of attention concerns the origin of the selective process. *Exogenous selection* is innately specified and therefore does not require learning. *Endogenous selection* involves learning and prior experience. Based on these distinctions, Enns and Trick (2006) proposed four modes of visual attention: reflexes, habits, exploration and deliberation. Reflexes and habits are both automatic, unconscious processes, but habits are learned whereas reflexes are innate. Exploration and deliberation are both conscious and controlled processes, but exploration is innately specified, whereas deliberation is learned and is typically the result of a specific goal (see Table 6.1). Based on evidence from studies on each mode of selection, Enns and Trick (2006) concluded that age-related changes are more evident in the two modes of selection that originate from learning (habit and deliberation) than in the two modes that originate from innate tendencies (reflex and exploration). Age changes are also more evident in the two controlled modes (exploration and deliberation) than in the two automatic modes (reflex and habit). When these two trends are combined, reflexes appear to show the greatest stability over the life course, while deliberation shows the greatest developmental change (Iarocci et al., 2009).

Table 6.1   Four modes of selective attention

Process		Origin	
		Exogenous	Endogenous
	Automatic	Reflex	Habit
	Controlled	Exploration	Deliberation

Adapted from Enns & Trick (2006), with permission of Oxford University Press.

Visual Reflexes

Reflexes involve unconscious, automatic processes that are triggered by specific environmental stimuli (Enns & Trick, 2006). Among the most universal visual reflexes of humans is orienting. *Orienting* alerts the observer to important novel and familiar events or objects in the environment that are relevant to achieving a particular goal. Thus, the observer must seamlessly coordinate his expectancies regarding an object of attention and control environmentally based or stimulus-driven processes that enhance the salience of task-irrelevant objects. Orienting is involved in coordinating shifts from an internal representation to the external object. An example is attending to an internal image of a familiar face as the visual field is scanned to locate a familiar person. The evidence on visual orienting is consistent in showing that the ability to orient, at least toward the location of an abrupt stimulus, changes little over the course of typical development (Plude, Enns, & Brodeur, 1994).

Visual Habits

Visual habits also involve unconscious, automatic processes, but unlike visual reflexes, are learned. Examples of habits within the visual selective attention literature can be found when examining the stimuli often used in these types of tasks. For example, for some individuals, directional symbols, such as arrows, are so well rehearsed and familiar that their meaning cannot be ignored (e.g., Hommel, Pratt, Colzato, & Godjin, 2001). This phenomena is supported by the findings on color naming Stroop tasks, in which younger school-aged children are more efficient than are older school-aged children at ignoring written words that are inconsistent with the color of the word (e.g., Schiller, 1966), as the younger children do not yet read as automatically as older children; thus, the written words do not interfere as readily with the color naming. This automaticity of visual habits was also supported in studies in which poor readers were less distracted by the irrelevant words than were good readers (Comalli, Wapner, & Werner, 1962; Fournier, Mazzarella, Ricciardi, & Fingeret, 1975). Ristic, Friesen, and Kingstone (2002) found that arrows were just as effective as eye gaze at influencing the direction of spatial attention in children as young as 4–5 years of age. They concluded that children of 4–5 years of age have already learned the visual habits associated with the meaning of an arrow. The age at which symbols, such as arrows, are processed automatically requires further research. However, the current research findings related to visual habits indicate

that the level of familiarity associated with the irrelevant information may play a role in the magnitude of the interference that results.

Visual Exploration

Visual exploration is a controlled process that is innately specified. Much of our visual processing is done in the absence of a specific goal. However, even when there is no specified goal to accomplish, some visual stimuli are processed preferentially over others (Enns & Trick, 2006). Thus, certain attributes can direct visual processing when the goal is primarily to explore. One important function of exploration is to alert the observer to change in the environment. The change detection task was devised to measure the response of an observer to various changes to the environment. This is a task in which two versions of the same scene are presented side by side, and the participant is asked to determine what is different in one scene. When this task was administered to typically developing 7-, 9-, 11-, and 21-year-olds, the findings showed that change detection improved between the ages of 7 and 9 years (Shore, Burack, Miller, Joseph, & Enns, 2006).

Visual Deliberation

Visual deliberation involves controlled, effortful processes, but unlike exploration, the origin of deliberation is not innately specified. Visual deliberation involves the deliberate selection of a specific goal. For example, deliberation is often measured in visual orienting tasks, when participants orient their response deliberately in response to a cue. This response is then compared to a response initiated when the orienting is reflexive in nature. Another aspect of visual selective attention that involves deliberation is switching from one visual task to another. The general conclusion on visual selective attention tasks that involve deliberation is that younger children are less developed in these areas than are older children and adults (e.g., Plude et al., 1994).

Methodological Considerations
ISSUES OF DEVELOPMENTAL LEVEL

The study of the efficiency of functioning in any domain among any group of persons with ID necessitates the consideration of issues related to developmental level (usually discussed with regard to MA) (Burack et al., 2002; Burack, Hodapp, & Zigler, 1998). Conceptually, the mapping of performance across levels of development is essential since certain problems are apparent earlier in life but not later. In other cases, development appears typical at younger ages, when all that is required are simple tasks indicative of lower MAs, but is deficient with more sophisticated tasks that reflect higher MAs (Burack, 1997; Burack, Pàsto, et al., 2001).

DEVELOPMENTAL ISSUES IN MATCHING AND ASSESSING PROFILES

A primary goal of matching in developmental research typically involves equating groups by MA rather than CA (Burack et al., 2002; Iarocci & Burack, 1998; Mervis & Robinson, 1999; Sigman & Ruskin, 1999). However, matching by MA is also not usually sufficient, as the measure may be too broad to reflect relative strengths and weaknesses that may affect the comparisons between groups (Burack, Pàsto, et al., 2001). For example, when two groups of persons with ID with different etiologies are matched on a measure of general MA, one might be considerably stronger on language skills and, therefore, likely to perform more successfully than another group with ID on tasks that require considerable verbal skills. Accordingly, the persons could be matched to the comparison groups on measures of verbal and nonverbal MA or other task-specific indices. The emphasis of these comparisons should be on developing profiles of development rather than on simple assessments of "stronger or weaker" (Burack, Iarocci, Flanagan & Bowler, 2004; Burack, Pàsto, et al., 2001).

Review of Studies on Attention and Syndromes of Intellectual Disability

This survey of attention studies included nine studies that were identified with an extensive search of the literature of the *American Journal of Mental Retardation* and other relevant journals of ID,

development, and developmental disabilities from 1970 to 2009. These studies included different processes or aspects of attention such as filtering, orienting, priming, sustained attention, and autonomic correlates of attention that were measured across modalities with a variety of research paradigms (refer to Table 6.2). However, we excluded paper-and-pencil studies of visual search or other attention processes so as not to confound motor performance with attentional performance.

Down Syndrome and Attentional Functioning

Two studies were found on visual orienting in persons with DS. Overall, the findings indicated similar performance between groups. Randolph and Burack (2000) examined visual filtering and reflexive orienting abilities among persons with DS compared to that of children matched on nonverbal MAs of 5–6 years. Task conditions varied with regard to the location of the target, the validity of a cue (flash of light) that preceded the target (valid, invalid, or neutral), and the absence or presence of distractors. Similar patterns of performance were found across groups. Reaction times (RTs) were faster when the target was preceded by a valid as compared to a neutral or invalid cue, and in the absence as compared to the presence of distractors. Randolph and Burack concluded that the filtering and reflexive orienting components of attention are intact among persons with DS at a MA level of approximately 5 years.

Goldman et al. (2005) examined voluntary (deliberate) visual orienting among children and adolescents with DS as compared to that of typically

Table 6.2   Summary of selective attention studies of fragile X, Williams, and Down syndromes

	Orienting	Sustained Attention	Selective Attention	Attentional Switching	Response Inhibition	Executive Functioning	Visual Search
FX		Cornish = impaired	Cornish = intact Tamn = impaired	Cornish = impaired Wilding = impaired	Cornish = intact Wilding = impaired	Cornish = impaired	Scerif = impaired
WS	Brown = impaired	Brown = intact					Scerif impaired
DS	Randolph = intact Goldman = intact Brown = intact	Brown = impaired	Randolph = intact	Wilding– impaired	Wilding– impaired		

developing children matched at a MA of 5.6 years. Task conditions varied with regard to the location of the target, the type of cue that preceded the target (valid, invalid, or neutral), and the interval (175 or 600 msec) between presentation of the cue and presentation of the target (SOA). Both groups showed similar patterns of cue effects under both short and long SOA conditions. Performance was enhanced with the valid as compared to the invalid cue, and with a SOA of 600 msec as compared to a SOA of 175 msec. The authors concluded that the efficiency of voluntary orienting among persons with DS is consistent with their developmental level. Thus, the two studies with persons with DS suggest intact functioning with regard to both reflexive visual orienting, thought to be innate and engaged without awareness, and voluntary visual orienting that is learned and requires cognitive effort.

Fragile X Syndrome and Attentional Functioning

Three studies of attention processing among persons with FXS were found. Cornish, Munir, and Cross (2001) compared the performance of adults with FXS, a heterogeneous group of adults with ID matched for CA and MA, and typically developing adults matched for MA, on a range of traditional, noncomputerized, attention tasks. The tasks tapped the selective and sustained aspects of attention. The task of selective attention demands deliberate attending that requires mental effort, and is, therefore, dependent on learning. Performance differed significantly between the groups on the tasks. On the task of selective attention (map search), the participants with ID performed less well than the participants with FXS and the typically developing adults, whereas on the task of sustained attention (elevator counting task), the participants with FXS and ID showed levels of performance that were similar and worse than that of the persons with typical development.

Wilding, Cornish, and Munir (2002) conducted a more detailed analysis of the attentional measures obtained in the original study by Munir et al. (2000). The performance of males with FXS was compared to the performance of boys with DS matched on CA and MA, and typically developing boys matched on MA. The participants were required to search a computer screen for target shapes. Task conditions varied with regard to the number of targets specified (1 vs. 2). Twenty-five target shapes were randomly presented on a computer

screen among 100 nontarget shapes. Once a target was selected, the color changed. Both the boys with FXS and DS made more repeated responses on targets than typically developing boys; however, these differences were stronger in the FXS group. In the dual-target condition, both the boys with FXS and the boys with DS had more difficulty than the typically developing boys to switch attention to a new target after a correct response. However, the boys with FXS showed more difficulty than the boys with DS at switching between targets. Wilding et al. concluded that the results provide further support for an executive attention deficit involving the deliberate inhibition of target repetition and switching attention between targets among persons with FXS.

Tamm, Menon, Johnson, Hessel, and Reiss (2002) also examined the process of inhibition by comparing the performance of 14 females with FXS and the performance of 14 age-matched, typically developing females on the counting Stroop task. The researchers used functional magnetic resonance imaging (fMRI) to chart differences in brain functioning between the two groups during this task. The task consisted of 12 alternating interference and neutral conditions. For both conditions, the participants were instructed to press the response key that corresponded to the number of words on the screen. During the neutral condition, the word "fish" was presented one, two, three, or four times. During the interference condition, the words "one," "two," "three," and "four" were presented one, two, three, or four times on the screen. Compared to typically developing participants, the females with FXS had longer RTs during the interference task and adopted a strategy that traded speed for accuracy. In addition, females with FXS demonstrated a different pattern of brain activation than typically developing females during the interference phase of the task.

Scerif, Cornish, Wilding, Driver, and Karmiloff (2004) examined the influence of target salience on the efficiency of visual search among typically developing toddlers and toddlers with FXS or WS. Target salience was manipulated by varying distractor size. Targets surrounded by smaller distractors are known to be more salient and can capture attention. All toddlers responded to the target using a computerized touch screen method. Participants were required to find ten target stimuli that remained on the screen throughout the task. The target changed in color once touched. Task conditions varied with regard to the number of distractors (0, 6, or 24) and the size of the distractors (small or medium). Search time per hit, mean distance between successive touches, total number of errors, and error types (touches on distractors or repetitions on previously found distractors) were influenced by distractor salience among typically developing toddlers. Toddlers with FXS and WS produced similar mean time and distance per touch as typically developing toddlers, but both also produced a larger number of errors. Toddlers with WS more than any other group were adversely affected by increasing the number of distractors, and they confused distractors with targets, whereas the toddlers with FXS perseverated on previously found targets. Scerif et al. (2004) concluded that these results reveal distinct search deficits for atypically developing toddlers, subtle visuoperceptual problems in those with WS, and executive control problems (e.g., inhibition) in those with FXS.

Similar executive control problems were also noted in adult women with FXS. Cornish, Swainson, Cunnington, Wilding, Morris, and Jackson (2004) measured the brain activity of three women with FXS using event related potentials (ERPs) and fMRI in a task that tapped both deliberate attention switching and response inhibition. The participants were required to respond to a centrally presented arrow by pressing a left or right response key depending on the direction of the arrow. They were instructed to respond immediately when the arrow was red and to respond at stimulus offset when the arrow was green. At a behavioral level, compared to typically developing females, the females with FXS were significantly slower and made more errors on trials that required an immediate response, and these errors were made mainly when both "GO" and "WAIT" trials were mixed in one block, indicating difficulty with switching attention. The performance of females with FXS was comparable to typically developing females on trials that required a delayed response, indicating that they were able to inhibit a response when sufficient time was provided. Neurophysiological data suggested that females with FXS recruit different areas of the brain than do typically developing females when inhibiting responses.

WILLIAMS SYNDROME

One study was found on orienting among persons with WS. Brown, Johnson, Paterson, Gilmore, Longhi, and Karmiloff-Smith (2003) examined visual orienting and sustained attention in toddlers with WS and DS, as compared to MA-matched

and CA-matched typically developing toddlers. The double-step saccade task was used in Experiment 1 as a measure of visual orienting. *Saccades* are rapid eye movements that move the foveal region of the retina between successive fixation points within the visual field; a double-step saccade involves two successive eye movements to target locations. The double-step saccade task trial began with a fixation stimulus, followed by the presentation of two targets presented consecutively with no overlap. Pairs of targets appeared opposite one another. Toddlers with WS made fewer looks to the first target and more looks to the center and other positions than any other group. Brown et al. (2003) concluded that toddlers with WS are impaired relative to toddlers with DS and both CA- and MA-matched typically developing toddlers in flexibly orienting to a target. In Experiment 2, three toys were placed in front of the children for 45 seconds each. The total duration of sustained attention to each toy and number of periods of sustained attention were coded. The toddlers with DS exhibited fewer periods of sustained attention than did MA-matched typically developing toddlers and less total duration of sustained attention than any other group. The toddlers with WS performed as well as typically developing toddlers with regard to sustained attention.

Conclusion ATTN TOPIC SENTENCE

The current review indicates a need for more research on specific aspects of attention, as well as more delineation with regard to the constructs of attention studied among persons with particular syndromes of mental retardation. The available evidence suggests that, rather than a generalized deficit of attention, different patterns of strengths and weaknesses in attention processing are present among persons with genetic syndromes. We propose that a more elaborative conceptual framework of attention is needed to further the study of attentional profiles among specific groups of persons with genetic syndromes. The proposed elaborated framework of attention was originally developed in the course of understanding the role of attention in automobile driving (Trick et al., 2004), and then later for understanding developmental change and stability in selective attention over the typical human lifespan (Enns & Trick, 2006). The Enns and Trick framework differentiates two dimensions of attention: awareness and origin. The dimension of awareness addresses the degree to which orienting occurs with conscious control and ranges from automatic to controlled. According to Enns and Trick, automatic selective attention is effortless, rapid, and is triggered by the presence of certain stimuli in the environment. In contrast, controlled selective attention is conscious or intentional. The second dimension of Enns and Trick's framework, origin, refers to the extent to which learning and experience play a role in attention. The dimension is comprised of two categories: exogenous and endogenous. Exogenous attention is innate, universal, and is initiated by a specific external stimulus (e.g., a flash of light). Conversely, endogenous selection of attention is influenced by an individual's goals and learning history. Based upon these two dimensions, four modes of visual selective attention are proposed, including how it is acquired, what the triggering stimuli are, the degree of conscious control that is possible, and the stability of each mode over time. Table 6.1 depicts the four modes of selective attention: Reflex, Habit, Exploration, and Deliberation.

According to Enns and Trick (2006), age-related changes are more evident in the two modes of selection that require learning (i.e., habit and deliberation) than in the two modes that originate from innate tendencies (i.e., reflex and exploration). Age changes are also more evident in the two controlled modes (i.e., exploration and deliberation) than in the two automatic modes (i.e., reflex and habit). When these two trends are combined, reflexes appear to show the greatest stability over the life course, whereas deliberation shows the greatest developmental change (Iarocci et al., 2009). Thus, if orienting and other "visual reflex" types of attention show little change over the course of typical development, the implication for research with individuals with different types of ID syndromes is that they might show spared or impaired abilities early on, and the same amount of impaired abilities later (vs. either MA, other ability match, or even CA), whereas with regard to visual deliberation, the pattern might be more varied over time since the greatest amount of developmental change is expected in this mode of attention.

Ultimately, this more elaborate specification of attentional profiles among persons with different genetic syndromes may contribute to our understanding of the etiology that underlies a particular syndrome of ID. In addition, the attentional profiles of persons with specific genetic disorders may provide useful endophenotypes in the search for relations between genetic susceptibility to the disorder and the behavioural expression of the syndrome. Endophenotypes are considered intermediate pathways in the developmental course that lead to a behavioural syndrome. Visual selective attention might operate as an endophenotype in at least two ways: over the course of the child's development, and at a single point in time as the child performs a particular task. Attentional processes that are theoretically or empirically linked to the phenotype of interest would be candidate endophenotypes. Genetic syndromes are known to display deficits or excesses in cognitive processes. A homogenous group with regard to known genetic deletions/mutations and a well-defined behavioural phenotype may provide clues about candidate genes involved in aspects of cognition that are abnormal in the group. For example, the attentional profile of individuals with WS may be related to their excessive fears and anxieties (Dykens, 2003; Dykens & Rosner, 2006) or to their intense interest in faces, and this may help us to uncover the genetic underpinnings of sociability (see Iarocci, Yager, & Elfers, 2008). Ultimately, cognitive profiles could be mapped onto genetic, neurophysiological, and behavioural profiles to provide insight into the commonalities, as well as the differences, across and within syndromes.

References

Brown, J. H., Johnson, M. H., Paterson, S. J., Gilmore, R., Longhi, E., & Karmiloff-Smith, A. (2003). Spatial representation and attention in toddlers with Williams syndrome and Down syndrome. *Neuropsychologia, 41(8)*, 1037–1046.

Burack, J. A. (1997). The study of atypical and typical populations in developmental psychopathology: The quest for a common science. In S. S. Luthar, J. A. Burack, D. Cicchetti, & J. R. Weisz, (Eds.), *Developmental psychopathology: Perspectives on adjustment, risk and disorder* (pp. 139–165). New York: Cambridge University Press.

Burack, J. A., Evans, D. W., Klaiman, C., & Iarocci, G., (2001). The mysterious myth of attention deficit and other defect stories: Contemporary issues in the developmental approach to mental retardation. *International Review of Research in Mental Retardation, 24*, 300–321.

Burack, J. A., Hodapp, R. M., & Zigler, E. (1998). *Handbook of mental retardation and development*. New York: Cambridge University Press.

Burack, J.A., Iarocci, G., Bowler, D., & Mottron L. (2002). Benefits and pitfalls in merging disciplines: The example of developmental psychopathology and the study of persons with autism. *Development and Psychopathology, 14*, 225–237.

Burack, J. A., Pastò, L., Porporino, M., Iarocci, G., Mottron, L., & Bowler, D. (2001). Applying developmental principles to the study of autism. In E. Schopler, N. Yirmiya, C. Shulman, & L. Marcus (Eds.), *The research basis of autism: Implications for Intervention*. New York: Kluwer Academic/Plenum.

Burack, Jacob A.; Iarocci, Grace; Flanagan, Tara D., Bowler, Dermot M. (2004). *Journal of Autism and Developmental Disorders, 34*, 65–73.

Comalli, P. E., Wapner, S., & Werner, H. (1962). Intereference effects of Stroop color-word test on childhood, adulthood, and aging. *Journal of Genetic Psychology,100*, 47–53.

Cornish, K., Swainson, R., Cunnington, R., Eilding, J., Morris, P., &Jackson, G. (2004). Do women with fragile X syndrome have problems in switching attention: Preliminary findings from ERP and fMRI. *Brain and Cognition, 54*(3), 235–239.

Dykens, E. M. (2003). Anxiety, fears, and phobias in persons with Williams syndrome. *Developmental Neuropsychology, 23*, 291–316.

Dykens, E. M., & Rosner, B. A. (2006). Psychopathology in persons with Williams syndrome. In C. A. Morris, P. P. Wang, & H. M. Lenhoff (Eds.), *Williams-Beuren syndrome: Research and clinical implications* (pp. 274–293). Baltimore: Johns Hopkins Press.

Enns, J. T. (1993). What can be learned about attention from studying its development?. *Canadian Psychology, 34*, 271–281.

Enns, J. T., & Trick, L. (2006). Four modes of selection. In E. Bialystok, & G. Craik (Ed.), *Lifespan cognition: Mechanisms of change* (pp. 43–56). New York: Oxford University Press.

Fournier, P. A., Mazzarella, M. M., Ricciardi, M. M., & Fingeret, A. L. (1975). Reading level and locus of interference in the Stroop color-word task. *Perceptual & Motor skills, 41*(1), 239–242.

Goldman, K. J., Flanagan, T., Shulman, C., Enns, J. T., & Burack, J. A. (2005). Voluntary orienting among children and adolescents with Down syndrome and MA-matched typically developing children. *American Journal on Mental Retardation, 110*(3), 157–163.

Hommel, B., Pratt, J., Colzato, L., & Godjin, R. (2001). Symbolic control of visual attention. *Psychological Science, 12*(5), 360–365.

Iarocci, G., & Burack, J.A. (1998). Understanding the development of attention in persons with mental retardation: Challenging the myths. In J.A. Burack, R.M. Hodapp, & E. Zigler (Eds.), *Handbook of mental retardation and development.* New York: Cambridge University Press.

Iarocci, G., Yager, J., & Effers, T. (2007). What gene-environment interactions can tell us about social competence in typical and atypical populations. *Brain and Cognition. 65*:112–127.

Iarocci, G., Enns, J. T., Randollph, B., & Burack, J. A. (2009). The modulation of visual orienting reflexes across the lifespan. *Developmental Science, 12*, 715–724.

Korbel, J. O., Tirosh-Wagner, T., Urban, A. E., Chen, X., Kasowski, M., Dai, L., et al. (2009). The genetic architecture of Down syndrome phenotypes revealed by high-resolution analysis of human segmental trisomies. *PNAS Proceedings of the National Academy of Sciences of the United States of America, 106*, 12031–12036.

Mervis, C. B., & Robinson, B. F. (1999). Metodological issues in cross-syndrome comparisons: Matching procedures, sensitivity (Se), and specificity (Sp). *Monographs of the Society for Re-search in Child development, 64*, 115–130.

Munir, F., Cornish, K. M., & Wilding, J. (2000). A neuropsychological profile of attention deficits in young male with fragile x syndrome. *Neuropsychologia, 38*, 1261–1270.

Plude, D., Enns, J. T., & Brodeur, D. A. (1994). The development of selective attention: A lifespan overview. *Acta Psychologica, 86*, 227–272.

Randolph, B., & Burack, J. A. (2000). Visual filtering and covert orienting in persons with Down syndrome. *International Journal of Behavioral Development, 24*, 167–172.

Ristic, J., Friesen, C. K., Kingstone, A. (2002). Are eyes special? It depends on how you look at it. *Psychonomic Bulletin & Review, 9*(3), 507–513.

Scerif, G., Cornish, k., Wilding, J., Driver, J., & Karmiloff-Smith, A. (2004). Visual search in typically developing toddlers and toddlers with Fragile X or Williams syndrome. *Developmental Science, 7*(1), 116–130.

Schiller, P. H. (1966). Developmental study of color-word interference. *Journal of experimental Psychology, 72*, 105–108.

Sigman, M., Ruskin, E. (1999). Continuity and change in the social competence of children with autism, down syndrome, and developmental delays. *Monographs of the Society for Research in Child Development, 64*, v–114.

Shore, D. I., Burack, J. A., Miller, D., Joseph, S., & Enns, J. T. (2006). The development of change detection. *Developmental Science, 9*, 490–497.

Tamm, L., Menon, V., Johnston, C. K., Hessl, D. R., & Reiss, A. L. (2002). FMRI study of cognitive interference processing in females with fragile X syndrome. *Journal of Cognitive Neuroscience. 14*(2), 160–171.

Trick, L., Enns, J. T., Mills, J., & Vavrik, J. (2004). Paying attention behind the wheel: A framework for studying the role of selective attention in driving. *Theoretical Issues in Ergonomic Science, 5*, 385–424.

Wilding, J., Cornish, K., Munir, F. (2002). Further delineation of the executive deficit in males with fragile X syndrome. *Neuropsychologia, 40*(8),1343–1344.

CHAPTER 7

Memory and Learning in Intellectual Disabilities

Stefano Vicari

Abstract

This chapter reviews the neuropsychological literature and recent experimental studies on long-term memory and learning development in intellectual disabilities (ID), particularly in genetic syndromes. The main goal is to report specific profiles of memory capacities (with some components more preserved and others more impaired) in people with ID of different etiologies but similar severity. Consistently with a neuropsychological approach, distinct memory profiles in ID and, more specifically, in genetic syndromes can be traced to the characteristics of their brain development and architecture. Therefore, the possible correlation between memory profiles and brain development will also be presented and discussed.

Keywords: Intellectual disability, long-term memory, short-term memory, learning, genetic syndromes

The study of memory and learning is an integral part of the behavioral sciences devoted to intellectual disabilities (ID). From the first reports at the beginning of the 1900s, memory dysfunction has been noted in people with ID (for reviews, see McPherson, 1948; Vicari & Carlesimo, 2002). Many authors have described how altered development of the memory function can seriously interfere with adequate maturation of general intellectual abilities and thus with the possibility of "learning" and modifying behavior on the basis of experience.

Based on this assumption, a large body of experimental literature is aimed at clarifying the qualitative characteristics and basic mechanisms of the memory deficit in ID. For example, in view of the multicomponential structure of the memory function (Squire, 1987; Tulving & Schacter, 1990), it is relevant to know whether the impairment in individuals with ID affects all components of the memory architecture or whether some components are more disrupted than others. Moreover, it is still a matter of debate whether a causal relationship exists between memory and ID, particularly from a psychometric point of view (e.g., are the reduced memory abilities usually reported in people with ID just an effect of lower IQ?). Finally, it has been hypothesized in recent studies that severity, qualitative features, and, possibly, basic mechanisms of the memory impairment are not homogeneous across all individuals with ID but may be differentiated (among other variables) by the etiology of the abnormal brain development. In this vein, a comparison of the qualitative profiles of the memory impairment exhibited by different etiological groups of ID persons, such as Down syndrome (DS), Prader-Willi syndrome, or Williams syndrome (WS), is crucial to obtain a better description of their neuropsychological deficit and gain new insights into the neural substrate underlying their memory impairment.

This chapter is dedicated to reviewing the neuropsychological literature and recent experimental studies on long-term memory and learning development in ID, particularly in genetic syndromes. The main goal is to report specific profiles of memory capacities (with some components more preserved and others more impaired) in people with ID of different etiology but similar severity. Consistent with a neuropsychological approach, distinct memory profiles in ID and, more specifically, in genetic syndromes can be traced to the characteristics of their brain development and architecture. Therefore, the possible correlation between memory profiles and brain development will also be presented and discussed.

Human Memory: A Multicomponential Function

According to structural approaches to memory, various regions of neuroarchitecture serve specific memory functions. This is supported by functional dissociations in healthy subjects and neuropsychological dissociations in brain-damaged patients that demonstrate that memory is fragmented into a series of functionally independent, but clearly interacting, systems and subsystems.

Squire (1987) elaborated a cognitive model of the memory function that has proved to be theoretically and practically useful. In agreement with Atkinson and Shiffrin (1971), Squire first distinguished between short-term memory (STM) and long-term memory (LTM). These two systems are characterized by their differences: one, *retention capacity*, which is limited to only a few items for STM and is practically unlimited for LTM; two, *information coding*, which is mainly phonological coding in the STM and is based on semantic processing of stimuli for LTM; and three, *mnesic trace deterioration rate*, which lasts for a few seconds without reiteration for STM and is variable but relatively slow for LTM.

Concerning LTM, the model distinguishes between explicit or declarative memory and implicit or procedural memory. *Explicit memory* is involved in intentional and/or conscious recall and recognition of experiences and informations. For example, when we study a chapter of geography knowing that we have to remember it to pass an exam, or when we learn the name of a new colleague and our appointment with her, or when we memorize the list of what we need before going to the market, we rely strongly on explicit memory resources. Conversely, *implicit memory* facilitates performance of perceptual, cognitive, and motor tasks, without any conscious reference to previous experiences (for a review, see Tulving & Schacter, 1990). In other words, implicit memory is acquired by experience: we need to use the keyboard of our laptop to become faster; likewise, in order to play a musical instrument, we need practice rather than study it in a theoretical way.

Explicit and implicit memory systems are not completely independent, but cooperate with each other. Nevertheless, the memory impairment profile observed in patients with pure amnesia is the strongest evidence supporting the dichotomy between implicit and explicit memory. Although these patients show normal procedural learning and have a normal repetition priming level, they are seriously deficient in intentionally recalling previously acquired information (Schacter, Chiu, & Ochsner, 1993). Squire also suggested that, in the context of implicit memory, distinct neural circuits are implicated in repetition priming, in learning visual–motor procedures and in operant conditioning. This additional fragmentation is also supported by neuropsychological evidence that some brain disorders (i.e., Alzheimer disease) are associated with impaired repetition priming without affecting procedural learning, whereas other pathological conditions (i.e., Huntington disease) compromise procedural learning but leave repetition priming intact (Heindel, Butters, & Salmon, 1988).

Long-term Memory in Intellectual Disabilities: A Diffuse and Pervasive Impairment?

Memory functioning was considered to be diffusely impaired in people with ID. As clearly summarized by Detterman (1979), in the "everything hypothesis," ID individuals are poor in virtually every type of memory task, so that any effort to find islands of relative weakness and strength in their memory performance is doomed to frustration.

The first reports of dissociable LTM performance in ID appeared only at the end of the1980s. Ellis and coworkers (Ellis & Allison, 1988; Ellis, Woodley-Zanthos, & Dulaney, 1989; Katz & Ellis, 1991) reported a series of experiments in which they compared the performance of ID and chronological age (CA)-matched typically developing individuals on memory tasks investigating effortful or automatic memory processes. According to Hasher and Zacks (1979, 1984), differences between effortful memory tasks, that is, the traditional free recall and recognition procedures, and automatic memory tasks, such as tests of frequency judgment and spatial location, reside in the amount of attentional resources and elaborative encoding implicated, which are maximal for the first type of memory tasks and minimal for the second. Hasher and Zacks (1979, 1984) suggested that performance levels on effortful and automatic memory tasks may be dissociated in several ways and, particularly, by comparing people with different overall levels of cognitive efficiency on the two kinds of tasks with intelligence expected to be related to performance on effortful but not on automatic memory tasks. Consistently with this latter claim, Ellis and Allison (1988) reported that individuals with ID performed significantly worse than a typically developing comparison group in the free recall of lists of words and pictures and in the frequency judgment of pictures, but were as accurate as the comparison group in the frequency judgment of words. Nevertheless, these findings were not definitively confirmed in different experimental paradigms (Dulaney, Raz, & Devine 1996; Ellis et al., 1989; Katz & Ellis, 1991; Uecker & Nadel, 1998). It is important to stress here that these pioneer studies compared memory performances obtained by individuals with ID and typically developing controls matched for CA. Consequently, the impact of the global cognitive development on performing memory tasks is substantially underestimated.

A different approach was used by Burack and Zigler (1990) in the search for LTM processes possibly spared in ID. These authors compared homogeneous groups of individuals with organic ID, familial ID, and mental age (MA)-matched individuals on episodic memory tests. The latter varied depending on whether the examiner's instructions during the study phase were aimed at producing intentional or incidental stimulus learning. In a free recall test of an intentionally learned word list, normal children scored higher than familial ID individuals who, in turn, scored higher than organic ID individuals. By contrast, in a paired-associate task in which no instruction to learn was given during the study phase (incidental learning), the two ID groups and the group of normal controls scored similarly.

Consistent with these pioneer studies, over the past 20 years, the literature on memory and ID has reported contrasting findings in support of the hypothesis of heterogeneous impairments in the intentional or explicit and the incidental or implicit memory domains. In the following sections, we will analyze these aspects more thoroughly.

Explicit Verbal Long-term Memory and Intellectual Disability

The evidence on the explicit memory performances of ID individuals and that of typically developing children conflicts. In fact, some authors documented comparable performances of ID and MA-matched typically developing children on verbal LTM tasks (Ellis, 1969; Schultz, 1983; Spitz, 1966), whereas others found reduced verbal (Cantor & Ryan, 1962; Iscoe & Semler, 1964) and visual (Burack & Zigler, 1990) LTM in individuals with ID. Parallel to uncertainties regarding the overall level of memory performances, studies on the qualitative aspects of memory impairment in ID children also provided discrepant findings. For example, Rossi (1963) reported a reduced use of semantic strategies by people with ID in a task involving free recall of related word lists, whereas subsequent studies reported opposite results (Spitz, 1966; Winters & Semchuk, 1986).

Two possible explanations for the discrepant results obtained by various authors are the methodological differences in the testing instruments used and the different levels of participants' ID severity. Another relevant explanation is the heterogeneity of the etiological groups included in the different ID samples. In fact, despite the large amount of experimental works on LTM functioning in persons with ID, only sporadic and relatively recent attempts have been made to look for possible qualitative differences in the memory profile of distinct ID etiological groups (Burack & Zigler, 1990; Vicari & Carlesimo, 2002). This initial lack of interest probably reflects a general skepticism about the possibility of showing behavioral differences in the various ID etiological groups (Ellis, 1969; Fisher & Zeaman, 1970). However, recent evidence suggests that, when appropriately investigated, qualitative differences in the memory performances of different ID groups are likely to emerge (Vicari & Carlesimo, 2002).

Due to its high incidence, DS is probably the ID etiological group most extensively investigated to discover possible qualitative peculiarities in memory profile (Vicari, 2006). In a study of individuals with DS, ID of unspecified etiology, and typically developing children matched for MA, Carlesimo, Marotta, and Vicari (1997) found that the DS group scored significantly worse than the other groups in tests that included a verbal list learning task. In this task, participants were presented with the same list of words and had to recall it repeatedly. They also had to recall a short story and to reproduce Rey's figure from memory. All these tests are considered reliable measures of explicit LTM functionality for verbal and visual–spatial material. Therefore, Carlesimo et al. (1997) concluded that the individuals with DS exhibited a severe impairment of explicit LTM. This is supported by findings from a number of studies (e.g., Nadel, 1999; Nichols et al., 2004; Pennington, Moon, Edgin, Stedron, & Nadel, 2003; Vicari, Bellucci, & Carlesimo, 2000, 2006), in which individuals with DS recalled fewer words than typically developing MA-matched controls. Apparently contrasting results were reported by Jarrold, Baddeley, and Phillips (2007), who assessed recall and recognition of verbal information in a group of 20 individuals with DS and found no deficits in verbal LTM. Note, however, that in Jarrold et al.'s study children with DS were not matched with typically developing children for MA. Consequently, as Jarrold et al. also observed, the interpretation of their findings is controversial, and an explicit LTM impairment in people with DS is still a possibility.

The diffuse impairment of explicit LTM reported in people with DS cannot be generalized to all individuals with ID. In the case of individuals with WS, studies on explicit LTM performance report more contradictory results. Udwin and Yule (1991) investigated performances on the Rivermead test in a group of children with WS and a comparison group of children with ID matched for age and verbal IQ. The children with WS showed unimpaired overall performance in the visuo-spatial tasks of the battery but were less efficient than the comparison group in the verbal test items. Udwin and Yule also noted that the individuals with WS performed particularly well on the face recognition task, which is a specific strength in WS (Bellugi, Lichtenberger, Jones, Lai, & St. George, 2000; Karmiloff-Smith et al., 1997). Therefore, the individuals with WS assessed in Udwin and Yule's study may have performed relatively worse on the remaining visuo-spatial memory tasks than on the verbal items.

Vicari, Carlesimo, Brizzolara, and Pezzini (1996) documented poor performance of children with WS compared to a group of typically developing children matched for MA in verbal LTM; namely, in the delayed free recall and recognition of a word list. Moreover, in the immediate recall of the same word list, Vicari et al. (1996) found comparable recall of the last items on the list in the two groups (recency effect) but reduced recall of the first items on the list in the WS group (primacy effect). According to the classical dual-store interpretation of the serial position curve in the immediate recall of word lists (e.g., Glanzer, 1972), the normal recency effect in the individuals with WS provides new support for the idea of relatively preserved verbal STM in these individuals (Vicari & Carlesimo, 2006). In contrast, the poor primacy

effect is indicative of difficulty in storing new verbal representations in the declarative LTM.

The hypothesis that language and auditory STM might be dissociated from long-term verbal memory in individuals with WS was also supported by Nichols et al. (2004). However, Brock, Brown, and Boucher (2006) reported contrasting findings; that is, LTM performance in children with WS was comparable to that of typically developing children. Using a free recall task, Brock et al. found similar long-term learning in participants with WS and in typically developing children, and no primacy effect in either group. Nonetheless, when the participants were encouraged to engage in overt, cumulative rehearsal in a second experiment, significant and comparable primacy effects were observed in both groups. Based on these findings, Brock et al. argued against the conclusions by Vicari et al. and Nichols et al., of a dissociation between short- and long-term verbal memory in WS. As different criteria were adopted in the reported studies to match WS and typically developing children (i.e., MA in Nichols et al. and Vicari et al. and overall verbal memory abilities in Brock et al.), no definitive conclusions can be drawn about the characteristics of verbal LTM in WS.

In summary, individuals with DS and WS appear to show an impairment of verbal LTM, although different patterns of long-term verbal memory abilities emerged. For example, individuals with DS showed a diffuse and general impairment relative to MA-matched, typically developing persons, whereas those with WS usually exhibited a less severe pattern, with some aspects of verbal LTM preserved relative to the typically developing groups of comparable MA.

Explicit Visual–Spatial Long-term Memory and Intellectual Disability

Differences in the etiological groups of people with ID also emerged in the few studies on explicit visual–spatial LTM. Although Ellis et al. (1989) documented relative preservation of this function in people with ID, a general impairment of visual–spatial LTM is reported in more recent studies (Carlesimo et al., 1997; Jarrold et al., 2007; Vicari et al., 1996).

Vicari, Bellucci, and Carlesimo (2005) investigated the performances of individuals with WS and those with DS in a visual–object test, concerning the physical characteristics of objects such as form and color, and a visual–spatial learning test, referring the position or motion in space of stimuli. In agreement with Moscovitch, Kapur, Kohler, and Houle (1995) visual–object LTM and visual–spatial LTM are thought to be mediated by different neural systems and, therefore, constitute two distinct aspects of the organization of explicit LTM. In Vicari et al. (2005), two tests distinctively exploring the visual–object and the visual–spatial LTM were adopted. Both tests were organized in two distinct parts: the study phase and the test phase. During the study phase of the visual–object test, 15 pictures of common objects (e.g., a tree) were shown to the participants. During the test phase, immediately after the study phase, four different versions of the same object (e.g., four trees) were depicted on each page; only one of the four was the same as the target object in the study phase; the other three were physically different distracters. Study and test phases were presented three consecutive times. In the visual–spatial learning test, the pages were divided into four quadrants and each figure was positioned in one of the quadrants. During the test phase, the target stimuli were presented and the participants were asked to indicate the position of the figure on an empty page divided into four quadrants. The entire test was administered three times. The results of this study showed poorer visual–spatial learning but analogous visual–object learning in the individuals with WS as compared to typically developing children matched by MA. The individuals with DS as compared to typically developing children matched for MA revealed the opposite profile, that is, analogous learning of visual–spatial sequences and poorer learning of visual–object patterns.

The performance of the WS participants seems to extend to the LTM domain the dissociation between a deficit in visual–spatial information processing and preserved processing of visual–object data described in this population in perceptual (Atkinson et al., 1997; Atkinson et al., 2003) and working memory (Vicari, Bellucci, & Carlesimo, 2003, 2006) tasks. Indeed, the learning level of WS persons was comparable to that of typically developing children matched for MA on the visual–object test but clearly poorer on the visual–spatial test. Note that what mainly distinguished the performance of the typically developing children from that of the WS persons on the visual–spatial test was the learning rate from the first to the third recognition trial. This finding is contrary to the reductionist hypothesis that the origin of the LTM deficit shown by individuals with WS is the effect of reduced perceptual processing and/or deficient working memory maintenance of visual–spatial data. According to the reductionist hypothesis, individuals with WS are likely to perform poorly on

any visual–spatial LTM task simply because of their generalized problems in visual–spatial functioning. However, our findings show that immediate recognition of items studied only once might also be heavily influenced by proficiency in perceptual analysis and working memory processing, although the reduced learning across successive trials seems to be a reliable index of the compromised ability to store new information in LTM. Individuals with DS showed dissociation between more preserved visual–spatial memory and greater impairment of visual–object learning ability. There is general agreement in the literature that the neuropsychological profile of people with DS is characterized by strengths in nonverbal abilities, as revealed by their performance in graphic, constructive, and spatial tests, which are generally less impaired than linguistic abilities (Martens, Wilson, & Reutens, 2008; Wang & Bellugi, 1994). A sparing of visual–spatial but not visual–object memory was found in people with DS (Ellis et al., 1989). Ellis et al. argued that memory for the spatial position of objects is characterized by greater automaticity than memory for visual and/or verbal content of information and is therefore less impaired in persons with DS. In our study, the comparison of two groups of individuals with known genetic syndromes suggests a different type of interpretation. Individuals with DS had greater difficulty in learning visual–object material and a substantial sparing of visual–spatial learning, and persons with WS showed the opposite pattern. Thus, not all people with ID have preserved visual–spatial memory, as Ellis seemed to suggest. Rather, different patterns can be observed in individuals with ID of different etiologies.

In summary, findings on visual–object and visual–spatial LTM in people with DS and WS suggest there are different patterns of memory performance in these two etiological groups, both characterized by ID. Consequently, the impairment exhibited by the WS group in the visual–spatial test cannot simply be attributed to the presence of ID, but must be considered a peculiar characteristic of this syndrome. Moreover, the pattern of performance of the WS group extends to the LTM domain, their difficulty in managing visual–spatial material, and their relative sparing of the ability to process visual–object material (Martens et al., 2008).

Implicit Long-term Memory and Intellectual Disability

In the past 15 years, implicit memory and learning has been investigated in people with ID, and some experimental data have indicated that the dissociation between explicit and implicit memory processes, which is so frequently described in brain-damaged adults with associated explicit and implicit memory disorders, might also extend to individuals with ID. Within the implicit memory domain, three distinct components have been hypothesized to be impaired: repetition priming, procedural learning, and operant conditioning (Schacter, Dobbins, & Schnyer, 2004; Squire, 1987). Repetition priming refers to a facilitation of the identification or production of an experimental item following prior experience with the item. Studies of facilitation in identifying perceptually degraded pictures due to previous exposure to the same pictures have consistently reported a comparable priming effect between individuals with ID and typically developing individuals matched for CA (Takegata & Futuruka, 1993; Wyatt & Conners, 1998) or, more precisely, for MA (Perrig & Perrig, 1995). Nevertheless, a rather complex and somewhat contradictory pattern of results emerged from studies of repetition priming for verbal material.

Most of these studies were based on the Stem Completion procedure, in which participants are required to complete a list of stems (i.e., the first three letters) with the first word that comes to mind. In this test, the priming effect is revealed by a bias in completing the stems with words that have been previously studied rather than with unstudied words. Using this procedure, Carlesimo et al. (1997) and Vicari, Bellucci, and Carlesimo (2000, 2001) investigated repetition priming in various groups of individuals with ID (etiologically unspecified, DS, and WS) and typically developing children matched for MA. Results showed comparable priming effects in all groups (etiologically unspecified, DS, WS, and typically developing children). However, using the same experimental paradigm, Mattson and Riley (1999), and Komatsu, Naito, and Fuke (1996) reported reduced priming in groups of ID individuals with DS or with an unspecified etiology. These contradictory results are likely due to the methodological differences between the studies. In fact, in contrast to the findings reported above (Carlesimo et al., 1997; Vicari et al., 2000, 2001), in the studies of Mattson and Riley (1999) and Komatsu et al. (1996), the two groups of ID individuals were matched for CA but not for MA. Moreover, Mattson and Riley's (1999) individuals with DS, who had deficient priming, had lower IQs than did individuals with fetal alcohol syndrome, who had normal priming. An interpretative hypothesis may be that

verbal repetition priming varies as a function of global intellectual efficiency and that it is spared in mildly retarded individuals and poor in moderately retarded ones. Komatsu et al. investigated the repetition priming evoked by a Word Fragment Completion procedure. The level of processing during the study phase was manipulated by giving half of the words to be read and half to be generated starting from a sentence in which they were embedded. Participants with ID displayed a priming level comparable to that of typically developing comparison subjects for the words that had been previously read but less than normal priming for the words that had been generated. These results suggest that there is dissociation in people with ID between normal perceptual priming, facilitation elicited by perceptually reprocessing an item in the same physical format as in a previous presentation, and deficient conceptual priming, produced by reprocessing the semantic identity of an item without any overlapping between the perceptual formats of the study and the test presentations.

Experimental studies devoted to investigating procedural learning in ID are few and relatively recent. In one study, Vakil, Shelef-Reshef, and Levy-Shiff (1997) compared the improvement in accuracy displayed by groups of individuals with ID and MA-matched typically developing children across successive trials of the Tower of Hanoi and the Proteus Maze tests. On both tests, the individuals with ID performed significantly less accurately than did the comparison participants. However, on the Tower of Hanoi test, the rate of trial-to-trial improvement (which is considered a measure of implicit learning) was higher in the typically developing than in the ID group. Conversely, in the Proteus Maze test, which requires solving a series of mazes with the least number of errors possible, the two groups improved at the same rate, showing in this task a comparable implicit learning between groups. Similar findings were reported more recently by Atwell, Conners, and Merrill (2003) and Vinter and Detable (2003).

Results of two studies by Vicari et al. (2000, 2001) suggest a different pattern in the skill learning abilities of individuals with DS and WS. In the first study (Vicari et al., 2000), a group of individuals with DS showed the same rate of improvement as a group of typically developing children matched for MA in successive trials of the Tower of London test and in the comparison of repeated versus random blocks of a facilitated version of the serial reaction time (SRT) test, which requires implicit learning of the sequential order of a series of visual events. By contrast, Vicari et al. (2001) found that children with WS showed significantly less procedural learning than did typically developing children in both of these tests.

Don, Schellenberg, Reber, DiGirolamo, and Wang (2003) reported different findings in a study of implicit learning in children and adults with WS and in a comparison group of typically developing individuals matched for CA. The two groups showed evidence of implicit learning on both artificial grammar learning paradigm and in a rotor pursuit task.

The results from implicit memory studies of individuals with WS are equivocal, also because these studies did not directly compare different groups of individuals with ID matched for MA (Don et al., 2003).

To overcome this limitation, Vicari, Verucci, and Carlesimo (2007) recently tested 32 individuals with WS, 26 with DS, and 49 with typical development using a traditional version of the SRT test. The WS and DS groups were matched for MA and CA, and the two groups of individuals with ID were matched with typically developing children on the basis of MA. The SRT was administered on a portable computer (Compaq LTE 5280) that controlled stimulus presentation and reaction times (RT) and stored data online. Participants sat facing the screen, on which a bar with four empty squares (size 3.3 cm) appeared. During the task, one of the four squares was colored red. Participants were instructed to put their left middle and index fingers on the C and V keys of the keyboard, respectively; to put their right index and middle fingers on the B and N keys, respectively; and to press the key corresponding to the red square when it appeared on the screen. Participants were asked to respond as quickly and accurately as possible. When they pressed a key, the red square disappeared and then reappeared in a new position. The position of the red square changed according to a pseudorandom pattern or to a pre-established sequence. Total randomness was limited only in the sense that the red square could not appear in the same position twice in a row. Six blocks of 80 stimulus–response pairs were given. Although colored (red) square presentation was random in blocks 1 and 6, in blocks 2–5, a five-item sequence of stimuli was repeated 16 times in each block. Participants were not informed about the repeating pattern. However, to verify whether participants had gained declarative knowledge of the sequence, at the end of the sixth block they were asked whether the red square presentation followed

a pattern. Each participant was also asked to reproduce the sequence on the keyboard. The degree of declarative knowledge gained was evaluated by calculating the percentage of items correctly reproduced in the ordered sequence. No differences between groups were found in the percentage of items reproduced ($p > 0.1$). Data were analyzed by computing RT and response accuracy in each trial.

Reaction time was calculated as the latency between the appearance of the stimulus on the screen and the key pressing, regardless of whether the correct key was pressed. Whether the participants implicitly learned the order in which the items alternated on the screen, their RTs in the ordered sequences should have gradually decreased with respect to the first random sequence and, more importantly, should have drastically increased during the last random sequence.

Averages of the median RTs of the two groups in the six consecutive blocks of the SRT test are shown in Figure 7.1.

Results documented different patterns of RT changes in the three groups across blocks and, crucially, the RTs of the three groups differed significantly passing from the fifth to the sixth block (Figure 7.1). This difference, which is usually considered the most reliable measure of visual–motor sequence learning, was highly significant in the controls ($p = 0.02$) and DS individuals ($p = 0.004$), but not in the WS individuals ($p = 1$). Note that the group effect was significant. In particular, in the first experimental block, when the participants did not know anything about the task, the WS group was faster than the other two groups, which in turn were quite similar ($p = 0.8$). Thus, although WS participants were faster than DS and typically developing children, two different RT curves were drawn throughout the blocks: Typically developing and DS participants exhibited the U-shaped learning curve usually observed in this type of task; WS participants performed similarly in both randomized and ordered blocks and, therefore, failed to exhibit a learning curve.

These findings document for the first time that procedural learning in individuals with ID depends on the etiology of the syndrome, and they provide support for the etiological specificity account of cognitive development in individuals with ID. This conclusion is reinforced by the fact that differences in procedural learning between the DS and WS groups could not be accounted for by differences in general level of cognitive development. In fact, the two groups of persons with ID were matched for

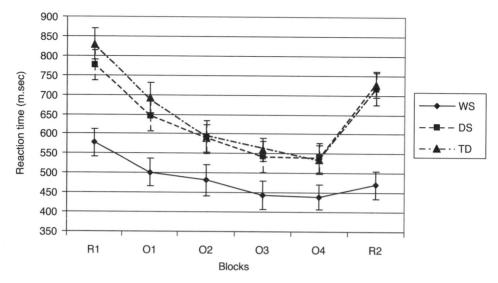

Fig. 7.1 Average reaction time performance and standard errors as a function of group and block, Ordered (O1, O2, O3, and O4 blocks) versus Random (R1 and R6 blocks) sequences (Vicari et al., 2007). Adapted with permission of John Wiley and Sons.

both CA and MA; moreover, no significant association was found between an overall index of procedural learning and measures of cognitive development, such as IQ and MA, either in the two groups of ID individuals or in the group of typically developing children.

In summary, the overall pattern of results emerging from the literature reviewed is quite inconsistent; indeed, some studies report normal performance and others deficient performance in ID individuals. However, much of the inconsistency may be related to the used CA-matched strategy of comparing participants; thus, the role also played by global cognitive efficiency in memory performances is underestimated. The overall level of cognitive efficiency of the ID groups investigated seems to be the main source of variability, with less compromised individuals usually reaching performance levels similar to those of the typically developing comparison participants, and more severely affected persons obtaining lower scores. In other cases, the nature of the information must be memorized (e.g., visuoperceptual vs. verbal) or the type of stimulus processing (perceptually driven vs. conceptually driven) could have made the difference. In any case, although these results are inconclusive, they permit rejecting Detterman's (1979) "everything hypothesis." Rather, a quite evident contrast emerges in the memory performances of ID individuals as a function of the experimental manipulation of both learning and retrieval conditions. On one side, there is absolute consistency in the experimental literature that, when the deliberate retrieval of intentionally

and/or effortfully encoded information is requested, the performance of ID individuals is poor in relation to CA- and MA-matched comparison groups. Conversely, when the memory of previously experienced procedures or information is tested implicitly, or when the task calls for the intentional retrieval of incidentally and/or automatically encoded information, the performance of ID individuals (at least those in the mild range of cognitive dysfunction) is frequently in the range of typically developing persons.

Memory and Learning in Intellectual Disability: A Neurobiological Perspective

The memory profile we described in people with ID is based on some specific characteristics of anomalous brain development. However, any attempt to identify which neuroanatomical structures are specifically involved in the memory impairment displayed by people with ID is speculative and must be based on qualitative comparisons of their deficits with those displayed by patients with acquired brain lesions.

Down Syndrome

According to autopsy observations, the brain weight of people with DS is lower than normal and their cerebellum, frontal, and temporal lobes are particularly small (Wisniewski, 1990). Consistent with this, evidence from volumetric magnetic resonance imaging (MRI) studies of individuals with DS suggests reduced overall brain volume, with disproportionately smaller volume in frontal, temporal (including uncus, amygdala, hippocampus, and parahippocampal gyrus), and cerebellar regions (Pinter, Eliez, Schmitt, Capone, & Reiss, 2001). By contrast, the brains of people with DS usually show relatively preserved volume of subcortical areas, such as lenticular nuclei (Bellugi, Mills, Jerningan, Hickok, & Galaburda, 1999) and posterior (parietal and occipital) cortical gray matter (Pinter et al., 2001). Based on these findings, the neuropsychological profiles we described in DS could be due to the differences observed in cortical and subcortical structures. For example, consistent with Fabbro, Alberti, Gagliardi, and Borgatti (2002), the reduced performance of people with DS on linguistic tasks may be partially explained as an impairment of the frontocerebellar structures involved in articulation and verbal working memory. In other words, the volumetric reduction of frontal and cerebellar areas in the brains of individuals with DS may determine the reduced efficiency of the cognitive processes usually sustained by the integrity of these cerebral regions, such as speech and phonological working memory (at least for the articulatory component). Likewise, reduced LTM capacity, which seems to be the most relevant characteristic of people with DS, may be related to temporal lobe dysfunction and, specifically, to hippocampal dysfunction (Pennington et al., 2003).

Concerning visual–spatial abilities, evidence from primates has shown that the extrastriate cortical areas are organized in two distinct functionally specialized systems: one is the dorsal stream (including the structures of the parietal cortex), which is involved in the visual processing of spatial localization, and the second is the ventral stream (including structures of the inferotemporal cortex) involved in processing information pertaining to the physical characteristics of objects (Mishkin & Ungerleider, 1982). The cortical structures involved in the perceptual processing of stimuli also participate in storage and recovery of the same information (Moscovitch et al., 1995). Concordantly, some experimental data deriving from studies on both humans and animals suggest that the maintenance and recovery of information pertaining to spatial position and the physical characteristics of the objects in LTM involve the ventral and the dorsal stream in different ways. For example, the inferotemporal regions of brain-injured patients are involved in remembering the visual characteristics of objects (Pigott & Milner, 1993). Similar investigations in monkeys have shown that bilateral ablation of these areas produces a serious deficit in recognition tests limited to the physical characteristics of the stimuli (Iwai & Osawa, 1990). In a positron emission tomography (PET) study evaluating the visual–object and visual–spatial abilities of LTM, Moscovitch et al. showed that the area most involved in the recovery of physical characteristics of objects is localized in the inferotemporal cortex, a region of the fusiform gyrus (area 37). In contrast, recovery of spatial localization primarily activates an area of the inferior parietal lobule in the region of the supramarginal gyrus (area 40). Consistent with the literature reported above, we may speculate that people with DS who perform relatively better in visual–object than in visual–spatial memory tests might present relatively preserved maturation of the dorsal compared to the ventral component of the visual system.

Neuropsychological (Molinari et al., 1997) and functional neuroimaging data (Van Der Graaf, De Jong, Maguire, Meiners, & Leenders, 2004) confirm the critical role of the basal ganglia and cerebellum in the implicit learning of visuo-motor skills. As reported above, the brains of individuals with DS exhibit severe cerebellar hypoplasia with normal morphology of basal ganglia (Jernigan, Bellugi, Sowell, Doherty, & Hesselink, 1993). Thus, in view of the normal skill learning displayed by individuals with DS, a prevalent role of basal ganglia development in the normal maturation of procedural memory can be suggested.

Williams Syndrome

The brains of individuals with WS usually exhibit specific, characteristic features that may be related to their atypical brain morphology (Martens et al., 2008). Specifically, remarkable atrophy of the posterior regions of the brain (Bellugi et al., 1999; Jernigan et al., 1993), as well as reduced volume in the posterior regions of the corpus callosum (Luders et al., 2007; Tomaiuolo et al., 2002) have been reported. The hypoplasia of the corpus callosum may determine defective callosal transfer of information, thus causing insufficient integration and coordination of the activity of posterior parts of both cerebral hemispheres. Furthermore, Van Essen et al. (2006) documented cortical folding abnormalities in individuals with WS that spread from the dorsoposterior to the ventroanterior regions bilaterally. Studies utilizing functional neuroimaging confirm a cortical dysfunction of posterior brain areas in WS. Namely, reduced resting blood flow has been shown in the anterior hippocampal formation and in the intraparietal/occipital sulcus (Meyer-Lindenberg et al., 2005), whereas hypoactivation during tasks of visual processing has been shown in the parietal region of the dorsal stream (Meyer-Lindenberg et al., 2004). All these findings support the hypothesis that the reduced posterior brain regions and corpus callosum may play a role in determining the visual–spatial difficulties of individuals with WS in both perceptual and memory domains.

The brain development of children with WS is also characterized by a remarkable atrophy of basal ganglia (Jernigan et al.,1993) and by a neurochemical alteration (reduction of the neurotransmitter N-acetylaspartate) in the cerebellum (Rae et al., 1998), thus suggesting a neurobiological substrate for the impaired maturation of procedural learning. At present, the relative contribution of abnormal basal ganglia and cerebellar development to the defective maturation of skill learning in WS children is only a matter of conjecture. Nevertheless, there are two reasons why the implicit memory disorders observed in WS may be associated with the volumetric reduction of the basal ganglia. First, the performance profile exhibited by WS children, which is characterized by impaired procedural learning of both visuo–motor and pure cognitive skills, resembles that of Huntington disease patients more than cerebellum-damaged patients. Second, as reported above, individuals with DS show severe atrophy of the cerebellum but normal procedural learning of both visuo-motor and cognitive tasks, which undermines the role of cerebellar circuit maturation in the development of skill learning.

Studies on genetic syndromes that describe their individual neuropsychological profiles in relation to specific brain characteristics are still sporadic, and there is no evidence that definitively demonstrates a causal relationship between brain features, cognitive abilities and behavior in individuals with DS and WS. Other studies directly evaluating the possible correlation between morphovolumetric and spectroscopic indexes of brain functioning and the ability of people with DS and WS to learn visuo-motor and cognitive procedures are needed to understand the relative contribution of the basal ganglia and abnormal cerebellar development to the impaired maturation of procedural memory in these people. This is a very fascinating challenge with great potential for clarifying the biological nature of behavior and, more specifically, for interpreting the differences observed in the cognitive and LTM functioning of people with DS, WS, and, more generally, etiologically well-defined forms of ID.

Conclusion

Memory is usually impaired in people with ID and occurs at different levels of memory articulation. Regarding LTM, differential patterns of impairment are confirmed across different etiological groups of ID individuals. For example, people with DS usually perform worse than typically developing comparisons matched for MA on verbal and visual–spatial explicit memory tasks, but similarly, in the implicit memory domain. It is noteworthy that the memory profile observed in DS is not the same as in persons with WS, who are characterized by relative strengths in visual LTM and by impairments in verbal and spatial memory, as well as in the implicit learning of new procedures.

In many persons with ID, memory profiles change with changes in etiology. The parallel evaluation of scores on neuropsychological tests and of morphovolumetric and neurofunctional data in specific etiological ID groups seems a promising avenue for establishing the possible correlates between impaired memory development and abnormal brain maturation.

Findings from the experimental literature reviewed in this chapter are relevant for people working in the fields of both normal memory development and of memory deficits following brain damage. The former can compare "normal" memory development with that of people with ID in an attempt to dissociate distinct functional components of the memory system on the basis of discrepant developmental trends. The latter can attempt to apply the same theoretical and experimental approaches used in the investigation of memory-disordered adults to the memory deficits exhibited by people with ID to gain new insights on the neural substrate and on the basic mechanisms of normal and pathological memory development.

Finally, these data can provide invaluable information for educational psychologists and teachers for planning evidence-based interventions to alleviate the learning difficulties of individuals with ID and to improve their quality of life.

Acknowledgments

The financial support of the Lejeune Foundation and Telethon (grant number GGP06122) are gratefully acknowledged. I would also like to thank Giovanni Augusto Carlesimo for his patient collaboration over the past 20 years.

References

Atkinson, J., Braddick, O., Anker, S., Curran, W., Andrew, R., Wattam-Bell, J., & Braddick, F. (2003). Neurobiological models of visuo-spatial cognition in children with Williams syndrome: Measures of dorsal-stream and frontal function. *Developmental Neuropsychology, 23*, 139–172.

Atkinson, J., King, J., Braddick, O., Nokes, L., Anker, S., & Braddick, F. (1997). A specific deficit of dorsal stream function in Williams syndrome. *NeuroReport, 8*, 1919–1922.

Atkinson, R. C., & Shiffrin, R. M. (1971). The control of short-term memory. *Scientific American, 225*, 82–90.

Atwell, J. A., Conners, F. A., & Merrill, E. C. (2003). Implicit and explicit learning in young adults with mental retardation. *American Journal on Mental Retardation, 108*, 56–68.

Bellugi, U., Lichtenberger, L., Jones, W., Lai, Z., & St. George, M. (2000). The neurocognitive profile of Williams syndrome: A complex pattern of strengths and weaknesses. *Journal of Cognitive Neuroscience, 12*(Suppl. 4), 7–29.

Bellugi, U., Mills, D., Jerningan, T., Hickok, G., & Galaburda, A. (1999). Linking cognition, brain structure, and brain function in Williams syndrome. In H. Tager-Flusberg (Ed.), *Neurodevelopmental disorders* (pp. 111–136). Cambridge, MA: MIT Press.

Brock, J., Brown, G. D. A., & Boucher, J. (2006). Free recall in Williams syndrome: Is there a dissociation between short and long term memory? *Cortex, 42*, 366–375.

Burack, J. A., & Zigler, E. (1990). Intentional and incidental memory in organically mentally retarded, familial retarded, and nonretarded individuals. *American Journal on Mental Retardation, 94*, 532–540.

Cantor, G. N., & Ryan, T. J. (1962). Retention of verbal pair-associated in normals and retardates. *American Journal of Mental Deficiency, 66*, 861–865.

Carlesimo, G. A., Marotta, L., & Vicari, S. (1997). Long-term memory in mental retardation: Evidence for a specific impairment in subjects with Down's syndrome. *Neuropsychologia, 35*, 71–79.

Detterman, D. K. (1979). Memory in the mentally retarded. In N. R. Ellis (Ed.), *Handbook of mental deficiency, psychological theory and research* (2nd ed., pp. 727–760). Hillsdale, NJ: Erlbaum.

Don, A. J., Schellenberg, E. G., Reber, A. S., DiGirolamo, K. M., & Wang, P. P. (2003). Implicit learning in children and adults with Williams syndrome. *Developmental Neuropsychology, 23*, 201–225.

Dulaney, C. L., Raz, N., & Devine, C. (1996). Effortful and automatic processes associated with Down syndrome and nonspecific mental retardation. *American Journal on Mental Retardation, 100*, 418–423.

Ellis, N. R. (1969). A behavioural research strategy in mental retardation: defense and critique. *American Journal of Mental Deficiency, 73*, 557–567.

Ellis, N. R., & Allison, P. (1988). Memory for frequency of occurrence in retarded and nonretarded persons. *Intelligence, 12*, 61–75.

Ellis, N. R., Woodley-Zanthos, P., & Dulaney, C. L. (1989). Memory for spatial location in children, adults, and mentally retarded persons. *American Journal on Mental Retardation, 93*, 521–527.

Fabbro, F., Alberti, A., Gagliardi, C., & Borgatti, R. (2002). Differences in native and foreign language repetition task between subjects with Williams and Down syndromes. *Journal of Neurolinguistics, 15*, 1–10.

Fisher, M., & Zeaman, D. (1970). Growth and decline of retardate intelligence. In N. R. Ellis (Ed.), *International review of research on mental retardation* Vol. 4 (pp. 151–191). New York: McGraw-Hill.

Glanzer, M. (1972). Storage mechanisms in recall. In G. H. Bower (Ed.), *The psychology of learning and motivation: Advances in research and theory* Vol. 5. New York: Academic Press.

Hasher, L., & Zacks, R. T. (1979). Automatic and effortful processes in memory. *Journal of Experimental Psychology: General, 108*, 356–388.

Hasher, L., & Zacks, R. T. (1984). Automatic processing of fundamental information. *American Psychologist, 39*, 1372–1388.

Heindel, W. C., Butters, N., & Salmon, D. P. (1988). Impaired learning of a motor skill in patients with Huntington's disease. *Behavioral Neuroscience, 102*, 141–147.

Iscoe, I., & Semler, I. J. (1964). Pair-associated in learning in normal and mentally retarded children as a function of four conditions. *Journal of Comparative Physiology and Psychology, 57*, 387–392.

Iwai, E., & Osawa, Y. (1990). *Vision memory and the temporal lobe*. New York: Elsevier.

Jarrold, C., Baddeley, A. D., & Phillips, C. (2007). Long-term memory for verbal and visual information in Down syndrome and Williams syndrome: Performance on the doors and people test. *Cortex, 43*, 233–247.

Jernigan, T. L., Bellugi, U., Sowell, E., Doherty, S., & Hesselink, R. (1993). Cerebral morphologic distinctions between WS and DS. *Archives of Neurology, 50*, 186–191.

Karmiloff-Smith, A., Grant, J., Berthoud, I., Davies, M., Howlin, P., & Udwin, O. (1997). Language and Williams syndrome: How intact is "intact." *Child Development, 68*, 274–290.

Katz, E. R., & Ellis, N. R. (1991). Memory for spatial location in retarded and nonretarded persons. *Journal of Mental Deficiency Research, 35*, 209–229.

Komatsu, S., Naito, M., & Fuke, T. (1996). Age-related and intelligence-related differences in implicit memory: Effects of generation on a word-fragment completion test. *Journal of Experimental Child Psychology, 62*, 151–172.

Luders, E., Di Paola, M., Tomaiuolo, F., Thompson, P. M., Toga, A. W., Vicari, S., et al. (2007). Effects of Williams syndrome on callosal thickness in scaled and native space. *Neuroreport, 18*, 203–207.

Martens, M. A., Wilson S. J., & Reutens, D. C. (2008). Research review: Williams syndrome: A critical review of the cognitive, behavioural, and neuroanatomical phenotype. *Journal of Child Psychology and Psychiatry, 49*, 576–608.

Mattson, S. N., & Riley, E. P. (1999). Implicit and explicit memory functioning in children with heavy prenatal alcohol exposure. *Journal International of Neuropsychological Society, 5*, 462–471.

McPherson, M. W. (1948). A survey of experimental studies of learning in individuals who achieve subnormal ratings on standardized psychometric measures. *American Journal of Mental Deficiency, 52*, 232–254.

Meyer-Lindenberg, A., Kohn, P., Mervis, C. B., Kippenhan, J. S., Olsen, R. K., Morris, C. A., & Berman, K. F. (2004). Neural basis of genetically determined visuo-spatial construction deficit in Williams syndrome. *Neuron, 43*, 623–631.

Meyer-Lindenberg, A., Mervis, C. B., Sarpal, D., Koch, P., Steele, S., Kohn, P., et al. (2005). Functional, structural, and metabolic abnormalities of the hippocampal formation in Williams syndrome. *Journal of Clinical Investigation, 115*, 1888–1895.

Mishkin, M., & Ungerleider, L. G. (1982). Contribution of striate inputs to the visuo-spatial functions of parieto-preoccipital cortex in monkeys. *Behavioral Brain Research, 6*, 57–77.

Molinari, M., Leggio, M. G., Solida, A., Ciorra, R., Misciagna, S., Silveri, M., & Petrosini, L. (1997). Cerebellum and procedural learning: Evidence from focal cerebellar lesions. *Brain, 120*, 1753–1762.

Moscovitch, C., Kapur, S., Kohler, S., & Houle, S. (1995). Distinct neural correlates of visual long-term memory for spatial location and object identity: A positron emission tomography study in humans. *Proceedings of the National Academy of Science, 92*, 3721–3725.

Nadel, L. (1999). Learning and memory in Down syndrome. In J. A. Rondal, D. L. J. Perera, & L. Nadel (Eds.), *Down syndrome: A review of current knowledge* (pp. 133–142). London: Whurr Publisher Ltd.

Nichols, S., Jones, W., Roman, M. J., Wulfeck, B., Delis, D. C., Reilly, J., & Bellugi, U. (2004). Mechanisms of verbal memory impairment in four developmental disorders. *Brain and Language, 88*, 180–189.

Pennington, B. F., Moon J., Edgin, J., Stedron, J., & Nadel, L. (2003). The neuropsychology of Down syndrome: Evidence for hippocampal dysfunction. *Child Development, 74*, 75–93.

Perrig, P., & Perrig, W. J. (1995). Implicit and explicit memory in mentally retarded, learning disabled and normal children. *Swiss Journal of Psychology, 54*, 77–86.

Pigott, S., & Milner, B. (1993). Capacity of visual short-term memory after unilateral frontal or anterior temporal-lobe resection. *Neuropsychologia, 31*, 1–15.

Pinter, J. D., Eliez, S., Schmitt, J. E., Capone, G. T., & Reiss, A. L. (2001). Neuroanatomy of Down's syndrome: A high-resolution MRI study. *American Journal of Psychiatry, 158*, 1659–1665.

Rae, C., Lee, M. A., Dixon, R. M., Blamire, A. M., Thompson, C. H., Styles, P., & Radda, G. K. (1998). Brain biochemistry in Williams syndrome: Evidence for a role of the cerebellum in cognition? *Neurology, 51*, 33–40.

Rossi, E. L. (1963). Associative clustering in normal and retarded children. *American Journal of Mental Deficiency, 67*, 700–704.

Schacter, D. L., Chiu, C. Y. P., & Ochsner, K. N. (1993). Implicit memory: A selective review. *Annual Review of Neuroscience, 16*, 159–182.

Schacter, D. L., Dobbins, I. G., & Schnyer, D. M. (2004). Specificity of priming: A cognitive neuroscience perspective. *Nature Review of Neuroscience, 5*, 853–862.

Schultz, E. E. (1983). Depth of processing by mentally retarded and MA-matched nonretarded individuals. *American Journal of Mental Deficiency, 88*, 307–313.

Spitz, H. H. (1966). The role of input organization in the learning and memory of mental retardates. In N. R. Ellis (Ed.), *International review on mental retardation* Vol. 2 (pp. 29–56). New York: Academic Press.

Squire, L. R. (1987). *Memory and brain.* Oxford, UK: Oxford University Press.

Takegata, R., & Furutuka, T. (1993). Perceptual priming effect in mentally retarded persons: Implicit and explicit remembering. *Japanese Journal of Educational, 41*, 176–182.

Tomaiuolo, F., Di Paola, M., Caravale, B., Vicari, S., Petrides, M., & Caltagirone, C. (2002). Morphology and morphometry of the corpus callosum in Williams syndrome: A magnetic resonance imaging analysis. *NeuroReport, 13*, 1–5.

Tulving, E., & Schacter, D. L. (1990). Priming and human memory systems. *Science, 247*, 301–306.

Udwin, O., & Yule, W. (1991). A cognitive and behavioral phenotype in Williams syndrome. *Journal of Clinical and Experimental Neuropsychology, 13*, 232–244.

Uecker, A., & Nadel, L. (1998). Spatial but not object memory impairments in children with fetal alcohol syndrome. *American Journal on Mental Retardation, 103*, 12–18.

Vakil, E., Shelef-Reshef, E., & Levy-Shiff, R. (1997). Procedural and declarative memory development. *American Journal on Mental Retardation, 102*, 147–160.

Van Der Graaf, F. H., De Jong, B. M., Maguire, R. P., Meiners, L. C., & Leenders, K. L. (2004). Cerebral activation related to skills practice in a double serial reaction time task: Striatal involvement in random-order sequence learning. *Brain Research and Cognitive Brain Research, 20*, 120–131.

Van Essen, D. C., Dierker, D., Snyder, A. Z., Raichle, M. E., Reiss, A. L., & Korenberg, J. (2006). Symmetry of cortical folding abnormalities in Williams syndrome revealed by surface-based analysis. *The Journal of Neuroscience, 26*, 5470–5483.

Vicari, S. (2006). Motor development and neuropsychological patterns in persons with Down syndrome. *Behavior Genetics, 36*, 355–364.

Vicari S., Bellucci S., & Carlesimo, G. A. (2000). Implicit and explicit memory: A functional dissociation in persons with Down syndrome. *Neuropsychologia, 38*, 240–251.

Vicari, S., Bellucci, S., & Carlesimo, G. A. (2001). Procedural learning deficit in children with Williams syndrome. *Neuropsychologia, 39*, 665–677.

Vicari, S., Bellucci, S., & Carlesimo, G. A. (2003). Visual and spatial working memory dissociation: Evidence from a genetic syndrome. *Developmental Medicine and Child Neurology, 45*, 269–273.

Vicari, S., Bellucci, S., & Carlesimo G. A. (2005). Visual and spatial long-term memory: Differential pattern of impairments in Williams and Down syndromes. *Developmental Medicine and Child Neurology, 47*, 305–311.

Vicari, S., Bellucci, S., & Carlesimo G. A. (2006). Evidence from two genetic syndromes for the independence of spatial and visual working memory. *Developmental Medicine and Child Neurology, 48*, 126–131.

Vicari, S., & Carlesimo, G. A. (2002). Children with intellectual disabilities. In A. Baddeley, B. Wilson, & M. Kopelman (Eds.), *Handbook of memory disorders* (pp 501–518). Chichester, UK: John Wiley & Sons, Ltd.

Vicari, S., & Carlesimo, G. A. (2006). Short-term memory deficits are not uniform in Down and Williams syndromes. *Neuropsychological review, 16*, 87–94.

Vicari, S., Carlesimo, G. A., Brizzolara, D., & Pezzini, G. (1996). Short-term memory in children with Williams syndrome: A reduced contribution of lexical-semantic knowledge to word span. *Neuropsychologia, 34*(9), 919–925.

Vicari, S., Verucci, L., & Carlesimo, G. A. (2007). Implicit memory is independent from IQ and age but not from etiology: Evidence from Down and Williams syndromes. *Journal of Intellectual Disability Research, 51*, 932–941.

Vinter, A., & Detable, C. (2003). Implicit learning in children and adolescents with mental retardation. *American Journal of Mental Retardation, 108*, 94–107.

Wang, P. P., & Bellugi, U. (1994). Evidence from two genetic syndromes for dissociation between verbal and visual-spatial short-term memory. *Journal of Clinical Experimental Neuropsychology, 16*, 317–322.

Winters, J. J., & Semchuk, M. T. (1986). Retrieval from long-term store as a function of mental age and intelligence. *American Journal of Mental Deficiency, 90*, 440–448.

Wisniewski, K. E. (1990). Down syndrome children often have brain with maturation delay, retardation of growth, and cortical digenesis. *American Journal of Medical Genetics (Suppl 7)*, 274–281.

Wyatt, B. S., & Conners, F. A. (1998). Implicit and explicit memory in individuals with mental retardation. *American Journal of Mental Retardation, 102*, 511–526.

Short-term Memory and Working Memory in Mental Retardation

Christopher Jarrold *and* Jon Brock

Abstract

This chapter provides an overview of the range of working memory impairments associated with learning disability, and the possible consequences of such deficits. In doing so, it raises a number of questions, notably: Are there aspects of short-term or working memory that are particularly vulnerable to mental retardation? Are there any syndrome-specific patterns of working memory impairments? And, how might these relate to educational outcomes and other aspects of cognitive and linguistic development? To properly interpret findings from studies involving individuals with mental retardation, the chapter begins by raising a number of general methodological points about the assessment of working memory, and by emphasizing the theoretical distinction between working memory and short-term memory.

Keywords: Working memory, cognitive development, memory impairment, learning disability, linguistic development, mental retardation

Working memory refers to the active maintenance of information while the same or other information is simultaneously processed (e.g., Baddeley & Logie, 1999; Engle, Tuholski, Laughlin, & Conway, 1999; Just & Carpenter, 1992) and is an important aspect of cognitive development. This is demonstrated by the fact that performance on measures of working memory is an excellent predictor of educational attainment (Bayliss, Jarrold, Gunn, & Baddeley, 2003; Daneman & Merikle, 1996; Hitch, Towse, & Hutton, 2001). Moreover, studies have consistently shown that working memory capacity is strongly related to intelligence—so-called psychometric *g*. Indeed, some researchers have argued that working memory is almost synonymous with *g* (Colom, Rebollo, Palacios, Juan-Espinosa, & Kyllonen, 2004; Kyllonen & Christal, 1990; see also Conway, Kane, & Engle, 2003; although see Ackerman, Beier, & Boyle, 2005 for a meta-analysis and critique of this field). For example, Süß, Oberauer, Wittman, Wilhelm, and Schulze (2002) have suggested that,

"at present, working memory capacity is the best predictor for intelligence that has yet been derived from theories and research on human cognition" (p. 284). It is unsurprising, therefore, that researchers should focus on working memory as a possible underlying cause of many different forms of learning disability.

Much of the research into working memory deficits associated with mental retardation has been guided by Baddeley's (1986) model. According to Baddeley, working memory involves the combined functioning of a central control system, the central executive, and two peripheral short-term memory (STM) systems, the phonological loop and the visuospatial sketch pad, that are specialized for the maintenance of verbal and visuospatial information respectively. Researchers have typically been interested in whether these different components of the model can be impaired selectively or differentially in particular developmental disorders (see Alloway & Gathercole, 2006). However, our focus in this chapter is less on specific disorders (although examples from specific syndromes will be covered where relevant); rather, our aim is to provide an overview of the range of working memory impairments associated with learning disability, and the possible consequences of such deficits. In doing this we ask a number of questions, notably: Are there aspects of short-term or working memory that are particularly vulnerable to mental retardation? Are there any syndrome-specific patterns of working memory impairments? And, how might these relate to educational outcomes and other aspects of cognitive and linguistic development? To properly interpret findings from studies involving individuals with mental retardation, we begin by raising a number of general methodological points about the assessment of working memory, and by emphasizing the theoretical distinction between working memory and STM.

Theoretical and Methodological Issues

Individuals with mental retardation or learning difficulties are often unable to comprehend long sentences and follow complicated instructions, and it may be necessary to break down tasks into smaller, more manageable chunks that can be processed step-by-step. In some cases, these difficulties can be attributed to basic memory problems. Thus, for example, by the end of a long sentence, the individual may have already forgotten the beginning. Often, however, difficulties in holding on to the information are exacerbated when the individual is required to engage in other activities, ignore extraneous information, or act upon the incoming information. For instance, in carrying out a set of instructions, the act of performing the initial operations may impede the ability to remember the remaining instructions (Gathercole & Alloway, 2006; Gathercole, Lamont, & Alloway, 2006). This distinction between basic memory processes and the ability to maintain information despite competing task requirements is fundamental to the distinction between STM and working memory. These two terms are often used interchangeably; however, in this chapter, we will limit the use of the term *working memory* to situations in which individuals not only have to maintain information, but also have to actively transform that material or engage in some other distracting activity. We use the term *short-term memory* to refer to cases in which maintenance only is required.

In line with these definitions, STM is typically assessed using so-called *simple span* tasks in which participants recall, usually in correct serial order, the list of just-presented items. For example, visuospatial STM is often assessed using the Corsi span task (cf. Milner, 1971), in which participants are required to recall series of spatial locations by recreating the just-presented spatial sequence. Similarly, in digit and word span tasks, participants are asked to repeat lists of varying lengths to determine the maximum number, or span, that they can accurately maintain.

Despite their structural similarity, many researchers would argue that digit and Corsi span tasks tap independent memory stores. This view follows directly from Baddeley's (1986) model, which, as noted above, suggests that independent mechanisms exist for storing verbal and visuospatial information in the short-term. Indeed, there is considerable evidence that aspects of verbal and visuospatial STM are dissociable, including data from the developmental literature. For example, Hale, Bronik, and Fry (1997) found that 8- and 10-year-old children's digit and Corsi spans were subject to selective interference from verbal and visuospatial dual tasks, respectively.

Similarly, factor analytic studies of children's STM have tended to produce separate verbal and visuospatial factors (e.g., Bayliss et al., 2003; Gathercole, Pickering, Ambridge, & Wearing, 2004). There are, nevertheless, apparent similarities between children's performance on verbal and visuospatial STM tasks, particularly in terms of the pattern of order errors observed (Pickering, Gathercole, & Peaker, 1998). Moreover, studies that have examined developmental changes in these measures have shown that they share substantial age-related variance (Bayliss, Jarrold, Baddeley, Gunn, & Leigh, 2005; Chuah & Maybery, 1999). One suggestion, therefore, is that the development of STM rests on changes in the efficiency of a domain-general maintenance process (cf. Jones, Farrand, Stuart, & Morris, 1995) that operates on dissociable content domains (Jarrold & Bayliss, 2007; Pickering et al., 1998).

In contrast to STM, working memory is often measured using *complex span* tasks, in which participants are again required to recall a series of items, usually in correct serial order, but also have to complete a subsidiary task before the presentation of each item. In many instances, the completion of the interleaved subsidiary processing tasks is what provides the participant with the to-be-remembered items. For example, in reading span tasks (e.g., Daneman & Carpenter, 1980), participants read a series of sentences, often judging them for veracity, and have to remember the final word of each sentence for subsequent recall. Other complex span measures have been developed that vary the modality of either the processing or storage component of the task (e.g., Case, Kurland, & Goldberg, 1982; Hitch & McAuley, 1991; Shah & Miyake, 1996) but all have in common the requirement to maintain target items in the face of the potentially distracting effects of concurrent processing operations.

Complex span tasks are not necessarily the only way of assessing working memory (see below) but, importantly, they have good construct validity insofar as they correlate well with higher-level abilities such as academic achievement and fluid intelligence (see Conway et al., 2005). Crucially, these correlations are typically stronger than those observed between higher-level abilities and simple span measures (Bayliss et al., 2003; Daneman & Merikle, 1996; Lépine, Barrouillet, & Camos, 2005; Oberauer, Schulze, Wilhelm, & Süß, 2005), indicating that working memory measures capture something more than STM tasks. Although both simple and complex span tasks share a storage component—namely, the requirement to hold in mind information in correct serial order—complex span tasks differ from their simple span counterparts in two important respects: First, they involve an additional processing component, and consequently, the efficiency with which one can complete this aspect of the task will affect overall performance. Second, the *combination* of processing and storage requirements in a complex span task introduces an additional element associated with the need to maintain storage items in the face of concurrent and potentially distracting processing. It is this element that is thought to correspond to the executive aspect of working memory (Engle et al., 1999; Engle, 2002), or, more specifically, the central executive within Baddeley's (1986) model.

Bayliss et al. (2003) examined these two aspects of complex span performance by assessing the extent to which it was related to separate measures of individuals' ability to carry out the storage and processing aspects of the task. Performance on the separate processing task predicted complex span scores even when performance on the separate storage task was controlled for. In addition, the remaining "residual" variance in complex span performance, over and beyond that attributable to the storage and processing components, was related to individuals' academic attainment and intelligence (see also Bayliss, Jarrold, Baddeley, Gunn, & Leigh, 2005). This finding, the authors argued, is consistent with the view that complex span performance depends on the additional, executive ability of combining storage and processing operations.

In sum, complex span tasks share storage requirements with simple span tasks, but are additionally affected by individuals' processing efficiency and their ability to combine processing and storage operations. Correspondingly, working memory can be viewed as an extension of STM, insofar as both abilities involve short-term storage, but working memory has additional processing and executive control aspects. Having clarified this distinction, the remainder of the chapter considers the extent to which mental retardation of various types is associated with deficits in short-term storage of information, and the executive aspects of working memory.

Short-term Memory

As noted in the preceding section, STM for verbal and visuospatial information is widely assumed to tap separable memory stores (Baddeley, 1986), although it is unclear to what extent common mechanisms support the retention of items in these systems. An important question, therefore, in the context of the study of learning disability and mental retardation is whether STM deficits dissociate along verbal and visuospatial lines and, if so, whether this reflects selective impairment to specific STM systems, or more general problems in the verbal or visuospatial domains. In the immediately following subsections, we examine these issues in relation to two developmental disorders, Down syndrome (DS) and Williams syndrome (WS). Having addressed this question, we consider possible underlying causes of any such deficits in terms of potential problems in rehearsal and in the representation of item and order information in STM. We conclude this section by looking at potential consequences of impaired STM.

Domain-specific Short-term Memory Impairments in Down and Williams Syndromes

Down syndrome and WS are genetic disorders associated with mental retardation, although this is often more marked in those with DS (e.g., Klein & Mervis, 1999). Cognitive profiles in both disorders are somewhat uneven; individuals with DS tend to have poorer verbal than nonverbal abilities (e.g., Chapman, 1997; Laws & Bishop, 2004), whereas WS is associated with specific deficits in visuospatial cognition (e.g., Farran & Jarrold, 2003; Mervis, Morris, Robinson, & Bertrand, 1999). This dissociation between verbal and visuospatial capabilities has been mirrored in studies comparing STM in the two disorders. In the first such study, Wang and Bellugi (1994) found that individuals with DS performed less well than did individuals with WS on a digit span task, whereas the opposite pattern was observed on the Corsi span task. Subsequent studies have largely replicated this pattern of findings (Klein & Mervis, 1999; Vicari et al., 2004). In particular, Jarrold, Baddeley, and Hewes (1999) reported that, relative to individuals with mental retardation of unspecified etiology, individuals with DS were selectively impaired on the digit span task, whereas individuals with WS were selectively impaired on the Corsi span task. It is important to note, however, that neither verbal STM in WS nor visuospatial STM in DS can be considered to be intact; in both disorders, STM is impaired relative to chronological age expectations. As such, the contrast between STM capabilities in WS and DS should not be portrayed as a "pure" double dissociation.

An important consideration here is whether apparently selective deficits in STM may in fact be caused by more general representational deficits; as noted above, poor STM performance can be characterized in terms of an impairment to a specific subsystem with Baddeley's (1986) working memory model, but it may reflect more general difficulties in dealing with verbal or visuospatial information. This issue is particularly relevant in this instance because WS is associated with severe deficits in visuospatial cognition. Indeed, Jarrold et al. (1999) found that the performance of individuals with WS on the Corsi span task was no worse than that of individuals with undifferentiated mental retardation when controlling for visuospatial skills. Thus, although visuospatial STM in WS may well be poorer than one would expect given individuals' overall level of ability, we cannot yet be certain that it is any poorer than expected, given the general visuospatial difficulties associated with the condition.

A similar argument could also be applied to verbal STM deficits in DS. As noted above, DS is associated with severe language deficits, and considerable evidence suggests that individuals' knowledge of the lexical, and perhaps also sublexical, properties of their language can support their performance on tests of verbal STM (see Brener, 1940; Majerus & Van der Linden, 2003; Thorn & Frankish, 2005). As Hulme and Roodenrys (1995) have pointed out, individuals with relatively impoverished language knowledge would be expected to perform less well on tests of verbal STM than would comparison groups with a richer language knowledge. In addition,

many individuals with DS have severe speech production difficulties that would be predicted to impact more on verbal tasks than on nonverbal tasks and may therefore contribute to poor verbal STM performance (cf. Cairns & Jarrold, 2005).

Our recent research in DS has explored the extent to which verbal STM deficits can be "explained away" in terms of more general speech and language difficulties. Our approach has been to use verbal STM measures that avoid the need to give a spoken response and then look at the impact of linguistic knowledge on performance. In our first study (Brock & Jarrold, 2004), we presented participants with an item recognition task, asking them to listen to two lists and then determine whether the items were the same or different. Unsurprisingly, performance was superior when the items were real words as opposed to made-up nonwords. Importantly, however, this "lexicality effect" was larger among individuals with DS than among control children, suggesting that, if anything, the DS group were more reliant on linguistic knowledge to support task performance. This was despite the fact that their overall performance was poorer. Participants were also given an order recognition task, in which the two lists always contained the same items, but with a change to the order of presentation of items in the second list on 50% of trials. Consistent with previous findings (Gathercole, Pickering, Hall, & Peaker, 2001; Thorn, Gathercole, & Frankish, 2002), the lexicality effect was minimized, indicating that word knowledge did not substantially affect performance. Nevertheless, individuals with DS still performed poorly on this task (see also Jarrold, Baddeley, & Phillips, 2002). In a second study (Brock & Jarrold, 2005), we showed that individuals with DS were significantly impaired on a digit reconstruction task in which they were required to point to numbers on a touch screen in response to a spoken list of digits. This was true, even when controlling for performance on a closely matched Corsi span task and the speed with which individuals could identify and search for spoken digits on the screen. Together, these findings suggest that the deficit seen among individuals with DS on traditional verbal STM tasks such as digit span is not caused by domain-general problems, but rather by specific difficulties in representing verbal information in STM.

Mechanisms of Verbal Short-term Memory Impairments

The above review of STM deficits associated with mental retardation shows that, although generalized visuospatial or linguistic difficulties can certainly account for poor STM performance in some cases, and may well play a part in accounting for deficits in others, developmental conditions appear to be associated with more fundamental impairments in the way information is represented in STM. This evidence is strongest in the case of verbal STM, and the following subsections consider the specific mechanisms that might underpin such deficits.

Rehearsal

Many studies investigating verbal STM deficits in mental retardation have been motivated by Baddeley's (1986) model of the phonological loop. This involves two components—a limited capacity phonological store and a rehearsal mechanism that is used for refreshing decayed phonological traces. According to the phonological loop model, the efficiency of rehearsal depends on the speed with which items can be rehearsed. This can explain why participants are better at recalling lists of short words than they are at recalling lists of long words, and why individuals with rapid speech rates (and presumably, therefore, faster rehearsal) perform better on serial recall tasks than do those with slower speech rates (Baddeley, Thomson, & Buchanan, 1975). The presence of word length effects has therefore been taken as an index of whether or not a certain group is engaging in rehearsal, and overt speech rate has been used to assess the speed or efficiency of that rehearsal.

Hulme and Mackenzie (1992) argued that verbal STM deficits may arise in various forms of mental retardation as a consequence of inefficient or even absent subvocal rehearsal processes. Indeed, studies have shown that a relative reduction in overt speech rate can account for observed verbal STM deficits in individuals with reading disability (Avons & Hanna, 1995; Swanson & Ashbaker, 2000), speech production difficulties (Raine, Hulme, Chadderton, & Bailey, 1991; White, Craft, Hale, & Park, 1994), and WS (Jarrold, Cowan, Hewes, & Riby, 2004). In a similar vein, a number of authors have argued that individuals with DS might show particularly poor verbal STM performance because of a failure to engage in articulatory rehearsal (Broadley & MacDonald, 1993; Comblain, 1994). Consistent with this view, Hulme and McKenzie (1992) found that individuals with DS did not demonstrate a reliable word length effect (although see Jarrold, Baddeley, & Hewes, 2000) or a reliable relationship between overt speech rate and STM performance (see also Jarrold, Cowan, et al., 2004). However, it appears unlikely that a failure to rehearse can entirely account for poor verbal STM performance in DS. Evidence suggests that typically developing children do not develop specific verbal rehearsal strategies until around the age of 7 years (Flavell, Beach, & Chinsky, 1966; Gathercole, Adams, & Hitch, 1994). Studies of DS usually involve typically developing children who are somewhat younger than this and are, therefore, unlikely to be rehearsing either. If this is the case, and these children still outperform individuals with DS, then this implies that the absence of rehearsal cannot account for verbal STM deficits in DS. Furthermore, verbal STM deficits have been observed among individuals with DS relative to comparison groups who have comparable speech rates, and who would therefore presumably have comparable rates of rehearsal were rehearsal taking place (Jarrold et al., 2000; Kanno & Ikeda, 2002).

In sum, although evidence is consistent with the view that failure to rehearse or a reduced efficiency of rehearsal can account for the difficulties that some individuals with mental retardation have on digit or word span tasks, this is not conclusive and certainly does not provide a complete explanation of all observed verbal STM deficits. From the point of view of the phonological loop model, one must conclude by default that DS is associated with an impaired phonological store (Jarrold, Purser, & Brock, 2006)—a deficit that may well also be present in other developmental disorders.

Item and Order Memory

The phonological loop model does not itself specify the mechanisms by which information is maintained in the phonological store. More recent models have, however, attempted to address this issue. Although they differ in the precise mechanisms involved, a common feature of these models is that they incorporate independent mechanisms for maintaining information about the items in a list and for encoding their serial order (see e.g., Brown, Preece, & Hulme, 2000; Burgess & Hitch, 1999; Page & Norris, 1998; see Burgess & Hitch, 2005, for a review). Such models raise the question of whether poor verbal STM in mental retardation is a reflection of impaired item memory or a deficit in serial order memory.

In general, the available evidence suggests that order memory mechanisms are more vulnerable in mental retardation (or at least that order memory deficits contribute most to group differences in verbal STM performance). For example, Brock,

McCormack, and Boucher (2005) reported that children with WS or with mental retardation of unknown etiology showed a selective deficit in order as opposed to item memory. Participants completed a probed serial recall task, in which they were presented with a list of words or nonwords and were then required to recall the single item that had occurred at a specified position in the list. The performance of these two groups of children was significantly poorer than that of a typically developing comparison group matched on receptive vocabulary knowledge. Importantly, however, error analyses revealed that group differences were driven almost exclusively by order errors (recalling an item that had occurred at a different position in the list), with no significant differences in item errors (recalling an item from outside the list or giving no response). A similar pattern of findings was observed in a more recent study of Velocardiofacial syndrome (VCFS) by Majerus, Van der Linden, Bressand, and Eliez (2006). Individuals with VCFS demonstrated significant impairments relative to controls on two serial order tasks—a test of order reconstruction and an order recognition task. However, there were no significant group differences on an item recognition task, in which participants were required to determine whether or not a single item was included in a just-presented list.

A slightly different pattern of results was found in our study of item and order memory in DS reviewed above (Brock & Jarrold, 2004). Although individuals with DS performed poorly on an order recognition task, they performed even less well on an item recognition task, in which they were required to decide whether a repeated list contained a single-phoneme change in one of the items. However, individuals with DS also showed a trend toward poorer performance on a simple phonological discrimination task that had minimal memory demands. This finding suggests that basic memory deficits may have been exacerbated by phonological discrimination difficulties that are perhaps related to hearing problems common in DS (e.g., Marcell & Cohen, 1992). As such, this study should not be taken as conclusive evidence that individuals with DS have selectively impaired item memory.

A number of studies have investigated STM for item information among individuals with developmental delay by assessing their ability to "scan" for targets within to-be-remembered lists (cf. Sternberg, 1966). More specifically, participants are given a list of target items to remember, followed by a series of individual probe items, and are asked to judge whether each probe item is a member of the target list. The typical finding from this task is that individuals' response times depend on the number of items in the target set, suggesting that a search of the target set occurs in response to each probe (Sternberg, 1966). Consequently, the slope of the search function with increasing target set size is thought to provide an index of efficiency of memory search (Hulme, Newton, Cowan, Stuart, & Brown, 1999; but see Monsell, 1978). Studies of individuals with mental retardation have provided evidence for increases in the *intercept* of the slope function but somewhat weaker evidence for increases in search slopes (Mosley, 1985; Phillips & Nettlebeck, 1984; Todman & Gibb, 1985). It is, therefore, possible that the reductions in speed of processing that one would expect to be associated with mental retardation lead to a fixed, general slowing in reaction times rather than a slower rate of search. However, the inconsistency observed across these studies may well be a reflection of heterogeneity in the samples employed, as this work has tended to focus on populations with relatively general learning difficulties rather than specific disorders. Consequently, there is a limit to what one can infer from these findings (cf. Burack, Iarocci, Flanagan, & Bowler, 2004).

In sum, there is more evidence of difficulties in the maintenance of serial order information among individuals with mental retardation than there is of difficulties in the representation of item information, although the latter may clearly be compromised by encoding difficulties associated with any particular condition. This suggests that serial order memory deficits in mental retardation may often reflect a reduction in the fidelity of a temporal ordering mechanism or a difficulty in making associations between items and their serial position (cf. Brown et al., 2000). What is less clear is whether such a deficit is specific to problems of serial ordering of verbal information, or rather reflects domain-general ordering difficulties. As noted above, there is evidence from typical development to suggest that a common mechanism is involved in the maintenance of order information in both verbal and visuospatial STM tasks (Bayliss, Jarrold, Baddeley, Gunn, & Leigh, 2005; Chuah & Mayberry, 1999; Pickering et al., 1998). However, Brock and Jarrold (2005) found specific deficits in the reconstruction of verbal serial order rather than visuospatial serial order in DS, thus raising the possibility that order information in these two domains may be supported by separable systems, which happen to develop in parallel in the typical case.

The Consequences of Short-term Memory Impairments

It has long been argued that STM plays an important role in aspects of long-term learning (Atkinson & Shiffrin, 1968). Baddeley (2000) has speculated that visuospatial STM may be involved in the learning of "spatial semantics," such as route finding, and there is some evidence from the adult neuropsychological literature to suggest that visuospatial STM deficits might cause problems of spatial learning (Hanley, Young, & Pearson, 1991). Farran, Blades, Tranter, and Boucher (2006) reported that individuals with WS had relative difficulties in retracing an unfamiliar route and also performed poorly on a small-scale maze task. Although it may be tempting to hypothesize that these difficulties are a result of visuospatial STM impairments, as noted above, it is impossible to be sure at present whether STM difficulties in WS are a cause or consequence of visuospatial impairments.

Researchers have paid considerably more attention to the possible causal relationship between STM and long-term learning in the verbal domain. Baddeley, Gathercole, and Papagno (1998) have proposed that STM capacity places an important constraint on language development and, more specifically, is critically involved in vocabulary acquisition, because the accuracy with which one maintains a representation of the phonological form of new items determines the ease of novel word learning. Consistent with this view, there is evidence from studies of typically developing children that early verbal STM skills predict later vocabulary development (Gathercole, Willis, Emslie, & Baddeley, 1992) as well as performance on word-learning tasks (Gathercole, Hitch, Service, & Martin, 1997). Somewhat less clear-cut results were reported in a study looking at the language capabilities of 8-year-old children who, 3 years previously, had been identified as having specific verbal STM deficits (Gathercole, Tiffany, Briscoe, Thorn, & The ALSPAC team, 2005). Vocabulary knowledge was unimpaired among a subgroup of children with persisting verbal STM problems but *was* impaired among a separate subgroup whose verbal STM problems had resolved over time.

Baddeley et al.'s (1998) account implies that STM impairments may contribute to deficits or delays in language development. However, proving causation is extremely difficult, as illustrated by research on specific language impairment (SLI). It has been widely argued that children with SLI have extremely poor verbal STM and that this may be an underlying cause of their language difficulties (see e.g., Gathercole & Baddeley, 1990; Kirchner & Klatzky, 1985). In fact, most of the evidence here comes from studies using tests of nonword repetition, in which participants are required to repeat exactly a series of nonsense words such as "perplisteronk" (e.g., Archibald & Gathercole, 2006; Dollaghan & Campbell 1998; Gathercole & Baddeley, 1990). Although such tasks clearly involve the recall of verbal material (e.g., Gathercole, Willis, Emslie, & Baddeley, 1994), the poor performance of individuals with SLI could equally be a reflection of difficulties in identifying phonemes or poor knowledge of the "phonotactic" constraints in their native language (e.g., Snowling, Chiat, & Hulme, 1991; van der Lely & Howard, 1993). Surprisingly few studies have directly measured performance on digit or word span tasks and, although these studies have shown that performance on such tasks is below age expectations (Briscoe, Bishop, & Norbury, 2001), the levels observed tend not to be significantly worse than those seen in language-matched comparison groups (Gathercole & Baddeley, 1990; van der Lely & Howard, 1993). It is, therefore, difficult to rule out the alternative hypothesis that language impairments lead to poor performance on verbal STM (cf. Hulme & Roodenrys, 1995).

Clearly, such arguments also have important implications for theories of language development in individuals with mental retardation. Jarrold, Baddeley, Hewes, Leeke, and Phillips (2004, Study 2) attempted to tease apart the alternative causal hypotheses by testing a large sample of children with mental retardation of unknown etiology, dividing them into two groups that were matched on receptive vocabulary knowledge at around the 5-year equivalent level, but were mismatched on age and therefore also on rate of vocabulary acquisition. If verbal STM deficits are simply a reflection of poor verbal abilities, then one would predict that the two groups, matched on verbal ability, would perform similarly on STM tasks. In fact, the younger group, who had acquired the same vocabulary knowledge at a much faster rate, outperformed the older group on a range of measures of verbal STM. This is consistent with the view that verbal STM skills determine the rate of vocabulary acquisition among such individuals. Once again, this study is open to the criticism that the sample was heterogeneous, and that different individuals may have had different underlying causes of their mental retardation. However, there is no reason to suspect that the two subsamples created from the larger group differed from one another in terms of their heterogeneity. It is also worth pointing out that similar patterns of performance have been observed in studies, reviewed above, showing that individuals with DS have poorer verbal STM than younger, typically developing children or children with other developmental disorders, even when vocabulary knowledge is controlled for. As noted previously, such findings are inconsistent with the view that poor vocabulary knowledge leads to poor STM performance, but are compatible with claims that impaired verbal STM leads to a slower rate of language acquisition (cf. Chapman, 1995; Jarrold, Baddeley, & Phillips, 1999; Laws, 1998).

In sum, the evidence to support the causal hypothesis that STM deficits lead to impaired language acquisition remains indirect. Given that Baddeley et al.'s (1998) account predicts that vocabulary learning in particular should be adversely affected by such a deficit, there is a surprising lack of studies investigating new word learning in individuals with language delay (Gathercole & Alloway, 2006). One study that looked explicitly at new word learning in DS using experimental measures found that individuals were unimpaired at producing the phonological label that they had been told applied to a novel item (Chapman, Kay-Raining Bird, & Schwartz, 1990), a finding at odds with the predictions of a verbal STM deficit account. However, in this study, participants were only required to learn one name of one object, and rather lenient scoring criteria for the accuracy of the production of this name were employed. Consequently, this test may have lacked the power to observe group differences. It is also important to note that receptive vocabulary is a relative strength among the various language functions in DS (Chapman, 1997; Vicari, Caselli, Gagliardi, Tonucci, & Volterra, 2002), which again calls into question the extent to which verbal STM deficits lead to problems of vocabulary acquisition in the condition. One possibility is that individuals with DS, and perhaps also SLI, acquire vocabulary in an atypical way and compensate for problems in verbal STM by relying more on lexical and semantic associations between novel words and existing lexical entries (cf. Baddeley, 1993). However, at present, this suggestion is only speculative, and remains to be verified empirically.

Working Memory

As noted above, working memory capacity—as opposed to STM—is strongly associated with intelligence and educational outcomes. It is perhaps unsurprising, therefore, that individuals with learning difficulties often show severe deficits on working memory tasks. For example, Henry (2001) compared simple and complex span performance in individuals who were matched for age, but who varied in degree of severity of their learning disability, and found that the various different IQ groups differed more in complex span than in simple span performance. Similarly, Gathercole and Pickering (2001) found that children in mainstream educational settings who had been identified as having special educational needs differed more from their peers on complex span tasks than on measures of STM. It is, however, worth noting that the task that most clearly distinguished the groups was backward digit recall. This task is assumed to tap working memory because it involves the manipulation of to-be-remembered information; in this case, to allow recall of the presented items in reverse order. Although this measure differs in form from complex span tasks, evidence suggests that it taps the same underlying construct (Conway et al., 2005).

Having said this, the analysis of complex span performance presented at the start of this chapter showed that individuals can perform poorly on working memory tasks for a number of reasons. Indeed, in a study in which individuals with generalized learning difficulties were given complex span tasks, as well as separate measures of storage ability and processing efficiency, Bayliss, Jarrold, Baddeley, and Leigh (2005) found that levels of complex span performance were unimpaired in this group. However, the individuals with learning difficulties performed less well than typically developing comparison individuals on simple span storage measures, while showing generally faster speed of processing. Although one must, again, be cautious in placing too much weight on data from a potentially heterogenous sample, these results do show that comparable levels of complex span performance can be reached in different ways; in this case, reflecting a different balance of strengths and weaknesses in the storage and processing aspects of the task.

More generally, when evaluating overall performance on complex span tasks, or indeed, many other working memory measures, one needs to ensure that poor performance is not simply a consequence of individuals having difficulty on the STM components that are necessarily embedded in these tasks. For example, it would not be at all surprising to find that individuals with DS performed poorly on a reading span task, given that one would expect them to find the verbal recall component of this task difficult (although see Pennington, Moon, Edgin, Stedron, & Nadel, 2003). Similarly, one would expect individuals to struggle on complex span tasks if they have particular difficulties in completing the processing components of such tasks (cf. Daneman & Tardif, 1987). For example, Siegel and Ryan (1989) found that individuals with mathematical learning difficulties performed poorly on a counting span working memory task in which they had to count the number of dots shown on a series of cards and remember these totals for subsequent recall (cf. Case et al. 1982). This finding was subsequently replicated by Hitch and McAuley (1991), who went on to show that, in their sample at least, this deficit in working memory performance was matched by a deficit in the time taken to carry out the processing component of the complex span task; that is, in counting the dots to generate the to-be-remembered totals. In other words, these findings indicate that individuals with learning difficulties might show poor working memory performance simply because they have difficulty in completing the component processing operations of the task. Crucially, one would not want to argue that this reflects an impairment to any executive aspect of working memory, because carrying out processing operations such as counting dots on cards is not necessarily executive in nature (Jarrold & Bayliss, 2007). Rather, to be certain that individuals are experiencing executively mediated deficits in combining the storage and processing operations of any working memory task, one needs to examine whether individuals have more difficulties on complex span tasks than one would expect, given their general storage capacity and processing efficiency (Bayliss et al., 2003; Engle et al., 1999; Kyllonen & Cristal, 1990). In other words, the stringent test of an executive account of working memory difficulties involves showing a reliably greater impairment in working memory performance than in STM or general speed of processing considered in isolation.

Executive Control and Working Memory

Few studies of working memory among individuals with mental retardation have properly applied such a stringent test and examined whether any deficits in performance exist over and beyond those attributable to deficits in STM capacity or processing efficiency. However, there are studies of developmental disorders that are not consistently associated with mental retardation, which nevertheless show how such an approach might be informative, and which indicate that the executive aspect of working memory might well be closely related to IQ differences among such individuals.

Attention Deficit Hyperactivity Disorder

Attention deficit hyperactivity disorder (ADHD) is associated with problems of executive control, although, perhaps unsurprisingly, deficits in inhibitory control appear to be the most marked feature of the executive impairments associated with the condition (Barkley, 1997; Pennington & Ozonoff, 1996). Although ADHD is not clearly associated with mental retardation, studies of working memory in the condition (reviewed comprehensively in Roodenrys et al., 2006) suggest that the extent of any deficit observed may depend on whether or not comparison groups are equated for IQ.

For example, two studies have shown evidence of deficits in working memory in ADHD that appear not to be attributable to problems in STM or processing efficiency, but which were observed relative to comparison groups who were of higher IQ. Karatekin (2004) examined both short-term and working memory among individuals with ADHD. Short-term memory was assessed using verbal and visuospatial versions of the scanning tasks described above, in which participants were presented with a memory set of a number of letters that were presented in different spatial locations on the screen. Following a variable delay, a probe letter was presented in a position on the screen, and participants were either asked to judge whether that letter (verbal condition) or that location (visuospatial condition) had been presented in the initial memory set. Individuals with ADHD were unimpaired, relative to an age-matched comparison group, in terms of accuracy on this task. However, these individuals were impaired on a separate, working memory dual task in which they were required to make speeded responses following the onset of a visual target, and, in one condition, simultaneously hold in mind a list of digits. Individuals with ADHD showed a reliably greater slowing of reaction times than the comparison individuals when simultaneously required to maintain a digit load, suggesting they suffered particularly from the combination of a memory load and a processing task.

Similar results were reported by Cornoldi et al. (2001, Study 1), who compared the performance of individuals with ADHD and an age-matched comparison group on a complex span task that required the inhibition of potentially distracting processing information, as well as on a control "dual" task in which processing material did not need to be inhibited.

In the complex span task, participants were presented with a series of sublists of nouns. They had to tap the table whenever an animal name was heard, and remember the last noun presented within each sublist. In the control task, participants still had to tap whenever an animal was presented, but had to remember all the items presented (fewer items in total were presented in this task). This control task therefore involved both processing and storage but, crucially, did not require individuals to resist interference from animal names they had responded to with a tap. There was a trend for individuals with ADHD to be impaired on the latter task, but the groups clearly differed on the complex span task. Moreover, when individuals with ADHD made errors, they were much more likely to respond with an animal name that they should have inhibited (a similar finding was reported in a second study which employed a visuospatial complex span task, but no control dual task).

These results are clearly consistent with the view that individuals with ADHD have difficulties in resisting interference in working memory due to their inhibitory difficulties. However, other studies that have examined complex span performance in the condition have found no evidence of deficits relative to comparison individuals matched for IQ (Siegal & Ryan 1989; Willcutt et al., 2001; see also Kunsti, Oosterlaan, & Stevenson, 2001). In fact this may not be so surprising given the evidence that variation in working memory capacity is closely related to variation in intelligence in the general population. In other words, if working memory capacity plays a role in determining IQ differences, and if, by extension, working memory deficits cause delayed IQ among individuals with mental retardation, then one will struggle to observe such deficits in studies in which comparison groups are IQ matched.

Autism

These points on IQ matching are also relevant to the question of whether autism is associated with working memory deficits, because although autism is not necessarily associated with mental retardation, many individuals with autism do have IQs outside the normal range (Bailey, Phillips, & Rutter, 1996). In addition, autism is a condition that is also associated with impaired executive functions (Hill, 2004), although Pennington and Ozonoff (1996) have suggested that there is less evidence of inhibitory difficulties in autism than there is in ADHD, and correspondingly more evidence of problems in

cognitive flexibility. Individuals with autism also perform poorly on planning tasks (e.g., Hughes, Russell, & Robbins, 1994), a deficit that might reflect problems in holding goal states in working memory (Ozonoff, Pennington, & Rogers, 1991; cf. Kimberg & Farah 1992). One might, therefore, expect that individuals with autism would have specific difficulties in working memory tasks, particularly given the need to switch flexibly between processing and memory requirements in such tasks. Importantly, there is evidence to indicate that individuals with autism may have no particular problems on either verbal or visuospatial STM measures (Bennetto, Pennington, & Rogers, 1996; Joseph, Steele, Meyer, & Tager-Flusberg, 2005; Russell, Jarrold, & Henry, 1996; Williams, Goldstein, & Minshew, 2006; although see Whitehouse, Maybery, & Durkin, 2006), and consequently, if working memory deficits are observed then they are unlikely to be explainable in terms of storage problems alone.

Most studies of working memory in autism have, in fact, reported little evidence of specific impairments. Indeed, some authors have explicitly argued that working memory is intact in autism (Ozonoff & Strayer, 2001). However, such claims may be premature, as many of the tasks used in studies of autism have questionable status as working memory measures. For example, Lopez, Lincoln, Ozonoff, and Lai (2005) reported unimpaired working memory among individuals with autism using a working memory index derived from performance on three subcomponents of the Wechsler Adult Intelligence Scale. One of these subtests was Arithmetic, which is at best partially determined by working memory ability, whereas another was the Digit Span subtest, which is itself a combination of forward and backward recall.

Ozonoff and Strayer (2001) similarly reported unimpaired performance in autism on three working memory tasks. The first of these was an n-back task, in which participants have to judge whether a presented item matches one presented n-back in a sequence (see also Williams et al., 2006). Although such tasks are often used as tests of working memory, particularly in neuroimaging studies, it is not clear that they necessarily involve the kind of manipulation of information that characterizes working memory (Conway et al., 2005; Jarrold & Towse, 2006; Ruiz, Elousúa, & Lechuga, 2005). Moreover, the maximum value of n in this study was 2, and some have suggested that n-back tasks place minimal working memory demands on participants when n is less than 3 (Hockey & Geffen, 2004; see Jarrold & Towse, 2006). The second task was a spatial memory task in which participants were simultaneously shown a set of different shapes in fixed spatial locations for a limited period, followed by a central probe that matched one of the previously presented shapes. The participants' task was to select the spatial position in which that item had appeared. Once again there is no clear sense in which this task, which is essentially a delayed recognition test, requires anything other than holding information in mind, although it may well require individuals to "bind" item and location information at encoding (Chalfonte & Johnson, 1996).

In the third task employed by Ozonoff and Strayer (2001), participants were presented with a computer screen displaying a series of colored boxes, some of which contained reward items. At the start of any trial, the participant was ignorant of which locations contained rewards and had to search each potential box in turn. After each search, the position of the boxes changed, and the participant therefore needed to keep track of the color of the boxes he had already visited. Individuals with autism did not differ from controls in the number of times they revisited previously searched boxes. Although this task does capture something of the "storage plus concurrent processing" aspect of accepted working memory measures, it is worth noting that a more recent study by Goldberg et al. (2005) found that a similar task was the only one of a number of potentially executive measures that clearly showed impaired performance among individuals with autism relative to typical controls (see also Joseph et al., 2005).

Studies that have examined complex span performance in autism have produced somewhat mixed results. Bennetto et al. (1996) found that their sample of high-functioning individuals with autism was impaired relative to controls on both reading and counting versions of complex span tasks. Crucially, the impairment in working memory remained even when potential differences in STM (digit span) were accounted for. The authors suggested that autism may be characterized by a general working memory deficit that prevents individuals from solving context-specific problems that require integration of multiple pieces of information over space and time. However, Bennetto et al. did not control for possible differences in reading and counting efficiency that might also account for the group difference in complex span performance. This concern was addressed by Russell et al. (1996), who gave individuals with autism, and comparison groups of equivalent verbal mental age, three complex span tasks: a counting span task; an operation span task, in which individuals complete a series of sums while remembering the successive totals; and an odd-man-out task in which participants had to locate successive targets that differed in form from their neighbors while remembering the positions of these targets (cf. Hitch & McAuley, 1991). Individuals with autism were found to be unimpaired on the latter two tasks but did show impaired counting span in one of two versions of the counting span task. However, this deficit could be directly attributed to the greater time taken by individuals with autism to count the dots within the processing episodes of this task (cf. Jarrold & Russell, 1997).

Taken together, the evidence for working memory deficits in autism currently appears rather weak. Having said this, few studies in the autism literature employ incontrovertible working memory measures and control for individuals' ability to complete the storage and processing components of such measures, to examine the executive requirements associated with combining them. Certainly, there is room for more work aimed at examining whether executive deficits in autism, and also in ADHD, lead to working memory impairments.

Conclusion

One of the points that comes out most clearly from the above review is that researchers differ in how they conceptualize working memory, with consequent inconsistencies in the tasks used to tap working memory function. Although the use of multiple measures to tap an underlying construct is, in theory, an informative research approach, this only holds if these measures have construct validity (cf. Conway et al., 2005). The ability of some of the measures just reviewed to tap working memory is questionable, and this alone could account for some of the inconsistency in findings highlighted in certain sections above. Baddeley's working memory model (Baddeley 1986, 2000) provides one but by no means the only (see Miyake & Shah, 1999) theoretical framework in which to interpret working memory deficits among individuals with mental retardation. This model has a number of strengths in this regard. In particular, the above review shows that individuals with different forms of mental retardation can differ in either their verbal or visuospatial STM performance, whereas other individuals show more deficits on working memory than on STM measures. This pattern of strengths and weaknesses supports the view that the verbal and visuospatial aspects STM should be dissociated, and that working memory needs to be conceptually distinguished from STM.

At the same time, our review indicates that poor STM or working memory performance can arise for a number of reasons, and that simply observing a deficit on either simple or complex tasks in a particular group is not in itself evidence of a fundamental short-term or working memory impairment. Individuals will perform poorly on these tasks if they struggle to encode or reproduce to-be-remembered items, or if they find it difficult to carry out any processing embedded in such tasks. Arguably, impaired performance that results from these effects does not reflect a fundamental memory deficit, and in the context of the study of mental retardation, poor memory performance may therefore be secondary to the more general learning difficulties that are associated with any given condition.

Having said this, it remains possible that fundamental short-term and working memory deficits themselves lie at the heart of some of the learning difficulties experienced by such individuals. As the above review has highlighted, STM deficits do appear to occur and would be expected to lead on to problems in long-term learning; in particular, the verbal STM deficits associated with conditions such as DS have been linked to problems in language acquisition. Similarly, given the close association between working memory performance and general intelligence seen in the general population, one might expect working memory deficits to play a causal role in constraining intellectual development among individuals with mental retardation. One clearly needs to be cautious in hypothesizing a single cause for all forms of mental retardation and in making the associated assumption that mental retardation is in itself a single, homogeneous entity (Burack, 1990). Nevertheless, the fact that working memory has been shown to be closely related to intelligence and reasoning (Kyllonen & Christal, 1990; Oberauer et al., 2005) means that working memory deficits are certainly a potential cause of mental retardation. Consequently, the extent of such deficits in these populations does deserve investigation, although this chapter has clearly shown the need for further work in this area.

However, one issue that needs to be borne in mind while carrying out such work is the extent to which matching groups, in order to determine whether deficits are specific or general, may risk "matching away" the deficit of interest. In particular,

if one hypothesizes that working memory impairments cause intellectual deficits and reduced IQ, then one will struggle to show working memory deficits among groups that are matched for IQ. Indeed, the above review of working memory skills in ADHD and autism suggests that any evidence of working memory problems in these populations tends to be seen when groups are not equated for IQ, and tends to disappear when IQ is controlled for. Although it is clearly important to question whether any observed working memory deficit is specific to a disorder—or rather is associated with general mental retardation that might also be associated with that condition—there is a very real sense in which one might never expect to see working memory deficits among groups matched for IQ. If so, then the most fruitful approach to future work in this area might involve assessing working memory skills within a group of individuals with a given developmental disorder, who themselves vary in IQ in order to determine whether this variation in intellectual ability is closely related to variance in working memory capacity.

References

Ackerman, P. L., Beier, M. E., & Boyle, M. O. (2005). Working memory and intelligence: The same or different constructs? *Psychological Bulletin, 131,* 30–60.

Alloway, T. P., & Gathercole, S. E. (2006). *Working memory in neurodevelopmental conditions.* Hove, UK: Psychology Press.

Archibald, L. M. D., & Gathercole, S. E. (2006). Short-term memory and working memory in specific language impairment. In T. P. Alloway, & S. E. Gathercole (Eds.), *Working memory in neurodevelopmental conditions* (pp. 139–160). Hove, UK: Psychology Press.

Atkinson, R. C., & Shiffrin, R. M. (1968). Human memory: A proposed system and its control processes. In K. W. Spence, & J. T. Spence (Eds.), *The psychology of learning and motivation* vol. 2 (pp. 89–105). New York: Academic Press.

Avons, S. E., & Hanna, C. (1995). The memory-span deficit in children with specific reading disability: Is speech rate responsible? *British Journal of Developmental Psychology, 13,* 303–311.

Baddeley, A. (1993). Short-term phonological memory and long-term learning: A single-case study. *European Journal of Cognitive Psychology, 5,* 129–148.

Baddeley, A. D. (1986). *Working memory.* Oxford: Oxford University Press.

Baddeley, A. (2000). The episodic buffer: A new component of working memory? *Trends in Cognitive Sciences, 4,* 417–423.

Baddeley, A., Gathercole, S., & Papagno, C. (1998). The phonological loop as a language learning device. *Psychological Review, 105,* 158–173.

Baddeley, A. D., & Logie, R. H. (1999). Working memory: The multiple-component model. In A. Miyake, & P. Shah (Eds.), *Models of working memory: Mechanisms of active maintenance and executive control* (pp. 28–61). Cambridge, UK: Cambridge University Press.

Baddeley, A. D., Thomson, N., & Buchanan, M. (1975). Word length and the structure of short-term memory. *Journal of Verbal Learning and Verbal Behavior, 14*, 575–589.

Bailey, A., Phillips, W., & Rutter, M. (1996). Autism: Towards an integration of clinical, genetic, neuropsychological, and neurobiological perspectives. *Journal of Child Psychology and Psychiatry, 37*, 89–126.

Barkley, R. A. (1997). Behavioral inhibition, sustained attention, and executive functions: Constructing a unifying theory of ADHD. *Psychological Bulletin, 121*, 65–94.

Bayliss, D. M., Jarrold, C., Baddeley, A. D., Gunn, D. M., & Leigh, E. (2005). Mapping the developmental constraints on working memory span performance. *Developmental Psychology, 41*, 579–597.

Bayliss, D. M., Jarrold, C., Baddeley, A. D., & Leigh, E. (2005). Differential constraints on the working memory and reading abilities of individuals with learning difficulties and typically developing children. *Journal of Experimental Child Psychology, 92*, 76–99.

Bayliss, D. M., Jarrold, C., Gunn, D. M., & Baddeley, A. D. (2003). The complexities of complex span: Explaining individual differences in working memory in children and adults. *Journal of Experimental Psychology: General, 132*, 71–92.

Bennetto, L., Pennington, B. F., & Rogers, S. J. (1996). Intact and impaired memory functions in autism. *Child Development, 67*, 1816–1835.

Brener, R. (1940). An experimental investigation of memory span. *Journal of Experimental Psychology, 26*, 467–482.

Briscoe, J., Bishop, D. V. M., & Norbury, C. F. (2001). Phonological processing, language, and literacy: A comparison of children with mild-to-moderate sensorineural hearing loss and those with specific language impairment. *Journal of Child Psychology and Psychiatry, 42*, 329–340.

Broadley, I., & MacDonald, J. (1993). Teaching short term memory skills to children with Down syndrome. *Down Syndrome: Research and Practice, 1*, 56–62.

Brock, J., & Jarrold, C. (2004). Language influences on verbal short-term memory performance in Down syndrome: Item and order recognition. *Journal of Speech, Language, and Hearing Research, 47*, 1334–1346.

Brock, J., & Jarrold, C. (2005). Serial order reconstruction in Down syndrome: Evidence for a selective deficit in verbal short-term memory. *Journal of Child Psychology and Psychiatry, 46*, 304–316.

Brock, J., McCormack, T., & Boucher, J. (2005). Probed serial recall in Williams syndrome: Lexical influences on phonological short-term memory. *Journal of Speech, Language, and Hearing Research, 48*, 360–371.

Brown, G. D. A., Preece, T., & Hulme, C. (2000). Oscillator-based memory for serial order. *Psychological Review, 107*, 127–181.

Burack, J. A. (1990). Differentiating mental retardation: The two-group approach and beyond. In R. M. Hodapp, J. A. Burack, & E. Zigler (Eds.), *Issues in the developmental approach to mental retardation* (pp. 27–48). Cambridge, UK: Cambridge University Press.

Burack, J., Iarocci, G., Flanagan, T., & Bowler, D. (2004). On mosaics and melting pots: Conceptual considerations of comparison and matching strategies. *Journal of Autism and Developmental Disorders, 34*, 65–73.

Burgess, N., & Hitch, G. J. (1999). Memory for serial order: A network model of the phonological loop and its timing. *Psychological Review, 106*, 551–581.

Burgess, N., & Hitch, G. (2005). Computational models of working memory: Putting long-term memory into context. *Trends in Cognitive Sciences, 9*, 535–541.

Cairns, P., & Jarrold, C. (2005). Exploring the correlates of impaired nonword repetition in Down syndrome. *British Journal of Developmental Psychology, 23*, 401–416.

Case, R., Kurland, D. M., & Goldberg, J. (1982). Operational efficiency and the growth of short-term memory span. *Journal of Experimental Child Psychology, 33*, 386–404.

Chalfonte, B. L., & Johnson, M. K. (1996). Feature memory and binding in young and older adults. *Memory and Cognition, 24*, 403–416.

Chapman, R. S. (1995). Language development in children and adolescents with Down syndrome. In P. Fletcher, & B. MacWhinney (Eds.), *Handbook of child language* (pp. 641–663). Oxford: Blackwell.

Chapman, R. S. (1997). Language development in children and adolescents with Down syndrome. *Mental Retardation and Developmental Disabilities Research Reviews, 3*, 307–312.

Chapman, R. S., Kay-Raining Bird, E., & Schwartz, S. E. (1990). Fast mapping of words in event contexts by children with Down syndrome. *Journal of Speech and Hearing Disorders, 55*, 761–770.

Chuah, Y. M. L., & Maybery, M. T. (1999). Verbal and spatial short-term memory: Common sources of developmental change? *Journal of Experimental Child Psychology, 73*, 7–44.

Colom, R., Rebollo, I., Palacios, A., Juan-Espinosa, M., & Kyllonen, P. C. (2004). Working memory is (almost) perfectly predicted by g. *Intelligence, 32*, 277–296.

Comblain, A. (1994). Working memory in Down's syndrome: Training the rehearsal strategy. *Down Syndrome: Research and Practice, 2*, 123–126.

Conway, A. R. A., Kane, M. J., Bunting, M. F., Hambrick, D. Z., Wilhelm, O., & Engle, R. W. (2005). Working memory span tasks: A methodological review and user's guide. *Psychonomic Bulletin and Review, 12*, 769–786.

Conway, A. R. A., Kane, M. J., & Engle, R. W. (2003). Working memory capacity and its relation to general intelligence. *Trends in Cognitive Sciences, 7*, 547–552.

Cornoldi, C., Marzocchi, G. M., Belotti, M., Caroli, M. G., De Meo, T., & Braga, C. (2001). Working memory interference control deficit in children referred by teachers for ADHD symptoms. *Child Neuropsychology, 7*, 230–240.

Daneman, M., & Carpenter, P. A. (1980). Individual differences in working memory and reading. *Journal of Verbal Learning and Verbal Behavior, 19*, 450–466.

Daneman, M., & Merikle, P. M. (1996). Working memory and language comprehension: A meta-analysis. *Psychonomic Bulletin and Review, 3*, 422–433.

Daneman, M., & Tardif, T. (1987). Working memory and reading re-examined. In M. Coltheart (Ed.), *Attention and performance XII* (pp. 491–508). Hillsdale, NJ: Erlbaum.

Dollaghan, C. A., & Campbell, T. F. (1998). Nonword repetition and child language impairment. *Journal of Speech, Language, and Hearing Research, 41*, 1136–1146.

Engle, R. W. (2002). Working memory capacity as executive attention. *Current Directions in Psychological Science, 11*, 19–23.

Engle, R. W., Tuholski, S. W., Laughlin, J. E., & Conway, R. A. (1999). Working memory, short-term memory, and general fluid intelligence: A latent-variable approach. *Journal of Experimental Psychology: General, 128*, 309–311.

Farran, E. K., & Jarrold, C. (2003). Visuospatial cognition in Williams syndrome: Reviewing and accounting for strengths and weaknesses. *Developmental Neuropsychology, 23,* 173–200.

Farran, E.K., Blades, M., Tranter, L., & Boucher, J. (2006). *How do individuals with Williams syndrome learn a route?* Paper presented at the British Psychological Society: Developmental Section Annual Conference, September. London, UK.

Flavell, J. H., Beach, D. R., & Chinsky, J. M. (1966). Spontaneous verbal rehearsal in a memory task as a function of age. *Child Development, 37,* 283–299.

Gathercole, S. E., Adams, A. M., & Hitch, G. J. (1994). Do young children rehearse? An individual differences analysis. *Memory and Cognition, 22,* 201–207.

Gathercole, S. E., & Alloway, T. P. (2006). Practitioner review: Short-term and working memory impairments in neurodevelopmental disorders: Diagnosis and remedial support. *Journal of Child Psychology and Psychiatry, 47,* 4–15.

Gathercole, S. E., & Baddeley, A. D. (1990). Phonological memory deficits in language disordered children: Is there a causal connection? *Journal of Memory and Language, 29,* 336–360.

Gathercole, S. E., Hitch, G. J., Service, E., & Martin, A. J. (1997). Phonological short-term memory and new word learning in children. *Developmental Psychology, 6,* 966–979.

Gathercole, S. E., Lamont, E., & Alloway, T. P. (2006). Working memory in the classroom. In S. Pickering (Ed.), *Working memory and education.* (pp. 219–240). New York: Elsevier Press.

Gathercole, S., & Pickering, S. (2001). Working memory deficits in children with special educational needs. *British Journal of Special Education, 28,* 89–97.

Gathercole, S. E., Pickering, S. J., Ambridge, B., & Wearing, H. (2004). The structure of working memory from 4 to 15 years of age. *Developmental Psychology, 40,* 177–190.

Gathercole, S. E., Pickering, S. J., Hall, M., & Peaker, S. M. (2001). Dissociable lexical and phonological influences on serial recognition and serial recall. *Quarterly Journal of Experimental Psychology, 54A,* 1–30.

Gathercole, S. E., Tiffany, C., Briscoe, J., Thorn, A., & The ALSPAC team. (2005). Developmental consequences of poor phonological short-term memory function in childhood: A longitudinal study. *Journal of Child Psychology and Psychiatry, 46,* 598–611.

Gathercole, S. E., Willis, C. S., Emslie, H., & Baddeley, A. D. (1992). Phonological memory and vocabulary development during the early school years: A longitudinal study. *Developmental Psychology, 5,* 887–898.

Gathercole, S. E., Willis, C., Emslie, H., & Baddeley, A. D. (1994). The Children's Test of Nonword Repetition: A test of phonological working memory. *Memory, 2,* 103–127.

Goldberg, M. C., Mostofsky, S. H., Cutting, L. E., Mahone, E. M., Astor, B. C., Denckla, M. B., et al. (2005). Subtle executive impairment in children with autism and children with ADHD. *Journal of Autism and Developmental Disorders, 35,* 279–293.

Hale, S., Bronik, M. D., & Fry, A. F. (1997). Verbal and spatial working memory in school-aged children: Developmental differences in susceptibility to interference. *Developmental Psychology, 33,* 364–371.

Hanley, J. R., Young, A. W., & Pearson, N. A. (1991). Impairment of the visuo-spatial sketch pad. *The Quarterly Journal of Experimental Psychology, 43A,* 101–125.

Henry, L. A. (2001). How does the severity of a learning disability affect working memory performance? *Memory, 9,* 233–247.

Hill, E. L. (2004). Executive dysfunction in autism. *Trends in Cognitive Sciences, 8,* 26–32.

Hitch, G. J., & McAuley, E. (1991). Working memory in children with specific arithmetical learning difficulties. *British Journal of Psychology, 82,* 375–386.

Hitch, G. J., Towse, J. N., & Hutton, U. (2001). What limits children's working memory span? Theoretical accounts and applications for scholastic development. *Journal of Experimental Psychology: General, 130,* 184–198.

Hockey, A., & Geffen, G. (2004). The concurrent validity and test-retest reliability of a visuospatial working memory test. *Intelligence, 32,* 591–605.

Hughes, C., Russell, J., & Robbins, T. R. (1994). Evidence for executive dysfunction in autism. *Neuropsychologia, 32,* 477–492.

Hulme, C., & Mackenzie, S. (1992). *Working memory and severe learning difficulties.* Hove, UK: Lawrence Erlbaum Associates.

Hulme, C., Newton, P., Cowan, N., Stuart, G., & Brown, G. (1999). Think before you speak: Pauses, memory search, and trace redintegration processes in verbal memory span. *Journal of Experimental Psychology: Learning, Memory, and Cognition, 25,* 447–463.

Hulme, C., & Roodenrys, S. (1995). Practitioner review: Verbal working memory development and its disorders. *Journal of Child Psychology and Psychiatry, 36,* 373–398.

Jarrold, C., Baddeley, A. D., & Hewes, A. K. (1999). Genetically dissociated components of working memory: Evidence from Down's and Williams syndrome. *Neuropsychologia, 37,* 637–651.

Jarrold, C., Baddeley, A. D., & Hewes, A. K. (2000). Verbal short-term memory deficits in Down syndrome: A consequence of problems in rehearsal? *Journal of Child Psychology and Psychiatry, 41,* 233–244.

Jarrold, C., Baddeley, A. D., Hewes, A. K., Leeke, T., & Phillips, C. (2004). What links verbal short-term memory performance and vocabulary level? Evidence of changing relationships among individuals with learning disability. *Journal of Memory and Language, 50,* 134–148.

Jarrold, C., Baddeley, A. D., & Phillips, C. (1999). Down syndrome and the phonological loop: The evidence for, and importance of, a specific verbal short-term memory deficit. *Down Syndrome Research and Practice, 6,* 61–75.

Jarrold, C., Baddeley, A. D., & Phillips, C. E. (2002). Verbal short-term memory in Down syndrome: A problem of memory, audition, or speech? *Journal of Speech, Language, and Hearing Research, 45,* 531–544.

Jarrold, C., & Bayliss, D. M. (2007). Variation in working memory due to typical and atypical development. In A. R. A. Conway, C. Jarrold, M. J. Kane, A. Miyake, & J. N. Towse (Eds.), *Variation in working memory* (pp. 134–161). New York: Oxford University Press.

Jarrold, C., Cowan, N., Hewes, A. K., & Riby, D. M. (2004). Speech timing and verbal short-term memory: Evidence for contrasting deficits in Down syndrome and Williams syndrome. *Journal of Memory and Language, 51,* 365–380.

Jarrold, C., Purser, H. R. M., & Brock, J. (2006). Short-term memory in Down syndrome. In T. P. Alloway, & S. E. Gathercole (Eds.), *Working memory and neurodevelopmental conditions* (pp. 239–266). Hove, UK: Psychology Press.

Jarrold, C., & Russell, J. (1997). Counting abilities in autism: Possible implications for central coherence theory. *Journal of Autism and Developmental Disorders, 27,* 25–37.

Jarrold, C., & Towse, J. T. N. (2006). Individual differences in working memory. *Neuroscience, 139*, 39–50.

Jones, D., Farrand, P., Stuart, G., & Morris, N. (1995). Functional equivalence of verbal and spatial information in serial short-term memory. *Journal of Experimental Psychology: Learning, Memory, and Cognition, 21*, 1008–1018.

Joseph, R. M., Steele, S. D., Meyer, E., & Tager-Flusberg, H. (2005). Self-ordered pointing in children with autism: Failure to use verbal mediation in the service of working memory? *Neuropsychologia, 43*, 1400–1411.

Just, M. A., & Carpenter, P. A. (1992). A capacity theory of comprehension: Individual differences in working memory. *Psychological Review, 99*, 122–129.

Kanno, K., & Ikeda, Y. (2002). Word-length effect in verbal short-term memory in individuals with Down's syndrome. *Journal of Intellectual Disability Research, 46*, 613–618.

Karatekin, C. (2004). A test of the integrity of the components of Baddeley's model of working memory in attention-deficit/hyperactivity disorder (ADHD). *Journal of Child Psychology and Psychiatry, 45*, 912–926.

Kimberg, D. Y., & Farah, M. J. (1992). A unified account of cognitive impairments following frontal lobe damage: The role of working memory in complex, organized behavior. *Journal of Experimental Psychology: General, 122*, 411–428.

Kirchner, D. M., & Klatzky, R. L. (1985). Verbal rehearsal and memory in language-disordered children. *Journal of Speech and Hearing Research, 28*, 556–565.

Klein, B. P., & Mervis, C. B. (1999). Cognitive strengths and weaknesses of 9- and 10-year-olds with Williams syndrome or Down syndrome. *Developmental Neuropsychology, 16*, 177–196.

Kuntsi, J., Oosterlaan, J., & Stevenson, J. (2001). Psychological mechanisms in hyperactivity: I. Response inhibition deficit, working memory impairment, delay aversion, or something else? *Journal of Child Psychology and Psychiatry, 42*, 199–210.

Kyllonen, P. C., & Christal, R. E. (1990). Reasoning ability is (little more than) working memory capacity?! *Intelligence, 14*, 389–433.

Laws, G. (1998). The use of nonword repetition as a test of phonological memory in children with Down syndrome. *Journal of Child Psychology and Psychiatry, 39*, 1119–1130.

Laws, G., & Bishop, D. V. M. (2004). Verbal deficits in Down syndrome and specific language impairment: A comparison. *International Journal of Language and Communication Disorders, 39*, 423–451.

Lépine, R., Barrouillet, P., & Camos, V. (2005). What makes working memory spans so predictive of high level cognition? *Psychonomic Bulletin and Review, 12*, 165–170.

Lopez, B. R., Lincoln, A. J., Ozonoff, S., & Lai, Z. (2005). Examining the relationship between executive functions and restricted, repetitive symptoms of autistic disorder. *Journal of Autism and Developmental Disorders, 35*, 445–460.

Majerus, S., & Van der Linden, M. (2003). Long-term memory effects on verbal short-term memory: A replication study. *British Journal of Developmental Psychology, 21*, 303–310.

Majerus, S., Van der Linden, M., Bressand, V., Eliez, S. (2006). *Verbal short-term memory in children and adults with a chromosome 22q11.2 deletion. A specific deficit in serial order retention capacities?* Manuscript submitted for publication.

Marcell, M. M., & Cohen, S. (1992). Hearing abilities of Down syndrome and other mentally handicapped adolescents. *Research in Developmental Disabilities, 15*, 533–551.

Mervis, C., Morris, C. A., Bertrand, J., & Robinson, B. F. (1999). Williams syndrome: Findings from an integrated program of research. In H. Tager-Flusberg (Ed.), *Neurodevelopmental disorders: Contribution to a new framework from the cognitive neurosciences* (pp. 65–110). Cambridge, MA: MIT Press.

Milner, B. (1971). Interhemispheric differences in the localisation of psychological processes in man. *British Medical Bulletin, 27*, 272–277.

Miyake, A., & Shah, P. (1999). *Models of working memory: Mechanisms of active maintenance and executive control.* Cambridge, UK: Cambridge University Press.

Monsell, S. (1978). Recency, immediate recognition memory, and reaction time. *Cognitive Psychology, 10*, 465–501.

Mosley, J. L. (1985). High-speed memory-scanning task performance of mildly mentally retarded and nonretarded individuals. *American Journal of Mental Deficiency, 90*, 81–89.

Oberauer, K., Schulze, R., Wilhelm, O., & Süß, H.-M. (2005). Working memory and intelligence–their correlation and their relation: Comment on Ackerman, Beier, and Boyle (2005). *Psychological Bulletin, 131*, 61–65.

Ozonoff, S., Pennington, B. F., & Rogers, S. J. (1991). Executive function deficits in high-functioning autistic individuals: Relationship to theory of mind. *Journal of Child Psychology and Psychiatry, 32*, 1081–1105.

Ozonoff, S., & Strayer, D. L. (2001). Further evidence of intact working memory in autism. *Journal of Autism and Developmental Disorders, 31*, 257–263.

Page, M. P. A., & Norris, D. (1998). The primacy model: A new model of immediate serial recall. *Psychological Review, 105*, 761–781.

Pennington, B. F., Moon, J., Edgin, J., Stedron, J., & Nadel, L. (2003). The neuropsychology of Down syndrome: Evidence for hippocampal dysfunction. *Child Development, 74*, 75–93.

Pennington, B. F., & Ozonoff, S. (1996). Executive functions and developmental psychopathology. *Journal of Child Psychology and Psychiatry, 37*, 51–87.

Phillips, C. J., & Nettlebeck, T. (1984). Effects of procedure on memory scanning of mild mentally retarded adults. *American Journal of Mental Deficiency, 88*, 668–677.

Pickering, S. J., Gathercole, S. E., & Peaker, S. M. (1998). Verbal and visuo-spatial short-term memory in children: Evidence for common and distinct mechanisms. *Memory and Cognition, 26*, 1117–1130.

Raine, A., Hulme, C., Chadderton, H., & Bailey, P. (1991). Verbal short-term memory span in speech-disordered children: Implications for articulatory coding in short-term memory. *Child Development, 62*, 415–423.

Roodenrys, S. (2006). Working memory function in attention deficit hyperactivity disorder. In T. P. Alloway, & S. E. Gathercole (Eds.), *Working memory in neurodevelopmental conditions* (pp. 187–211). Hove, UK: Psychology Press.

Ruiz, M., Elousúa, M. R., & Lechuga, M. T. (2005). Old-fashioned responses in an updating memory task. *The Quarterly Journal of Experimental Psychology, 58A*, 887–908.

Russell, J., Jarrold, C., & Henry, L. (1996). Working memory in children with autism and with moderate learning difficulties. *Journal of Child Psychology and Psychiatry, 37*, 673–686.

Shah, P., & Miyake, A. (1996). The separability of working memory resources for spatial thinking and language processing: An individual differences approach. *Journal of Experimental Psychology: General, 125*, 4–27.

Siegel, L. S., & Ryan, E. B. (1989). The development of working memory in normally achieving and subtypes of learning disabled children. *Child Development, 60*, 973–980.

Snowling, M., Chiat, S., & Hulme, C. (1991). Words, nonwords, and phonological processes: Some comments on Gathercole, Willis, Emslie, and Baddeley. *Applied Psycholinguistics, 12*, 369–373.

Sternberg, S. (1966). High-speed scanning in human memory. *Science, 153*, 652–654.

Süß, H.-M., Oberauer, K., Wittmann, W. W., Wilhelm, O., & Schulze, R. (2002). Working-memory capacity explains reasoning ability–and a little bit more. *Intelligence, 30*, 261–288.

Swanson, H. L., & Ashbaker, M. H. (2000). Working memory, short-term memory, speech rate, word recognition and reading comprehension in learning disabled readers: Does the executive system have a role? *Intelligence, 28*, 1–30.

Thorn, A. S. C., & Frankish, C. R. (2005). Long-term knowledge effects on serial recall of nonwords are not exclusively lexical. *Journal of Experimental Psychology: Learning, Memory, and Cognition, 31*, 729–735.

Thorn, A. S. C., Gathercole, S. E., & Frankish, C. R. (2002). Language familiarity effects in short-term memory: The role of output delay and long-term knowledge. *The Quarterly Journal of Experimental Psychology, 55A*, 1363–1383.

Todman, J., & Gibb, C. M. (1985). High speed memory scanning in retarded and non-retarded adolescents. *British Journal of Psychology, 76*, 49–57.

Van der Lely, H. K. J., & Howard, D. (1993). Children with specific language impairment: Linguistic impairment or short-term memory deficit? *Journal of Speech and Hearing Research, 36*, 1193–1207.

Vicari, S., Bates, E., Caselli, M. C., Pasqualetti, P., Gagliardi, C., Tonucci, F., & Volterra, V. (2004). Neuropsychological profile of Italians with Williams syndrome: An example of a dissociation between language and cognition? *Journal of the International Neuropsychological Society, 10*, 862–876.

Vicari, S., Caselli, M. C., Gagliardi, C., Tonucci, F., & Volterra, V. (2002). Language acquisition in special populations: A comparison between Down and Williams syndromes. *Neuropsychologia, 40*, 2461–2470.

Wang, P. P., & Bellugi, U. (1994). Evidence from two genetic syndromes for a dissociation between verbal and visual-spatial short-term memory. *Journal of Clinical and Experimental Neuropsychology, 16*, 317–322.

White, D. A., Craft, S., Hale, S., & Park, T. S. (1994). Working memory and articulation rate in children with spastic cerebral palsy. *Neuropsychology, 8*, 180–186.

Whitehouse, A. J. O., Maybery, M. T., & Durkin, K. (2006). Inner speech impairments in autism. *Journal of Child Psychology and Psychiatry, 47*, 857–865.

Willcutt, E. G., Pennington, B. F., Boada, R., Ogline, J. S., Tunick, R. A., Chhabildas, N. A., et al. (2001). A comparison of the cognitive deficits in reading disability and attention-deficit/hyperactivity disorder. *Journal of Abnormal Psychology, 110*, 157–172.

Williams, D. L., Goldstein, G., & Minshew, N. J. (2006). The profile of memory function in children with autism. *Neuropsychology, 20*, 21–29.

Executive Function Across Syndromes Associated with Intellectual Disabilities: A Developmental Perspective

Natalie Russo, Tamara Dawkins, Mariëtte Huizinga, *and* Jacob A. Burack

Abstract

Executive function (EF) is a general construct used to represent brain functions related to the conscious control of thought and action. This chapter reviews literature that supports the notion of a componential view of EF, as some disorders were associated with developmentally appropriate performance on some areas of EF, but not others. For example, individuals with Down syndrome were as able as developmentally matched peers in areas related to working memory and inhibition, but were clearly impaired in their abilities to switch flexibly between mental sets. This sparing of certain areas (in relation to developmental level) is inconsistent with the notion of a unitary view, which would imply that difficulty in one area of EF would mean difficulty in all areas of EF. Although the findings reviewed here still leave open the question of whether some combination of unitary and componential views is correct, the chapter provides evidence to suggest that a purely unitary view is unlikely.

Keywords: Executive function, componential view, brain function, brain development, thought control, action control

Executive function (EF) is a general construct used to represent brain functions related to the conscious control of thought and action (e.g., Zelazo & Muller, 2001). It is needed, for example, to evaluate alternatives and decide on a course of action, or to flexibly change plans or actions. Improvement in EF is considered to be related to development in a wide range of intellectual and social behaviors as children grow older (Case, 1985; Flavell, 1971; Siegler, 1983). For example, EF is related to school performance, reading, and mathematical and problem solving skills (Bayliss, Jarrold, Gunn, & Baddeley, 2003; Cowan, Saults, & Elliott, 2002), as well as to social-emotional development (Blair, 2003; Eslinger, Flaherty-Craig, & Benton, 2004; Hill & Frith, 2003).

The historical roots of research on EF can be traced back to clinical neuropsychological investigations of lesioned patients (e.g., the case of Phineas Gage; Tranel, 2002), in which, despite intact performance on IQ tests, adults with damage to the prefrontal cortex (PFC) show performance deficits on classic EF tasks, such as the Wisconsin Card Sorting Task (WCST; Heaton et al., 1983) and the Tower of Hanoi (Simon, 1975). On the WCST, patients with PFC lesions commit more errors of perseveration as compared to typically developing individuals (e.g., Anderson, Damasio, Jones, & Tranel, 1991; Stuss et al., 2000), whereas on the Tower of Hanoi, they fall short at recognizing the ultimate goal and resolving short-term goal conflicts (e.g., Goel & Grafman, 1995).

The performance of children on measures of EF reflects the slow maturation of the PFC (Dempster, 1992; Stuss, 1992). As children grow older, they become better able to control EF functions, giving rise to improvements in performance on laboratory measures such as the WCST and the Tower of Hanoi. At first glance, the performance of school-aged children appears to resemble that of adult patients with PFC lesions in some ways. For example, similarly to patients with PFC lesions, school-aged children perseverate and have difficulty with set maintenance on the WCST (e.g., Chelune & Baer, 1986; Huizinga & Van der Molen, 2007; Welsh, Pennington, & Groisser, 1991), as well as with planning toward the goal on the Tower of Hanoi task (e.g., Bull, Espy, & Senn, 2004; Welsh et al., 1991). Of course, children are not PFC lesion patients, and EF difficulties in childhood are related to maturational processes within the PFC as well as to those that enhance neuronal transmission within the PFC, such as synaptic pruning and myelination (Giedd et al., 1999; Gogtay et al., 2004; Huttenlocher, 1979; Sowell, Delis, & Stiles, 2001). Thus, brain maturation leads to developmental changes in EF abilities.

The Organization of Executive Function

The attempt to understand the organization of EF is complicated by inconsistent neuropsychological studies. In some studies, PFC patients show impairments on the WCST or the Tower of Hanoi, but not on both. In others, persons with different brain lesions show impaired performance on both tasks (for a review, see Stuss, 2006). These inconsistencies led to two general schools of thought, with some authors considering EF to be a group of multifaceted processes that include distinct subfunctions, with focal neural correlates (Stuss, Shallice, Alexander, & Picton, 1995; see Garon, Bryson, & Smith, 2008 for a review) and others that consider it a unitary construct (Baddeley, 1986; Cohen & Servan-Schreiber, 1992; Kimberg, D'Esposito, & Farah, 1997; Norman & Shallice, 1986).

There is evidence for both the unitary and componential views of EF. For example, behavioral (Brocki & Bohlin, 2004; Lehto, 1996; Lehto, Juujaervi, Kooistra, & Pulkkinen, 2003; Welsh et al., 1991) and neuroimaging (e.g., Aron, Robbins, & Poldrack, 2004; Narayanan et al., 2005; Rushworth, Walton, Kennerley, & Bannerman, 2004) studies with a variety of EF tasks have indicated low or nonsignificant correlations between tasks, thus supporting the componential view, whereas factor-analytic studies have tended to yield multiple EF factors that have some common variance, thus supporting the unitary view. In one factor analytic study, Miyake et al. (2000) used confirmatory factor analysis to assess common variance across experimental tasks thought to assess both similar (e.g., multiple inhibition tasks) and different (set shifting and inhibition tasks) EF components. They found three unique factors that they identified as inhibition of prepotent responses, working memory, and set shifting, but these were all moderately correlated

with each other. The underlying relationship between variables reflected in the correlations between factors may be related to an important function of the PFC—the regulation of perception, thoughts, and behaviors carried out through the inhibition or excitation of other brain areas (e.g., Shallice, 2002).

The practical distinctions between unitary versus multifaceted approaches to EF are especially relevant to the study of genetic syndromes. If EF is a unitary construct, such that its components are interdependent and have concordant developmental trajectories, then any organic insult or injury that impacts one EF process should affect all EF processes. In contrast, if EF is a dissociable process, then each EF subcomponent would have its own unique developmental trajectory, and an insult or injury to one area of functioning could selectively impact one process in ways different from the impact on the other processes. In addition to providing information regarding profiles of performance among persons with intellectual disability (ID), the study of EF in these populations is useful for understanding how, when, and what factors are necessary and sufficient to develop a mature, typical EF processing system.

The Development of Executive Function Among Typically Developing Children

Overall, the general development of EF is characterized as an inverted U-shaped curve, with important periods of development occurring in childhood and adolescence, hitting a plateau in young adulthood, and beginning a steady decline in later adulthood (Zelazo & Muller, 2001). Its development is characterized by an increased ability to control one's thoughts, behaviors, and actions, and to override reflexive actions. The notion of EF as a developing process (in both unitary and componential perspectives) is evident in infancy, when behavior is a simple reaction to internal or external cues. The adage "it's easy to take candy from a baby" exemplifies this, as all one must do is to provide another salient stimulus (e.g., a toy), and the infant's attention is automatically captured by this new stimulus, forgetting the old (the candy). This stage does not last long, and very soon, toddlers acquire "will" and the ability to formulate (simple) goals, such as wanting a specific cup or toy and showing impressive tenacity until their goal is attained (much to the dismay of their parents, at times). This ability to represent a problem, formulate a plan, and act on this plan continues to develop into the childhood years, with great transformations occurring in the preschool period (e.g., Carlson, 2005; Espy, 1997; Kirkham, Cruess, & Diamond, 2003; Munakata & Yerys, 2001; Zelazo, Müller, Frye, & Marcovitch, 2003).

Adult-level performance on the various components of EF appears to be attained at different ages during childhood and adolescence (e.g., Huizinga et al., 2006; Luciana & Nelson, 1999). More specifically, adult-like EF is generally in place around age 12 for set shifting and inhibition, and matures a little later in adolescence for working memory (see e.g., Cepeda, Kramer, & Gonzalez de Sather, 2001 and Kray, Eber, & Linderberger, 2004, for studies on the development of task/set shifting; Bunge, Dudukovic, Thomason, Vaidya, & Gabrieli, 2003, and Van den Wildenberg & Van der Molen, 2004, for studies on the development of inhibition; and Gathercole, Pickering, Ambridge, & Wearing, 2004, and Luna, Garver, Urban, Lazar, & Sweeney, 2004, for studies of the development of working memory). The observed improvement of EF during development has been attributed to PFC activation that becomes less diffuse and more focal as children grow older (e.g., Casey & Jones, 2010; Casey, Tottenham, Liston, & Durston, 2005). Of course, this description of different developmental trajectories for different facets of EF seems, on the surface, to support the componential view of EF but is really a question of definition. If one adheres to the notion that EF is one construct, then it cannot really be broken down into subcomponents. However, one of the most common ways of studying a construct (such as EF) is to deconstruct it into its parts and study each of these separately. Therefore, the notion of a protracted development of different EF components can only emerge from a componential view of the construct. For those who think that EF is one thing, then these distinctions between subcomponents are attempts by researchers to break things down into manageable, rather than meaningful parts.

A "different" kind of EF, characterized as "hot" EF, is mediated by ventromedial areas of the PFC and is related to the notion that people are not always able to act accordingly, even when they are able to cognitively determine the correct answer to a problem. Thus, hot EF is concerned more with emotionally related decision making and is thought to have a different, more protracted developmental trajectory than "cold" EF. The construct of hot EF is mentioned here for the sake of completeness, although no studies of hot EF of persons with ID have yet been published, and this distinction will thus not be discussed further.

Experimental Tracking of the Development of Executive Function

The developmental sequence of EF is often tracked with experimental paradigms that are sensitive to changes with regard to speed and accuracy of performance over time or as a function of age, but are generally only appropriate for finite age ranges (e.g., Diamond, 1995; Zelazo, Muller, Frye, & Marcovitch, 2003). Based on adult paradigms, in which multiple EF processes need to be recruited for successful performance, tasks used in the study of the development of EF are designed to isolate a specific component of EF. This allows for a more precise developmental profile across the individual components of EF, but is based on the artificial scenario in which the components act independently, rather than in some integrated, systematic way that is more typical of general developmental processes. In many cases, the utility of the experimental tasks are limited for the study of development, as they are usually only appropriate for limited age ranges, although developmental progression can be assessed in some cases with incremental decreases or increases in the difficulty of the experimental task that help minimize floor and ceiling effects in performance.

An example of a successful downward extension of an EF task from the adult literature to the preschool and infant literature concerns the process of set shifting—the ability to flexibly shift from one sorting rule to another (Miyake et al., 2000). In the WCST, which is commonly used to assess set shifting among adults, especially those with brain damage or injuries, participants are presented with cards that match targets on several dimensions (e.g., color, number of elements on a card, and shape) and are asked to sort the cards according to an undetermined rule (e.g., color). They are only told whether their sort was correct or incorrect, and after ten correct trials, the rule is changed (e.g., shape), and the participants must then switch their mindset and figure out the new sorting rule. This complex task relies mostly on set shifting, but also to a certain extent on other EF components, such as working memory—the ability to keep track of the sorting rules (Huizinga et al., 2006)—and inhibition, the ability to inhibit the desire to sort the cards according to a now-incorrect but learned dimension. However, as this task is too difficult for very young children and entails multiple EF processes that are potentially confounded (Huizinga et al., 2006, 2007; Miyake et al., 2004), the establishment of norms has only occurred for children over the age of 6.5 years. Downward extensions of this task have been developed to allow for a more specific focus on the set shifting component and can be used with infants as young as 6 months.

The Dimensional Change Card Sort Task (DCCS; Frye, Zelazo, & Palfai, 1995) was designed as a simplified, child-friendly version of the WCST to assess set shifting in children between the ages of 3 and 6 years. It is a three-level task that requires sorting first by one rule (e.g., color, pre-switch phase), and then switch and sort by a second rule (e.g., shape, post-switch phase). In a third level, children are presented with cards that either do or do not have a black border around them and are asked to sort by the color (or shape) rule if they see a card with a black border and sort by shape (or color) if the card has no black border (complex version). In using this task, Frye et al. (2005) and others (e.g., Zelazo, Mueller, Frye, & Marcovitch, 2003) were able to show that 3-year-old children were able to sort by the first dimension presented (e.g., color) but could not shift to the second rule, despite being reminded of the appropriate sorting rule on every trial. The perseveration, or lack of set shifting, noted in the 3-year-olds is particularly striking since the children are specifically told that they will no longer be playing the color game and that they must now sort by shape. Despite stating that they understood the rule and frequently telling the experimenter to stop repeating the instructions, the children continued to sort by the previously established color rule. However, children between the ages of 4 and 5 years were able to switch flexibly to the second rule, but were unable to complete a more complex version of the task with an extra layer of rules (see also Smidts, Jacobs, & Anderson, 2004 for similar findings using a different task).

In a further downward extension of the WCST, set shifting among children even younger than 3 years of age is generally measured with typical A-not-B tasks (for infants 6 months and up) (Piaget, 1954) and its variants (e.g., Kaufman, Leckman, & Ort, 1989). In an example of an A-not-B task, infants are shown two wells; a toy is placed in one of the wells in front of the infant, and the infant is prompted to retrieve it. After the toy has been correctly chosen by the infant for several consecutive trials, the toy is placed in the second well, again in full view of the infant, and the infant is prompted to search for the toy again. Variations on the A-not-B require infants to flexibly shift their search between wells or locations and are appropriate for toddlers over 23 months of age. For example, the multilocation search task, utilizes three rather than two wells, and in the spatial reversal task, the toddler does not see where the treat is placed initially, nor that a change in the location of the treat has occurred (e.g., Espy, Kaufman, & Glisky, 1999). Although here we have provided an example of a downward extension of set shifting tasks, similar simplified versions of adult tasks have been developed in the areas of planning, inhibition and working memory.

Executive Function in Intellectual Disability

In the remainder of this chapter, we examine EF among persons with specific etiologies associated with an ID, including Down syndrome (DS), fragile X syndrome (FXS), Prader-Willi syndrome (PWS), and phenylketonuria (PKU). In so doing, we structure our interpretations of findings to fit within the context of a developmental framework and consider the methodological issues inherently related to the study of EF in persons with ID. Briefly, the methodological challenges, which are not specific to the study of EF but which apply more broadly to studying any cognitive process among persons with ID, stem from the basic notion that by definition, a diagnosis of ID implies an inherent difference between chronological age (CA) and developmental level (mental age, MA). This raises the questions of whom, and on what basis, one should compare the performance of persons with ID to determine whether skills are intact, delayed, or deficient in some way, and how one accounts for this CA/MA discrepancy when making comparisons and interpreting research findings.

This review is not exhaustive, as we have chosen to include only those studies in which meaningful comparisons are made between persons with ID and another group of comparison participants. More specifically, studies were included in this review if the group of children with ID were the primary group of interest (rather than if they served as the comparison group for another population), and if the authors made a general effort to compare their groups on the basis of developmental level, be it to a group of other persons with intellectual impairments matched on CA or a group of typically developing individuals matched on the basis of MA. All studies that were included in this review were published before 2008, and were found either via PubMed, Eric, or MeSH searches by entering the term "executive function" and each of the four specific IDs that are being reviewed. Studies in which working memory was the primary EF studied were also excluded as these are being reviewed in another chapter (see Jarrold & Brock, 2011, Chapter 8, this volume). These inclusion and exclusion criteria yielded three studies of EF among persons with DS, four studies of persons with FXS, one among persons with PWS, and two among persons with PKU.

Executive Function among persons with Down Syndrome

As a result of the increased rates of Alzheimer disease among adults with DS, working memory has been the primary EF studied among this population (see Jarrold & Brock, 2011, Chapter 8, this volume). The literature on EF in areas other than working memory, in which persons with DS are the primary participants, includes only three behavioral studies. In all three studies, the participants were adults with DS, and the studies varied with respect to both the component of EF and methodology. Differences in matching methodology and the emphasis of different facets of EF in DS limit the conclusions that can be drawn from these studies, although they provide some convergent evidence that the development of set shifting, but not all other facets of EF, may be delayed in their development among persons with DS.

Planning, Inhibition, and Fluency in Down Syndrome

Pennington, Moon, Edgin, Stedron, and Nadel (2003) administered multiple measures of prefrontal executive functioning and hippocampal functioning in a study of 28 children and adolescents with DS and IQ matched typically developing children. The goals were to see if evidence of reduced cerebral volume in prefrontal and hippocampal regions, which are noted in postmortem studies of persons with DS, could be seen in functional developmental delays on tasks assessing these areas. The participants with DS were between the ages of 11 and 19 years (mean CA 14.7 years) and had mean MAs of 4.5 years, whereas the typically developing children were on average 4.92 years old. Pennington et al. included tasks that converged on EF processes requiring the "holding [of] information in active or working memory to guide action selection" (p. 80). Their experiments were thus biased toward assessing working memory, but also included other EF processes such as planning, fluency, and inhibition.

The hippocampal measures included verbal and spatial long-term memory (LTM), a test of pattern recognition, and a test of associated pair learning

taken from either the NEPSY (Korman, Kirk, & Kemp, 2001) or the CANTAB (e.g., Luciana & Nelson, 2002) which are both well-normed and validated neuropsychological test batteries assessing multiple functional domains such as memory, language, and learning. Specifically, Pennington et al. (2003) assessed verbal memory with a list learning task, in which participants are presented with a list of 15 words and asked to recall as many as possible on five successive trials, after which an interfering list is presented (which must also be recalled) before the memory of the target list is assessed again both immediately and after 30 minutes, thus assessing LTM for words. The spatial memory task was a water maze presented on a computer, in which participants had to use spatial cues learned with visual prompts to navigate to a target location in the absence of those visual prompts. In their measure of pattern recognition, the participants were required to view a series of 12 abstract patterns (two different trials were presented) for 3 seconds each, and then make a forced-choice response on which of two patterns had already been presented. They also completed a paired associates test that required that they associate an abstract pattern with its spatial location. Finally, Pennington et al. included their own ecological LTM task using a questionnaire in which the participants were asked to recall events (18 in all), such as what they had eaten for lunch, what time they had gotten up that morning, the date of their birthday, and the name of the examiner.

The prefrontal measures of planning, fluency, inhibition, and working memory were similar to the hippocampal measures, also taken from the NEPSY and the CANTAB. Planning was measured via the two-, three-, four-, and five-move problems from the Stockings of Cambridge, on which participants are required to move target balls one at a time in order to match a model in the shortest number of moves possible. The fluency tasks consisted of verbal and design fluency tasks from the NEPSY. On the verbal fluency task, participants were asked to generate as many words of animals and foods as they could in 1 minute, and in the design fluency task, the participants were asked to make as many designs as possible by joining two or more of five dots using straight lines. On one trial, the participants were presented with dots configured to resemble the way a 5 is presented on a dice, and in a second trial they were presented with a random configuration. The inhibition task entailed pressing one button when participants saw an "X" and another button when they saw an "O," but to refrain from pressing any button when a tone was presented with the letter. The span tasks, which assess working memory, included a spatial working memory task in which participants searched for a target in an increasingly complex spatial array. To succeed on this task, the participants needed to remember the spatial locations they chose on earlier trials because they were told that the target would never be presented in the same spatial location twice. A similar measure was used to test working memory for numbers.

Pennington et al. (2003) found that the performance of the participants with DS was worse than that of the typically developing children on the hippocampal, but not the prefrontal measures, suggesting that some aspects of EF, including planning and inhibition, are not impaired in younger populations of persons with DS. Rather, they found that the persons with DS were better (although nonsignificantly) on the prefrontal tasks than the typically developing children, which might be related to their higher CAs. Although neuroanatomical findings of prefrontal microcephaly may lead one to conclude that inhibition and planning would be impaired in this population as a result of a general decrease in brain size affecting the whole brain, the results from this study suggest typical developmental trajectories for planning and inhibition abilities. Perhaps difficulties appear later on or would appear on more complex tasks, but it would seem that inhibition and planning abilities develop in relation to general MA among persons with DS, at least up until an MA level of around 4.5 years.

Set-shifting in Down Syndrome

Zelazo, Burack, Benedetto, and Frye (1996) examined the relationship between set shifting and theory of mind (ToM) among adults with DS whose MAs ranged from 3 to 6 years as measured by the Peabody Picture Vocabulary Test (PPVT; mean MA was 5.1) and whose CAs were around 22 years. The researchers compared their performance to typically developing preschoolers of the same MA (MA = 5.2 years). They found that individuals with DS performed less well than their typically developing peers on both the measures of EF and ToM. Zelazo et al. used two deception-based ToM tasks, the crayon box task and the red cellophane task, and asked similarly structured questions for both. As an example, on the crayon box task, a participant was initially shown a crayon box containing straws. He or she was then presented with a crayon and a straw and was asked to point or respond verbally to the question: "What is in the box?" (reality question). After the experimenter put the box away, a puppet was introduced to the participant, who was asked three questions: "What does the puppet think is in the box, straws or crayons?" (false-belief question); "What is truly and really in the box, straws or crayons?" (reality question); and "What does this look like it has in it right now, straws or crayons?" (appearance question). To assess set shifting, the pre-, post-, and complex phases of the DCCS were administered after a set of practice trials in each of the two sorting conditions (color and shape) were introduced. Zelazo et al. (1999) found that the individuals with DS performed worse than the MA-matched typically developing children on all of the tasks. Persons with DS had difficulty abstracting what another person might think and perseverated on the first sorting dimension (e.g., color) of the DCCS, suggesting a difficulty in switching mental sets. Zelazo et al. concluded that individuals with DS showed delays in the development of both set shifting and ToM, which was reflected in a floor effect in performance for the participants with DS.

Zelazo et al. (1996) went a step further with their data analysis by characterizing participants' individual performance on a 5-point scale intended to reflect a participant's ability to use increasingly complex rules and rule structures. A score of 0 meant individuals were unable to learn the rules in the practice phase of the task, a score of 1 meant they learned the rules in the practice phase but could not use them during the test phase. Scores of 2, 3, and 4 meant participants passed the pre-, post-, and complex phases respectively. The typically developing children displayed performance that was concordant with their developmental level, as most passed the post-switch phase of the task. In contrast, the participants with DS frequently displayed difficulty simply learning the rules. Four of the 12 participants with DS scored 0, whereas five participants scored 1. Only two of the participants with DS were able to pass the post-switch phase, and only one was able to pass the complex version of the task. The inability to correctly complete even the pre-switch phase was particularly surprising as the MAs of the participants with DS (MA = 5.2 years) suggested that these tasks were developmentally appropriate. The findings that individuals with DS were unable to learn the sorting rules on the DCCS and were thus below developmental expectations, suggest a fundamental delay in the development of rule learning, a precursor to flexible rule use. The finding that three of the participants with DS were able to show some flexibility in their use of rules suggests that there may be individual differences in the level of achievement reached in the area of cognitive flexibility, and may also support the notion that, among persons with DS, there is a significant delay, rather than a complete deficit, in set shifting in this group.

In another study of set shifting, Rowe, Lavender, and Turk (2006) compared the performance of adults with DS with adults with an unspecified ID matched on the basis of age (mean CA = 33 years) and verbal abilities as measured by the British version of the Peaboby Picture Vocabulary Test (no descriptive information regarding the mean MAs of their participants were provided). The authors administered a series of EF and attention measures that included tests of set shifting and planning to a group of persons with DS and a heterogeneous group of individuals with ID. The set shifting task was the Weigl Color-Form Sort (Weigl, 1941), which is similar to the DCCS used by Zelazo et al. (1996), except that three rather than two test cards (circles, squares, and triangles of three different colors) need to be sorted first according to one dimension (e.g., color) and then to another (e.g., shape). The number of cards does not impact the difficulty level in typically developing children (see Zelazo et al., 2003), but the Weigl is more complex than the DCCS because the sorting rules are not explicitly stated on each trial. Scoring on the Weigl is based on a point system similar to the one used by Zelazo et al. (1996), although participants are given more points for sorting by form than by color without prompting. The planning measure the authors used was the Tower of London, which is similar to the Stockings of Cambridge task that was used by Pennington et al. (2003). After correcting for multiple comparisons, the only difference that remained between the groups was on the measure of set shifting.

Since the set shifting task and the scoring system used by Zelazo et al. (1996) and Rowe et al. (2003) were similar, the findings of the two studies can be compared. In both studies, the participants with DS were able to sort by both shape and form, but had difficulty applying these rules to the experimental tasks, suggesting a general difficulty with both flexible rule use and set shifting. There were, however, three major drawbacks to the Rowe study that lead us to interpret their findings with caution. The first issue relates to the use of a mixed group of persons with unidentified ID, which is problematic because the composition of the mixed group is impossible to replicate and thus findings of strengths or weaknesses

in relation to this group are not replicable (see e.g., Burack, Hodapp, & Zigler, 1990; Burack, Evans, Klaiman, & Iarocci, 2001b; Burack, Iarocci, Bowler, & Mottron, 2002,Burack, Iarocci, Flanagan & Bowler, 2004) for a more in-depth discussion of these issues). The second issue related to the authors' choice of matching procedure, as they matched their groups on the basis of receptive language abilities, as measured by the British Peabody Picture Vocabulary Test, but neither administered nor scored this test according to the standardized guidelines outlined in the manual, as they had all participants start at the first item. Third, they did not provide any indication of the MAs of their participants, such that their results are impossible to frame within the context of development.

Conclusions about Executive Function in Down Syndrome

The findings reviewed provide preliminary evidence that rule use and set shifting may be particularly delayed among persons with DS, whereas other components of EF, such as inhibition and planning, might follow a more typical developmental trajectory in this group, at least until an MA of 4.5 years. Pennington et al. (2003) found that the performance of persons with DS was slightly better than that of matched typically developing children on some components of EF, including working memory, planning, and inhibition, whereas both Zelazo et al. (1996) and Rowe et al. (2006) found impairments in set shifting. One main difference between the Pennington studies and those of Zelazo and Rowe relates to the nature of the tasks used, as the authors chose to examine completely different facets of EF. Second, both the DCCS (used by Zelazo) and the Weigl (used by Rowe) are heavily reliant on language abilities: The presentation of rules requires participants to understand what is being asked of them and to potentially use verbal rehearsal strategies to guide their placements of the target cards, even if no verbal response is required. In contrast, Pennington et al. (2003) specifically chose tasks that were nonverbal in nature. As individuals with DS show specific strengths in nonverbal areas relative to weaknesses in verbal areas, differences in findings might in part be attributable to their language content. One way to better tease apart the relationship between language and EF would be to design verbal and nonverbal versions of the same task that assesses the same facet of EF, to determine whether unevenness in cognitive profile among persons with DS might be related to findings of impaired or intact EFs. The preliminary evidence, however, suggests that persons with DS show impairments on measures of set shifting that have a strong verbal component, while their inhibition, planning, and fluency abilities are consistent with their developmental level.

Executive Function Among Persons with Fragile X Syndrome

Increased numbers of cytosine-guanine-guanine (CGG) repeats are associated with the presence, classification (i.e., full vs. premutation), and severity of deficits among persons with fragile X. Increased CGG repeats lead to diminished levels of fragile X mental retardation protein (FMRP), a protein influential in embryonic development and regulation of synaptic activity (e.g., Pierreti et al., 1991; Tassone et al., 2000), and are directly related to the degree of impairment observed in cognitive and executive functioning (e.g., Thompson et al., 1994) among persons with FXS. For example, females with a full mutation show greater deficits in inhibitory functioning and set shifting ability as compared to females with a permutation (e.g., Bennetto, Taylor, Pennington, Porter, & Hagerman, 2001; Cornish et al., 2001; Mazzocco, Pennington, & Hagerman, 1993; Sobesky, Pennington, Porter, Hull, & Hagerman, 1994; Sobesky, Taylor, Pennington, Riddle, & Hagerman, 1996). In addition, females with the full mutation show less severe impairments in relation to males with the full mutation, and females with the premutation are likely to show similar developmental trajectories to typically developing females (e.g., Baily, Hutton, & Skinner, 1998; Rousseau, et al., 1994). Thus, analyses of EF among persons with FXS must include, in addition to all of the other developmental factors outlined in this chapter, the number of CGG repeats in their interpretation of findings.

Inhibition in Fragile X Syndrome

Inhibition is notably impaired throughout childhood and adulthood among persons with FXS, and may represent a significant and persistent area of weakness. For example, in a study of children with FXS, Munir, Cornish, and Wilding (2000b) investigated the inhibitory functioning of boys with FXS with a mean CA of 10.88 years and verbal mental ages (VMA) of 6.77 years; they contrasted their performance with that of groups of boys with DS (mean CA 11.17 years; VMA 6.09 years), typically developing boys with poor attention skills (mean CA 7.58 years; VMA 6.96 years), and typically

developing boys with good attention skills (mean CA 7.97 years; VMA 7.77 years) matched on verbal mental ability as measured by the short form of the British Picture Vocabulary Scale (BPVS). Inhibition ability was measured using the walk task and the same–opposite task from the Test of Everyday Attention for children (Robertson, Ward, Ridgeway, & Nimmo-Smith, 1994). In the walk task, children are asked to mark dots along a column of printed feet. Two tones, each representing a rule the children must follow, are presented at intervals. One tone indicates that the child should place a mark on the next step, and the other tone indicates that the child should refrain from responding, thus measuring the ability to both follow rules and inhibit a prepotent response. In the same–opposite task, the children are timed as they follow a path and name the digits 1 and 2 presented along the path. During the second part of the task, the children are asked to say "one" when they see a 2 and say "two" when they see a 1, again measuring inhibitory processing. Munir et al. found that the children with FXS were less able to inhibit or delay their responses on the walk task in relation to all of the comparison groups, and were significantly slower when performing the same–opposite task in relation to the two groups of typically developing children. These findings are consistent with the behavioral phenotype of persons with FXS, who show impulsivity and hyperactivity and suggest a deficit in inhibitory functioning among children with FXS that is more pronounced than MA-matched typically developing children with poor attentional abilities.

Among adults with FXS, inhibitory function has mainly been studied with the contingency naming task (CNT), which requires the naming of designs based on a given rule (Bennetto et al., 2001; Sobesky et al.,1996). On the CNT, the participants are presented with red and blue triangles and squares and asked to name either the color or the shape of the stimulus. Difficulties in inhibitory processing appear to persist into adulthood in females with full mutation but not in females with the permutation form of FXS, who perform similarly to their typically developing counterparts from childhood into adulthood (Bennetto et al., 2001; Sobesky et al., 1996).

Set-shifting in Fragile X Syndrome

Individuals with FXS also show difficulties in the ability to switch between mental sets (Cornish et al., 2001) in relation to individuals with DS and typically developing children, with the severity of impairment seemingly related to the severity of the disorder.

For example, a positive relationship between the number of perseverative responses on the Wisconsin Card Sorting Task (with higher perseveration related to worse performance) and the number of repeats of the CGG sequence was found in a series of studies of women with the full mutation and those with the premutation (Mazzocco et al., 1993; Sobesky et al., 1994; Thomspon et al., 1994), However, these findings need to be interpreted with caution as the IQs of the women with the premutation were higher than those with the full mutation, and the higher cognitive abilities of the permutation group may have accounted for the group differences.

Conclusions About Persons with Fragile X Syndrome and Executive Function

The initial evidence of EF in persons with FXS provides an example of the link between genotypic and phenotypic expression and the relationship between genetics and outcome. Among individuals with FXS, the number of CGG repeats and FMRP levels are intrinsically linked with the severity of the disorder, as well as with the specific severity of deficits across at least one area of EF, inhibition. These findings highlight the need to further assess the extent to which genetic abnormalities lead to delays and deficits in EF within syndromes and between subgroups within each syndrome.

Phenylketonuria

Phenylketonuria is one of the most treatable causes of ID, and since the development of early screening measures, most individuals with PKU have been spared from the major effects of the disorder. However, a large proportion of females with PKU are now entering childbearing age, and this presents new risks, as elevated levels of phenylamine in the mother are harmful to the developing fetus. Maternal PKU (MPKU) arises when mothers with PKU are not treated adequately during pregnancy, and leads to ID in 97% of offspring, with microcephaly (73%), low birth weight (40%), and congenital heart disease (12%) being the most common comorbid problems (Lenke & Levy, 1980; Levy & Ghavami, 1996). Although the toxic elements of PKU and MPKU are the same, differences in the timing of children's exposure to this toxicity in turn lead to differences in the expression of cognitive strengths and weaknesses (Antshel & Waisbren, 2003). In metabolic disorders, neurochemical aberration and the timing of exposure can be measured, which may help shed light on how metabolic factors can disrupt the pathogenesis of EF at specific pointes

in development (Antshel & Waisbren, 2003). For this reason, most studies of persons with PKU measure phenylamine levels and correlate these with the level of impairment.

Executive Function in Phenylketonuria

Even in the absence of the global cognitive impairment among persons with early-treated PKU, difficulties across several EF components that include visuospatial memory and planning are still present. For example, Leuzzi et al. (2004) studied EF among 14 early- and continuously treated children with PKU whose average age was 10 years, relative to a comparison group of typically developing children matched on overall IQ as measured by Wechsler Intelligence Scale for Children-Revised (WISC-R), gender, CA, and socioeconomic status. Both groups were administered several measures of EF, including set shifting, maze learning, sorting, searching, planning, and visuospatial memory tasks. Despite being matched on the basis of IQ, the individuals with PKU performed worse than the typically developing children on the Tower of London, Elithorn's Perceptual Maze Test, and the copy section of the Rey-Osterreich Complex Figures Test, which all suggest specific deficits in planning abilities. This deficit was related to dietary control, with the participants with PKU with worse dietary control performing worse than those whose PKU was better controlled.

Inhibition in Phenylketonuria

To compare differences in the EF abilities of persons with different subtypes of PKU, Antshel and Waisbren (2003) compared the performance of children and adolescents with inherited PKU, those with MPKU, and a group of typically developing participants on measures of inhibition of return, auditory/verbal learning, visuospatial visuoconstruction, visual memory and organization skills, word retrieval, and visuomotor integration. Executive function and attention were also assessed by parent report using the BRIEF, a questionnaire designed to assess EF difficulties as they would appear in everyday activities, and which yields indices of Behavioral Regulation, Metacognition, and a Global Executive Composite; and the ADHD rating scale, which is an 18-item questionnaire that differentiates between attention difficulties that would be classified as inattentive at one end and impulsive at the other. Groups of 46 children with PKU, 15 with MPKU and 18 typically developing participants, all between the ages of 7 and 16 years, were matched on the basis of IQ as measured by two subtests (Block Design and Vocabulary) of the WISC-III. Levels of phenylamine were measured subsequent to the completion of the testing battery to assess the relationship between test performance and level of phenylamine for all groups.

The participants with PKU and those with MPKU shared similar score profiles in some areas but not others. Both groups had similar word reading speeds, as measured by the Stroop word reading score. However, the individuals with MPKU displayed greater difficulties with EF aspects reflecting behavioral regulation when compared to both typically developing participants and those with PKU. The results from this study indicated that individuals with MPKU were more severely affected as they displayed symptoms of inattention, hyperactivity, and had behavioral regulation difficulties, whereas the children with inherited PKU only showed symptoms of inattention. These findings suggest that the type of EF difficulty that is evident among persons with PKU is related to how the disorder was acquired and as a function of the level of toxicity.

Conclusions About Persons with Phenylketonuria and Executive Function

The findings from studies of PKU provide an example of the link between genetics, environment, and outcome. Individuals with early- and continuously treated PKU tend to have generally positive outcomes, with only minor attentional issues. In contrast, untreated or poorly controlled PKU can have important consequences that significantly interfere with both the day-to-day functioning and the general outcome of these children.

Executive Function in Prader-Willi Syndrome

Preliminary support for differences in EF skills between persons with PWS and typically developing individuals is based on behavioral descriptions of persons with PWS that include rigidity and difficulty dealing with change (Clarke et al., 1996; Dykens & Kasari, 1997). Only one study was found in which the EF performance of persons with PWS was compared to another group on the basis of developmental level, rather than CA. Although their comparison group consisted of a group of persons with ID of mixed etiology, which as we know is problematic, it is nonetheless reported here. Walley and Donaldson (2005) did not find any significant EF differences on measures of initiating, planning,

set shifting, inhibition, and working memory ability between 12 persons with deletion PWS and six with uniparental disomy (UPD) PWS (caused by maternal uniparental disomy of chromosome 15, which results in the inheritance of two copies of maternal chromosome 15 and an absence of a paternal copy of chromosome 15; Nicholls, 1993) and a matched group of persons with ID of various etiologies. Participants were all between the ages of 16 and 49 with VIQs (verbal IQs; as measured by the vocabulary and similarities subtests of the Wechsler Adult Intelligence Scale–Revised) between 51 and 93. These findings provide some initial support for developmentally appropriate maturation of EF processes among persons with PWS.

Conclusions About Persons with Prader-Willi Syndrome and Executive Function

The preliminary data presented here indicate that among persons with PWS, EF appears intact in relation to MA-matched participants. However, more research will need to be conducted to substantiate this claim and investigate the pattern of strengths and weaknesses in EF ability of persons with PWS. These include making comparisons between persons with PWS and a homogeneous group of persons with ID, as well as making comparisons to typically developing individuals matched on the basis of MA. A second consideration in the study of EF among persons with PWS is that under the general umbrella of PWS are several different subtypes that seem to differentiate individuals' performance on EF tasks. For example, persons with different subtypes of PWS, such as those with the deletion and UPD subtypes, demonstrate different patterns of strengths and weaknesses in EF performance. As such, comparisons between different subtypes and typically developing persons are warranted and necessary for understanding how subtle changes in a disorder are acquired and can impact brain development and functional outcomes. Profiles of EF development will need to be developed for both groups separately and in relation to both typically developing persons and persons with other genetic syndromes.

Conclusion

The literature reviewed here supports the notion of a componential view of EF, as some disorders were associated with intact performance on some areas of EF, but not others. For example, individuals with DS were as able as developmentally matched peers in areas related to working memory and inhibition (Pennington et al., 2003), but were clearly impaired in their abilities to switch flexibly between mental sets (Zelazo et al., 1996). This sparing of certain areas (in relation to developmental level) is inconsistent with the notion of a unitary view, which would imply that difficulty in one area of EF would mean difficulty in all areas of EF. Although the findings reviewed here still leave open the question of whether some combination of unitary and componential views is correct, we provide evidence to suggest that a purely unitary view is not likely.

As the origin of more genetic disorders is uncovered, the number of cognitive and EF profiles of different groups that can be gathered will multiply. The development of dynamic, etiologically specific profiles of cognitive and executive functioning will allow for a developmental perspective on genetic disorders related to intellectual impairments, and will also serve to inform the typically developing literature by providing initial links between genetic markers and neurocognitive functioning. The confluence of findings from studies of persons with genetic syndromes is also relevant to a more specific, precise understanding of the relationship between cognitive abilities and EF among typically developing individuals, for whom the development of these processes is inextricably intertwined. The study of EF profiles among persons with ID allows us to understand not only the limits of development that are related to a specific etiology, but also informs us about the malleability and boundaries of typical trajectories of development. The evidence presented in this chapter suggests that general ID is not unilaterally related to overall EF deficit, but rather can be expressed in intact, delayed, or impaired performance.

References

Anderson, S. W., Damasio, H, Jones, R. D., & Tranel, D. (1991). Wisconsin Card Sorting Test performance as a measure of frontal love damage. *Journal of Clinical and Experimental Neuropsychology, 13* (6), 909–22.

Antshel, K. M., & Waisbren, S. E. (2003). Timing is everything: Executive functions in children exposed to elevated levels of phenylalanine. *Neuropsychology, 17,* 458–468.

Aron, A. R., Robbins, T. W., & Poldrack, R. A. (2004). Inhibition and right inferior frontal cortex. *Trends in Cognitive Neurosciences, 8* (4), 170–7.

Baddeley, A, (1986). Modularity, mass-action and memory. *Quarterly Journal of Experimental Psychology, 38* (4), 527–33.

Bailey, D. B., Hatton, D. D., & Skinner, M. (1998). Early developmental trajectories of males with fragile X syndrome. *American Journal on Mental Retardation, 103,* 29–39.

Bayliss, D. M., Jarrold, C., Gunn, D. M., & Baddeley, A. D. (2003). The complexities of complex span: explaining individual differences in working memory in children and adults. *Journal of Experimental Psychology, General, 132* (1), 71–92.

Bennetto, L., Taylor, A. K., Pennington, B. F., Porter, D., & Hagerman, R. J. (2001). Profile of cognitive functioning in women with the fragile X mutation. *Neuropsychology, 15,* 290–299.

Blair, C. (2003). Behavioral inhibition and behavioral activation in young children: relations with self-regulation and adaptation to preschool in children attending Head Start. *Developmental Psychobiology, 42*(3), 301–11.

Brocki, K. C., & Bohlin, G. (2004). Executive functions in children aged 6 to 13: a dimensional and developmental study. *Developmental Neuropscyhology, 26* (2), 571–93.

Bull, R., Espy, K. A., & Senn, T. E. (2004). A comparison of performance on the Towers of London and Hanoi in young children. *Journal of Child Psychology and Psychiatry, 45,* 743–754.

Bunge, S. A., Dudukovic, N. M., Thomason, M. E., Vaidya, C. J., & Gabrieli, J. D. (2003). Immature frontal lobe contributions to cognitive control in children: evidence from fMRI. *Neuron, 33* (2), 301–11.

Burack, J. A., Evans, D. W., Klaiman, C., & Iarocci, G. (2001). The mysterious myth of attentional deficit and other defect stories: Contemporary issues in the developmental approach to mental retardation. *International Review of Research in Mental Retardation, 24,* 300–321.

Burack, J. A., Hodapp, R., & Zigler, E. (1990). Towards a more precise understanding of mental retardation. *Journal of child Psychology and Psychiatry, 31(3),* 471–5.

Burack, J. A., Iarocci, G., Bowler, D. M., & Mottron, L. (2002). Benefits and pitfalls in the merging of disciplines: The example of developmental psychopathology and the study of persons with autism. *Development and Psychopathology, 14,* 225–237.

Burack, J. A., Iarocci, G., Flanagan, T., & Bowler, D. M. (2004). On melting pots and mosaics: Conceptual considerations for matching strategies. *Journal of Autism and Developmental Disorders, 34,* 65–73.

Carlson, S. M. (2005). Developmentally sensitive measures of executive function in preschool children. *Developmental Neuropsychology, 28*(2). 595–616.

Case, R. (1985). *Intellectual development: Birth to Adulthood.* Orlando, FL: Academic Press.

Casey, B. J., & Jones, R. M. (2010). Neurobiology of the adolescent brain and behavior: implications for substance use disorders. *Journal of the American Academy of Child and Adolescent Psychiatry, 49*(12), 1189–201.

Casey, B. J., Tottenham, N., Liston, C., & Durston, S. (2005). Imaging the developing brain: what have we learned about cognitive development? *Trends in Cognitive Science, 9*(3), 104–110.

Cepeda, N. J., Kramer, A. F., & Gonzalez de Sather, J. C. (2001). Changes in executive control across the life span: examination of task-switching performance. *Developmental Psychology, 37*(5), 715–30.

Chelune, G. J., & Baer, R. A. (1986). Developmental norms for the Wisconsin Card Sorting test. *Journal of Clinical and Experimental Neuropsychology, 8,* 3, 219–228.

Cohen, J. D., & Servan-Schreiber, D. (1992). Context, cortex and dopamine: a connectionist approach to behavioral and biology in schizophrenia. *Psychological Review, 99*(1), 45–77.

Cornish, K. M., Munir, F., & Cross, G. (2001). Differential impact of the FMR-1 full mutation on memory and attention functioning: A neuropsychological perspective. *Journal of Cognitive Neuroscience, 13,* 144–150.

Cowan, N., Saults, J. S., & Elliott, E. M. (2002). The search for what is fundamental in the development of working memory. *Advances in Child Development and Behavior, 29*, 1–49.

Dempster F. (1992) The rise and fall of the inhibitory mechanism: Toward a unified theory of cognitive development and aging. *Developmental Review, 12*, 45–75.

Diamond, A. (1995). Evidence of robust recognition memory early in life even when assessed by reaching behavior. *Journal of Experimental Child Psychology, 59*, 419–456.

Dunst, C. J. (1990). Sensorimotor development of infants with Down syndrome. In D. Cicchetti, & M. Beeghly (Eds.), *Children with Down syndrome* (pp. 180–230). New York: Cambridge University Press.

Dykens E. M., & Kasari, C. (1997). Maladaptive behavior in children with Prader-Willi syndrome, Down syndrome and nonspecific mental retardation. *American Journal of Mental Retardation, 102* (3), 228–37.

Eslinger, P. J., Flaherty-Craig, C. V., & Benton, A. L. (2004). Developmental outcomes after early prefrontal cortex damage. *Brain and Cognition, 55*(1), 84–103.

Espy, K. A. (1997). The Shape School: Assessing executive function in preschool children. *Developmental Neuropsychology, 13*, 495–99.

Espy, K., Kaufmann, P., & Glisky, M. (1999). Neuropsychologic function in toddlers exposed to cocaine in utero: A preliminary study. *Developmental Neuropsychology, 15*, 447–460.

Flavell, J. H. (1971). First discussant's comments: What is memory development the development of? *Human Development, 14*, 272–278.

Fowler, A. E., Gelman, R., & Gleitman, L. R. (1994). The course of language learning in children with Down syndrome: Longitudinal and language level comparisons with young normally developing children. In H. Tager-Flusberg (Ed.), *Constraints in language acquisition* (pp. 91–140). Hillsdale: NJ: Lawrence Erlbaum Associates.

Frye, D., Zelazo, P. D., & Palfai, T. (1995). Theory of mind and rule-based reasoning. *Cognitive Development, 10*, 483–527.

Garon, N., Bryson, S. E., & Smith, I. M. (2008). Executive function in preschoolers: a review using an integrative framework. *Psychological Bulletin, 134*(1), 31–60.

Gathercole, S. E., Pickering, S. J., Ambridge, B., & Wearing, H. (2004). The structure of working memory from 4 to 15 years of age. *Developmental Psychology, 40*(2). 177–190.

Giedd, J. N., Blumenthal, J., Jeffries, N. O., Castellanos, F. X., Liu, H., Zijdenbos, A., Paus, T., Evans, A. C., & Rappaport, J. L. (1999). Brain development during childhood and adolescence: a longitudinal MRI study. *Nature Neuroscience, 2*(10), 861–3.

Goel, V., & Grafman, J. (1995). Are the frontal lobes implicated in 'planning' functions? Interpreting data from the Tower of Hanoi. *Neuropsychologia, 33*(5), 623–42.

Gogtay, N., Giedd, J. N., Lusk, L., Hayashi, K. M., Greenstein, D., Vaituzis, A. C., Nugent, T. F. 3rd, Herman, D. H., Clasen, L. S., Toga, A. W., Rapoport, J. L., & Thompson, P. M. (2004). Dynamic mapping of human cortical development during childhood through early adulthood. *Proceedings from the National Academy of Science, 101*(21), 8174–9.

Heaton, R. K., Chelune, G. J., Talley, J. L., Kay G. G., & Curtiss, G. (1993). *Wisconsin Card Sorting Test manual: Revised and expanded, Psychological Assessment Resources*, Odessa, FL.

Hill, E., & Frith, U. (2003). Understanding autism: insights from mind and brain. *Philosophical Transactions of the Royal Society of London. Series B. Biological Sciences, 358*(1430), 281–9.

Huizinga, M., & Van der Molen, M. W. (2007). Age-group differences in set-shifting and set-maintenance on the Wisconsin Card Sorting Task. *Developmental Neuropsychology, 31*(2) 193–215.

Huttenlocher, P. R. (1979). Synaptic density in human frontal cortex-developmental changes and effects of aging. *Brain Research, 163*(2), 195–205.

Jarrold, C., & Brock, J. (2011). Short-term memory and working memory in mental retardation. In J. A. Burack, R. M. Hodapp, G. Iarocci, & E. Zigler (Eds.), *The Oxford handbook of intellectual disability and development*, 2nd ed. New York: Oxford University Press.

Kaufmann, P., Leckman, J. M., & Ort, S. I. (1989). Delayed response performance in males with Fragile-X. *Journal of Clinical and Experimental Neuropsychology, 12*, 69.

Kimberg, D. Y., D'Esposito, M., & Farah, M. J. (1997). Effects of bromocriptine on human subjects depend on working memory capacity. *Neuroreport, 8*(16), 3581–5.

Kirkham, N., Cruess, L., & Diamond, A. (2003). Helping children apply their knowledge to their behavior on a dimension-switching task. *Developmental Science, 6*, 449–476.

Korman, M, Kemp, S. L., & Kirk, U. (2001). Effects of age on neurocognitive measures of children ages 5 to 12: a cross-sectional study on 800 children from the United States. *Developmental Neuropsychology, 20* (1), 331–54.

Kray, J. Eber, J., & Linderberger, U. (2004). Age differences in executive functioning across the lifespan: the role of verbalization in task preparation. *Acta Psychologica, 115*(2–3), 143–65.

Lehto, J. (1996). Are executive function tests dependent upon working memory capacity? *Quarterly Journal of Experimental Psychology, 49*, 29–50.

Lehto, J., Juujarvi, P., Kooistra, L., & Pulkkinen, L. (2003). Dimensions of executive functioning: Evidence from children. *British Journal of Developmental Psychology, 21*, 59–80.

Lenke, R. R., & Levy, H. L. (1980). Maternal phenylketonuria and hyperphenylalaninemia. An international survey of the outcome of untreated and treated pregnancies, *The New England Journal of Medicine, 303*, 1202–1208.

Levy, H. L., & Ghavami, M. (1996). Maternal phenylketonuria: A metabolic teratogen. *Teratology, 53*, 176–184.

Leuzzi, V., Pansini, M., Sechi, E., Chiarotti, F., Carducci, C. I., Levi, G., & Antonozzi, I. (2004). Executive function impairment in early-treated PKU subjects with normal mental development. *Journal of Inherited Metabolic Disease, 27*, 115–125.

Luciana, M., & Nelson, C. A. (1998). The functional emergence of prefrontally-guided working memory systems in four-to-eight -year-old children. *Neuropsychologia, 36*(3), 273–93.

Luciana, M., & Nelson, C. A. (2002). Assessment of neuropsychological function through use of the Cambridge Neuropsychological Testing Automated Battery: performance in 4-to12-yer old children. *Developmental Neuropsychology 22*(3), 595–624.

Luna, B., Garver, K. E., Urban, T. A., Lazar, N. A., & Sweeney, J. A. (2004). Maturation of cognitive processes from late childhood to adulthood. *Child Development, 75*(5), 1357–72.

Mazzocco, M. M., Pennington, B. F., & Hagerman, R. J. (1993). The neurocognitive phenotype of female carries of fragile X: Additional evidence for specificity. *Journal of Developmental and Behavioral Pediatrics, 14*, 328–325.

Miyake, A., Friedman, N. P., Emerson, M. J., Witzki, A. H., Howerter, A., & Wager, T. D. (2000). The unity and diversity of executive functions and their contributions to complex "Frontal Lobe" tasks: a latent variable analysis. *Cognitive Psychology, 41*(4), 49–00.

Munakata, Y., & Yerys, B. E. (2001). All together now: when dissociations between knowledge an action disappear. *Psychological Science, 12*(4), 335–7.

Munir, F., Cornish K. M., & Wilding J. (2000b). A neuropsychological profile of attention deficits in young males with fragile X syndrome. *Neuropsychologia, 38*, 1261–1270.

Narayanan, N. S., Prabhakaran, V., Bunge, S. A., Christoff, K., Fine, E. M., & Gabrieli, J. D. E. (2005). The role of the prefrontal cortex in the maintenance of verbal working memory: An event-related fMRI analysis. *Neuropsychology, 19*(2), 223–232.

Nicholls, R. D. (1993). Genomic imprinting and uniparental disomy in Angelman and Prader-Willi syndromes: A review. *American Journal of Medical Genetics, 46*, 16–25.

Norman W, Shallice T. 1986. Attention to action. In: Davidson R. J, Schwartz G. E, Shapiro D., editors. *Consciousness and self regulation: Advances in research and theory*, Vol. 4, (pp. 1–18). New York: Plenum.

Pennington, B. F., Moon, J., Edgin, J., Stedron, J., & Nadel, L. (2003). The neuropsychology of Down syndrome: Evidence for hippocampal dysfunction. *Child Development, 74*, 75–93.

Piaget, J. (1954). *Construction of Reality in the Child*. Basic Books.

Piaget, J. (1963). *The origins of intelligence in children*. New York: W.W. Norton.

Pieretti, M., Zhang, F., Ying-Hui, F., Warren, S. T., Oostra, B. A., Caskey, C. T., & Nelson, D. L. (1991). Absence of expression of the FMR-1 gene in fragile X syndrome. *Cell, 66*, 817–822.

Robertson, I. H., Ward, T., Ridgeway, V., & Nimmo-Smith, I. (1994). The structure of normal human attention: the Test of Everyday Attention. *Journal of International Neuropsychological Society, 2*(6), 525–34.

Rousseau, F., Bonaventure, J., Legeai-Mallet, L., Pelet, A., Rozet, J.-M., Maroteaux, P., et al. (1994). Mutations in the gene encoding fibroblast growth factor receptor-3 in achondroplasia. *Nature, 6*, 318–321.

Rowe, J., Lavender, A., & Turk, V. (2006). Cognitive executive function in Down's syndrome. *British Journal of Clinical Psychology, 45*(1), 5–17.

Rushworth, M. F., Walton, M. E., Kennerley, S. W., Bannerman, D. M. (2004) Action sets and decisions in the medial frontal cortex. *Trends in Cognitive Sciences, 8*(9), 410–7.

Siegler, R. S. (1983). Five generalizations about cognitive development. *American Psychologist, 38*, 263–277.

Simon H. A. (1975). The functional equivalence of problem solving skills. *Cognitive Psychology, 7*, 268–288.

Smidts, D. P., Jacobs, R., Anderson, V. (2004) The Object Classification Task for Children (OCTC): a measure of concept generation and mental flexibility in early childhood. *Developmental Neuropsychology, 26*(1) 385–401.

Sobesky, W. E., Pennington, B. F., Porter, B., Hull, C. E., & Hagerman, R. J. (1994). Emotional and neurocognitive deficits in fragile X. *American Journal of Medical Genetics, 51*, 378–385.

Sobesky, W. E., Taylor, A. K., Pennington, B. F., Bennetto, L., Porter, D., Riddle, J., & Hagerman, R. J. (1996). Molecular/clinical correlations in females with fragile X. *American Journal of Medical Genetics, 64*, 340–345.

Sowell, E. R., Delis, D., Stiles, J., Jernigan, T. L. (2001) Improved memory functioning and frontal lobe maturation between childhood and adolescence: a structural MRI study. *Journal of the International Neuropsychological Society, 7*(3) 312–22.

Stuss, D.T. (1992) Biological and psychological development of executive functions. *Brain and Cognition, 20*(1) 8–23.

Stuss, D. T. (2006) Frontal lobes and attention: processes and networks, fractionation and integration. *Journal of the International Neuropsychological Society, 12*(2) 261–71.

Stuss, D. T., Levine, B., Alexander, M. P., Hong, J., Palumbo, C., Hamer, L., Murphy, K. J., Izukawa, D. (2000) Wisconsin Card Sorting Test performance in patients with focal frontal and posterior brain damage: effects of lesion location and test structure on separable cognitive processes. *Neuropsychologia. 38*(4) 388–402.

Stuss, D. T., Shallice, T., Alexander, M. P., Picton, T. W. (1995) A multidisciplinary approach to anterior attentional functions. *Annals of the New York Academy of Sciences, 15*(769) 191–211.

Swanson, H. L. (2006). Cross-sectional and incremental changes in working memory and mathematical problem solving. *Journal of Educational Psychology, 98*(2), 265–281.

Tassone, F., Hagerman, R. J., Taylor, A. K., Mills, J. B., Harris, S. W., Gane, L. W., & Hagerman, P. J. (2000). Clinical involvement and protein expression in individuals with the FMR1 premutation. *American Journal of Medical Genetics, 91*, 144–152.

Thompson, N. M., Gulley, M. L., Rogeness, G. A., Clayton, R. J., Johnson, C., Hazelton, B., et al. (1994). Neurobehavioral characteristics of CGG amplification status in fragile X females. *American Journal of Medical Genetics, 54*, 378–383.

Tranel, D. (2002). Emotion, decision-making and the ventromedial prefrontal cortex. In D. T. Stuss & R. T. Knight (Eds.). *Principles of frontal lobe function*. New York: Oxford University Press.

Van den Wildenberg, W. P., & van der Molen, M. W., (2004) Developmental trends in simple and selective inhibition of compatible and incompatible responses. *Journal of Experimental Child Psychology, 8*(3) 201–20.

Walley, R. M., & Donaldson, M. D. C. (2005). An investigation of executive function abilities in adults with Prader-Willi syndrome. *Journal of Intellectual Disability Research, 49*, 613–625.

Weigl, E. (1941). On the psychology of so-called processes of abstraction. *Journal of Abnormal and Social Psychology, 36*, 3–33.

Welsh, M., Pennington, B., & Groisser, D. (1991). A normative developmental study of executive function: A window on prefrontal function in children. *Developmental Neuropsychology, 7*, 131–149.

Zelazo, P. D., Burack, J., Beneddeto, E., & Frye, D. (1996). Theory of mind and rule use in individuals with Down syndrome: A test of the uniqueness and specificity claims. *Journal of Child Psychology and Psychiatry, 37*, 479–484.

Zelazo, P. D., & Muller, U. (2001). Executive function in typical and atypical development. In U. Goswami (Ed.), *Handbook of childhood cognitive development*. Oxford, UK: Blackwell.

Zelazo, P. D., Mueller, U., Frye, D., & Marcovitch, S. (2003). The development of executive function in early childhood. *Monographs of the Society for Research in Child Development, 68*(3), Serial No. 274.

Zelazo, P. D., Sommerville, J. A., & Nichols, S. (1999). Age-related changes in children's use of external representations. *Developmental Psychology, 35*, 1059–1071.

Musical Ability and Developmental Disorders

Anjali K. Bhatara, Eve-Marie Quintin, *and* Daniel J. Levitin

Abstract

This chapter begins by discussing the link between intelligence and musical ability. It then presents the currently available data on the musical abilities and behaviors of individuals with Williams syndrome (WS), Down syndrome (DS), fragile X syndrome, tuberous sclerosis complex, and Rett syndrome. Evidence to date suggests that individuals with developmental disorders such as WS, tuberous sclerosis complex, and possibly DS, have musical abilities that are relatively spared as compared to their other cognitive and perceptual deficits. Musical appreciation and enjoyment does not seem to be dependent on cognitive faculties, and can be useful as a means of establishing communication and influencing behavior, even in individuals with severe mental retardation.

Keywords: Musical ability, intelligence, William syndrome, Down syndrome, fragile X syndrome, tuberous sclerosis complex, Rett syndrome

Music is one of the clearest examples of a cultural universal. It is characterized by both its ubiquity and its antiquity—no known culture now or anytime in the past has lacked music (Huron, 2001). Unlike another human universal, language, music appears to be relatively robust in the face of developmental delay, mental retardation, and other cognitive deficits (Miller, 1989). This may suggest a possible evolutionary origin for music, that music may have been an evolutionary adaptation that preceded even language (Levitin, 2006; Miller, 2000; Mithen, 2006). For decades, most of what the scientific community knew about musical ability among those with cognitive deficits came from anecdotal reports and case studies. Recent improvements in digital audio technology (for the accurate storage and manipulation of music) have made it increasingly possible to conduct controlled studies on special populations, and the results are helping to round out the picture of musical behaviors among individuals with cognitive, perceptual, and emotional deficits.

In the first part of this chapter, the link between intelligence and musical ability will be discussed.

Next, we present the currently available data on the musical abilities and behaviors of individuals with Williams syndrome (WS), Down syndrome (DS), fragile X syndrome (FXS), tuberous sclerosis complex, and Rett syndrome. Although WS has been the most researched in this field, we do not restrict our discussion of musical behaviors to these individuals, although more space will be devoted to this disorder than to the others. Musical skills in WS will be discussed in terms of music production, sensitivity to music in the context of absolute pitch, musical aptitude and ability, response to musical emotions, and auditory and musical processing as measured by neuroimaging. For DS, musical responsiveness, musical abilities, and auditory processing will be described. Musical responsiveness in tuberous sclerosis complex will also be reviewed, and auditory processing will be addressed for both tuberous sclerosis complex and Rett syndrome. As will become evident throughout this chapter, much work remains to be done. We will discuss some music therapy work, but this is not a main focus of the chapter, so we focus on laboratory studies, controlled experiments, and a few case studies. Finally, we conclude with remarks concerning the use of music with individuals with mental retardation or developmental disorders.

Part of the initial research interest in musical abilities in developmental disorders and mental retardation has arisen from studies of individuals with autism spectrum disorders who exhibit savant skills. These are impressive islets of ability made all the more striking by the individuals' impairments in other areas. The abilities can include calendar calculation, art, music, hyperlexia, outstanding spatial ability (e.g., architectural drawing), or mnemonistics (e.g., Sloboda, Hermelin, & O'Connor, 1985). The presence of savant skills in a few individuals has inspired researchers to study general populations of individuals with mental retardation or developmental delay. Perhaps these abilities are relatively spared even in those individuals who do not exhibit extraordinary talents.

For musical savants, one frequently reported ability is absolute pitch (AP). For the present discussion, AP will be defined as the ability to correctly identify pitches by name (Levitin & Rogers, 2005). Of the normal population, approximately 1 in 10,000 is believed to possess this ability (Levitin & Rogers, 2005; Takeuchi & Hulse, 1993). Miller (1989) reports several case studies of individuals with AP-like abilities. Research on AP has shown that one is very unlikely to develop absolute pitch after a certain critical or sensitive period (Levitin & Zatorre, 2003). Musicians often become efficient at making relative pitch judgments, which means that they learn to identify intervals (the distance between two notes), and they can rely on these judgments to identify the pitches of the melody. Thus, relative pitch can sometimes impersonate absolute pitch ability, and careful procedures are required to distinguish the two (Levitin & Rogers, 2005).

Note on Methodologies

When studying musical ability and auditory processing in individuals with mental retardation, certain methods may be more useful than others. For nonverbal individuals, observation of behavior may be one of the only methods available. For more verbally able individuals, self-report of musical preferences and experiences, musical cognitive tests, and tests of ability may be used. To examine the brain bases of music and auditory processing, the temporal resolution of electroencephalography (EEG) and

magnetoencephalography (MEG) has potential to make these methods more useful than functional magnetic resonance imaging (fMRI) and positron emission tomography (PET).

Intelligence and Musical Ability

One interesting question that pertains to mental retardation and musical ability is the extent to which musical ability is dependent on intellectual ability. Braswell, Decuir, Hoskins, Kvet, and Oubre (1988) found some evidence of independence; in their study, the group of participants with moderate mental retardation scored lower than the group with profound mental retardation on the rhythm subtest of the Primary Measures of Music Audiation (PMMA), and lower than the group with severe mental retardation on the tonal subtest of the PMMA. Studies of musical savants also point to the independence of musical ability and general intelligence (Hermelin, O'Connor, & Lee, 1987; Miller, 1999; O'Connor & Hermelin, 1988), although these savant skills may be closely associated with behavioral traits of autism, even without the presence of the full disorder (Anastasi & Levee, 1960, Heaton & Wallace, 2004). In addition, a study of typically developing children showed no correlation between the PMMA scores and IQ (Norton, 1980), and a study of children with mental retardation showed no correlations between any of the subtests of the Musical Aptitude Profile (Gordon, 1965, rev. 1995) and mental age (MA; Rice, 1970). However, a study of a group of adults with mental retardation showed that PMMA rhythm subtest (but not tonal) scores were correlated with expressive language ability (Hoskins, 1985), scores on the Seashore music battery (Seashore, Emil, Saetveit, & Lewis, 1960) were correlated with IQ (although not MA) for a group of children with mental retardation (McLeish & Higgs, 1982), and a study of functional music skills (such as operating a record player or playing an instrument) in individuals with mental retardation showed these skills to be negatively correlated with severity of mental retardation (DiGiammarino, 1990).

Williams Syndrome
Music Production

The musical abilities of people with WS tend to be relatively preserved compared to their other cognitive functions. In addition to preserved musical abilities, they show heightened perceptual and emotional responses to sound, both musical and nonmusical (Levitin, Cole, Lincoln, & Bellugi, 2005) and frequently report heightened musical interests (Carrasco, Castillo, Aravena, Rothhammer, & Aboitiz, 2005; Levitin, Cole, Chiles, Lai, Lincoln, & Bellugi, 2004). During their leisure time, children with WS perform fewer visuospatial activities and more musical activities than do children with Prader-Willi syndrome (Sellinger, Hodapp, & Dykens, 2006).

Individuals with WS have demonstrated rhythmic production abilities at a level equivalent to MA-matched controls (Levitin & Bellugi, 1998), and music perceptual abilities (although not melodic production abilities) at a level equivalent to chronological age (CA)-matched controls (Levitin, 2005). Lenhoff (1996) and Levitin and Bellugi (1998) observed that music camp attendees displayed heightened facility for learning complex rhythms, excellent memory for lyrics, ease in composing song lyrics, and ability with harmony, and an unusual number had absolute pitch. This is, of course, a biased sample, but it demonstrates that these musical abilities are at least somewhat spared in a number of children with WS.

Musical Sensitivity and Absolute Pitch

Some of the studies of heightened responses to sound have employed the term *hyperacusis*, but this term has not been used consistently—depending on the researcher, it has been used at varying times to refer to four separate phenomena. Levitin et al. (2005) classify these persons as having *true hyperacusis* (lowered hearing thresholds and higher detectability of soft sounds); *odynacusis* (lowered pain threshold for loud sounds); *auditory allodynia* (fear of certain types of sounds at normal volume, not because they are too loud); and *auditory fascinations* (strong attraction to certain types of sounds), which often grow out of auditory aversions. In the groups surveyed, those with WS reported the highest prevalence of symptoms in all four categories when compared with people with autism, DS, and controls.

Gothelf, Farber, Raveh, Apter, and Attias (2006) surveyed the mothers of 49 children with WS about "auditory allodynia," although the authors did not differentiate among the four phenomena just discussed. The researchers performed auditory testing on 21 of the 41 children reported to have auditory allodynia to screen for true odynacusis and hearing loss. However, as has been the norm in the literature, these results were all reported together as being measures of "hyperacusis," and the researchers

concluded that 84% of the children in their study demonstrated this broadly defined hyperacusis. A study of individuals with WS in Sweden found that fears, as measured by the Fear Survey for Children—Revised (Ollendick, 1983; Svensson & Öst, 1999), were correlated with hyperacusis (the authors' definition of hyperacusis fit under the headings of auditory allodynia and odynacusis), but neither was correlated with musicality (Blomberg, Rosander, & Andersson, 2006).

As mentioned previously, the prevalence of AP in the neurotypical population is approximately 1 in 10,000. Lenhoff, Perales, and Hickok (2001) tested five children with WS at a music camp, and found that all five demonstrated AP. Four of these five had begun formal musical training after the age of 6, whereas the critical period for normal children is thought to occur between the ages of 3 and 6. The authors suggest that the prevalence of AP among WS individuals may be higher than in the normal population, but more supporting evidence is needed.

Although some of their musical abilities seem to be relatively spared, there is evidence that individuals with WS may not demonstrate the global preference for music that unimpaired individuals do. This local–global distinction has been extensively studied in the literature on autism spectrum disorders but may also be relevant for WS. The individual pitches of a melody can be considered as *local* attributes of music, as opposed to contour and melody, which are considered as *global* attributes of music. Contour is defined as the patterns of rises and falls; that is, the direction of pitch movement without regard to the distance of movement. Melody is the direction *and* the distance of movement; in other words, the general musical theme of a musical piece, what we hum and remember (Levitin, 2006). Global processing relies on the attribution of meaning to a gestalt or perceptual whole (Kubovy, 1981; Navon, 1977), whereas local processing would be more reliant on perception of surface features. Deruelle, Schön, Rondan, and Mancini (2005) performed a study in which children with WS and unimpaired CA-matched controls listened to 24 tonal melodies followed by a comparison melody, which was either the same, differed in contour, or differed in one interval, and they were asked to judge if the two melodies were the same or different. Overall, the children with WS performed more poorly than did the controls. The controls were more accurate in detecting contour violations than interval violations, which, according to the authors, can be attributed to a global precedence of perception in the controls. However, the WS group showed no difference between the two conditions, which may indicate a global deficiency in music perception in WS.

Musical Aptitude and Ability: Pitch, Rhythm, and Melody

Other ways of measuring musical abilities in WS are with musical aptitude tests. Hopyan, Dennis, Weksberg, and Cytrynbaum (2001) tested 14 children and adolescents with WS on pitch (tonal subtest), rhythm, melodic imagery (containing a musical questions and answers, participants decided if the question and answer went together), phrasing, and musical affect. The first four tests were taken from subtests in the PMMA and the Musical Aptitude Profile (Gordon, 1965, rev. 1995; 1986), whereas the fifth was developed for the study.

In the tonal and rhythm tests from Hopyan et al. (2001), both of which were taken from the PMMA, the WS group was impaired relative to CA-matched controls. Don, Schellenberg, and Rourke (1999) measured WS children's musical abilities using the same subtests and found that they performed less well than did controls on the rhythmic subtests, and below the mean for their CAs on both subtests. The authors suggest that this shows that musical ability may not be completely spared, but is relatively strong when compared with other abilities (especially visuospatial abilities). They also found that musical abilities were significantly correlated with verbal abilities. However, Levitin (2005) tested a group of WS participants on these same PMMA subtests (although resynthesized to remove tape static and artifacts) and found no differences between the scores of participants with WS and those from 20 Juilliard (a renowned music college) students.

On a separate rhythm task, that of rhythmic completion, Levitin and Bellugi (1998) found that the WS individuals between the ages of 9 and 20 performed equally as well as MA-matched controls aged 5–7. This is somewhat unsurprising because it shows that their musical abilities are at the same level as the rest of their abilities, although it is in contrast to Kaplan (1977), who showed that developmentally disabled children performed worse than MA-matched controls on a similar task. One interesting aspect of these results is that the mistakes made by the individuals with WS were three times more likely to be "creative" or "musical" mistakes than those made by the control children. This may be due to greater CA in the WS group, which would

mean they have more years of musical listening experience.

Huron (2001) suggests a connection between the hypersociability demonstrated by people with WS and musicality, perhaps because of purported evolutionary connections between music and social bonding. This connection is controversial, although sociability and musicality may be connected indirectly through the lack of inhibition demonstrated by individuals with WS. This lack of inhibition would lead to greater sociability and make them more likely to sing or play music in public without fear. This greater frequency of "practice," then, would lead to relatively greater musical abilities.

Musical Affect

Individuals with WS have also been shown to have strong emotional connections with music. Dykens, Rosner, Ly, and Sagun (2005) examined the relationship between music and anxiety in WS. They compared the WS group to age-matched groups with Prader-Willi syndrome or DS, and included IQ as a covariate. Those in the WS group were more likely to take music lessons and play an instrument, and they had higher ratings of musical skills. They found that the WS group had more intense levels of involvement with music than did the other groups with mental retardation, and the WS group's emotional response to negative music and to producing music included fewer externalizing symptoms (as measured by the Child Behavior Checklist; Achenbach, 1991), less anxiety, and fewer fears when compared with the other mental retardation groups.

It is difficult to disentangle the fact that the WS group has taken more lessons and demonstrates a higher level of musical proficiency than the other groups from their higher ratings on the emotional responses to music. Since these data are purely correlational, further study is warranted.

As mentioned above, Hopyan et al. (2001) developed a musical affect test to more quantitatively examine the perception of emotion in music in individuals with WS. Participants were asked to decide whether each of several musical excerpts went best with a happy, sad, or scary face. The WS group performed more poorly than did the CA-matched control group on pitch, rhythm, and musical affect (they were equal on judgments of happy, but poorer at judging sad or scary excerpts), but they performed as well as the controls on melodic imagery and phrasing judgments, perhaps demonstrating a stronger melodic than rhythmic ability.

These results are challenging to interpret because their difficulty with this task may reflect difficulty in matching the semantic labels to the emotions rather than a lack of perception of the expressiveness in the music.

Auditory and Musical Processing: Evidence from Neuroimaging

Levitin et al. (2003) scanned participants with WS and controls during a passive music listening task. They found strikingly different patterns of neural organization. Regions supporting noise and music processing in normal subjects (superior and medial temporal gyri, for example) were not consistently activated in the WS participants. The WS participants also showed reduced activation in temporal lobes. However, during music processing, they also showed significantly greater activation in the right amygdala and a widely distributed network of activation in cortical and subcortical structures, including the brainstem, which the controls did not show. There is also evidence for increased connectivity between the primary auditory cortex and the limbic system in individuals with WS, which could be thought to contribute to increased emotional involvement with music or hypersensitivity to sounds in individuals with WS (Holinger et al., 2005).

Some studies have reported a high proportion of individuals with WS who demonstrated sensorineural hearing loss (Cherniske et al., 2004), with a higher-than-normal prevalence in children (Marler, Elfenbein, Ryals, Urban, & Netzloff, 2005), suggesting a connection between the genetic deletions in WS and auditory function. There are also numerous abnormalities in the auditory cortex of individuals with WS when compared with controls (Holinger et al., 2005), including reduced leftward asymmetry of the planum temporale and atypical right Sylvian fissure patterning (Eckert et al., 2006). In addition, auditory brainstem response, as measured by the brainstem auditory evoked response (BAER), has shown significantly prolonged latency in participants with WS compared with controls (Gothelf et al., 2006).

Summary

In summary, evidence to date suggests that music production and perception abilities in individuals with WS are spared relative to other abilities, such as visuospatial ability. However, more objective measures of musical ability with carefully chosen control groups are needed to establish how their musical abilities compare to those of typical controls and to individuals with other developmental disorders.

Down Syndrome
Musical Responsiveness

Many writers have observed that a trait common among children with DS is to show a fondness for music and rhythmic movements (Brousseau & Brainerd, 1928; Brushfield, 1924; Stratford & Ching, 1983). However, empirical evidence to support this is scarce. Anecdotal reports suggest that music is a useful tool for behavioral management, such as assuring successful dental treatment of children with DS (Desai, 1997). When compared with other groups of individuals with developmental disorders, individuals with DS do not always differ in their musical responsiveness or enjoyment. They tend to perform fewer visuospatial activities and more musical activities in their leisure time than do individuals with Prader-Willi syndrome, and they do not differ from individuals with WS (Sellinger et al., 2006). An early observation study of a group of children with DS and a group of comparison children with mental retardation showed no difference in pleasure exhibited in response to music or rhythmic ability (Blacketer-Simmonds, 1953). Stratford and Ching (1989) tested groups of children with DS and with other mental retardation etiologies on their movement responses to music. They found no difference among groups in type or number of movements used to respond to music. However, Dykens et al. (2005) showed that, when compared with Prader-Willi and WS groups, the DS group showed more movement in response to the music, and they were more likely than the others to respond that negative-toned excerpts made them feel happy. Additionally, in a survey study of musical interest and experience, Levitin et al. (2004) found that the musical interest of individuals with DS was equivalent to the amount of musical interest of individuals with WS, and higher than that of typically developing children.

Musical Ability

Few studies have explored the musical abilities of individuals with DS, but the available evidence suggests preserved musical abilities for their MA. In a test of rhythmic tapping ability among children with DS, children with other mental retardation, and typically developing controls (all matched on MA), the DS and typically developing groups did not differ, whereas the mental retardation group was impaired relative to the other two groups (Stratford

& Ching, 1983). Individuals with DS were found to be impaired in melodic repetition when compared with individuals with WS and CA but not MA-matched controls, but were no different from the WS group in a melodic completion task (Levitin, 2005).

Auditory Processing

A comparison of adolescents with DS and adolescents with other mental retardation on peripheral hearing measures showed that children with DS were less sensitive across most pure tone frequencies, had poorer speech reception thresholds, and showed a stronger tendency toward conductive/middle ear difficulties, and high-frequency loss (Marcell & Cohen, 1992). Measures of central auditory processing using EEG and MEG have shown abnormalities in components of signals evoked by auditory stimuli, including abnormally accelerated brainstem potentials and delays in cortical electrical evoked potentials and their magnetic counterparts (Diaz & Zurron, 1995; Pekkonen, Osipova, Sauna-Aho, & Arvio, 2007; Seidl et al., 1997; Squires, Aine, Buchwald, Norman, & Galbraith, 1980). This indicates some impairment in preattentive auditory processing, which would affect stimulus discrimination in individuals with DS (Pekkonen et al., 2007). Their auditory processing differs from children with fetal alcohol syndrome also; using discriminant function analysis, one study showed that children with DS can be differentiated from control children, as well as from children with fetal alcohol syndrome, by examining the latency and amplitude of the P300 EEG component in response to an infrequent tone stimulus (Kaneko, Ehlers, Philips, & Riley, 1996).

Fragile X Syndrome

Boys with FXS can show typical enjoyment of music; Hatton et al. (2000) reports that music is one of the activities young boys with FXS enjoy, and it can be used as a calming influence and an incentive to assist with teaching.

Studies of general auditory processing frequently demonstrate some abnormalities in neural responses to sound. Individuals with FXS can show hyperarousal to auditory stimuli (Hagerman, 1999). Rojas et al. (2001), using MEG, found that the amplitude of the N100m auditory evoked field component in response to 1kHz sine tones was higher for adults with FXS than for typical controls, and the individuals with FXS also had reduced left versus right hemisphere asymmetry in N100m location along the x-axis. The authors suggest that this may be indicative of relatively more neurons being activated for individuals with FXS in response to auditory stimuli, consistent with subjectively more intense experience of the auditory stimuli. Studies of lower-level auditory function in FXS, as measured by auditory brainstem responses (ABR), have shown mixed results: Arinami, Sato, Nakajima, and Kondo (1988) showed that the participants with FXS had prolonged interpeak latencies. However, later research has shown no difference in ABR latencies between individuals with FXS and typical controls (Miezejeski et al., 1997; Roberts et al., 2005), and Miezejeski et al. (1997) proposes that the differences found previously can be attributed to sedation, which causes longer ABR latencies.

Structural neuroanatomical work has shown decreases in the size of lobules VI and VII of the posterior cerebellar vermis in individuals with autism and FXS (Courchesne, Yeung-Courchesne, Press, Hesselink, & Jernigan, 1988; Reiss, Aylward, Freund, Joshi, & Bryan, 1991; Reiss, Patel, Kumar, & Freund, 1988). The cerebellum may be important for many aspects of music perception and performance, including timing and discrimination of auditory intervals (Peretz & Zatorre, 2005) and emotional processing of music (Pallesen et al., 2005). However, the direct implication of cerebellar abnormalities in musical processing in FXS remains to be studied.

Tuberous Sclerosis Complex

One study has examined the musical responsiveness of children with tuberous sclerosis complex, and no diagnosis of autistic disorder using the Nonverbal Measure of the Measurement of the Musical Responsiveness of Children (MMRC; Matsuyama, 2005; Matsuyama, Ohsawa, & Ogawa, 2007). The authors found a significant correlation among normal children and children with autism between the scores on the Nonverbal MMRC and developmental age, but no such correlation was found for the children with tuberous sclerosis complex, who showed high musical responsiveness at young developmental ages. This suggests to the author that music may be a nondelayed domain for the children with tuberous sclerosis complex (Matsuyama et al., 2007). However, other authors have also found no evidence of correlation between musical batteries scores and MA among individuals with mental retardation (McLeish & Higgs, 1982; Rice, 1970), so further study of this phenomenon is required.

There is some evidence of abnormal ABRs in children with tuberous sclerosis complex, although the study to show this tested only four participants with tuberous sclerosis complex (Ferri, Elia, Musumeci, & Bergonzi, 1993). Auditory abnormalities in tuberous sclerosis complex may also be correlated with autistic behavior. In a study of electrical evoked responses to pitches, the children with tuberous sclerosis complex and autistic behavior showed longer latencies and lower amplitude on the N1 component, as well as a mismatch negativity, with a longer latency when compared with the children with tuberous sclerosis complex but no autistic behavior (Seri, Cerquiglini, Pisani, & Curatolo, 1999).

Rett Syndrome

Research in auditory processing in Rett syndrome has shown abnormal brainstem frequency-following responses, with patterns more similar to infants than to adults, suggesting developmental arrest of the auditory system (Galbraith, Philippart, & Stephen, 1996). Evidence from a longitudinal study suggests no degeneration of white matter in the auditory brainstem (Pillion & Naidu, 2000). Cortical event-related potential measures of auditory functioning show overall longer latencies and smaller amplitudes, suggesting slower information processing and reduced brain activity (Stauder, Smeets, van Mil, & Curfs, 2006). Peripheral hearing loss does not appear to be a common problem in individuals with Rett syndrome (Stach, Stoner, Smith, & Jerger, 1994) or correlated with the type of genetic mutation (Pillion & Naidu, 2000), but abnormal middle latency responses and late vertex responses suggest that they may have a central auditory disorder (Stach et al., 1994). Even with these auditory impairments, music therapy has been shown to be useful in enhancing communication abilities and/or as a source of pleasure and relaxation in case studies with girls with Rett syndrome (Kerr, Archer, Evans, Prescott, & Gibbon, 2006; Wigram & Lawrence, 2005; Yasuhara & Sugiyama, 2001).

Music in Behavior Modification

Regardless of the musical ability of the individual with mental retardation, music may be useful in many ways. For example, it has been shown to be useful as a reinforcer to help severely disabled individuals learn to perform tasks (Gutowski, 1996), help less severely disabled children improve arithmetic skills (Miller, 1977), or decrease crying and other challenging behaviors among individuals with mental retardation (Allen & Bryant, 1985; Davis, Wieseler, & Hanzel, 1980), and it has been found to be as effective as juice at influencing behavior

(Saperston, Chan, Morphew, & Carsrud, 1980). When combined with auditory behavior prompts, it has also been shown to be effective at reducing aberrant behaviors in social situations (Alberto, Taber, & Fredrick, 1999).

The effect of background music on the behaviors of individuals with mental retardation is less clear; some studies have found no effect of non-contingent background music on worker productivity (Wentworth, 1991) or general activity level (Kaufman & Sheckart, 1985), whereas others find a positive effect on worker productivity (Groeneweg, Stan, Celser, MacBeth, & Vrbancic, 1998) or exercise output (Caouette & Reid, 1991). More study of differing tempi, loudness, and genre type is needed before background music can be used reliably to alter behavior. As an illustration of this, a study investigating one child and two adults with mental retardation found that music with a fast beat decreased challenging behaviors in all three individuals, whereas music with a slow beat increased these behaviors in two of the three individuals (Durand & Mapstone, 1998). Loudness is also important to consider; louder or more active music may decrease the need for self-stimulatory behavior among individuals with mental retardation. Cunningham (1986) found that loud music decreased vocalization rate among a group of individuals with severe mental retardation, whereas soft music increased this self-stimulatory behavior. In a similar vein, Reardon and Bell (1970) found that stimulative rock music led to decreases in stereotyped behavior when compared with more sedative Bach chorales. Tierney, McGuire, and Walton (1978) found an increase in body-rocking behaviors in response to a radio broadcast of pop music, but they did not regulate the type of pop music, so no strong conclusions can be drawn from this. This may also be due to the complexity of the task the individuals were performing; for more complex tasks, the music may cause interference and decrease productivity, or it may simply be ignored (Groeneweg et al., 1998).

Conclusion

Evidence to date suggests that individuals with developmental disorders such as WS, tuberous sclerosis complex, and possibly DS, have musical abilities that are relatively spared as compared to their other cognitive and perceptual deficits. Musical appreciation and enjoyment does not seem to be dependent on cognitive faculties, and it can be useful as a means of establishing communication and influencing behavior even in individuals with severe mental retardation. Individuals with WS show heightened sensitivities to music when compared with controls, as well as higher levels of odynacusis, hyperacusis, and auditory allodynia and fascinations, suggesting that the auditory world is more interesting to them as well as more intrusive into their perceptions than it is to controls.

Taken together, the available evidence so far from empirical studies suggests that music can function as a distinct mental faculty (Gardner, 1983; Levitin & Bellugi, 1998). In spite of sometimes gross impairments in other cognitive domains, such as language, spatial cognition, mathematical ability, and reasoning, individuals can demonstrate relatively preserved musical ability, and IQ seems to be at least partly independent of musical ability. This challenges traditional notions about the unity of intelligence and supports so-called "multiple-intelligence" theories (e.g., Gardner, 1983).

It is important to keep in mind that people with neurodevelopmental disorders frequently have impaired peripheral and/or central auditory processing, which could affect their experience of music. Additionally, it is important to recognize also that what we consider to be music is itself composed of several differentiable subabilities, including (but not limited to) rhythm perception, rhythm production, pitch perception, pitch production, performance ability, composition ability, and emotional sensitivity to musical passages. A complete understanding of music and cognition requires that we fractionate musical ability into its subcomponents and look for integral and separable neuroanatomical substrates, as well as for their behavioral correlates.

Encouragingly, the literature is rife with anecdotal evidence and case studies indicating numerous beneficial uses and effects of music for individuals with developmental disorders. It is clear that music can be important for people of all levels of intellectual functioning. However, there is still a need for more empirical behavioral studies of music and various types of developmental disorders using larger groups of participants and carefully selected control groups. In addition, there is ample room for more neuroimaging studies in auditory processing with all of these populations with developmental disorders.

References

Achenbach, T. M. (1991). *Manual for the Child Behavior Checklist/4–18 and 1991 Profile*. Burlington, VT: University of Vermont Department of Psychiatry.

Alberto, P. A., Taber, T. A., & Fredrick, L. D. (1999). Use of self-operated auditory prompts to decrease aberrant behaviors in students with moderate mental retardation. *Research in Developmental Disabilities, 20*(6), 429–439.

Allen, L., & Bryant, M. C. (1985). A multielement analysis of contingent versus contingent-interrupted music. *Applied Research in Mental Retardation, 6*(1), 87–97.

Anastasi, A., & Levee, R. F. (1960). Intellectual defect and musical talent: A case report. *American Journal of Mental Deficiency, 64,* 695–703.

Arinami, T., Sato, M., Nakajima, S., & Kondo, I. (1988). Auditory brain-stem responses in the fragile X syndrome. *American Journal of Human Genetics, 43*(1), 46–51.

Blacketer-Simmonds, D. A. (1953). An investigation into the supposed differences existing between mongols and other mentally defective subjects with regard to certain psychological traits. *Journal of Mental Science, 99,* 702–719.

Blomberg, S., Rosander, M., & Andersson, G. (2006). Fears, hyperacusis and musicality in Williams syndrome. *Research in Developmental Disabilities, 27,* 668–680.

Brousseau, K., & Brainerd, H. G. (1928). *Mongolism: A study of the physical and mental characteristics of mongolian imbeciles.* Baltimore: The Williams & Wilkins Company.

Brushfield, T. (1924). Mongolism. *British Journal of Childhood Diseases, 21,* 241–243.

Braswell, C., Decuir, A., Hoskins, C., Kvet, E., & Oubre, G. (1988). Relation between musical aptitude and intelligence among mentally retarded, advantaged, and disadvantaged subjects. *Perceptual and Motor Skills, 67*(2), 359–364.

Caouette, M., & Reid, G. (1991). Influence of auditory stimulation on the physical work output of adults who are severely retarded. *Education and Training in Mental Retardation, 26*(1), 43–52.

Carrasco, X., Castillo, S., Aravena, T., Rothhammer, P., & Aboitiz, F. (2005). Williams syndrome: Pediatric, neurologic, and cognitive development. *Pediatric Neurology, 32*(3), 166–172.

Cherniske, E. M., Carpenter, T. O., Klaiman, C., Young, E., Bregman, J., Insogna, K., et al. (2004). Multisystem study of 20 older adults with Williams syndrome. *American Journal of Medical Genetics, 131A,* 255–264.

Courchesne, E., Yeung-Courchesne, R., Press, G. A., Hesselink, J. R., & Jernigan, T. L. (1988). Hypoplasia of cerebellar vermal lobules VI and VII in autism. *New England Journal of Medicine, 318*(21), 1349–1354.

Cunningham, T. (1986). The effect of music volume on the frequency of vocalizations of institutionalized mentally retarded persons. *Journal of Music Therapy, 23*(4), 208–218.

Davis, W. B., Wieseler, N. A., & Hanzel, T. E. (1980). Contingent music in management of rumination and out-of-seat behavior in a profoundly mentally retarded institutionalized male. *Mental Retardation, 18*(1), 43–45.

Deruelle, C., Schön, D., Rondan, C., & Mancini, J. (2005). Global and local music perception in children with Williams syndrome. *Neuroreport: For Rapid Communication of Neuroscience Research, 16*(6), 631–634.

Desai, S. S. (1997). Down syndrome: A review of the literature. *Oral surgery, Oral Medicine, Oral Pathology, Oral Radiology and Endodontics, 84,* 279–285.

DiGiammarino, M. (1990). Functional music skills of persons with mental retardation. *Journal of Music Therapy, 27*(4), 209–220.

Diaz, F., & Zurron, M. (1995). Auditory evoked potentials in Down's syndrome. *Electroencephalography and Clinical Neurophysiology, 98,* 526–537.

Don, A. J., Schellenberg, E., & Rourke, B. P. (1999). Music and language skills of children with Williams syndrome. *Child Neuropsychology, 5*(3), 154–170.

Durand, V. M., & Mapstone, E. (1998). Influence of "mood-inducing" music on challenging behavior. *American Journal on Mental Retardation, 102*(4), 367–378.

Dykens, E. M., Rosner, B. A., Ly, T., & Sagun, J. (2005). Music and anxiety in Williams syndrome: A harmonious or discordant relationship? *American Journal on Mental Retardation, 110*(5), 346–358.

Eckert, M. A., Galaburda, A. M., Karchemskiy, A., Liang, A., Thompson, P., Dutton, R. A., et al. (2006). Anomalous sylvian fissure morphology in Williams syndrome. *NeuroImage, 33*, 39–45.

Ferri, R., Elia, M., Musumeci, S. A., & Bergonzi, P. (1993). Brainstem auditory evoked potentials in tuberous sclerosis. *Italian Journal of Neurological Sciences, 14*(4), 311–316.

Galbraith, G. C., Philippart, M., & Stephen, L. M. (1996). Brainstem frequency-following responses in Rett syndrome. *Pediatric Neurology, 15*(1), 26–31.

Gardner, H. (1983). *Frames of mind: The theory of multiple intelligences.* New York: Basic Books.

Gordon, E. E. (1965, rev. 1995). *Musical aptitude profile [Audio recording and book].* Boston: Houghton Mifflin.

Gordon, E. E. (1986). *Primary measures of music audiation [Audio recording and book].* Chicago: G.I.A. Publications.

Gothelf, D., Farber, N., Raveh, E., Apter, A., & Attias, J. (2006). Hyperacusis in Williams syndrome: Characteristics and associated neuroaudiologic abnormalities. *Neurology, 66*, 390–395.

Groeneweg, G., Stan, E. A., Celser, A., MacBeth, L., & Vrbancic, M. I. (1998). The effect of background music on the vocational behavior of mentally handicapped adults. *Journal of Music Therapy, 25*(3), 118–134.

Gutowski, S. (1996). Response acquisition for music or beverages in adults with profound multiple handicaps. *Journal of Developmental and Physical Disabilities, 8*(3), 221–231.

Hagerman, R. J. (1999). *Neurodevelopmental disorders: Diagnosis and treatment.* New York: Oxford University Press.

Hatton, D. D., Bailey, D. B., Roberts, J. P., Skinner, M., Mayhew, L., Clark, R. D., et al. (2000). Early intervention services for young boys with fragile X syndrome. *Journal of Early Intervention, 23*(4), 235–251.

Heaton, P., & Wallace, G. L. (2004). Annotation: The savant syndrome. *Journal of Child Psychology and Psychiatry, 45*(5), 899–911.

Hermelin, B., O'Connor, N., & Lee, S. (1987). Musical inventiveness of five idiot-savants. *Psychological Medicine, 17*(3), 685–694.

Holinger, D. P., Bellugi, U., Mills, D. L., Korenberg, J. R., Reiss, A. L., Sherman, G. F., et al. (2005). Relative sparing of the primary auditory cortex in Williams syndrome. *Brain Research, 1037*, 35–42.

Hopyan, T., Dennis, M., Weksberg, R., & Cytrynbaum, C. (2001). Music skills and the expressive interpretation of music in children with Williams-Beuren syndrome: Pitch, rhythm, melodic imagery, phrasing, and musical affect. *Child Neuropsychology, 7*(1), 42–53.

Hoskins, C. (1985). Relationship between expressive language ability and rhythm perception, pitch perception, vocal range, and vocal midpoint among mentally retarded adults. *Perceptual and Motor Skills, 60*, 644–646.

Huron, D. (2001). Is music an evolutionary adaptation? *Annals of the New York Academy of Sciences, 930*, 43–61.

Kaneko, W. M., Ehlers, C. L., Philips, E. L., Riley, E. P. (1996). Auditory event-related potentials in fetal alcohol syndrome and Down's syndrome children. *Alcoholism: Clinical and Experimental Research, 20*(1), 35–42.

Kaplan, P. R. (1977). *A criterion-referenced comparison of rhythmic responsiveness in normal and educable mentally retarded children.* Unpublished doctoral dissertation, University of Michigan, Ann Arbor.

Kaufman, F. M., & Sheckart, G. R. (1985). The effects of tempo variation and white noise on the general activity level of profoundly retarded adults. *Journal of Music Therapy, 22*(4), 207–217.

Kerr, A. M., Archer, H. L., Evans, J. C., Prescott, R. J., & Gibbon, F. (2006). People with MECP2 mutation-positive Rett disorder who converse. *Journal of Intellectual Disability Research, 50*(Pt. 5), 386–394.

Kubovy, M. (1981). Integral and separable dimensions and the theory of indispensable attributes. In M. Kubovy, & J. Pomerantz (Eds.), *Perceptual organization.* Hillsdale, NJ: Erlbaum.

Lenhoff, H. M. (1996). *Music and Williams syndrome: A status report and goals.* Paper presented at the Seventh International Professional Williams Syndrome Conference, Valley Forge, PA.

Lenhoff, H. M., Perales, O., & Hickok, G. (2001). Absolute pitch in Williams syndrome. *Music Perception, 18*(4), 491–503.

Levitin, D. J. (2005). Musical behavior in a neurogenetic developmental disorder: Evidence from Williams syndrome. *Annals of the New York Academy of Sciences, 1060*, 325–334.

Levitin, D. J. (2006). *This is your brain on music: The science of a human obsession.* New York: Dutton-Penguin.

Levitin, D. J., & Bellugi, U. (1998). Musical abilities in individuals with Williams syndrome. *Music Perception, 15*(4), 357–389.

Levitin, D. J., Cole, K., Chiles, M., Lai, Z., Lincoln, A., & Bellugi, U. (2004). Characterizing the musical phenotype in individuals with Williams syndrome. *Child Neuropsychology, 10*(4), 223–247.

Levitin, D. J., Cole, K., Lincoln, A., & Bellugi, U. (2005). Aversion, awareness, and attraction: Investigating claims of hyperacusis in Williams syndrome phenotype. *Journal of Child Psychology and Psychiatry, 46*(5), 514–523.

Levitin, D. J., Menon, V., Schmitt, J. E., Eliez, S., White, C. D., Glover, G. H., et al. (2003). Neural correlates of auditory perception in Williams syndrome: An fMRI study. *NeuroImage, 18*, 74–82.

Levitin, D. J., & Rogers, S. E. (2005). Absolute pitch: Perception, coding, and controversies. *Trends in Cognitive Sciences, 9*(1), 26–33.

Levitin, D. J., & Zatorre, R. J. (2003). On the nature of early music training and absolute pitch: A reply to Brown, Sachs, Cammuso, and Folstein. *Music Perception, 21*(1), 105–110.

Marcell, M. M., & Cohen, S. (1992). Hearing abilities of Down syndrome and other mentally handicapped adolescents. *Research in Developmental Disabilities, 13*, 533–551.

Marler, J. A., Elfenbein, J. L., Ryals, B. M., Urban, Z., & Netzloff, M. L. (2005). Sensorineural hearing loss in children and adults with Williams syndrome. *American Journal of Medical Genetics, 138A*, 318–327.

Matsuyama, K. (2005). Correlation between musical responsiveness and developmental age among early age children as assessed by the Non-Verbal Measurement of the Musical Responsiveness of Children. *Medical Science Monitor, 11*(10), 485–492.

Matsuyama, K., Ohsawa, I., & Ogawa, T. (2007). Do children with tuberous sclerosis complex have superior musical skill?—A unique tendency of musical responsiveness in children with TSC. *Medical Science Monitor, 13*(4), 156–164.

McLeish, J., & Higgs, G. (1982). Musical ability and mental subnormality: An experimental investigation. *British Journal of Educational Psychology, 52*(Pt 3), 370–373.

Miezejeski, C. M., Heaney, G., Belser, R., Brown, W. T., Jenkins, E. C., & Sersen, E. A. (1997). Longer brainstem auditory evoked response latencies of individuals with fragile X syndrome related to sedation. *American Journal of Medical Genetics, 74*, 167–171.

Miller, D. M. (1977). Effects of music-listening contingencies on arithmetic performance and music preference of EMR children. *American Journal of Mental Deficiency, 81*(4), 371–378.

Miller, G. (2000). Evolution of human music through sexual selection In N.L. Wallin, B. Merker, & S. Brown (Eds.), *The Origins of Music*, (pp 329–360). Cambridge, MA: MIT Press.

Miller, L. K. (1989). *Musical savants: Exceptional skill in the mentally retarded*. Hillsdale, NJ: Lawrence Erlbaum Associates.

Miller, L. K. (1999). The savant syndrome: Intellectual impairment and exceptional skill. *Psychological Bulletin, 125*(1), 31–46.

Mithen, S. (2006). *The Singing Neanderthals: The origin of music, language, mind and body*. Cambridge, MA: Harvard University Press.

Navon, D. (1977). Forest before trees: The precedence of global features in visual perception. *Cognitive Psychology, 9*, 353–383.

Norton, D. (1980). Interrelationships among music aptitude, IQ, and auditory conservation. *Journal of Research in Music Education, 28*(4), 207–217.

O'Connor, N., & Hermelin, B. (1988). Low intelligence and special abilities. *Journal of Child Psychology and Psychiatry, 29*(4), 391–396.

Ollendick, T. H. (1983). Reliability and validity of the revised fear survey schedule for children (FSSC-R). *Behaviour Research and Therapy, 21*, 685–692.

Pallesen, K. J., Brattico, E., Bailey, C., Korvenoja, A., Koivisto, J., Gjedde, A., et al. (2005). Emotion processing of major, minor, and dissonant chords: A functional magnetic resonance imaging study. *Annals of the New York Academy of Sciences, 1060*, 450–453.

Pekkonen, E., Osipova, D., Sauna-Aho, O., & Arvio, M. (2007). Delayed auditory processing underlying stimulus detection in Down syndrome. *NeuroImage, 35*(4), 1547–1550.

Peretz, I., & Zatorre, R. J. (2005). Brain organization for music processing. *Annual Review of Psychology, 56*, 89–114.

Pillion, J. P., & Naidu, S. (2000). Auditory brainstem response findings in Rett syndrome: Stability over time. *Journal of Pediatrics, 137*(3), 393–396.

Reardon, D. M., & Bell, G. (1970). Effects of sedative and stimulative music on activity levels of severely retarded boys. *American Journal of Mental Deficiency, 75*(2), 156–159.

Reiss, A. L., Aylward, E., Freund, L. S., Joshi, P. K., & Bryan, R. N. (1991). Neuroanatomy of fragile X syndrome: The posterior fossa. *Annals of Neurology, 29*(1), 26–32.

Reiss, A. L., Patel, S., Kumar, A. J., & Freund, L. (1988). Preliminary communication: Neuroanatomical variations of the posterior fossa in men with the fragile X (Martin-Bell) syndrome. *American Journal of Medical Genetics, 31*(2), 407–414.

Rice, J. A. (1970). Abbreviated Gordon Musical Aptitude Profile with EMR children. *American Journal of Mental Deficiency, 75*(1), 107–108.

Roberts, J., Hennon, E. A., Anderson, K., Roush, J., Gravel, J., Skinner, M., et al. (2005). Auditory brainstem responses in young males with fragile X syndrome. *Journal of Speech, Language, and Hearing Research, 48*, 494–500.

Rojas, D. C., Benkers, T. L., Rogers, S. J., Teale, P. D., Reite, M. L., & Hagerman, R. J. (2001). Auditory evoked magnetic fields in adults with fragile X syndrome. *Neuroreport, 12*(11), 2573–2576.

Saperston, B. M., Chan, R., Morphew, C., & Carsrud, K. B. (1980). Music listening versus juice as a reinforcement for learning in profoundly mentally retarded individuals. *Journal of Music Therapy, 17*, 174–183.

Seashore, C., Emil, C. E., Saetveit, J. G., & Lewis, D. (1960). *Seashore measures of musical talents*. New York: The Psychological Corporation.

Seidl, R., Hauser, E., Bernert, G., Marx, M., Freilinger, M., & Lubec, G. (1997). Auditory evoked potentials in young patients with Down syndrome. Event-related potentials (P3) and histaminergic system. *Cognitive Brain Research, 5*, 301–309.

Sellinger, M. H., Hodapp, R. M., & Dykens, E. M. (2006). Leisure activities of individuals with Prader-Willi, Williams and Down syndromes. *Journal of Developmental and Physical Disabilities, 18*(1), 59–71.

Seri, S., Cerquiglini, A., Pisani, F., & Curatolo, P. (1999). Autism in tuberous sclerosis: Evoked potential evidence for a deficit in auditory sensory processing. *Clinical Neurophysiology, 110*(10), 1825–1830.

Sloboda, J. A., Hermelin, B., & O'Connor, N. (1985). An exceptional musical memory. *Music Perception, 3*(2), 155–170.

Squires, N., Aine, C., Buchwald, J., Norman, R., & Galbraith, G. C. (1980). Auditory brain stem response abnormalities in severely and profoundly retarded adults. *Electroencephalography and Clinical Neurophysiology, 1980*(50), 192–185.

Stach, B. A., Stoner, W. R., Smith, S. L., & Jerger, J. F. (1994). Auditory evoked potentials in Rett syndrome. *Journal of the American Academy of Audiology, 5*(3), 226–230.

Stauder, J. E. A., Smeets, E. E. J., van Mil, S. G. M., & Curfs, L. G. M. (2006). The development of visual- and auditory processing in Rett syndrome: An ERP study. *Brain and Development, 28*(8), 487–494.

Stratford, B., & Ching, E. (1983). Rhythm and time in the perception of Down's syndrome children. *Journal of Mental Deficiency Research, 27*(Pt. 1), 23–38.

Stratford, B., & Ching, E. (1989). Response to music and movement in the development of children with Down's syndrome. *Journal of Mental Deficiency Research, 33*(1), 13–24.

Svensson, L., & Öst, L.-G. (1999). Fears in Swedish children. A normative study of the Fear Survey Schedule for Children—Revised. *Scandinavian Journal of Behaviour Therapy, 28*, 23–36.

Takeuchi, A. H., & Hulse, S. H. (1993). Absolute pitch. *Psychological Bulletin, 113*(2), 345–361.

Tierney, I. R., McGuire, R. J., & Walton, H. J. (1978). The effect of music on body-rocking manifested by severely mentally deficient patients in ward environments. *Journal of Mental Deficiency Research, 22*(4), 255–261.

Wentworth, R. (1991). The effects of music and distracting noise on the productivity of workers with mental retardation. *Journal of Music Therapy, 28*(1), 40–47.

Wigram, T., & Lawrence, M. (2005). Music therapy as a tool for assessing hand use and communicativeness in children with Rett Syndrome. *Brain & Development, 27,* S95–S96.

Yasuhara, A., & Sugiyama, Y. (2001). Music therapy for children with Rett syndrome. *Brain & Development, 2001,* S82–S84.

Brain-based Methods in the Study of Developmental Disabilities: Examples from Event-related Potentials and Magnetic Resonance Imaging Research

Alexandra P.F. Key *and* Tricia A. Thornton-Wells

Abstract

Numerous technologies are available for studying the brain basis of developmental disabilities, each of which has its advantages and disadvantages. These include electroencephalography (EEG), event-related potentials (ERP), magnetoencephalography (MEG), near-infrared optical tomography (NIROT), positron emission tomography (PET), magnetic resonance imaging (MRI), and magnetic resonance spectroscopy (MRspect). This chapter focuses on two technologies—ERP and MRI—which are increasingly being used in research on developmental disabilities. It discusses how each methodology works and what kinds of research questions each is well suited to answer. It illustrates the application of these methods in four specific genetic disorders: Down syndrome, Prader-Willi syndrome, Williams syndrome, and fragile X syndrome. Finally, the chapter discusses gaps in current research, issues of experimental design, and suggests directions for future studies.

Keywords: Brain imaging, developmental disabilities, event-related potentials, ERP, magnetic resonance imaging, MRI

Over the past 20 years, research in the area of developmental disabilities, particularly those with a known genetic basis, has expanded from reliance almost entirely on behavioral assessments to inclusion of brain-based measures. The search is on to find brain correlates of behaviors or traits characteristic of specific diagnoses. Brain measures can identify structures or processes associated with typical and atypical functioning at various developmental stages. Differences in brain mechanisms underlying developmental disabilities might not be easily observable in behavior either because of a limited behavioral repertoire of the person (e.g., infants, persons with severe intellectual disabilities) or due to the insufficient sensitivity of the behavioral tools (e.g., even significant delays in the speed of information processing might not be captured by the traditional reaction time measures). Yet, by studying the brain, we have a greater chance of identifying specific markers of atypical functioning and linking those to genetic etiology. These brain-based findings could then translate into targets for pharmacologic or early behavioral interventions, or lead to gene therapy development.

Brain-based research methods provide information about which areas of the brain are involved in performing particular types of tasks or behaviors (e.g., recognizing letters or listening to music) and how these brain structures differ between individuals with typical development and those with a particular developmental disability. It is also possible to assess how efficiently various brain regions function and how well they communicate with other parts of the brain. Such detailed information can provide crucial insights into whether a particular behavioral pattern or cognitive difficulty is related to anatomical or functional brain characteristics. Brain-based measures can also help disambiguate the contributions of sensory processes, attention, motivation, emotion regulation, response selection and execution, or higher cognitive functions to the cognitive and behavioral profiles of persons with developmental disability.

Numerous technologies are available for studying the brain basis of developmental disabilities, each of which has its advantages and disadvantages. These include but are not limited to electroencephalography (EEG), event-related potentials (ERP), magnetoencephalography (MEG), near-infrared optical tomography (NIROT), positron emission tomography (PET), magnetic resonance imaging (MRI), and magnetic resonance spectroscopy (MRspect). These methods differ in their procedures of data acquisition (e.g., recording of electrical, magnetic, or biochemical signals) and the type of the information provided, with some being more sensitive to the timing of brain activity (e.g., EEG/ERP, MEG) whereas others are better suited for identifying specific brain regions involved in task performance (e.g., PET, MRI; see Papanicolaou, 1998, for a more detailed overview of the imaging methods). In this chapter, we focus on two of these technologies—ERP and MRI—which are increasingly being used in research on developmental disabilities. We will briefly discuss how each methodology works and what kinds of research questions each is well-suited to answer. We will also illustrate how these methods have been used in four specific genetic disorders: Down syndrome (DS), Prader-Willi syndrome (PWS), Williams syndrome (WS), and fragile X syndrome (FXS). Finally, we will discuss gaps in current research, issues of experimental design, and suggest directions for future studies.

Brief Overview of the Selected Neuroimaging Techniques
Electrophysiology

Electroencephalogram recordings have long been used as an indicator of ongoing brain activity. They allow one to examine general brain characteristics, such as levels of arousal and degree of functional connectivity among various brain regions, as well as specific processes underlying temperament, attention, perception, and working memory. A brief temporary change in the EEG in response to a particular external or internal event (e.g., hearing a sound, making a decision) is known as an *event-related potential*. Because their millisecond-level resolution is comparable to the speed of many cognitive processes, ERPs are widely used to examine both automatic (e.g., sensory; reflected mainly within the first 200 msec after stimulus onset) and controlled (e.g., memory, attention, inhibition; 200+ msec after stimulus onset) stages of information processing (Key, Dove, & Maguire, 2005; Russeler, Nager, Mobes, & Munte, 2005; Zani &

Proverbio, 2003). Furthermore, ERP waveform shapes and specific peak characteristics (e.g., amplitude, latency, scalp distribution) change with age and thus allow for tracking of maturation- and learning-related effects, making them an excellent tool for studying typical and atypical development (e.g., Jing & Benasich, 2006; Ponton et al., 2000; Sharma, Dorman, & Kral, 2005).

In addition to the excellent temporal sensitivity, advantages of ERPs also include their noninvasive nature (e.g., no injections as in PET, no confinement to small spaces as in MRI), flexibility in acquisition (e.g., can be recorded in participant's home or at hospital bedside), fast acquisition time (EEG sensors can be applied within 2–5 minutes), and ability to provide information about cognition even in the absence of verbal or other overt behavioral responses. These characteristics make ERPs especially valuable for studying infants, as well as children and adults with physical and/or communicative limitations, who might also be highly anxious or present a host of sensory and behavioral issues that make traditional behavioral assessments difficult to complete.

One limitation of the ERP technique is that it does not offer the detailed spatial resolution needed to directly link activity recorded on the scalp to specific brain regions. Even with high-density electrode arrays, not all brain electrical activity is captured due to variations in signal strength, distance from various cortical areas to the scalp, and the orientation of cortical columns generating the signal. Also, although modern analysis approaches allow researchers to model potential brain sources of scalp-recorded activity, a shortage of standardized age- and syndrome-specific head models makes identifying brain sources of EEG/ERP data in persons with developmental disabilities even more complicated, as many genetic syndromes are associated with alterations in brain size, structure, and organization relative to a typical adult brain. However, other techniques for documenting brain structures and their activity, such as an MRI, can offer the needed spatial resolution.

Magnetic Resonance Imaging

Magnetic resonance imaging uses strong magnetic fields and radio waves to detect differences in tissue structure and function. Structural MRI (sMRI) can provide very high spatial resolution (down to 1 mm for 3 Tesla scanners) of brain tissue, allowing for quantification and analysis of the shape, density, and volume of specific brain structures. Anatomical differences in specific brain regions might implicate specific developmental time points, environmental factors, or genes involved in particular neurotransmitter systems (e.g., frontal lobe regions mature relatively late in development and can be influenced by dopaminergic and serotoninergic function). Diffusion tensor imaging (DTI) uses MRI technology to examine the structure and integrity of white matter, which is made up of myelinated neurons providing high speed connections between gray matter (both cortical and subcortical) regions of the brain. Abnormalities in white matter might impact cognitive functions that require coordination or integration across multiple, sometimes distal, regions of the brain (e.g., episodic memory function requires coordination of frontal, temporal, and parietal cortices with higher-order association areas). Functional MRI (fMRI) can provide information about the brain areas involved in performing a specific function by detecting changes in oxygen use during a given task (vs. a control condition). Individual and group differences in brain activation patterns might reflect deficits, compensatory mechanisms (e.g., increased activation of the language-related left inferior parietal lobe during numerical tasks in persons with dyscalculia), or enhanced functioning (e.g., increased bilateral activation of temporal and inferior frontal lobes during melodic or rhythmic discrimination in musicians).

When looking for high specificity with regard to which brain structures (particularly deep brain structures) are involved in certain tasks, fMRI is perhaps the best technology currently available. In addition, the recent development of rapid event-related experimental designs for fMRI allows for the analysis of temporal sequence, or the relative timing of brain activation, thus bringing the temporal resolution closer to that of the EEG/ERP methods. It is sometimes possible to design experiments amenable to both ERP and fMRI, in which findings from each method could be jointly analyzed for converging evidence (Cornish et al., 2004). Furthermore, multimodal systems are being implemented that allow for simultaneous measurement of both ERPs and MRI (Laufs, Daunizeau, Carmichael, & Kleinschmidt, 2008).

The application of MRI methods to the study of developmental disabilities is a very young but promising enterprise that has the potential to yield great insights into the brain basis of diagnosis-specific strengths and weaknesses. However, it can be challenging to identify adequate numbers of participants with rare genetic disorders who are willing to participate in MRI research. Despite the "open"

physical design of newer MRI machines, some individuals do experience feelings of claustrophobia, have difficulty tolerating the loud noises the MRI machine makes during scanning, or simply cannot remain still for several minutes at a time, as is necessary for longer scans. Creative solutions are often required to facilitate desensitization and to reduce head motion artifacts during scanning. For instance, prospective participants might be asked to listen to a recording of scanner noises several days prior to scanning and can participate in a practice scan using a mock scanner, which looks and sounds exactly like a real MRI machine but does not have a magnet in it. Also, individuals might be assigned a scanning "buddy" who remains in continuous social and/or physical contact (e.g., holding hands, talking, etc.) during the scan to help ease anxiety. Although developing scanning protocols for use in populations with developmental disabilities might appear a daunting task, it is important to recognize that such studies are being conducted successfully and are yielding otherwise unattainable information about the specific phenotypes.

Application of Neuroimaging Methods to the Study of Developmental Disabilities
Down Syndrome
EVENT-RELATED POTENTIAL STUDIES

The only longitudinal ERP study in DS that could be located by a computerized search of a number of databases (e.g., PubMed, Google Scholar) was done in the context of a larger study examining developmental changes in visual evoked responses during the first 6 months of life. In a sample of seven infants with DS (trisomy 21), Ellingson (1986) observed subtle and transient differences in brain responses to stroboscopic stimuli. At 1 week of age, there was a 30-msec delay in the occipital P2 response (the only component consistently identified in all participants) of infants with DS compared to typical full-term infants, suggesting slightly slower cortical response to stimulation. However, by 6 months, no group differences reached significance. Given the small sample size for the DS group and the high variability typical for ERPs recorded in young infants, it is not possible to conclusively determine whether the group differences at the younger age were sample-specific or reflected early brain differences that later disappeared due to possible compensatory mechanisms.

Cross-sectional ERP studies are more common and provide information about brain functioning at a particular developmental stage. A number of studies examined sensory processing and habituation in DS and observed similarly atypical brain responses from infancy through adulthood. Barnet and Lodge (1967) were among the first to report that, between 0–14 months of age, infants with DS (*n* = 15; 14 trisomy 21, one translocation) demonstrated an exaggerated vertex P2–N3 response to sensory stimulation (suggesting a larger than typical number of neurons firing in synchrony) that did not follow the typical pattern of reduction in size with repeated stimulation, indicative of altered inhibitory mechanisms that support habituation and learning. Increased amplitudes and lack of habituation were also reported in children with DS between 2 and 12 years of age (Dustman & Callner, 1979; Lichy, Vesely, Adler, & Zizka, 1975). In a study comparing visual (flashes), auditory (clicks), and somatosensory (shocks) ERPs in persons with DS aged 5–62 years, Callner et al. (1978) found that, regardless of sensory modality and across all age groups, the amplitude of ERP components over frontal and central areas was substantially larger for all participants with DS than for the typically developing persons matched on sex. These findings suggest that development of neural inhibitory processes in DS is not delayed but rather never fully emerges (see also Callner et al., 1978; Lichy et al., 1975), thus impacting the basic learning mechanisms and the higher-order cognitive processes that rely on them.

In a series of studies using more complex and socially salient visual stimuli (faces), Karrer et al. (1995, 1998) demonstrated that habituation in 6-month-old infants with DS is possible, but it occurs at a significantly slower rate. In an oddball paradigm, in which one stimulus is presented infrequently (10%–30% of total trials) among frequent presentations (70%–90% of trials) of another stimulus, a frontal Nc response (400–800 msec) thought to reflect recognition of familiar stimuli or detection of novelty, did not differ between frequent and novel trials due to increased amplitudes for the frequent stimuli. However, when the number of frequent trials was doubled (from 80 to 160), and thus provided a much more extended experience with the stimuli, ERPs of infants with DS demonstrated the expected amplitude reduction for repeated stimulation, suggesting that impaired habituation might be contributing to less efficient memory processes. Furthermore, infants with DS were able to detect the rare stimulus, but ERP evidence of stimulus discrimination was observed at atypical scalp locations, indicating reliance on atypical neural processes or altered connectivity among the brain areas supporting novelty detection in DS.

Deficits in basic stimulus discrimination reflected in the amplitude of brain responses might be associated with more complex behavioral deficits as well. In a study of ten 4- to 8-year-old children with DS, Yoder et al. (2006) demonstrated that impaired differentiation of speech syllables might be among the factors underlying poor grammatical comprehension frequently reported in persons with DS. Specifically, smaller differences between ERP amplitudes elicited by contrasting consonant-vowel syllables (e.g., /da/ vs. /ga/) correlated with lower scores on the Test of Auditory Comprehension of Language (TACL-3) measuring the degree of morphological comprehension.

In addition to atypical amplitudes, ERPs of persons with DS have also been consistently characterized by prolonged latencies, suggesting slower information processing. In the auditory domain, delays for several peaks within 0–500 msec after stimulus onset were reported in children and adults with DS (4–15 year-olds: Kaneko, Ehlers, Philips, & Riley, 1996; 11–20 years: Seidl et al., 1997; Diaz & Zurron, 1995; adults: Pekkonen, Osipova, Sauna-Aho, & Arvio, 2007; St. Clair & Blackwood, 1985; Vieregge, Verleger, Schulze-Rava, & Kompf, 1992). For the P2 and N2 responses that reflect processing of basic stimulus features and detection of differences, such delays remained significant even after controlling for mental age (Diaz & Zurron, 1995), suggesting not delayed maturation but altered brain responsiveness and organization associated with preattentive auditory processing (see also Lincoln, Courchesne, Kilman, & Galambos, 1985). Concordantly, delayed sensory processing was also reported for somatosensory (Chen & Fang, 2005) and olfactory (Wetter & Murphy, 1999) stimuli, indicating that alterations in brain responsiveness are not limited to a particular modality but reflect a more general slowing of information processing, possibly due to structural changes in the brain.

Similar to the brain–behavior connections observed for the ERP amplitudes, prolonged latency has been associated with attention and memory processes in DS. Delays in the auditory P3 response (thought to reflect memory updating and target detection) have been reported in adults with DS who also have early-onset dementia. Blackwood et al. (1988) examined auditory ERPs in 89 individuals with DS, aged 16–66 years, and reported a marked increase in P3 latency starting around 37 years (see also St. Clair & Blackwood, 1985) compared to the 54-year onset for typically developing persons, a 17-year difference that was due to the

16 participants with DS showing signs of dementia. In a follow-up study, Muir et al. (1988) recorded auditory ERPs in 65 adults from the original sample. Seven of the nine individuals (78%) who demonstrated clinical deterioration during the 2 years between the first and second ERP assessment had pronounced delays in P3 latency (up to 3 standard deviations (SD) or greater than the group mean; Muir et al., 1988). These findings suggest that ERPs might be useful in identifying early markers of cognitive decline in persons with DS.

Because P3 latency in a target detection task often overlaps in time with the behavioral response to the stimuli, it could be reflecting processes associated with motor preparation for a response in addition to the cognitive functions. However, Lalo et al. (2005) demonstrated that observed delays in the latency of an auditory P3 in adults with DS are not directly related to difficulties with motor functioning. Twenty adults with DS (18–31 years) completed one passive (i.e., no behavioral response required) and two active (simple vs. complex motor response) versions of the auditory oddball task. Although the movement complexity of the motor response did not affect behavioral or ERP data among the sex-matched, typically developing comparison group, the participants with DS displayed longer reaction times but shorter P3 latencies in the simple (i.e., pushing a button under the finger) compared to the complex response condition (pointing to a target on one's chest), suggesting that motor preparation processes do not necessarily interact with the attention processes in individuals with DS.

Latency and amplitude characteristics of ERPs in persons with DS might also index alterations in underlying neurochemistry. Seidl et al. (1997) examined whether characteristics of the P3 response might be affected in part by the histaminergic system, reported to be atypical in persons with DS (Epstein, 1995). Administering antihistaminergic treatment to typically developing participants resulted in ERPs that resembled those of persons with DS in terms of the increased P3 latency and delayed amplitude reduction. However, the treatment had no effect on the earlier N1–P2–N2 peaks in the typical group, suggesting that some but not all aspects of cognitive functioning in DS might be due to histaminergic impairment.

MAGNETIC RESONANCE IMAGING STUDIES

Structural MRI studies in DS have reported numerous volumetric differences in the brain (Teipel & Hampel, 2006). The majority of these studies have focused on early-onset dementia, which affects over one-third of persons with DS who are 55 or older. In this context, DS has been studied as a more predictable model of Alzheimer disease (AD). Studies have shown that, similar to typically developed participants with AD, middle-aged adults with DS who do not yet have clinical symptoms of dementia already have decreased hippocampal volume and increased lateral ventricles (Emerson, Kesslak, Chen, & Lott, 1995; Pearlson et al., 1998; Teipel et al., 2004). More recently, early preclinical signs of dementia were shown to correlate with a combination of decreased gray matter volume (as measured by sMRI) and an increase in glucose metabolic rate (as measured by PET) in the hippocampus, thalamus, caudate, and inferior frontal lobe (Haier, Head, Head, & Lott, 2008).

Other studies not focused on AD have shown that, compared to typically developing age-matched persons, participants with DS have decreased volume of the brain overall, including the cerebellum and cerebral gray and white matter, and specifically in the hippocampus (Pinter, Eliez, Schmitt, Capone, & Reiss, 2001; Weis, Weber, Neuhold, & Rett, 1991) and in frontal and occipital lobes (Jernigan, Bellugi, Sowell, Doherty, & Hesselink, 1993). However, persons with DS also showed increased volume of the parahippocampal gyrus that might be related to developmental abnormalities in neurogenesis (Kesslak, Nagata, Lott, & Nalcioglu, 1994; Raz et al., 1995). The one fMRI study published to-date investigated speech and language processing and showed that persons with DS have different brain activation patterns during passive story listening when compared to age-matched participants with typical development. Typically developing participants showed greater activation to forward versus backward speech in receptive language areas of the superior and middle temporal gyri, whereas subjects with DS showed similar activation to forward and backward speech, which also included the cingulated gyrus, parietal lobe, and precuneus, perhaps as a compensatory mechanism (Losin, Rivera, O'Hare, Sowell, & Pinter, 2009).

SUMMARY

Structural imaging data available for adults with DS indicate volumetric changes in a number of brain areas supporting a wide range of cognitive functions. However, the lack of fMRI data and the absence of MRI studies involving children and adolescents with DS makes it difficult to determine whether these findings reflect general syndrome-specific brain alterations or differences specific to atypical, early aging changes on the brain. Event-related potential studies have included a wider range of participants with DS, but the majority of the research has focused on comparing brain responses of persons with DS to those of typical comparison groups using basic sensory stimuli. Only a small number of studies addressed the connection between the brain processes and behavioral phenotypes, identifying delayed habituation, reduced stimulus discrimination, and slower information processing as the potential mechanisms contributing to observed behavioral characteristics. Examining contributions of brain chemistry and motor processes to the observed brain and behavioral responses has further improved our understanding of the mechanisms of cognitive functioning in DS and broadened the range of possible targets for future interventions.

Prader-Willi Syndrome

EVENT-RELATED POTENTIAL STUDIES

Event-related potential studies in PWS have focused mainly on documenting the cognitive profile and phenotypic differences within this diagnostic group. Stauder et al. (2002) examined ERPs of adults (n = 10) with PWS during a visual and auditory oddball tasks. The visual task required detection of a face with a direct versus averted gaze, and the auditory task targeted discrimination of a higher-pitched tone from two lower-pitch sounds. Although there were no group differences in the early ERP peaks, the P3 response to targets in both modalities showed a typical scalp distribution but had smaller amplitudes in persons with PWS compared to typically developing participants (no criteria for sample matching reported). The decrease was most significant in the auditory oddball task, although behavioral performance between the persons with PWS and the typically developing group was comparable (70% vs. 78% correct, respectively), and P3 responses to the nontarget stimuli did not differ between the groups. The results were interpreted to reflect a specific weakness in auditory short-term memory processes for adults with PWS.

Difficulties in elucidating a cognitive profile associated with PWS could be due to phenotype variability within the syndrome, directly related to differences in the genetic subtypes, as approximately 70% of individuals with PWS have paternal deletions at 15q (q11–q13), and 25% show maternal uniparental disomy (UPD). Stauder et al. (2005)

compared the brain activity of adults with PWS due to paternal deletion (n = 11) or maternal UPD (n = 11) to sex- and age-matched typically developed persons during a response inhibition task (Continuous Performance Test-AX) in which a participant had to respond to a letter "X" only when it was preceded by an "A" and not by any other letter. Persons with both PWS subtypes did not show the expected increase in N2 amplitude for trials requiring withholding of the response, suggesting impairment in early inhibitory processes. Subtype differences were reflected in the later-occurring P3 component associated with general inhibition. Although the typically developed and deletion groups showed a clear P3 response, with larger amplitudes to the inhibition trials, the ERPs of the UPD group reflected a delayed and reduced P3, consistent with their lower accuracy and increased reaction times, suggesting that these participants might have a particular difficulty monitoring their performance and following task instructions.

Genetic subtype differences were also observed in an ERP study examining food preferences among eight adults with UPD and nine adults with deletion subtypes of PWS. Key and Dykens (2008) demonstrated that initial evaluation of food stimuli (within 130 msec after stimulus onset) in persons with UPD appears similar to that of typical adults matched on age and sex, as both groups categorized food stimuli first in terms of general suitability for consumption (i.e., contaminated vs. not). Conversely, the ERPs of persons with the deletion subtype reflected a focus on quantity of food elements that only later shifted to the examination of food's suitability for consumption.

MAGNETIC RESONANCE IMAGING STUDIES

Structural MRI studies in persons with PWS have found multiple brain abnormalities. Miller et al. (2007) compared persons with PWS (17 with paternal deletion; six with UPD) to their typically developing siblings and to unrelated individuals with early-onset morbid obesity (EMO) and observed that ventriculomegaly (enlarged lateral ventricles), which has been reported in other disorders involving intellectual disability (Soto-Ares, Joyes, Delmaire, Vallee, & Pruvo, 2005), was present in all 20 participants with PWS but in none of the 21 typically developed siblings or the 16 persons with EMO (Miller et al., 2007). Abnormalities of the Sylvian fissure (specifically polymicrogyria), which have been previously associated with language disorders (Guerreiro et al., 2002), were found in 60% of participants with PWS but in none of the typically developed siblings or persons with EMO. Individuals with PWS were also characterized by decreases in gray matter volume in the parietal-occipital lobe, which might be related to obsessive-compulsive (OCD) behaviors. One DTI study involving eight participants with PWS (all with a paternal deletion) and eight age- and gender-matched typically developed participants found indications of white matter abnormalities in fronto-thalamic regions, possibly related to various psychiatric dysfunction (e.g., psychosis, OCD behaviors), and in the posterior limb of the internal capsule, which might be related to decreased muscle tone in PWS (Yamada, Matsuzawa, Uchiyama, Kwee, & Nakada, 2006).

Most of the functional neuroimaging research in PWS has focused on hyperphagia and related early-onset obesity aspects of the phenotype. Dimitropoulos and Schultz (2008) reported that participants with PWS ($n = 9$; seven deletion, one UPD, one translocation) showed greater brain activation to pictures of high-calorie versus low-calorie foods in areas related to hunger and motivation versus a typically developed comparison group ($n = 10$). Holsen et al. (2006) investigated the brain oxygen level dependent (BOLD) response of participants with PWS ($n = 9$; seven deletion, two UPD) and of healthy-weight, typically developing individuals ($n = 9$) while looking at pictures of food before and after eating a meal. Areas of the brain that drive eating behavior and those that suppress food intake were activated more in the PWS versus the typically developed group. In a follow-up study using the same fMRI paradigm, Holsen et al. (2009) found differential patterns of activation among participants with PWS depending on genetic etiology (maternal UPD, $n = 9$; versus paternal deletion, $n = 9$). Post-meal, PWS participants with UPD showed greater activation (vs. the deletion group) in areas related to cognitive control over food-related decision making—dorsolateral prefrontal cortex and para-hippocampal gyrus. In both pre- and post-meal conditions, the deletion group showed greater activation (vs. the UPD group) in areas involving emotion processing and food motivation—medial prefrontal cortex and amygdala. Notably, there are no published fMRI studies investigating OCD behaviors in PWS.

SUMMARY
Structural MRI studies have documented differences in brain structure possibly related to language deficits and OCD behaviors. Functional MRI and

ERP studies investigating genetic subtype differences within PWS have focused primarily on feeding-related behaviors, which are a major part of the PWS phenotype, and these studies are just beginning to shed light on the specific strengths and weaknesses associated with various forms of PWS. Although obtained in small samples of adults, results suggest that persons with the deletion subtype might be at greater risk for food-related behavioral problems because they do not appear to have the automatic skill to categorize food stimuli in terms of safe versus unsafe to eat. On the other hand, persons with the UPD subtype might have greater difficulties with attention and inhibition of the prepotent response. Combined with existing behavioral data, these findings can be useful for formulating more subtype-specific research questions, thus leading to improved understanding of PWS in general. Also, there is a clear lack of brain-based studies involving children with PWS, and future research studies should include a wider range of ages.

Williams Syndrome
EVENT-RELATED POTENTIAL STUDIES
Event-related potential studies in WS have spanned a wide range of phenotypic characteristics, such as auditory sensitivity, speech and language processing, and visuospatial skills. In a study of mechanisms underlying hyperacusis frequently reported in adults with WS, Neville and colleagues (1989) observed that, although auditory brainstem evoked responses were typical, cortical activation to auditory stimuli in adults with WS was less refractory than in the typical comparison sample. In response to spoken words, the pattern of ERPs included larger than typical P1 (50 msec) and P2 (200 msec) responses and a smaller N1, most pronounced over temporal brain regions. The group differences were specific to auditory stimuli as no group differences in ERPs were present in the visual modality.

Unusual ERP responses were also observed in persons with WS during lexical tasks requiring semantic processes, such as listening to spoken sentences in which the last word matched or did not match the preceding context (Neville, Mills, & Bellugi, 1994). In typical individuals, the semantically anomalous final word elicits an N400 response with greater amplitude over the right than the left hemisphere. Persons with WS generated a more symmetrical N400 response due to a larger than typical amplitude over the left hemisphere. Bellugi (1999) demonstrated a similar lack of hemispheric asymmetry in response to closed-class words, which typically convey information about grammatical relations (e.g., articles, prepositions, conjunctions). Although in typical populations these words are associated with increased negativity over left than right anterior scalp, present by about 7 years of age (Mills, Coffey, & Neville, 1993), this response remained of equal amplitude among adults with WS, suggesting that relatively preserved language abilities in persons with WS might rely on atypical brain mechanisms as reflected in the lack of lateralization of observed brain activity across a variety of language-related tasks.

In the area of visuospatial processing, a weakness for the WS phenotype, Grice et al. (2003) demonstrated that difficulties with such tasks might be at least in part associated with atypical early perceptual processing. In a perceptual completion task that targeted the ability to perceive illusory contours created by a spatial arrangement of geometric shapes, participants with WS demonstrated behavioral evidence of being able to perceive the illusion (correctly tracing the illusory figure with a finger), but their ERP responses were different from typically developed persons matched on age and sex. Although the overall size of the N1 response in the WS group was normal and demonstrated the expected difference between the actually drawn and illusory shapes, absent were the typical differences between the N1 amplitudes to illusory contours and the no-contour random arrangement of the geometric shapes. Grice at al. noted that the latter discrimination might have been performed at a different time, outside of the restricted analysis window used in the study, potentially reflecting a slower visual analysis process that might include additional stages or rely on atypical brain pathways compared to those of the typically developed persons.

Atypical attention to local (part) versus global (whole) visual information may be another reason for visuospatial difficulties in persons with WS. Key and Dykens (2011) presented 21 young adults with WS and 16 age- and sex- matched typically developing controls with big letters made of small letters (e.g., small S's arranged into the overall shape of an H) and asked to note when a target letter was presented. The target could appear randomly as a big (global) or a small (local) letter with equal probability (20% of trials), but no specific instructions directing attention to a particular perceptual level were given. Persons with WS and typical participants were similar in their early perceptual analyses and involuntary orienting to global targets as reflected by modulation of the occipital P1/N1 and frontal P3a responses. However, differently from typical persons, no increases in the amplitudes of N1 or P3a in response to local targets were observed for persons with WS, suggesting altered ability to notice local elements. At the more advanced stage of visual processing involving voluntary attention, participants with typical development demonstrated the expected increase in the centro-parietal P3b amplitude for local and global targets. In the persons with WS, this effect was absent, mainly due to the increased P3b amplitude in response to the distracters. Together, these findings in persons with WS were interpreted to reflect over-engaged attention to all stimuli, greater than typical global-to-local interference, and inability to allocate sufficient attentional resources to local information when not explicitly required to do so.

Despite difficulties with many basic visuospatial perceptual tasks, persons with WS appear to be very proficient at face perception, which typically relies heavily on configural processing. However, ERP evidence suggests that even face processing is performed using atypical brain mechanisms in adults with WS. In a face matching task in which participants viewed pairs of upright or inverted faces and indicated whether the second face in a pair matched the first (Mills et al., 2000), ERPs of 18 adults (aged 18–38 years) with WS were characterized by reduced amplitudes of the N1 and P170 components and a pronounced N2 response that was absent or attenuated in the typically developing sample (n = 23, matched on age). The increase in amplitude of the N2 was correlated with better performance on the Benton Test of Facial Recognition. These ERP patterns were not observed in two participants who had a clinical diagnosis of WS but did not have the corresponding genetic deletion (Mills et al., 2000). Furthermore, participants with WS did not show the expected differences in the morphology, latency, and distribution of the match–mismatch ERP effects to upright compared to inverted faces. Although an upright face presents an expected configuration of two eyes above a nose and a mouth, inverting a face is assumed to disrupt the relationship among the facial elements, making the task of matching faces in a pair rely to a greater extent on feature comparison. In the typically developing sample, mismatched upright faces elicited an anterior N320 response that was larger over the right than the left hemisphere, whereas inverted mismatched faces were associated with a symmetrical posterior P500 peak. The participants with WS showed a N320 response with reversed hemisphere asymmetry for both upright and inverted mismatches, although the latter was associated with reduced amplitudes, suggesting that the orientation of the stimuli modulated the amplitude of the N320, but did not result in engagement of distinct neural systems for upright and inverted faces.

MAGNETIC RESONANCE IMAGING STUDIES

Both structural and functional neuroimaging have been used successfully to investigate the neural basis of the WS phenotype. Structural MRI studies have identified abnormalities in brain structures such as the corpus callosum (Schmitt, Eliez, Warsofsky, Bellui, & Reiss, 2001; Wang, Doherty, Hesselink, & Bellugi, 1992) and the hippocampal formation (Meyer-Lindenberg et al., 2005b), as well as reduced cortical brain volume (Reiss et al., 2000; Thompson et al., 2005) and altered gyral patterns (Gaser et al., 2006; Kippenhan et al., 2005). Using DTI, Marenco et al. (2007) examined five high-functioning WS adults (IQ: mean ± SD = 87 ± 6) and five IQ-matched typically developed persons (IQ: mean ± SD = 92 ± 4) and found that participants with WS showed white matter integrity increases in longitudinal tracts, coursing along the anterior-posterior axis, and decreases in transverse fibers, coursing right-to-left (Marenco et al., 2007). Hoeft et al. (2007) presented results from a larger group (*n* = 20) of adults with WS whose intellectual disability range was more similar to population statistics for WS (IQ: mean ± SD = 65 ± 11), and these individuals were compared to an age-matched typically developed group (IQ: mean ± SD = 114 ± 13). Similar to Marenco et al. (2007), Hoeft et al. found evidence of increased fiber coherence in the inferior longitudinal fasciculus that connects the temporal and occipital lobes, which the authors suggest might be related to relative strengths in face recognition and/or the relatively spared verbal abilities in WS (Hoeft et al., 2007; Marenco et al., 2007).

Functional MRI studies have identified differential activation patterns in multiple brain regions related to specific aspects of the phenotype. Meyer-Lindenberg et al. (2004) showed that individuals with WS (*n* = 13) had decreased activation of areas of the visual cortex related to the dorsal stream ("where") pathway that has been strongly implicated in the visuospatial deficits of participants with WS compared to those with typical development (*n* = 11) (Meyer-Lindenberg et al., 2004). Levitin et al. (2003) found that, in comparison to typically developed adults (*n* = 5), participants with WS (*n* = 5)

had a more widely distributed pattern of activation when listening to music (vs. a silent condition) (Levitin et al., 2003). Also, when comparing music and noise conditions, participants with WS failed to modulate brain activity in the auditory cortex and showed more similar activation between conditions than did the typically developed group (Levitin et al., 2003). In further examining the auditory phenotype of WS, Thornton-Wells et al. (2010) reported that individuals with WS had substantial activation of the visual cortex to musical and nonmusical sounds in the absence of visual stimuli, suggesting enhanced structural and/or functional connectivity between these sensory cortices in participants with WS versus typically developed (*n* = 13 per group) (Thornton-Wells et al., 2010).

An fMRI study of social cognition showed decreased activation of the amygdala to the viewing of threatening faces in participants with WS (*n* = 13) versus a typically developed comparison group (*n* = 13), possibly related to the decreased fear of strangers reported in WS (Meyer-Lindenberg et al., 2005a). Participants with WS also showed increased activation of the amygdala to threatening scenes and a failure to activate frontal regions as part of the normal inhibitory feedback loop that keeps fear, perseveration, and anxiety in check. Thus, these results might be related to increased fears and nonsocial anxiety (e.g., fear of thunderstorms, heights, or death) experienced by many with WS (Dykens, 2003). Finally, Mobbs et al. (2007) found that participants with WS (*n* = 11) showed decreased activation in brain regions related to response inhibition in comparison to typically developed participants (*n* = 11), possibly explaining the impulsivity and lack of behavioral inhibition seen in WS (Mobbs et al., 2007).

SUMMARY

Magnetic resonance imaging and ERP studies in WS provide consistent findings indicating atypical patterns of brain activation in response to auditory stimuli, alterations in brain connectivity that might contribute to observed atypical lateralization of responses, and differences in the structure and function of areas supporting visuospatial processes. Furthermore, neuroimaging studies demonstrate that not all aspects of visual processing are uniformly atypical in WS, and observed behavioral deficits are often task- or stimulus-specific, thus providing a more precise documentation of strengths and weaknesses associated with the syndrome. Future MRI/ERP studies involving younger children with WS will expand our current understanding of the observed differences and determine whether the observed alterations in brain mechanisms are a product of atypical developmental trajectory or specific changes in the brain due to genetic factors.

Fragile X Syndrome

EVENT-RELATED POTENTIAL STUDIES

Behaviorally, persons with FXS are often described as anxious and highly sensitive to sensory stimulation (Hagerman, Hills, Scharfenaker, & Lewis, 1999; Merenstein et al., 1996; Miller et al. 1999). Event-related potential evidence demonstrates that such overreactions might stem from abnormal sensory processing in the brain that can be present throughout the lifespan. Castren et al. (2003) examined sound discrimination and auditory habituation in four boys (7–13 years) with FXS and age-matched typically developing children. The amplitude of the N1 component to tones was significantly larger in males with FXS, and response to repeated tones did not demonstrate habituation of N1 or N2 amplitude. Similar observations of the enhanced brain responses to sensory inputs have been reported for somatosensory and auditory modalities in adults with FXS (Ferri et al., 1994; Ragazzoni et al. 1999; Rojas et al., 2001). A greater than typical number of neurons firing in synchrony might lead to subjective experiences of increased stimulus intensity, heightened state of arousal, and changes in alertness and/or attentiveness to the external world, and thus might be the mechanism underlying anxiety and sensory hypersensitivity in FXS.

Using an active oddball task in which the participants were asked to detect the presence of a high-pitched target tone among low-pitched distracters, St. Clair et al. (1987) observed that, in addition to enlarged N1 and P2 responses (reflecting increased processing of a stimulus' sensory features), adults with FXS (*n* = 28; 16–66 years, 26 males) also demonstrated delayed N2 and P3 latencies and reduced P3 amplitude, suggesting less efficient stimulus evaluation and comparison processes. Furthermore, a sizeable P3 response was present in response to both frequent and infrequent stimuli, which was interpreted as reflecting poor attention to the task rather than a decrease in auditory discrimination ability, as behavioral data revealed reasonably good target detection. Abnormalities in the P3 response were independent of age, percentage cell fragility, or intellectual ability, suggesting a more general impairment in brain structure and functioning, most likely in medial temporal regions and hippocampus, identified in prior studies as the likely generators of the scalp P3 response and reported to be atypical in persons with FXS.

Difficulties with attention were also observed in females with FXS during a task requiring response switching and inhibition. Cornish et al. (2004) used ERPs to examine attentional control (see also Munir, Cornish, & Wilding, 2000; Wilding, Cornish, & Munir, 2002) in three women with the *FMR1* full mutation (aged 19–32 years) who were asked to respond immediately to some visual stimuli (Go trials) or to delay their response until stimulus offset for other stimuli (Wait trials). Relative to the typically developing comparison group (*n* = 18), the females with FXS were significantly slower and made more errors on Go trials but were comparable on Wait trials. Inhibition-sensitive N2 responses to Wait trials of the FXS group were similar to those of the typically developing participants. However, differences in the brain activity between Go and Wait trials were less pronounced in the FXS group, suggesting a weakness in inhibiting the activation of the wrong type of response in each condition.

MAGNETIC RESONANCE IMAGING STUDIES

Most neuroimaging studies investigating FXS have focused on anatomical differences and have found a complex pattern of changes in brain volume within specific regions. In a study of 101 boys aged 1 to 3 years, Hoeft et al. (2008) reported that the superior temporal gyrus, hippocampus, and orbitofrontal cortex had decreased gray matter volume in participants with FXS (*n* = 51) relative to a typically developing comparison group (*n* = 32) and participants with idiopathic (of unknown origin) developmental delay (*n* = 18). Other regions, such as the caudate, fusiform gyrus, and thalamus, had increased gray matter volume relative to typically developing persons (Hoeft et al., 2008). The caudate is thought to be involved in the stereotyped behaviors of FXS. Within the sample of children with FXS, caudate volume was significantly correlated with levels of FMR1 protein, such that reduced production of FMR1 was associated with a larger caudate (Hoeft et al., 2008). Similarly, there appears to be a gene dosage effect, with those persons who have more severe (longer repeat) mutations also having larger caudate volumes (Eliez, Blasey, Freund, Hastie, & Reiss, 2001). In addition, white matter abnormalities were found in the medial prefrontal region that might be related to deficits in executive function in FXS (Hoeft et al., 2008).

Using fMRI, Kwon et al. (2001) found evidence for an inability to modulate brain activity for increasingly difficult working memory tasks, which might be directly related to decreased levels of FMR1 protein (Kwon et al., 2001). More recently, Hagan et al. (2008) showed that in high-functioning female participants with FXS, an emotion circuit involving the anterior cingulate cortex, caudate, and insula for processing emotional face stimuli might be disrupted (Hagan, Hoeft, Mackey, Mobbs, & Reiss, 2008). Also related to social deficits in FXS, Watson et al. (2008) reported that, when viewing faces with direct versus averted eye gaze, male participants with FXS had decreased activation in prefrontal regions and increased activation in the left insula, compared to comparison groups with either typical development or idiopathic developmental delay (Watson, Hoeft, Garrett, Hall, & Reiss, 2008). In a study of executive control that also used ERPs (see above section), Cornish et al. (2004) reported that participants with FXS had problems with switching between Go and Wait trials and that brain areas involved in response suppression (bilateral ventral prefrontal cortex) and response conflict (anterior cingulate) were activated in all task conditions, perhaps indicating compensatory strategies for task performance (Cornish et al., 2004).

SUMMARY

Magnetic resonance imaging and ERP studies provide consistent findings reflecting difficulties with executive functioning in males and females with FXS, particularly in the area of attentional control. Additional ERP evidence that brains of persons with FXS tend to overrespond to sensory stimulation provides at least a partial explanation for the anxiety and sensory hypersensitivity common to the FXS phenotype. Together, these findings can be used to develop new pharmacological and/or behavioral intervention procedures.

Conclusion

In this chapter, we demonstrate the value of brain-based methods for studying developmental disabilities. Our review of the available ERP and MRI studies in four genetic syndromes provides examples of how neuroimaging methods offer noninvasive, in vivo means of documenting the brain basis of neurodevelopmental disorders. Because these measures are closer to the underlying biology of a condition than many behavioral assessments, they have the potential to identify structural and functional features that are very specific to a particular etiology,

even when behavioral features might be similar across etiologically distinct disorders. However, it is important to acknowledge the limitations of the existing studies and to consider ways to maximize the utility of future research endeavors.

Lack of Longitudinal Studies

The vast majority of ERP and MRI studies in atypical populations have been cross-sectional in nature, thereby limiting our inferences about the developmental trajectory of these disorders and their implications for typical development. Therefore, although they are more difficult in practice, there is undoubtedly a critical need for more longitudinal studies in developmental disabilities. For example, it is largely unknown whether the brains of individuals with developmental disabilities are any more or less plastic in general or during specific critical periods for development compared to those of persons with typical development. Future brain-based studies are needed to address this question by including paradigms targeting learning and examining the role of environmental factors (e.g., availability and diversity of stimulation, etc.) on outcomes in developmental disabilities. Also, studies focusing on early as well as late developmental stages are needed to better understand the lifetime developmental course of genetic disorders.

Differences in numbers of developmental neuroimaging studies in persons with genetic conditions compared to the number of similar studies in typical populations have been attributed to challenges in recording neuroimaging data in children with developmental disabilities (Kaneko et al., 1996) and the difficulty of ensuring participants' cooperation and comprehension of instructions due to lower IQ levels (Prasher, 1994). However, the sizeable number of existing ERP and MRI studies involving persons with a variety of genetic conditions indicates the feasibility of obtaining quality data in infants, children, and adults with developmental disabilities using these brain-based methods.

Comparison Group Issues

Despite their unique contributions to the study of developmental disabilities, brain-based studies are not immune to the concerns reported in the behavioral research, such as the issue of appropriately chosen comparison participants for a developmental disability study group. A typically developing group is often the comparison of choice. Recently, large longitudinal fMRI studies in typical participants have been conducted (Marsh, Gerber, & Peterson, 2008;

Shaw et al., 2008), and age-appropriate structural templates are being developed to ameliorate problems with comparing brain function between groups with gross differences in brain structure, but these are in various stages of development and are not in widespread use (Kazemi, Moghaddam, Grebe, Gondry-Jouet, & Wallois, 2007; Wilke, Holland, Altaye, & Gaser, 2008; Yoon, Fonov, Perusse, & Evans, 2009). Furthermore, for some neuroimaging methods, such as fMRI, the choice of comparison participants might be limited at younger ages as the techniques for conducting such studies in infants are still developing.

Sometimes the use of a chronological age-matched, typically developing comparison group is questioned and matching on mental age is recommended instead. As a result, individuals with very different chronological ages and developmental, behavioral, and cognitive profiles will be compared, in order to match them on IQ, and therefore, to control for intellectual disability. For instance, individuals with WS might be compared with individuals of similar IQ who have DS or autism spectrum disorder. However, such matching might also present problems, as the resulting group differences might be attributed to changes in brain structures associated with different genetic abnormalities.

Alternatively, in disorders for which some individuals have normal or near-normal overall intelligence, the opportunity exists for selection of participants based on normal IQ, such that intellectual disability is effectively removed as a confounder, and participants can be matched to typically developing comparison groups also with normal IQ. This option has the advantage that individuals could participate in more difficult or complex experiments. However, it has the distinct disadvantage that results might not be generalizable to the larger population of individuals with the disorder.

Experimental Paradigm Choices

The careful choice of the experimental paradigms and testing procedures might also help increase the utility and success rates of brain-based studies in the field of developmental disability. Evidence from developmental studies in typical (Kushnerenko, Cepoiene, Balan, Fellman, & Naatanen, 2002; Jing & Benasich, 2006) and atypical (e.g., Key & Dykens, 2008; Yoder et al., 2006) populations indicates that passive assessment paradigms, which do not require the participant to provide an overt behavioral response and therefore have very low cognitive load, can yield valuable information.

Utilizing such seemingly simple paradigms would also facilitate longitudinal studies in developmental disabilities as the same task could be administered to infants, children, and adults, enabling researchers to obtain systematic documentation of syndrome-specific brain development complementing data from standardized behavioral assessments.

Interdisciplinary Connections

Finally, there is also a need for greater interdisciplinary integration of brain-based, genetic, and behavioral research studies to improve our understanding of the various relationships among genes, proteins, brain structure, brain function, and behavior. The reviewed studies clearly demonstrate that brain-based measures have strong associations with behavioral, neurochemical, and genetic data. By further studying disorders with a known genetic etiology, we can learn how a mutation or loss of specific genes can impact neurodevelopment and, by extension, how normal variation in these genes can lead to the immense variability in what is considered "typical development." In the recent years, a number of "imaging genetics" studies have been conducted that directly test for association of genetic variants with structural or functional neuroimaging measures (Glahn, Paus, & Thompson, 2007; Hariri, Drabant, & Weinberger, 2006; Potkin et al., 2009). As analogous studies looking for genetic association with levels of biomarkers are also becoming more common, combining multiple levels of phenotypic measurement is more feasible and would be a very powerful approach.

Also, a dearth of neuroimaging research is translational in nature. In part, this is related to the immaturity of the field and the fact that many researchers are still trying to answer basic science questions. However, whenever possible, brain-based research studies should attempt to identify specific targets for behavioral or pharmacological intervention, and then monitor the effects of the intervention, as is already being done in typical populations.

Acknowledgments

The authors would like to thank Dr. Robert Hodapp and all the editors for their feedback and guidance on the manuscript.

References

Barnet, A. B., & Lodge, A. (1967). Click evoked EEG responses in normal and developmentally retarded infants. *Nature, 214*, 252–255.

Bellugi, U., Lichtenberger, L., Mills, D., Galaburda, A., & Korenberg, J. R. (1999). Bridging cognition, the brain and molecular genetics: Evidence from Williams syndrome. *Trends in Neurosciences, 22*, 197–207.

Blackwood, D. H., St. Clair, D. M., Muir, W. J., Oliver, C. J., & Dickens, P. (1988). The development of Alzheimer's disease in Down's syndrome assessed by auditory event-related potentials. *Journal of Mental Deficiency Research, 32*(Pt 6), 439–453.

Callner, D. A., Dustman, R. E., Madsen, J. A., Schenkenberg, T., & Beck, E. C. (1978). Life span changes in the averaged evoked responses of Down's syndrome and nonretarded persons. *American Journal of Mental Deficiency Research, 82*, 398–405.

Castren, M., Paakkonen, A., Tarkka, I. M., Ryynanen, M., & Partanen, J. (2003). Augmentation of auditory N1 in children with fragile X syndrome. *Brain Topography, 15*, 165–171.

Chen, Y. J., & Fang, P. C. (2005). Sensory evoked potentials in infants with Down syndrome. *Acta Paediatrica, 94*, 1615–1618.

Cornish, K., Swainson, R., Cunnington, R., Wilding, J., Morris, P., & Jackson, G. (2004). Do women with fragile X syndrome have problems in switching attention: Preliminary findings from ERP and fMRI. *Brain and Cognition, 54*, 235–239.

Diaz, F., & Zuron, M. (1995). Auditory evoked potentials in Down's syndrome. *Electroencephalography and Clinical Neurophysiology, 96*, 526–537.

Dimitropoulos, A., & Schultz, R. T. (2008). Food-related neural circuitry in Prader-Willi syndrome: Response to high- versus low-calorie foods. *Journal of Autism and Developmental Disorders, 38*, 1642–1653.

Dustman, R. E., & Callner, D. A. (1979). Cortical evoked responses and response decrement in nonretarded and Down's syndrome individuals. *American Journal of Mental Deficiency Research, 83*, 391–397.

Dykens, E. M. (2003). Anxiety, fears, and phobias in persons with Williams syndrome. *Developmental Neuropsychology, 23*, 291–316.

Eliez, S., Blasey, C. M., Freund, L. S., Hastie, T., & Reiss, A. L. (2001). Brain anatomy, gender and IQ in children and adolescents with fragile X syndrome. *Brain, 124*, 1610–1618.

Ellingson, R. J. (1986). Development of visual evoked potentials and photic driving responses in normal full term, low risk premature, and Trisomy-21 infants during the first year of life. *Electroencephalography and Clinical Neurophysiology, 63*, 309–316.

Emerson, J. F., Kesslak, J. P., Chen, P. C., & Lott, I. T. (1995). Magnetic resonance imaging of the aging brain in Down syndrome. *Progress in Clinical and Biological Research, 393*, 123–138.

Epstein, C. J. (1995). Down syndrome Trisomy 21. In C. R. Scriver, W. S. Beaudet, W. S. Sly, & D. Valle (Eds.), *The metabolic and molecular bases of inherited disease* (pp. 749–794). New York: McGraw-Hill.

Ferri, R., Musumeci, S. A., Elia, M., Del, G. S., Scuderi, C., & Bergonzi, P. (1994). BIT-mapped somatosensory evoked potentials in the fragile X syndrome. *Neurophysiologie Clinique, 24*, 413–426.

Gaser, C., Luders, E., Thompson, P. M., Lee, A. D., Dutton, R. A., Geaga, J. A., et al. (2006). Increased local gyrification mapped in Williams syndrome. *Neuroimage, 33*, 46–54.

Glahn, D. C., Paus, T., & Thompson, P. M. (2007). Imaging genomics: Mapping the influence of genetics on brain structure and function. *Human Brain Mapping, 28*, 461–463.

Grice, S. J., Haan, M. D., Halit, H., Johnson, M. H., Csibra, G., Grant, J., et al. (2003). ERP abnormalities of illusory contour perception in Williams syndrome. *Neuroreport, 14*, 1773–1777.

Guerreiro, M. M., Hage, S. R., Guimaraes, C. A., Abramides, D. V., Fernandes, W., Pacheco, P. S., et al. (2002). Developmental language disorder associated with polymicrogyria. *Neurology, 59*, 245–250.

Hagan, C. C., Hoeft, F., Mackey, A., Mobbs, D., & Reiss, A. L. (2008). Aberrant neural function during emotion attribution in female subjects with fragile X syndrome. *Journal of the American Academy of Child and Adolescent Psychiatry, 47*, 1443–1354.

Hagerman, R. J., Hills, J., Scharfenaker, S., & Lewis, H. (1999). Fragile X syndrome and selective mutism. *American Journal of Medical Genetics, 83*, 313–317.

Haier, R. J., Head, K., Head, E., & Lott, I. T. (2008). Neuroimaging of individuals with Down's syndrome at-risk for dementia: Evidence for possible compensatory events. *Neuroimage, 39*, 1324–1332.

Hariri, A. R., Drabant, E. M., & Weinberger, D. R. (2006). Imaging genetics: Perspectives from studies of genetically driven variation in serotonin function and corticolimbic affective processing. *Biological Psychiatry, 59*, 888–897.

Hoeft, F., Barnea-Goraly, N., Haas, B. W., Golarai, G., Ng, D., Mills, D., et al. (2007). More is not always better: Increased fractional anisotropy of superior longitudinal fasciculus associated with poor visuospatial abilities in Williams syndrome. *Journal of Neuroscience, 27*, 11960–11965.

Hoeft, F., Lightbody, A. A., Hazlett, H. C., Patnaik, S., Piven, J., & Reiss, A. L. (2008). Morphometric spatial patterns differentiating boys with fragile X syndrome, typically developing boys, and developmentally delayed boys aged 1 to 3 years. *Archives of General Psychiatry, 65*, 1087–1097.

Holsen, L. M., Zarcone, J. R., Brooks, W. M., Butler, M. G., Thompson, T. I., Ahluwalia, J. S., et al. (2006). Neural mechanisms underlying hyperphagia in Prader-Willi syndrome. *Obesity (Silver Spring), 14*, 1028–1037.

Holsen, L. M., Zarcone, J. R., Chambers, R., Butler, M. G., Bittel, D. C., Brooks, W. M., et al. (2009). Genetic subtype differences in neural circuitry of food motivation in Prader-Willi syndrome. *International Journal of Obesity, 33*, 273–283.

Jernigan, T. L., Bellugi, U., Sowell, E., Doherty, S., & Hesselink, J. R. (1993). Cerebral morphologic distinctions between Williams and Down syndromes. *Archives of Neurology, 50*, 186–191.

Jing, H., & Benasich, A. A. (2006). Brain responses to tonal changes in the first two years of life. *Brain & Development, 28*, 247–256.

Kaneko, W. M., Ehlers, C. L., Philips, E. L., & Riley, E. P. (1996). Auditory event-related potentials in fetal alcohol syndrome and Down's syndrome children. *Alcoholism, Clinical and Experimental Research, 20*, 35–42.

Karrer, J. H., Karrer, R., Bloom, D., Chaney, L., & Davis, R. (1998). Event-related brain potentials during an extended visual recognition memory task depict delayed development of cerebral inhibitory processes among 6-month-old infants with Down syndrome. *International Journal of Psychophysiology, 29*, 167–200.

Karrer, R., Wojtascek, Z., & Davis, M. G. (1995). Event-related potentials and information processing in infants with and without Down syndrome. *American Journal of Mental Retardation, 100*, 146–159.

Kazemi, K., Moghaddam, H. A., Grebe, R., Gondry-Jouet, C., & Wallois, F. (2007). A neonatal atlas template for spatial normalization of whole-brain magnetic resonance images of newborns: Preliminary results. *Neuroimage, 37,* 463–473.

Kesslak, J. P., Nagata, S. F., Lott, I., & Nalcioglu, O. (1994). Magnetic resonance imaging analysis of age-related changes in the brains of individuals with Down's syndrome. *Neurology, 44,* 1039–1045.

Key, A., Dove, G., & Maguire, M. (2005). Linking brainwaves to the brain: An ERP primer, *Developmental Neuropsychology, 27,* 183–215.

Key, A., & Dykens, E. M. (2008). "Hungry Eyes": Visual processing of food images in adults with Prader-Willi syndrome. *Journal of Intellectual Disability Research, 52,* 536–546.

Key, A. & Dykens, E. (2011). Electrophysiological study of local/global processing in Williams syndrome. *Journal of Neurodevelopmental Disorders, 3,* 28–38.

Kippenhan, J. S., Olsen, R. K., Mervis, C. B., Morris, C. A., Kohn, P., Meyer-Lindenberg, A., et al. (2005). Genetic contributions to human gyrification: Sulcal morphometry in Williams syndrome. *Journal of Neuroscience, 25,* 7840–7846.

Kushnerenko, E., Ceponiene, R., Balan, P., Fellman, V., & Naatanen, R. (2002). Maturation of the auditory change detection response in infants: A longitudinal ERP study. *Neuroreport, 13,* 1843–1848.

Kwon, H., Menon, V., Eliez, S., Warsofsky, I. S., White, C. D., Dyer-Friedman, J., et al. (2001). Functional neuroanatomy of visuospatial working memory in fragile X syndrome: Relation to behavioral and molecular measures. *American Journal of Psychiatry, 158,* 1040–1051.

Lalo, E., Vercueil, L., Bougerol, T., Jouk, P. S., & Debu, B. (2005). Late event-related potentials and movement complexity in young adults with Down syndrome. *Neurophysiology Clinique, 35,* 81–91.

Laufs, H., Daunizeau, J., Carmichael, D. W., & Kleinschmidt, A. (2008). Recent advances in recording electrophysiological data simultaneously with magnetic resonance imaging. *Neuroimage, 40,* 515–528.

Levitin, D. J., Menon, V., Schmitt, J. E., Eliez, S., White, C. D., Glover, G. H., et al. (2003). Neural correlates of auditory perception in Williams syndrome: An fMRI study. *Neuroimage, 18,* 74–82.

Lichy, J., Vesely, C., Adler, J., & Zizka, J. (1975). Auditory evoked cortical responses in Down's syndrome. *Electroencephalography and Clinical Neurophysiology, 38,* 440.

Lincoln, A. J., Courchesne, E., Kilman, B. A., & Galambos, R. (1985). Neuropsychological correlates of information-processing by children with Down syndrome. *American Journal of Mental Deficiency Research, 89,* 403–414.

Losin, E. A., Rivera, S. M., O'Hare, E. D., Sowell, E. R., & Pinter, J. D. (2009). Abnormal fMRI activation pattern during story listening in individuals with Down syndrome. *American Journal of Intellectual and Developmental Disabilities, 114,* 369–380.

Marenco, S., Siuta, M. A., Kippenhan, J. S., Grodofsky, S., Chang, W. L., Kohn, P., et al. (2007). Genetic contributions to white matter architecture revealed by diffusion tensor imaging in Williams syndrome. *Proceedings of the National Academy of Sciences U.S.A., 104,* 15117–15122.

Marsh, R., Gerber, A. J., & Peterson, B. S. (2008). Neuroimaging studies of normal brain development and their relevance for understanding childhood neuropsychiatric disorders.

Journal of the American Academy of Child and Adolescent Psychiatry, 47, 1233–1251.

Merenstein, S. A., Sobesky, W. E., Taylor, A. K., Riddle, J. E., Tran, H. X., & Hagerman, R. J. (1996). Molecular-clinical correlations in males with an expanded FMR1 mutation. *American Journal of Medical Genetics, 64,* 388–394.

Meyer-Lindenberg, A., Hariri, A. R., Munoz, K. E., Mervis, C. B., Mattay, V. S., Morris, C. A., et al. (2005a). Neural correlates of genetically abnormal social cognition in Williams syndrome. *Nature Neuroscience, 8,* 991–993.

Meyer-Lindenberg, A., Kohn, P., Mervis, C. B., Kippenhan, J. S., Olsen, R. K., Morris, C. A., et al. (2004). Neural basis of genetically determined visuospatial construction deficit in Williams syndrome. *Neuron, 43,* 623–631.

Meyer-Lindenberg, A., Mervis, C. B., Sarpal, D., Koch, P., Steele, S., Kohn, P., et al. (2005b). Functional, structural, and metabolic abnormalities of the hippocampal formation in Williams syndrome. *Journal of Clinical Investigation, 115,* 1888–1895.

Miller, J. L., Couch, J. A., Schmalfuss, I., He, G., Liu, Y., & Driscoll, D. J. (2007). Intracranial abnormalities detected by three-dimensional magnetic resonance imaging in Prader-Willi syndrome. *American Journal of Medical Genetics Part A, 143,* 476–483.

Miller, L. J., McIntosh, D. N., McGrath, J., Shyu, V., Lampe, M., Taylor, A. K., et al. (1999). Electrodermal responses to sensory stimuli in individuals with fragile X syndrome: A preliminary report. *American Journal of Medical Genetics, 83,* 268–279.

Mills, D., Coffey, S. A., & Neville, H. J. (1993). Changes in cerebral organization during primary language acquisition. In G. Dawson, & K. W. Fischer (Eds.), *Human behavior and the developing brain.* New York: Guilford Publications.

Mills, D. L., Alvarez, T. D., St. George, M., Appelbaum, L. G., Bellugi, U., & Neville, H. (2000). III. Electrophysiological studies of face processing in Williams syndrome. *Journal of Cognitive Neuroscience, 12*(Suppl 1), 47–64.

Mobbs, D., Eckert, M. A., Mills, D., Korenberg, J., Bellugi, U., Galaburda, A. M., et al. (2007). Frontostriatal dysfunction during response inhibition in Williams syndrome. *Biological Psychiatry, 62,* 256–261.

Muir, W. J., Squire, I., Blackwood, D. H., Speight, M. D., St Clair, D. M., Oliver, C., et al. (1988). Auditory P300 response in the assessment of Alzheimer's disease in Down's syndrome: A 2-year follow-up study. *Journal of Mental Deficiency Research, 32*(Pt 6), 455–463.

Munir, F., Cornish, K. M., & Wilding, J. (2000). Nature of the working memory deficit in fragile-X syndrome. *Brain and Cognition, 44,* 387–401.

Neville, H. J., Holcomb, P. J., & Mills, D. M. (1989). Auditory, sensory and language processing in Williams syndrome: An ERP study. *Journal of Clinical and Experimental Neuropsychology, 11,* 52.

Neville, H. J., Mills, D. L., & Bellugi, U. (1994). Effects of altered auditory sensitivity and age of language acquisition on the development of language-relevant neural systems: Preliminary studies of Williams syndrome. In S. Broman, & J. Grafman (Eds.), *Atypical cognitive deficits in developmental disorders: Implications for brain function* (pp. 67–83). Hillsdale, NJ: Lawrence Erlbaum Associates.

Papanicolaou, A. C. (1998). *Fundamentals of functional brain imaging.* The Netherlands: Swets & Zeitlinger.

Pearlson, G. D., Breiter, S. N., Aylward, E. H., Warren, A. C., Grygorcewicz, M., Frangou, S., et al. (1998). MRI brain changes in subjects with Down syndrome with and without dementia. *Developmental Medicine and Child Neurology, 40*, 326–334.

Pekkonen, E., Osipova, D., Sauna-Aho, O., & Arvio, M. (2007). Delayed auditory processing underlying stimulus detection in Down syndrome. *Neuroimage, 35*, 1547–1550.

Pinter, J. D., Eliez, S., Schmitt, J. E., Capone, G. T., & Reiss, A. L. (2001). Neuroanatomy of Down's syndrome: A high-resolution MRI study. *American Journal of Psychiatry, 158*, 1659–1665.

Ponton, C., Eggermon, J., Don, M., Waring, M., Kwong, B., Cunningham, J., & Trautwein, P. (2000). Maturation of the mismatch negativity: Effects of profound deafness and cochlear implant use. *Audiology & Neuro-Otology, 5*, 167–185.

Potkin, S. G., Turner, J. A., Guffanti, G., Lakatos, A., Fallon, J. H., Nguyen, D. D., et al. (2009). A genome-wide association study of schizophrenia using brain activation as a quantitative phenotype. *Schizophrenia Bulletin, 35*, 96–108.

Prasher, V. P., Krishnan, V. H. R., Blake, A., Clarke, D. J., & Corbett, J. A. (1994). Visual evoked potential in the diagnosis of dementia in people with Down syndrome. *International Journal of Geriatric Psychiatry, 9*, 473–478.

Ragazzoni, A., Ferri, R., Di, R. F., Del, G. S., Barcaro, U., & Navona, C. (1999). Giant somatosensory evoked potentials in different clinical conditions: Scalp topography and dipole source analysis. *Electroencephalography and Clinical Neurophysiology Supplement, 49*, 81–89.

Raz, N., Torres, I. J., Briggs, S. D., Spencer, W. D., Thornton, A. E., Loken, W. J., et al. (1995). Selective neuroanatomic abnormalities in Down's syndrome and their cognitive correlates: Evidence from MRI morphometry. *Neurology, 45*, 356–366.

Reiss, A. L., Eliez, S., Schmitt, J. E., Straus, E., Lai, Z., Jones, W., et al. (2000). IV. Neuroanatomy of Williams syndrome: A high-resolution MRI study. *Journal of Cognitive Neuroscience, 12*(Suppl 1), 65–73.

Rojas, D. C., Benkers, T. L., Rogers, S. J., Teale, P. D., Reite, M. L., & Hagerman, R. J. (2001). Auditory evoked magnetic fields in adults with fragile X syndrome. *Neuroreport, 12*, 2573–2576.

Russeler, J., Nager, W., Mobes, J., & Munte, T. F. (2005). Cognitive adaptations and neuroplasticity: Lessons from event-related brain potentials. In R. Konig, P. Heil, E. Budinger, & H. Scheich (Eds.), *The auditory cortex: A synthesis of human and animal research* (pp, 467–485). Mahwah, NJ: Lawrence Erlbaum Associates.

Schmitt, J. E., Eliez, S., Warsofsky, I. S., Bellugi, U., & Reiss, A. L. (2001). Corpus callosum morphology of Williams syndrome: Relation to genetics and behavior. *Developmental Medicine and Child Neurology, 43*, 155–159.

Seidl, R., Hauser, E., Bernert, G., Marx, M., Freilinger, M., & Lubec, G. (1997). Auditory evoked potentials in young patients with Down syndrome. Event-related potentials P3 and histaminergic system. *Brain Research: Cognitive Brain Research, 5*, 301–309.

Sharma, A., Dorman, M., & Kral, A. (2005). The influence of a sensitive period on central auditory development in children with unilateral and bilateral cochlear implants. *Hearing Research, 203*, 134–143.

Shaw, P., Kabani, N. J., Lerch, J. P., Eckstrand, K., Lenroot, R., Gogtay, N., et al. (2008). Neurodevelopmental trajectories of the human cerebral cortex. *Journal of Neuroscience, 28*, 3586–3594.

Soto-Ares, G., Joyes, B., Delmaire, C., Vallee, L., & Pruvo, J. P. (2005). [MR imaging in mental retardation]. *Journal of Neuroradiology, 32*, 224–238.

St. Clair, D., & Blackwood, D. (1985). Premature senility in Down's syndrome. *Lancet, 2*, 34.

St. Clair, D. M., Blackwood, D. H., Oliver, C. J., & Dickens, P. (1987). P3 abnormality in fragile X syndrome. *Biological Psychiatry, 22*, 303–312.

Stauder, J. E., Brinkman, M. J., & Curfs, L. M. (2002). Multi-modal P3 deflation of event-related brain activity in Prader-Willi syndrome. *Neuroscience Letters, 327*, 99–102.

Stauder, J., Boer, H., Gerits, R., Tummers, A., Whittington, J., Curf, L. (2005). Differences in behavioural phenotype between parental deletion and maternal uniparental disomy in Prader–Willi syndrome: an ERP study. *Clinical Neurophysiology, 116*, 1464–1470.

Teipel, S. J., Alexander, G. E., Schapiro, M. B., Moller, H. J., Rapoport, S. I., & Hampel, H. (2004). Age-related cortical grey matter reductions in non-demented Down's syndrome adults determined by MRI with voxel-based morphometry. *Brain, 127*, 811–824.

Teipel, S. J., & Hampel, H. (2006). Neuroanatomy of Down syndrome in vivo: A model of preclinical Alzheimer's disease. *Behavioral Genetics, 36*, 405–415.

Thompson, P. M., Lee, A. D., Dutton, R. A., Geaga, J. A., Hayashi, K. M., Eckert, M. A., et al. (2005). Abnormal cortical complexity and thickness profiles mapped in Williams syndrome. *Journal of Neuroscience, 25*, 4146–4158.

Thornton-Wells, T. A., Kim, C. Y., Cannistraci, C. J., Eapen, M., Anderson, A., Gore, J. C., et al. (2010). Auditory attraction: Activation of visual cortex to music and sound in Williams syndrome. *American Journal of Intellectual and Developmental Disabilities, 115*, 172–189.

Vieregge, P., Verleger, R., Schulze-Rava, H., & Kompf, D. (1992). Late cognitive event-related potentials in adult Down's syndrome. *Biological Psychiatry, 32*, 1118–1134.

Wang, P. P., Doherty, S., Hesselink, J. R., & Bellugi, U. (1992). Callosal morphology concurs with neurobehavioral and neuropathological findings in two neurodevelopmental disorders. *Archives of Neurology, 49*, 407–411.

Watson, C., Hoeft, F., Garrett, A. S., Hall, S. S., & Reiss, A. L. (2008). Aberrant brain activation during gaze processing in boys with fragile X syndrome. *Archives of General Psychiatry, 65*, 1315–1323.

Weis, S., Weber, G., Neuhold, A., & Rett, A. (1991). Down syndrome: MR quantification of brain structures and comparison with normal control subjects. *American Journal of Neuroradiology, 12*, 1207–1211.

Wetter, S., & Murphy, C. (1999). Individuals with Down's syndrome demonstrate abnormal olfactory event-related potentials. *Clinical Neurophysiology, 110*, 1563–1569.

Wilding, J., Cornish, K., & Munir, F. (2002). Further delineation of the executive deficit in males with fragile-X syndrome. *Neuropsychologia, 40*, 1343–1349.

Wilke, M., Holland, S. K., Altaye, M., & Gaser, C. (2008). Template-O-Matic: A toolbox for creating customized pediatric templates. *Neuroimage, 41*, 903–913.

Yamada, K., Matsuzawa, H., Uchiyama, M., Kwee, I. L., & Nakada, T. (2006). Brain developmental abnormalities in

Prader-Willi syndrome detected by diffusion tensor imaging. *Pediatrics, 118,* e442–e448.

Yoder, P. J., Camarata, S., Camarata, M., & Williams, S. M. (2006). Association between differentiated processing of syllables and comprehension of grammatical morphology in children with Down syndrome. *American Journal of Mental Retardation, 111,* 138–152.

Yoon, U., Fonov, V. S., Perusse, D., & Evans, A. C. (2009). The effect of template choice on morphometric analysis of pediatric brain data. *Neuroimage, 45,* 769–777.

Zani, A., & Proverbio, A. M. (2003). Cognitive electrophysiology of mind and brain. In A. Zani, & A. M. Proverbio (Eds.), *The cognitive electrophysiology of mind and brain* (pp. 3–12). San Diego: Academic Press.

PART 4

Language Development

Language Development in Childhood, Adolescence, and Young Adulthood in Persons with Down Syndrome

Robin S. Chapman *and* Elizabeth Kay-Raining Bird

Abstract

This chapter summarizes the strengths and weaknesses of the emerging language profile in children, adolescents, and young adults with Down syndrome (DS). It reviews in detail studies of expressive language skill in vocabulary, speech–motor skill, syntax, and pragmatics, and includes a section on studies of receptive language skill in vocabulary and syntax. Finally, the chapter considers proposed causes of the behavioral language phenotype and individual variation in its expression, and discusses the implications of the findings.

Keywords: Down syndrome, language profile, language skill, speech-motor skill, syntax, pragmatics

Research on specific populations with developmental disabilities has much to teach us about our models of normal development of language and communication, our understanding of persons with intellectual disability (Cicchetti, 1984), and our approach to language intervention. Comparisons between groups matched on mental age (MA) offer useful tests of our theories of what can go wrong in developmental disorders of language and communication, and their genetic and environmental causes (Burack, 2004). The fractionation of language and communication skills that we encounter offers an important empirical test of our acquisition theories (Abbeduto & Chapman, 2005; Bates, 2004; Chapman, 2000, 2003; Cunningham, Glenn, Wilkinson, & Sloper, 1985) and provides a rationale for intervention programming (Abbeduto & Boudreau, 2004; Fidler, Philofsky, & Hepburn, 2007; Kaiser, Hester, & McDuffie, 2001).

Historically, language learning in children with developmental disabilities was often confounded with cognitive development more generally, as vocabulary comprehension tests were used as a quick short-cut estimation of IQ. Early accounts believed language learning to proceed at the same rate as other developing skills. In the last 20 years, the emergence of genetic and environmental markers for specific syndromes and the longitudinal, detailed psychometric assessment of nonverbal cognitive and language skills have altered these assumptions radically (Carr 1995, 2000).

Research on language acquisition in Down syndrome (DS) and comparisons with other developmentally delayed populations has pursued the questions of whether evidence exists for a specific deficit in language learning, beyond that in general learning; and, if so, the configuration of the deficit, its developmental course, and its causes. To anticipate the answer, research has revealed a behavioral phenotype specific to children with DS of expressive language deficit in vocabulary, syntax (word order), grammatical morphology (inflections), and phonology (speech sounds), but not in pragmatics (uses of language) (Abbeduto, et al., 2003, Abbeduto & Chapman, 2005, Chapman et al., 2006; Chapman & Hesketh, 2000; Nadel, 2003; Miller, 1987, 1988, 1999; Rice, Warren, & Betz, 2005; Roberts, Chapman, & Warren, 2007; Roizen, 2002). The process of language expression is more affected than that of language comprehension, or receptive language. The details of the phenotype have emerged over time as limitations of earlier assessment practices have become apparent.

In this chapter, we summarize the strengths and weaknesses of the emerging language profile in children, adolescents, and young adults with DS. We then review in more detail studies of expressive language skill in vocabulary, speech–motor skill, syntax, and pragmatics. This is followed by a section on studies of receptive language skill in vocabulary and syntax. Finally, we consider proposed causes of the behavioral language phenotype and individual variation in its expression, and discuss the implications of the findings.

Down Syndrome: The Genetic Basis

Down syndrome results from the triplication of chromosome 21 in some 96% of cases and, uncommonly, from mosaic triplication in only some cells (2%) or partial triplication of the chromosome (2%). Chromosome 21, sequenced in 2000, is the next-to-smallest human chromosome with now over 400 identified genes (Gardiner & Costa, 2006; Hattori et al., 2000). The cascade of gene overexpression and shifts in regulation of expression that accompany the syndrome result in a wide range of changes in fetal brain development and later cognitive impairment. IQs range from 36 to 90. This is accompanied by a phenotypical developmental pattern of behavioral strengths and deficits in cognition, communication, and language (Chapman & Hesketh, 2000; Dykens, Hodapp, & Evans, 2006). A variable range of physical effects are found in children and adolescents (Saenz, 1999). Ultimately, the language differences reviewed in this chapter will be traceable to the combination of differences in genetic expression and language learning experience in the children's lives, but the account will not be as simple as a single-gene cause.

Evidence for a Specific Phenotype of Language Learning in Children with Down Syndrome

Overview

When we evaluate language learning, the evidence for a phenotypically specific pattern of language and cognitive skills in children with DS emerges early (see Table 12.1), with delays in expressive vocabulary relative to expectations based on nonverbal MA (Fidler, Hepburn, & Rogers, 2006; Miller, 1995), but not, initially, in comprehension vocabulary. As children with DS age from 2 to 4 years, the proportion of children showing expressive vocabulary

deficits increases (Miller, 1995). Delays in expressive language extend to mean length of utterance (MLU), when children begin putting two words together (Miller, 1995), and to the syntactic forms acquired with increasing utterance length (Thordardottir, Chapman, & Wagner, 2002). The order of acquisition of complex sentences shows that typical of normal development for MLU. Acquisition of expressive grammatical morphemes (the, –ing, noun plural and possessive, locative prepositions, past tense, auxiliary verbs, pronouns, and conjunctions) is the most delayed, proceeding in the developmental order found in children acquiring language typically, and delayed relative to both comprehension and MLU (Vicari, Caselli, & Tonucci, 2000).

Although syntax comprehension may approximate levels expected on the basis of nonverbal MA in young children, rates of development of syntax comprehension are slower than measures of nonverbal cognition that exclude visual short-term memory (STM; Chapman, Schwartz, & Kay-Raining Bird, 1991; Price, Roberts, Vandergrift, & Martin, 2007), and actual losses in syntax comprehension skill arise in longitudinal study of individuals in late adolescence and young adulthood (Chapman, Hesketh, & Kistler, 2002).

Studies of Expressive Language Development

The different developmental trajectories of expressive and receptive language acquisition in individuals with DS make it useful to review the literature separately for the two domains. In this section, we take up expressive language skills as they emerge developmentally: early communication, babbling and phonological development, emergence of signed and spoken words, later expressive vocabulary use, acquisition of expressive syntax and grammatical morphology, the question of whether expressive syntax plateaus, and expressive pragmatics and discourse development. In a section to follow, we will review the findings for receptive language development across the domains that have been principally studied, vocabulary comprehension and syntax comprehension.

Early Communication

Infants with DS show a delayed and more prolonged period of attending to faces through eye contact, and less time spent in object-directed activity (Berger & Cunningham, 1981, 1983). Thus, their preferred activities and experience may encompass a greater

Table 12.1 Developmental emergence of the behavioral phenotype of Down syndrome (DS)

Age	Domain	Behavioral phenotype
Infancy	Cognition	Learning delays at ages 0–2 accelerating at ages 2–4
(0–4 years)	Speech	Slower in transition from babbling to speech; poorer intelligibility
	Language Comprehension	Comparable to nonverbal cognition or lower
	Language Production	Delay relative to cognition and comprehension in rate of expressive language development, in vocabulary and mean length of utterance (MLU)
	Adaptive behavior	Less frequent nonverbal requesting
Childhood	Cognition	Selective deficit in auditory–verbal short-term memory (STM)
(5–12 years)	Speech	Longer period of phonological errors and more variability; poorer intelligibility
	Language Comprehension	Comparable to cognition or lower
	Language Production	Expressive language delay relative to comprehension and cognition
	Adaptive behavior	Poorer recognition of fear emotion. Fewer behavior problems than other groups with cognitive disability; more than siblings without DS. Anxiety, depression, and withdrawal increase with age
Adolescence	Cognition	Deficits in auditory and visual STM
(13–18 years)	Speech	More variability in fundamental frequency, rate control, and placement of sentential stress
	Language Comprehension	Size of word comprehension vocabulary, but conceptual level, exceeds cognitive level
		Syntax comprehension equals or lags cognition
	Language Production	Expressive language acquisition continues throughout adolescence and complex syntax, although it lags nonverbal cognition
	Adaptive Behavior	Fewer behavior problems than other groups with cognitive disability
		Anxiety, depression, and withdrawal increase with age
Young Adulthood	Cognition	Deficits in auditory and verbal STM
	Speech	Higher incidence of stuttering and hypernasality
	Language Comprehension	Longitudinal loss of syntax comprehension skill
		Continued increase in size of receptive vocabulary
	Language Production	Expressive language acquisition continues, although it lags cognition
	Adaptive Behavior	Fewer maladaptive behaviors than other groups with cognitive disability
		Higher rates of depression with increased age
Older Adulthood	Cognition	Changes in personality precede Alzheimer dementia
	Adaptive Behavior	Dementia in DS is not associated with increased rates of aggression

Adapted from Chapman & Hesketh (2000) with permission of John Wiley and Sons.

range of face-to-face communication games and fewer routines engaging objects (Abbeduto & Chapman, 2005; Kasari, Mundy, Yirmiya, & Sigman, 1990). When they reach the stage of jointly attending to objects and the other person, their gestural communication includes communication games, pointing, and protesting with frequencies similar to typically developing children, but fewer nonverbal requests (Mundy, Kasari, Sigman, & Ruskin, 1995; Mundy, Sigman, Kasari, & Yirmiya, 1988; Murphy & Abbeduto, 2005). Requesting might appear more frequently if the setting incorporates face-to-face communication games than object-centered play. Sign language is often taught in these early play contexts to bridge the delays in early vocabulary associated with speech motor, hearing, and intelligibility problems (Sterling & Warren, 2007).

Babbling and Phonological Development
More similarities than differences have been identified in the prelinguistic speech sound use of infants with DS relative to same-age peers (Stoel-Gammon, 2001). Similarities include frequency of vocalization; developmental progression from vegetative sounds to vowel to consonant use; the more frequent initial use of back consonants, followed by an increasing use of bilabial and alveolar consonants; a predominance of stops, glides, and nasals in consonant manner of production; and vowel quality (Dodd, 1972; Smith & Oller, 1981; Smith & Stoel-Gammon, 1996; Steffens, Oller, Lynch, & Urbano, 1992). Nonetheless, on average, infants with DS are delayed by 2 months in the onset of canonical babbling as measured through parent report or direct observations, and are less stable in their canonical productions over time (Lynch, Oller, Steffens, Levine, Basinger, & Umbel, 1995).

Emergence of Signed and Spoken Words
Comprehension of words precedes word use, as for typically developing children. First spoken words are reported to appear between 1 and 6 years for children with DS (Gillham, 1990), with a range of 0 to 85 words at 3 years (Strominger, Winkler, & Cohen, 1984). Gestures are used more frequently in the group with DS than by typically developing children, especially pretending gestures and symbolic gestures (*gone, hot, be quiet*), once children have a comprehension vocabulary of more than 100 words (Caselli et al., 1998); spoken words may still be fewer than 50 in number.

The milestone of at least 50 spoken words emerges between 3.5 and 6 years (Gillham, 1990).

In most studies, the growth of spoken vocabulary appears slower than one might expect, given nonverbal MA (Berglund & Eriksson, 2000; Berglund, Eriksson, & Johansson, 2001; Caselli et al., 1998; Mervis & Robinson, 2000; Miller, 1995). A large-scale study of parents' report of word learning in 330 Swedish children with DS suggests that the typical performance of 3-year-olds with DS is similar to typically developing children of 16 months; at 4 years, average performance is similar to typically developing children of 20 months (Berglund et al. 2001). In Miller's (1995, 1999) longitudinal study of expressive spoken and signed vocabulary learning of preschoolers, the rate of acquisition was slower than expected based on MA measured by the Bayley (1969) test; although it was faster than the growth of expressive syntax. Individual variation is also considerable, although 35% of the children with DS that Miller studied had expressive vocabulary sizes consistent with expectations based on MA.

Later Expressive Vocabulary Use
School-aged children and adolescents with DS show expressive vocabulary deficits relative to nonverbal cognitive levels and comprehension (Chapman, Seung, Schwartz, & Kay-Raining Bird, 1998; Laws & Bishop, 2003; Roberts et al., 2007). Verbs of emotion and mental state are less frequent in language samples obtained from children and adolescents with DS than one would expect on the basis of their MA (Beeghly & Cicchetti, 1997) or expressive language level indexed by MLU (Hesketh & Chapman, 1998). Labeling of the emotions of fear and anger is also a deficit relative to other expressive skills (Kasari, Freeman, & Hughes, 2001). The number of different words produced in language samples of DS conversation and narration is significantly lower than that produced by typically developing children matched for nonverbal MA (Chapman et al., 1998; Roberts, Hennon, Dear, Anderson, & Vandergrift, 2007).

Speech Production
Phonological delays (Smith & Stoel-Gammon, 1983) and phonetic difficulties resulting from neuromotor, anatomical, and physiological differences (Brown-Sweeney & Smith, 1997; Van Borsel, 1996) are present in individuals with DS. Intelligibility problems are frequent (Barnes, Roberts, Mirrett, Sideris, & Misenheimer, 2006; Dodd & Thompson, 2001; Kumin, 1994, 1996, 2001; Kumin, Councill, & Goodman, 1994; Miller & Leddy, 1998). Indeed, over 95% of 937 parents surveyed reported that

their children with DS experienced some difficulty being understood, although parents of older children reported fewer speech intelligibility problems. However, measures of the intelligibility of language transcripts, in which listeners can replay speech and have knowledge of the speaking task, are not related to measures of number of different words or MLU (Chapman et al., 1998; Miles, Chapman, & Sindberg, 2006).

Prelinguistically, speech sound productions of infants with DS and typical development differ little in quantity or quality (Oller & Siebert; 1988; Smith & Oller, 1981; Smith & Stoel-Gammon, 1996), although there is some evidence that the onset of canonical babbling may be delayed and less stable in DS (Lynch et al., 1995). Speech sounds emerge in words for children with DS in a therapy context, on average, as early as 2 years and for /p/ (pat), and as late as 4 years 3 months for the voiced "th" (there) (Kumin et al., 1994). Children with DS are more variable than typically developing controls in their speech sound productions (Dodd & Thompson, 2001). Speech sound errors continue through adulthood for many individuals with DS, with adolescents and adults exhibiting more speech sound omissions than 3-year-old typically developing controls (Van Borsel, 1996).

Acquisition of Expressive Syntax and Grammatical Morphology

Expressive syntax is even more delayed than expressive vocabulary (Chapman et al., 1991). Emergence of two-word utterances is delayed in many children with DS, relative to nonverbal MA expectations, with a longer period in which single words and gestures co-occur (Iverson, Longobardi, & Caselli, 2003, in a study of 4-year-olds). When matched to typically developing children by expressive vocabulary size, preschool children with DS lag slightly on expressive grammar scales (Berglund & Eriksson, 2000; Berglund et al., 2001). When matched to typically developing children on nonverbal MA, individuals with DS aged 5–20 years show significantly lower MLU in narrative tasks without the presence of visual support (Chapman et al., 1998; Boudreau & Chapman, 2000). The sentence structures associated with MLU are increasingly complex in comparable ways among typically developing and DS speakers matched for MLU (Thordardottir et al., 2002). There is, of course, wide individual difference in the rate of syntax acquisition associated with differences in rates of cognitive development (Chapman et al., 1998).

Studies show that grammatical morphology is an area of particular deficit in expressive syntax development (Chapman et al., 1998; Eadie, Fey, Douglas, & Parsons, 2002; Fabbretti, Pizzuto, Vicari, & Volterra, 1997). For example, when matched by MLU on expressive sentence length of language samples, the participants with DS are more likely to omit grammatical function words (e.g., articles, prepositions, forms of be, past tense –ed, third person singular –s, noun plurals) (Chapman et al., 1998). They are also likely to use fewer modal auxiliaries (e.g., can, may, will) (Hesketh & Chapman, 1998). Although grammatical morphology is particularly delayed in acquisition, the order in which grammatical morphemes are acquired is the same as that in typically developing children (Eadie et al., 2002).

Plateauing of Expressive Syntax?

Fowler and colleagues reported that the acquisition of expressive syntax plateaued in adolescence (Fowler, Gelman, & Gleitman, 1994). They suggested a *critical period* for language acquisition for individuals with DS, with a cut-off at the onset of adolescence; or, alternately, a limitation of language learning to *simple syntax* (sentences containing only one verb). The language samples on which Fowler's based her report of a plateau were conversational (question–answer and comment during free play with the examiner), and her findings of plateauing for younger adolescents were confirmed in our own conversational samples (Chapman et al., 1998). Our narrative language samples from the same adolescents, in contrast, revealed a different developmental pattern, one of ongoing increases in utterance length with age throughout adolescence and young adulthood, with increasingly complex syntactic structure associated with longer utterances (Chapman et al., 1998; Chapman et al., 2002; Thordardottir et al., 2002). Narrative language samples offer a better method than conversational samples for revealing more advanced syntactic development. By narrative measures, expressive language learning continues in adolescence and young adulthood for individuals with DS. The implications for educational practice are clear: Educational support for language learning should be continued in adolescence, rather than withdrawn because a plateau has been reached.

Expressive Pragmatics and Discourse Development

Pragmatic development is an area of both strengths and some differences (see Cebula & Wishart, 2007, for review). Although nonverbal requesting of objects may be less frequent in infancy, the social skills of children with DS serve them well in the subsequent development of communicative functions (Johnston & Stansfield, 1997). Toddlers with DS show strengths in social interaction (Dykens et al. 2006) that extend to use of the same range of communication functions in mother–child conversation as that found in typically developing children matched for language level (Coggins, Carpenter, & Owings, 1983), including the repair of communication breakdowns when clarification is requested (Coggins & Stoel-Gammon, 1982). Preschoolers with DS stay on topic with their mothers as often as children matched for MA (Tannock, 1988), but are less likely to introduce new topics or make requests (Beeghly, Weiss-Perry, & Cicchetti, 1990). Compared to children matched for expressive language level, these children stayed on topic for more turns and gave more appropriate conversational responses to adults.

In a study of conversational interactions of boys with DS in comparison with typically developing boys matched for nonverbal MA, Roberts et al. (2007) found that the boys with DS were less elaborative when maintaining topics and produced a higher proportion of turns that were only adequate in quality. Referential communication tasks reveal problems for adolescents with DS both in the quality of expressive language and in taking the point of view of others (Abbeduto et al., 2006). A factor compromising the success of conversational interactions is the presence of more frequent dysfluencies in the speech of individuals with DS (Ferrier, Bashir, Maryash, Johnston, & Wolff, 1991).

Narrative language samples reveal the diverging skills of individuals with DS. The content attempted in narrative is as advanced as MA-matched comparison groups of typically developing children (Boudreau & Chapman, 2000; Miles & Chapman, 2002) when wordless films or picture books are narrated. Mention of salient events, themes, and plot elements in narratives based on wordless picture books occur with frequencies comparable to groups matched for nonverbal MA or syntax comprehension (Miles & Chapman, 2002). In contrast, these narratives show deficits in MLU, sentence complexity, and vocabulary use, and individuals with DS show deficits even in relation to the MLU of their narratives in producing the grammatical bound morphemes required by English. When narrative samples are based on the recall of verbally rather than visually presented stories, children and adolescents with DS recall less in their retellings than the MA-matched children (Kay-Raining Bird, Chapman, & Schwartz, 2004), reflecting their specific problems in auditory-verbal STM.

Interactive trade-offs in the construction of spoken narratives are also evident when visual support for the story is provided. When narratives are obtained from wordless picture books, adolescents and young adults with DS show measures of narrative and utterance length and lexical diversity (although not grammatical morpheme use) that are comparable to comparison groups matched for syntax comprehension, and better than groups matched for MLU on the narratives obtained without visual support, in contrast to previous findings (Miles, Chapman, & Sindberg, 2006). This finding underscores the importance of considering sampling methods when evaluating language. Variation as a function of sampling method can also reveal the conditions that would lead to improved expressive language for those with language deficits as identified by usual methods.

Picture support is one particularly helpful aid to storytelling for individuals with DS. Miles, Sindberg, Bridge, and Chapman (2002) and Miles, Chapman, and Sindberg (2004) investigated whether adult prompting for more talk or provision of specific questions (adult scaffolding) additionally improved storytelling from wordless picture books. The effect of scaffolding across time was examined by asking adolescents with DS to practice telling the same stories from picture books six times, with sessions separated by 1 to 2 weeks. The low scaffolding condition included the pictures, the adult's repetition of the participant's story content with the addition of missing grammatical morphemes, and nonspecific prompts to "tell me more." For a second story, the high scaffolding condition included all the elements of the low scaffolding condition plus specific "WH" questions (who, what, where, what's happening, when) for missing simple sentence content. Scoring of the setting information for the story showed that almost all the participants mentioned the protagonist on all tellings, few mentioned the time of day on any telling, and both persons with DS and typically developing children matched for MLU increased their mention of spatial location in the high scaffolding condition over repeated tellings.

A follow-up study of full story content (Miles & Chapman, 2005) indicated that both plot line/theme expression and MLU increased across tellings for adolescents with DS as well as for MLU-matched and syntax comprehension-matched typically developing children, with narrative content and semantic diversity being higher in the high scaffolding condition with question prompts. An analysis of storytelling strategies (Miles et al., 2004) in the narratives revealed that almost all the participants approached the task as one of telling related story events. The adolescents with DS, however, were more likely to use multiple utterances in commenting on a page and to include character voice in their narration, compared to the typically developing group matched for syntax comprehension.

Acquisition of Receptive Language

The studies just reviewed all bear on the expressive communication skills of children and adolescents with DS, from nonverbal communication acts to first words and vocabulary use, sentence syntax and grammatical morphology, pragmatics, and discourse skills. The development of receptive language comprehension, in contrast to the expressive language deficits in vocabulary, syntax, and morphology previously reported, show a different developmental trajectory. Here, we consider findings for the same series of language skills from the perspective of receptive, rather than expressive, language learning.

Vocabulary Comprehension

One-year-old infants with DS prefer to listen to nursery rhymes sung by a female voice rather than played on a musical instrument, as do the MA-matched typically developing comparison group, but show longer response durations (Glenn, Cunningham, & Joyce, 1981). In childhood, vocabulary comprehension shows both strengths and some specific weaknesses in individuals with DS. Children with DS show early vocabulary comprehension typical of expectations based on MA, as reported by parents on the MacArthur Communicative Development Inventory (Miller, 1995). Chapman et al. (1991) also reported vocabulary levels commensurate with nonverbal MA in children aged 5–12 years with DS.

However, specific word classes may show decrements. Comprehension of emotion words for fear is a problem for children and adolescents with DS (Williams, Wishart, Pitcairn, & Willis, 2005). Comprehension of mental state verbs, as well as others' states of mind on theory of mind tasks, also show deficits in adolescents with DS in comparison to typically developing children matched on MA (Abbeduto et al., 2001; Zelazo, Burack, Benedetto, & Fry, 1996).

In adolescence, general vocabulary comprehension levels on the Peabody Picture Test of Vocabulary (PPVT; Dunn & Dunn, 1981, 1997), a test based on sampling words on the basis of frequency of occurrence and picturability, exceed MA measures (Chapman et al., 1991). Vocabulary comprehension tests based on difficulty of conceptual content, such as subtest one of the Test of Auditory Comprehension of Language (Carrow-Woolfolk, 1985, 1999), show equivalence in adolescence with nonverbal MA measures (Miolo, Chapman, & Sindberg, 2005). The apparent conflict in these results can be resolved by noting that the PPVT typically tests higher than nonverbal cognitive level in adolescents with intellectual disabilities from a variety of syndromes (Facon, Facon-Bollengier, & Grubar, 2002; Facon, Grubar, & Gardez, 1998; Glenn & Cunningham 2005; Chapman, 2006). The adolescents in these studies have in common an extended number of years and more varied experiences for vocabulary learning than do MA-matched controls. Thus, adolescents with DS appear to have a larger, but not a conceptually more advanced, comprehension vocabulary, with significant difficulties in comprehension of mental state words.

Other investigators, however, report vocabulary comprehension levels among adolescents with DS that are lower than comparison groups matched for nonverbal MA levels (Hick, Botting, & Conti-Ramsden, 2005; Price et al., 2007; Roberts, Hennon, et al., 2007). These investigators used cognitive matching procedures, such as the Leiter International Performance Scale—Revised (Roid & Miller, 1997), that did not include visual short-term tasks, in contrast to Chapman's studies operationalizing nonverbal cognition as the mean of the pattern analysis test of visual cognition and the bead memory test of visual STM (Stanford Binet 4th ed.; Thorndike, Hagen, & Sattler, 1986). Because visual STM scores show a significant decline in adolescence (Chapman et al. 1991), the matched cognitive level was probably lower for the Chapman studies than for those studies that used the Leiter and reported a vocabulary comprehension decrement. If visual STM is excluded from the operational definition of nonverbal MA, then adolescents with DS may show a decrement in vocabulary comprehension.

Syntax Comprehension

Syntax comprehension, the understanding of meaning conveyed by sentence structure, is a strength relative to syntax production in children and adolescents with DS, but a weakness relative to nonverbal MA (Chapman et al., 1991; Chapman et al., 2002; Price et al., 2007). Syntax comprehension shows a slower rate of development than does the rate of nonverbal cognitive development, especially if the nonverbal MA measures exclude visual STM. A longitudinal study over 6 years indicates actual loss of syntax comprehension skills in late adolescence and early adulthood, even as the same individuals are improving in expressive sentence length (Chapman et al., 2002). Why the developmental trajectory for syntax comprehension declines in adolescence, in contrast to the increasing developmental trajectory for syntax production, is unknown. The measures of the syntax comprehension depend crucially on auditory STM for the sentence, and visual STM for the picture alternatives inspected, and both STM systems are compromised in adolescence (visual STM is MA-equivalent in younger children). Most language sample measures that operationalize expressive syntax, in contrast, do not depend on these STM systems. One hypothesis would be that both visual and auditory STM in adolescence are sensitive to early effects of Alzheimer disease, associated with the overproduction of amyloid precursor protein (APP) on chromosome 21.

Predicting Individual Differences in Language Skills

We have discussed the developmental emergence of the specific behavioral phenotype that characterizes individuals with DS, but there are wide individual differences in their rates of development. Predictors of these individual differences in DS language performance have been extensively studied (see Abbeduto & Chapman, 2005, and Roberts, Chapman, & Warren, 2007, for reviews). Individual differences in cognitive function generally are as great as the range of variability in typically developing children, albeit at a lower level of function. Individual differences in language skills are also great within domains, including comprehension and production of vocabulary, syntax, discourse, communication functions, and phonology. The predictors of variability in these domains that have been evaluated include chronological age (CA), nonverbal MA, auditory–verbal STM, visual STM, hearing status, and pattern and amount of language input.

Chronological Age

As Table 12.1 and the previously reviewed developmental trajectories illustrate, specific language impairment emerges with increasing CA in DS.

Cognitive Development

Infants and toddlers with DS show an initial delay in early sensorimotor learning from 1 to 2 years that widens from 2 to 4 years; they also show a wide range of individual difference, with IQs ranging from 30 to 90, with a mean of about 50 (Beeghly et al., 1990). Visual STM shows impairment relative to visual cognition in adolescents with DS (Chapman et al., 1991; Vicari, Bellucci, & Carlesimo, 2006; see Chapman & Hesketh, 2000, for review). Chapman et al. (1991) operationalized nonverbal MA as the mean of the two visual cognition tasks (bead memory and pattern analysis from Stanford-Binet 4th ed.) and found that nonverbal MA and CA accounted for a substantial amount of variance in language comprehension and language production in individuals between 5 to 21 years of age (Chapman et al., 1998). In a subsequent analysis of longitudinal data over a 6-year period for 33 of these participants, evaluating the two visual cognition predictors separately, Chapman et al. (2002) found that bead memory, the visual STM task, together with auditory STM and CA, explained both initial variation and subsequent trajectory of syntax comprehension performance (Chapman et al., 2002). In turn, syntax comprehension predicted the most variance in MLU from narrative language productions.

Auditory–Verbal Working Memory and Language Acquisition

Auditory–verbal STM is impaired relative to visual STM (Lanfranchie, Cornoldi, & Vianello, 2004) and relative to nonverbal cognitive skills in children and adolescents with DS (see Gathercole & Alloway, 2006, for review). Evidence for a selective deficit in auditory–verbal working memory, as opposed to nonverbal visual cognition, has been repeatedly confirmed for digit span in children and adolescents with DS (Brock & Jarrold, 2005; Kay-Raining Bird & Chapman, 1994; Lanfranchi et al., 2004; Marcell & Weeks, 1988; Marcell, Ridgeway, Sewell, & Whelan, 1995; Vicari, Marotta, & Carlesimo, 2004), even when the response required was to touch, rather than to say, the number (Brock & Jarrold, 2005). Nonword repetition, a task understood as a purer measure of phonological working memory, also shows deficits in DS, even when lenient scoring is adopted to allow for articulation problems (Laws, 1998; Laws & Gunn, 2004).

Baddeley's Model of Working Memory

Baddeley's model of working memory has been adopted as one general framework in which the auditory STM deficit in DS can be understood (Baddeley & Jarrold, 2007; Jarrold & Baddeley, 2001; Jarrold, Baddeley, & Phillips, 1999). In its early versions, working memory was treated as a single component, but multiple components are currently recognized. The version of the model that Baddeley and Jarrold (2007) adopt for DS has four components: the *phonological loop*, the *visuospatial sketch pad*, the *central executive*, and a new component, the *episodic buffer*. The phonological component is responsible for maintaining speech-based information in a passive phonological store of approximately 2 seconds capacity. This is refreshed by the phonological, or articulatory, loop, which maintains the information through overt or covert rehearsal or repetition of the loop. The visuospatial sketchpad holds visual information in working memory store. The central executive acts as an attentional control system, allocating attentional resources to input and rehearsal. The episodic buffer is a temporary, multidimensional store that forms an interface between the various subsystems of working memory, long-term memory, and perception, allowing long-term knowledge and episodic context to influence the recognition and chunking of information in the working memory stores.

The Baddeley model allows auditory–verbal working memory tasks to be fractionated into the roles of episodic buffer, phonological loop, and central executive. Episodic memory presumably contributes improved auditory working memory recall for known language items versus nonwords, and, to a lesser degree, for nonwords that follow the sequences of sounds typical in the local language, as compared to nonwords containing sounds or sound sequences not encountered in the individual's language. Children with DS are similar to typically developing children in showing poorer auditory–verbal working memory for nonwords, as measured by the Nonword Repetition Task (Laws, 1998).

Central executive functions include the allocation of attentional resources to the task through selective attention and the use of learning strategies, but it is not clear whether central executive function is selectively impaired in children with DS (i.e., poorer performance than expected for nonverbal cognitive level). Deficits in central executive function are typically assessed with dual processing or backward digit span tasks that require attention to be reallocated. These tasks, typically at 5- or 6-year-old levels at a minimum, are too difficult for most children and adolescents with DS to perform

(Miolo et al., 2005). Measures of central executive function with developmental levels of 2–4 years, rather than 5- to 6-year levels, would be an appropriate level of difficulty to assess this aspect of working memory in most children and adolescents with DS (e.g., Espy, Bull, Martin, & Stroup, 2006; Zelazo, 2006). The assessment of working memory in middle-aged people with DS, although it reveals deficits in the phonological loop compared to individuals with a mixed etiology of cognitive impairment, shows no evidence of a deficit in the central executive component of working memory (Numminen, Service, Ahonen, & Ruoppila, 2001). Training of verbal working memory skills improves task performance but shows limited transfer (Conners, Rosenquist, & Taylor, 2001).

The phonological loop, on the evidence previously reviewed, is clearly compromised for children and adolescents with DS. Digit span tasks reveal, typically, span lengths of 2–4 digits, performance worse than would be expected for nonverbal MA. The auditory–verbal STM deficit is not attributable to distraction (Marcell, Harvey, & Cothran, 1988), hearing loss (Laws, 2004), or impaired comprehension (Miolo et al., 2005). Nor is it attributable to a slower speaking rate, with consequent impairment of the size of chunk that could be rehearsed; children with DS speak faster than typically developing MA matches (Kanno & Ikeda, 2002; Seung & Chapman, 2000, 2004). Neither children and adolescents with DS nor MA-matched controls show overt rehearsal in memory span tasks, suggesting that overt rehearsal is not a factor determining span length (Jarrold, Baddeley, & Hewes, 2000; Vicari et al., 2004). Speech–motor difficulties do not seem to correlate with span length (Jarrold et al., 2002). Nor is there evidence that the auditory–verbal STM deficit can be attributed to atypically rapid forgetting of information in phonological STM (Purser & Jarrold, 2005). Rather, Jarrold, Baddeley, and Phillips (1999) have attributed the deficit to a capacity limitation in phonological store.

In an alternative view of the capacity limitation to phonological store, Seung and Chapman (2004) hypothesize that the capacity limitation arises dynamically, through reduced activity in an automatic articulatory loop that connects receptive language to language production and back again—a "rehearsal" loop for speech that is automatic and covert, rather than intentional and overt. Such a loop would also allow listening experience to subserve the acquisition of expressive language. Seung and Chapman hypothesized that the diminishment of such a loop in children with DS is responsible for both the auditory–verbal STM deficit and the expressive language deficit observed. Such a circuit has been identified in adults through diffusion tensor imaging, operating through the arcuate fasciculus, linking the temporal language cortex where comprehension takes place to premotor area (Glasser & Rilling, 2008). Imaging evidence for a compromised auditory–articulatory loop has not yet been sought among children with DS. Imaging evidence for the forwarding of cortical activity from the left temporal (receptive language) area to left premotor areas while listening to words has been reported for adults (Price et al., 1996) and for typically developing toddlers (Imada, Zhang, Cheour, Taulu, Ahonen, & Kuhl, 2006). The developmental necessity for a link between sound perception and sound production in infancy has been argued by Kent and Vorperian (2007). Because the vocal tract and muscles governing speech production are growing rapidly and at differing rates, the infant must constantly revise motor instructions on the basis of his perceptual outcome, and a perceptual–articulatory loop allows such revision; it would also account for the shift, in the second half of the first year, to babbled sounds drawn from the language encountered by the infant in his environment.

Relation Between the Auditory–Verbal Working Memory Deficit and Expressive Language Impairment

Evidence from hierarchical linear modeling and correlational studies clearly establish the association between auditory–verbal STM skill and expressive language skill both cross-sectionally (Laws, 2004) and longitudinally (Chapman et al., 2002), after nonverbal cognition has been taken into account. Hearing did not explain variance in these analyses, although in Laws (2004), those individuals with hearing loss were less likely to be able to produce an intelligible narrative.

Both children with DS and children with specific language impairment show deficits in auditory–verbal STM, as compared to typically developing children matched on MA (Laws & Bishop, 2003), with subsequent deficits in both receptive and expressive vocabulary compared to a typically developing group (Hick et al., 2005, Laws & Gunn, 2004). Some exceptional cases of spared language production and reading skill were reported in individuals with DS (Groen, Laws, Nation, & Bishop, 2006; Rondal, 1998; Vallar & Papagno, 1993), but these individuals were also reported to have unusually good skills in auditory–verbal short-term working memory.

Hearing Status

Conductive or sensorineural hearing loss occurs in almost two-thirds of children with DS (Roizen, 2002), but the presence of mild hearing impairment explains only an additional 4% of the variance (after MA and CA) in syntax comprehension (Chapman et al., 1991). It also shows a significant relationship, in adolescents, to grammatical morphology comprehension (Miolo et al., 2005) and fast-mapping of words in comprehension (Chapman, 2003; Chapman, Sindberg, Bridge, Gigstead, & Hesketh, 2006; McDuffie, Sindberg, Hesketh, & Chapman, 2007). Hearing status does show a significant relation to intelligibility of narratives, but not to sentence length of lexical diversity of narratives (Chapman et al., 1991; Laws, 2004).

Language Input

The amount of language encountered from parents and others during language learning years will affect the rate of language learning in this as in other populations. Mothers of preschool-aged children with DS are more directive, but equally supportive, of their children in their interactions, compared to parents of children matched for communication level (Tannock, 1988). Parents of 5- to 20-year-old children and adolescents with DS communicate as frequently as parents of typically developing children matched for MA with their children in a task involving play with novel toys (Johnson-Glenberg & Chapman, 2004). The complexity of the DS parents' language is consistent with their children's comprehension, rather than production, levels. Because comprehension and production levels diverge for children and adolescents with DS, sentence models provided at comprehension levels may be less useful for the support of expressive language learning, although helpful for further receptive language learning. Whether children with DS would benefit from additional responsive input modeled at the current level of their expressive language is a question that warrants further research.

Dual Language Development in Individuals with Down Syndrome

The existence of problems in phonological working memory and the problems in acquisition of expressive language in individuals with DS suggest that bilingual acquisition might constitute a particular problem for them, because the time available for encountering each language is necessarily reduced; such views have led to recommendations that children with DS not learn a second language (Thordardottir, 2002). The evidence, however, suggests no additional problems in acquisition. Case studies demonstrate that at least some individuals with DS become highly functional in two or more languages (Vallar & Papagno, 1993; Woll & Grove, 1996). Kay-Raining Bird, Cleave, Trudeau, studied the language development of four groups of children matched on developmental level (monolingual and bilingual children with DS, and monolingual and bilingual typically developed children). They showed that bilingual children with DS perform at least as well in their dominant language as their monolingual counterparts with DS, suggesting that bilingualism does not disadvantage these individuals. As would be expected, expressive morphosyntactic difficulties were evident in both groups with DS, showing that bilingualism does not change the profile of language strengths and weaknesses in this population. A detailed comparison of the semantic and syntactic abilities of a subgroup of these children confirmed the findings of the group study (Feltmate & Kay-Raining Bird, 2008).

Implications for Future Research

The research reviewed here establishes evidence for an expressive language learning deficit in children with DS, accompanied by problems in intelligibility and loss, in late adolescence and young adulthood, of syntax comprehension skills. Predictors of variation in these three areas—expressive language, intelligibility, and syntax comprehension—differ, suggesting that the causes of deficit in each of these three domains may be different. Future research can fruitfully pursue the characteristics of trisomy 21 that are related to variation in each domain.

For example, the role of auditory–verbal working memory skills in expressive language acquisition in DS deserves further investigation, including the contributions of phonological store, the phonological loop, central executive functions, and contributions of phonotactic and linguistic knowledge from long-term memory (episodic store). Imaging methods can establish whether experience in listening to language is accompanied by activation in premotor planning areas, thus establishing evidence for a possible deficit in the phonological loop that could be related to both auditory–verbal working memory deficits and expressive language learning deficits. Developmentally simplified tasks to test central executive functions can probe their contribution to

sentence production. The biochemical events underlying phonological store can be examined. Recently, theorists have proposed that working memory is sustained by calcium-mediated synaptic facilitation in the recurrent connections of neocortical networks (Mongillo, Barak, & Tsodyks, 2008). If so, dysfunction of calcium-mediated synaptic facilitation should be demonstrable in DS, associated with gene dosage effects on chromosome 21.

Problems in intelligibility are a second area in need of research; the contributions of DS-related facial structure, muscle function, motor learning, and hearing impairment to achievement of intelligible speech need to be examined and related to gene dosage effects. Intervention methods for improving intelligibility need to be evaluated, and improved conditions for hearing and speech need to be established at home and in classrooms.

The loss of syntax comprehension skills in young adulthood constitutes an acquisition pattern unique to individuals with DS, and its cause is an important question for study. One possibility is that the loss is an early consequence of Alzheimer disease. Another possibility is that it is the consequence of reduced educational programming for language learning in adolescence and reduced access to environments of extensive language use in young adulthood. If Alzheimer disease is the cause, then drug therapies useful in Alzheimer disease may be helpful; if changes in educational environments are the cause, then these can be revised. The particular pattern of strengths and weaknesses in learning in DS also suggest the importance of further research on the temporal fractionation of learning: roles of axon growth, dendritic growth and stability, synaptic plasticity, long-term memory consolidation in sleep, and their relation to gene dosage effects in DS are all candidates for further work.

The longitudinal studies of cognitive and language development in individuals with DS yield individual measures of rate of acquisition in multiple domains; genome scans for the dosage-affected metabolic pathways underlying this developmental variability are now possible and would reveal fundamental mechanisms of learning in all children.

Implications for Intervention

The research just reviewed has a number of important implications for speech–language intervention with DS individuals. These include the importance of recognizing that individuals with DS face both general learning challenges and specific deficits in expressive language acquisition.

Thus, speech–language pathology services are important to provide throughout the language learning period—which, research shows, runs from infancy through the third decade of life in persons with DS. Support for speech–language learning should include speech therapy for intelligibility, audiological consultation to manage recurrent otitis media and hearing loss, and language therapy that provides service both to the child and her family. Intervention programs based on developmental principles are important to provide in both family and school settings. These programs provide a linguistically responsive language learning environments, elaborate social interaction into communication games and imaginative play, emphasize communicative success through the use of signing or other augmentative means if the child has intelligibility problems, and continue language learning in conversational contexts (Paul, 2007). Goals for language learning should include both comprehension skills and production skills; these are likely to be at different levels for children with DS because of their expressive language deficit. Grammatical morphology will require additional goal setting, as it is an area of greatest expressive language deficit. For those children in bilingual language learning environments, therapy should be offered in both languages, and learning opportunities should be enriched in both languages.

Conclusion

In this chapter on language in children, adolescents, and young adults with DS, we have shown that a typical pattern of language learning emerges, with strengths and weaknesses. Comprehension skills are better than expressive language skills, which show a deficit; and, within the expressive domain, lexical skills are better than syntactic skills, with use of grammatical morphology the most developmentally delayed. The pattern of fractionation of language skills is consistent with emergent, interactionist theories of language acquisition, rather than modular ones, and requires a developmental framework for their interpretation. Social skills are a strength in communication patterns, and phonological working memory a deficit correlated with deficits in expressive language acquisition. Mild hearing loss plays a role in impairing comprehension of grammatical morphology, in reducing the fast-mapping of novel words encountered one or a few times, and in impairing speech intelligibility, which is a frequent problem in DS. In late adolescence and young adulthood, persons with DS show actual loss of sentence comprehension skill; but throughout the period from early adolescence through young adulthood, language production skills continue to improve, contrary to the claims of critical period or simple syntax hypotheses. Children and adolescents with DS can become bilingual without causing additional delays in spoken language acquisition, and with consequent expansion of language for learning and use.

Acknowledgments

The preparation of this chapter was supported by NIH Grant R01-HD23353 to the first author, with additional support from the National Down Syndrome Society, and by NIH Grant P30HD03352 awarded to the Waisman Center. Preparation was also supported by grants to the second author from the Social Sciences and Humanities Research Council of Canada (#410–2000-1409 and #410–2003-1875).

References

Abbeduto, L., & Boudreau, D. (2004). Theoretical influences on research on language development and intervention in individuals with mental retardation. *Mental Retardation and Developmental Disabilities Research Reviews, 10,* 184–192.

Abbeduto, L., & Chapman, R. (2005). Language and communication skills in children with Down Syndrome and Fragile X. In P. Fletcher & J. Miller, Eds., *Trends in language acquisition research, vol. 4: Developmental theory and language disorders.* (pp. 53–72). Amsterdam, NL: John Benjamins.

Abbeduto L., Murphy M., Richmond E., Amman, A., Beth, P., Weissman, M., et al. (2006). Collaboration in referential communication: Comparison of youth with Down syndrome or fragile X syndrome. *American Journal on Mental Retardation, 3,* 170–183.

Abbeduto L., Murphy M., Cawthon S., Richmond E., Weissman M., Karadottir S., & O'Brien A. (2003). Receptive language skills of adolescents and young adults with mental retardation: A comparison of Down syndrome and fragile X syndrome. *American Journal on Mental Retardation, 108,* 149–160.

Abbeduto, L., Pavetto, M., Kesin, E. Weissman, M., Karadottir, S., O'Brien, A., & Cawthon, S. (2001). The linguistic and cognitive profile of Down syndrome: Evidence from a comparison with fragile X syndrome. *Down Syndrome Research and Practice, 7,* 9–16.

Baddeley, A., & Jarrold, C. (2007). Working memory and Down syndrome. *Journal of Intellectual Disability Research, 51,* 925–931.

Barnes, E. F., Roberts, J., Mirrett, P., Sideris, J., & Misenheimer, J. (2006). A comparison of oral structure and oral-motor function in young males with fragile X syndrome and Down syndrome. *Journal of Speech, Language, and Hearing Research, 49,* 903–917.

Bates, E. A. (2004). Explaining and interpreting deficits in language development across clinical groups: Where do we go from here? *Brain and Language, 88,* 248–253.

Bayley, N. (1969). *Manual for Bayley scales of infant development.* New York: Psychological Corporation.

Beeghly, M., & Cicchetti, D. (1997). Talking about self and other: Emergence of an internal state lexicon in young children with Down syndrome. *Development and Psychopathology, 9,* 729–748.

Beeghly, M., Weiss-Perry, B., & Cicchetti, D. (1990). Beyond sensorimotor functioning: Early communicative and play development of children with Down syndrome. In D. Cicchetti & M. Beeghly (Eds.), *Children with Down syndrome: A developmental perspective* (pp. 329–368). New York: Cambridge University Press.

Berger, J., & Cunningham, C. C. (1981). Development of eye contact between mothers and normal versus Down syndrome infants. *Developmental Psychology, 17,* 678–689.

Berger, J., & Cunningham, C. C. (1983). Early social interactions between infants with Down's syndrome and their parents. *Health Visit, 56,* 58–60.

Berglund, E., & Eriksson, M. (2000). Communicative development in Swedish children 16–28 months old: the Swedish early communicative development inventory—words and sentences. *Scandinavian Journal of Psychology, 41,* 133–144.

Berglund, E., Eriksson, M., & Johansson, I. (2001). Parental reports of spoken language skills in children with Down syndrome. *Journal of Speech, Language, and Hearing Research, 44,* 179–191.

Boudreau, D., & Chapman, R. (2000).The relationship between event representation and linguistic skill in narratives of children and adolescents with DS. *Journal of Speech, Language, and Hearing Research, 43,* 1146–1159.

Brock, J., & Jarrold, C. (2005). Serial order reconstruction in DS: Evidence for a selective deficit in verbal short-term memory. *Journal of Child Psychology and Psychiatry, 46,* 304–316.

Brown-Sweeney, S. G., Smith, B. L. (1997). The development of speech production abilities in children with Down syndrome. *Clinical Linguistics and Phonetics, 11,* 345–362.

Burack, J. (2004). Editorial Preface, *Journal of Autism and Developmental Disorders, 34,* 3–5.

Carr, J. (1995). *Down's syndrome: Children growing up.* New York: Cambridge University Press.

Carr, J. (2000). Intellectual and daily living skills of 30-year-olds with Down's syndrome: Continuation of a longitudinal study. *Journal of Applied Research in Intellectual Disabilities, 13,* 1–16.

Carrow-Woolfolk, E. (1985). *Test for Auditory Comprehension of Language-Revised.* Allen, TX: DLM Teaching Resources.

Carrow-Woolfolk, E. (1999). *Test for Auditory Comprehension of Language - Third Edition.* Circle Pines, MN: AGS.

Caselli, M. C., Vicari, S., Longobardi, E., Lami, L., Pizzoli, C., & Stella, G. (1998). Gestures and words in early development of children with Down syndrome. *Journal of Speech, Language, and Hearing Research, 41,* 1125–1135.

Cebula, K. R., & Wishart, J. G. (2007). Social cognition in children with Down syndrome. (pp. 43–86). In L.M. Glidden, Ed., *International Review of Research in Mental Retardation,* vol. 35, Academic Press.

Chapman, R. (2000). Children's language learning: An interactionist perspective. *Journal of Child Psychology and Psychiatry, 41,* 33–54.

Chapman, R. (2003). Language and communication in individuals with Down syndrome. (pp. 1–34) In L. Abbeduto (Ed.,), *International Review of Research in Mental Retardation: Language and Communication, 27.* Academic Press.

Chapman, R. (2006). Language learning in Down syndrome: The speech and language profile compared to adolescents with cognitive impairment of unknown origin. *Down Syndrome Research and Practice, 10.*

Chapman, R., & Hesketh, L. (2000). Behavioral phenotype of individuals with Down syndrome. *Mental Retardation and Developmental Disability Research Reviews, 6,* 84–95.

Chapman, R., Hesketh, L., & Kistler, D. (2002). Predicting longitudinal change in language production and comprehension in individuals with Down syndrome: Hierarchical linear modeling. *Journal of Speech, Language, and Hearing Research, 45,* 902–915.

Chapman, R., Schwartz, S., & Kay-Raining Bird, E. (1991). Language skills of children and adolescents with DS: I. Comprehension. *Journal of Speech and Hearing Research, 34,* 1106–1120.

Chapman, R. S., Seung, H. K., Schwartz, S. E., & Kay-Raining Bird, E. (1998). Language skills of children and adolescents with Down syndrome: II. Production deficits. *Journal of Speech, Language, and Hearing Research, 41,* 861–873.

Chapman, R., Sindberg, H., Bridge, C., Gigstead, K., & Hesketh, L. J. (2006). Effect of memory support and elicited production on fast-mapping of new words by adolescents with DS. *Journal of Speech, Language, & Hearing Research, 49,* 3–15.

Cicchetti, D. (1984). The emergence of developmental psychopathology. *Child Development, 55,* 1–7.

Conners, F. A., Rosenquist, C. J., & Taylor, L. S. (2001). Memory training for children with Down syndrome. *Downs Syndrome Research and Practice, 7,* 25–33.

Coggins, T. E., Carpenter, R. L., & Owings, N. O. (1983). Examining early intentional communication in Down's syndrome and nonretarded children. *International Journal of Language & Communication Disorders, 18,* 98–106.

Coggins, T. E. and Stoel-Gammon, C. (1982). Clarification strategies used by four Down's Syndrome children for maintaining normal conversational interaction. *Education and Training of the Mental and Retarded, 16,* 65–67.

Cunningham, C. C., Glenn, S. M., Wilkinson, P., & Sloper, P. (1985). Mental ability, symbolic play and receptive and expressive language of young children with Down' s syndrome. *Journal of Child Psychology and Psychiatry, 26,* 255–265.

Dodd, B. (1972). Comparison of babbling patterns in normal and Down syndrome infants. *Journal of Mental Deficiency Research, 16,* 35–40.

Dodd, B., & Thompson, L. (2001). Speech disorder in children with Down syndrome. *Journal of Intellectual Disability Research, 45,* 308–316.

Dunn, L., & Dunn, L. (1981). *Peabody Picture Vocabulary Test-Revised.* Circle Pines: MN. American Guidance Service.

Dunn, L., & Dunn, L. (1997). *Peabody Picture Vocabulary Test-3rd Edition.* Circle Pines: MN. American Guidance Service.

Dykens, E. M., Hodapp, R. M., & Evans, D. W. (2006). Profiles and development of adaptive behavior in children with Down syndrome. *Down's Syndrome Research and Practice, 9,* 45–50.

Eadie, P., Fey, M., Douglas, J., & Parsons, C. (2002). Profiles of grammatical morphology and sentence imitation in children with specific language impairment and DS. *Journal of Speech, Language, and Hearing Research, 45,* 720–732.

Espy, K. A., Bull, R., Martin, J., & Stroup, W. (2006). Measuring the development of executive control with the shape school. *Psychological Assessment, 18,* 373–381.

Fabbretti, D., Pizzuto, E., Vicari, S., & Volterra, V. (1997). A story description task in children with Down's syndrome: Lexical and morphosyntactic abilities. *Journal of Intellectual Disabilities Research, 41,* 165–179.

Facon, B., Facon-Bollengier, T., & Grubar, J. (2002). Chronological age, receptive vocabulary, and syntax comprehension in children and adolescents with mental retardation. *American Journal on Mental Retardation, 107,* 91–98.

Facon, B., Grubar, J., & Gardez, C. (1998). Chronological age and receptive vocabulary of persons with DS. *Psychological Reports, 82,* 723–726.

Feltmate, K., & Kay-Raining Bird, E. (2008). Language learning in four bilingual children with Down syndrome: A detailed analysis of vocabulary and morphosyntax. *Canadian Journal of Speech-Language Pathology and Audiology, 32,* 6–20.

Ferrier, L., Bashir, A., Meryash, D., Johnston, J., & Wolff, P. (1991). Conversational skill of individuals with fragile X syndrome: A comparison with autism and DS. *Developmental Medicine and Child Neurology, 33,* 776–788.

Fidler, D. J., Hepburn, S., & Rogers, S. (2006). Early learning and adaptive behaviour in toddlers with Down syndrome: Evidence for an emerging behavioural phenotype? *Down Syndrome Research and Practice, 9,* 37–44.

Fidler, D. J., Philofsky, A., & Hepburn, S. L. (2007). Language phenotypes and intervention planning: Bridging research and practice. *Mental Retardation and Developmental Disabilities Research Review, 13,* 47–57.

Fowler, A., Gelman, R., & Gleitman, L. (1994). The course of language learning in children with Down syndrome. In H. Tager-Flusberg (Ed.), *Constraints on language acquisition studies of atypical children.* Hillsdale, NJ: Lawrence Erlbaum Associates.

Gardiner, K., & Costa, A.C. (2006). The proteins of human chromosome 21. *American Journal of Medical Genetics C, Seminar in Medical Genetics, 142,* 196–205.

Gathercole, S. E., & Alloway, T. P. (2006). Practitioner review: Short-term and working memory impairments in neurodevelopmental disorders: Diagnosis and remedial support. *Journal of Child Psychology and Psychiatry, 47,* 4–15.

Gillham, B. (1990). First words in normal and Down syndrome children: A comparison of content and wordform categories. *Child Language Teaching and Therapy, 6,* 25–32.

Glasser, M. F., & Rilling, J. K. (2008). DTI tractography of the human brain's language pathways. *Cerebral Cortex,* Advance Access published online on February 14, 2008.

Glenn, S., & Cunningham, C. (2005). Performance of young people with Down syndrome on the Leiter-R and British picture vocabulary scales. *Journal of Intellectual Disability Research 49,* 239–244.

Glenn, S., Cunningham, C., & Joyce, P. (1981). A study of auditory preferences in nonhandicapped infants and infants with Down's syndrome. *Child Development, 52,* 1303–1307.

Groen, M. A., Laws, G., Nation, K., & Bishop, D. V. M. (2006). A case of exceptional reading accuracy in a child with Down syndrome: Underlying skills and the relation to reading comprehension. *Cognitive Neuropsychology, 23,* 1190–1214.

Hattori, M., Fujiyama, A., Taylor, T. D., Watanabe, H., Yada, T., Park, H. S., et al., for Chromosome 21 mapping and sequencing consortium. (2000). The DNA sequence of human chromosome 21. (2000). *Nature, 405,* 311–319.

Hesketh, L., & Chapman, R. (1998). Verb use by individuals with DS. *American Journal on Mental Retardation, 103,* 288–304.

Hick, R. F., Botting, N., & Conti-Ramsden, G. (2005). Short-term memory and vocabulary development in children with Down syndrome and children with specific language impairment. *Developmental Medicine and Child Neurology, 47,* 532–538.

Imada, T., Zhang, Y., Cheour, M., Taulu, S. Ahonen, A., & Kuhl, P. K. (2006). Infant speech perception activates Broca's area: A developmental magnetoencephalography study. *Neuroreport, 17,* 957–962.

Iverson, J.M., Longobardi, E., & Caselli, M.C. (2003). Relationship between gestures and words in children with Down's syndrome and typically developing children in the early stages of communicative development. *International Journal of Language and Communication Disorders, 38,* 179–197.

Jarrold, C., & Baddeley, A. D. (2001). Short-term memory in Down syndrome: Applying the working memory model. *Down's Syndrome Research and Practice, 7,* 17–23.

Jarrold, C., Baddeley, A. D., & Hewes, A. K. (2000). Verbal short-term memory deficits in Down syndrome: A consequence of problems in rehearsal? *Journal of Child Psychology and Psychiatry, 41,* 233–244.

Jarrold, C., Baddeley, A. D., & Phillips, C. E. (2002). Verbal short-term memory in Down syndrome: A problem of memory, audition, or speech? *Journal of Speech, Language, and Hearing Research, 45,* 531–544.

Jarrold, C., Baddeley, A. D., & Phillips, C. (1999). Down syndrome and the phonological loop: The evidence for, and importance, of, a specific verbal short-term memory deficit. *Down's Syndrome Research and Practice, 6,* 61–75.

Johnson-Glenberg, M., & Chapman, R. (2004). Predictors of parent-child language during novel task play: A comparison between children who are typically developing and individuals with DS. *Journal of Intellectual Disabilities Research, 48,* 225–238.

Johnston, F., & Stansfield, J. (1997). Expressive pragmatic skills in pre-school children with and without Down's syndrome: Parental perceptions. *Journal of Intellectual Disability Research, 41* (1), 19–29.

Kaiser, A. P., Hester, P. P., & McDuffie, A. S. (2001). Supporting communication in young children with developmental disabilities. *Mental Retardation & Developmental Disabilities Research Review, 7,* 143–150.

Kanno, K., & Ikeda, Y. (2002). Word-length effect in verbal short-term memory in individuals with Down's syndrome. *Journal of Intellectual Disabilities Research, 46,* 613–618.

Kasari, C., Freeman, S. F. N., & Hughes, M. A. (2001). Emotion recognition by children with Down syndrome. *American Journal on Mental Retardation, 106,* 59–72.

Kasari, C., Mundy, P., Yirmiya, N., & Sigman, M. (1990). Affect and attention in children with Down syndrome. *American Journal on Mental Retardation, 95,* 55–67.

Kay-Raining Bird, E., & Chapman, R. S. (1994). Sequential recall in individuals with Down syndrome. *Journal of Speech and Hearing Research, 37,* 1369–1380.

Kay-Raining Bird, E., Chapman, R., & Schwartz, S. (2004). Fast-mapping of words and story recall by children with DS. *Journal of Speech, Language, and Hearing Research, 47,* 1286–1300.

Kay-Raining Bird, E., Cleave, P. L., Trudeau, N., Thordardottir, E., Sutton, A., & Thorpe, A. (2005). The language abilities of bilingual children with Down syndrome. *American Journal of Speech-language Pathology, 14,* 187–199.

Kent, R. D., & Vorperian, H. K. (2007). In the mouths of babes: Anatomic, motor, and sensory foundations of speech development in children. In Rhea Paul (Ed.), *Language disorders from a developmental perspective: Essays in honor of Robin S. Chapman* (pp. 55–82). Mahwah, NJ: Lawrence Erlbaum Associates.

Kumin, L. (1994). Intelligibility of speech in children with Down syndrome in natural settings: Parents' perspectives. *Perceptual and Motor Skills, 78,* 307–313.

Kumin, L. (1996). Speech and language skills in children with Down syndrome. *Mental Retardation and Developmental Disabilities Research Reviews, 2,* 109–115.

Kumin, L. (2001). Speech intelligibility in individuals with Down syndrome: A framework for targeting specific factors for assessment and treatment. *Down Syndrome Quarterly, 6,* 1–8.

Kumin, L., Councill, C., & Goodman, M. (1994). A longitudinal study of the emergence of phonemes in children with Down syndrome. *Journal of Communication Disorders, 27,* 293–303.

Lanfranchie, S., Cornoldi, C., & Vianello, R. (2004). Verbal and visuospatial working memory deficits in children with DS. *American Journal on Mental Retardation, 109,* 456–466.

Laws, G. (1998). The use of nonword repetition as a test of phonological memory in children with DS. *Journal of Child Psychology and Psychiatry, 39,* 119–1130.

Laws, G. (2004). Contributions of phonological memory, language comprehension and hearing to the expressive language of adolescents and young adults with Down syndrome. *Journal of Child Psychology and Psychiatry, 45,* 1085–1095.

Laws, G., & Bishop, D. (2003). A comparison of language abilities in adolescents with DS and children with specific language impairment. *Journal of Speech, Language, and Hearing Research, 46,* 1324–1339.

Laws, G., & Gunn, D. (2004). Phonological memory as a predictor of language comprehension in DS: A five-year follow-up study. *Journal of Child Psychology and Psychiatry, 45,* 326–337.

Lynch, M. P., Oller, K., Steffens, M. L., Levine, S. L., Basinger, D. L., & Umbel, V. (1995). Onset of speech-like vocalizations in infants with Down syndrome. *American Journal on Mental Retardation, 100,* 68–86.

Marcell, M., Harvey, C., & Cothran, L. (1988). An attempt to improve auditory short-term memory in Down's syndrome individuals through reducing distractions. *Research in Developmental Disabilities, 9,* 405–417.

Marcell, M., Ridgeway, M., Sewell, D., & Whelan, M. (1995). Sentence imitation by adolescents and young adults with Down's syndrome and other intellectual disabilities. *Journal of Intellectual Disability Research, 39,* 215–232.

Marcell, M., & Weeks, S. (1988). Short-term memory difficulties and Down's syndrome. *Journal of Mental Deficiency Research, 32,* 153–162.

McDuffie, A., Sindberg, H., Hesketh, L., & Chapman, R. (2007). Use of speaker intent and grammatical cues in fast-mapping by adolescents with DS. *Journal of Speech, Language, and Hearing Research, 50,* 1546–1561.

Mervis, C. B., & Robinson, B. F. (2000). Expressive vocabulary ability of toddlers with Williams syndrome or Down syndrome: A comparison. *Developmental Neuropsychology, 17,* 111–126.

Miles, S., & Chapman, R. (2002). Narrative content as described by individuals with DS and typically developing children. *Journal of Speech, Language, and Hearing Research, 45,* 175–189.

Miles, S., Chapman, R., & Sindberg, H. (2004). A microgenetic study of storytelling by adolescents with DS and typically developing children matched for syntax comprehension. Poster presented at the Symposium for Research on Child Language Disorders, Madison, WI, June.

Miles, S., & Chapman, R. (2005). The relationship between adult scaffolding and narrative expression by adolescents with DS. Poster presented at the Symposium on Research in Child Language Disorders, Madison, WI, June 10.

Miles, S., Chapman, R., & Sindberg, H. (2006). Sampling context affects MLU in the language of adolescents with DS. *Journal of Speech, Language, and Hearing Research, 49,* 325–337.

Miller, J. (1987). Language and communication characteristics of children with DS. In S. Pueschel, S. Tingley, J. Rynders, A. Crocker, & D. Crutcher (Eds.), *New perspectives on DS* (pp. 233–263). Baltimore: Paul H. Brookes.

Miller, J. F. (1988). The developmental asynchrony of language development in children with Down syndrome. In L. Nadel (Ed.), *The Psychobiology of Down Syndrome,* Cambridge: MIT Press, pp. 167–198.

Miller, J. F. (1995). Individual differences in vocabulary acquisition in children with Down syndrome. *Progress in Clinical Biology Research, 393,* 93–103.

Miller, J. F. (1999). Profiles of language development in children with Down syndrome. In J. F. Miller, M. Leddy, & L. A. Leavitt (Eds.), *Improving the communication of people with Down Syndrome* (pp.11–40). Baltimore: Paul H Brookes.

Miller, J. F., & Leddy, M. (1998). Down syndrome: The impact of speech production on language development. In R. Paul (Ed.), *Communication and Language Intervention: Vol. 8. Exploring the Speech-Language Connection* (pp. 163–177). Baltimore: Brookes Publishing.

Miolo, G., Chapman, R., & Sindberg, H. (2005). Sentence comprehension in adolescents with DS and typically developing children: Role of sentence voice, visual context, and auditory-verbal short-term memory. *Journal of Speech, Language, and Hearing Research, 48,* 172–188.

Mongillo, G., Barak, O., & Tsodyks, M. (2008). Synaptic theory of working memory. *Science, 319,* 1543–1546.

Mundy, P., Kasari, C., Sigman, M., & Ruskin, E. (1995). Nonverbal communication and early language acquisition in children with Down syndrome and in normally developing children. *Journal of Speech and Hearing Research, 38,* 157–167.

Mundy, P., Sigman, M., Kasari, C., & Yirmiya, N. (1988). Nonverbal communication skills in Down syndrome children. *Child Development, 59,* 235–249.

Murphy, M., & Abbeduto, L. (2005). Indirect genetic effects and the early language development of children with genetic mental retardation syndromes: The role of joint attention. *Infants and Young Children, 18,* 47–59.

Nadel, L. (2003). Down's syndrome: A genetic disorder in biobehavioral perspective. *Genes, Brain, & Behavior 2,* 156–166.

Numminen, H., Service, E., Ahonen, T., & Ruoppila, I. (2001). Working memory and everyday cognition in adults with Down's syndrome. *Journal of Intellectual Disabilities Research, 45,* 157–168.

Oller, D. K., & Siebert, J. M. (1988). Babbling of prelinguistic mentally retarded children. *American Journal on Mental Retardation, 92,* 369–375.

Paul, R. (2007). *Language Disorders from Infancy Through Adolescence: Assessment and Intervention*. St. Louis, MO: Mosby-Year Book.

Price, C. J., Wise, R. J. S., Warburton, E. A., Moore, C. J., Howard, D., Patterson, K., Frackowiak, R. S. J., & Friston, K. J. (1996). Hearing and saying: The functional neuroanatomy of auditory word processing. *Brain, 119*, 919–931.

Price, J., Roberts, J., Vandergrift, N., & Martin, G. (2007). Language comprehension in boys with fragile X syndrome and boys with Down syndrome. *Journal of Intellectual Disability Research, 51*, 318–326.

Purser, H. R., & Jarrold, C. (2005). Impaired verbal short-term memory in Down syndrome reflects a capacity limitation rather than atypically rapid forgetting. *Journal of Experimental Child Psychology, 91*, 1–23.

Rice, M. L., Warren, S. F., & Betz, S. K. (2005). Language symptoms of developmental language disorders: An overview of autism, Down syndrome, fragile X, specific language impairment, and Williams syndrome. *Applied Psycholinguistics, 26*, 7–27.

Roberts, J. E., Chapman, R. S., & Warren, S. (Eds.). (2007). *Speech and language development and intervention in Down syndrome and fragile X Syndrome*. Brookes Publishing.

Roberts, J., Hennon, E., Dear, E., Anderson, K., & Vandergrift, N. A. (2007). Expressive language during conversational speech in boys with fragile X syndrome. *American Journal on Mental Retardation, 112*, 1–15.

Roberts, J., Martin, G. E., Moskowitz, L., Harris, A. A., Foreman, J., Nelson, L. (2007). Discourse skills of boys with fragile X syndrome in comparison to boys with Down syndrome. *Journal of Speech, Language, and Hearing Research*, 50, 475–492.

Roberts, J., Price, J., Nelson, L., Burchinal, M., Hennon, E. A., Barnes, E. et al. (2007). Receptive vocabulary, expressive vocabulary, and speech production of boys with fragile X syndrome in comparison to boys with Down syndrome. *American Journal on Mental Retardation, 112*, 177–193.

Roberts, J. E., Price, J., & Malkin, C. (2007). Language and communication development in Down syndrome. *Mental Retardation and Developmental Disabilities Research Reviews, 13*, 26–35.

Roid, G. H., & Miller, L. J. (1997). Leiter International Performance Scale-Revised. Los Angeles, CA: Western Psychological Association.

Roizen, N. (2002). Down syndrome. In M. Batshaw (Ed.), *Children with disabilities (5th Ed.)*. Baltimore, MD: Brookes Publishing.

Rondal, J. A. (1998). Cases of exceptional language in mental retardation and Down syndrome: Explanatory perspectives. *Down Syndrome Research and Practice, 5*, 1–15.

Saenz, R. B. (1999). Primary care of infants and young children with Down syndrome. *American Family Physician, 59*, 395–396.

Seung, H-K., & Chapman, R. (2000). Digit span in individuals with DS and typically developing children: Temporal aspects. *Journal of Speech, Language, and Hearing Research, 43*, 609–620.

Seung, H-K., & Chapman, R. (2004). Sentence memory in individuals with DS and typically developing children. *Journal of Intellectual Disability Research, 48*, 160–171.

Smith, B. L., & Oller, K. (1981). A comparative study of premeaningful vocalizations produced by normally developing and Down's syndrome infants. *Journal of Speech and Hearing Disorders, 46*, 46–51.

Smith, B.L., & Stoel-Gammon, C. (1983). A longitudinal study of the development of stop consonant production in normal and Down's syndrome children. *Journal of Speech and Hearing Disorders, 48*, 114–118.

Smith, B. L., & Stoel-Gammon, C. (1996). A quantitative analysis of the reduplicated and variegated babbling in vocalizations by Down syndrome infants. *Clinical Linguistics and Phonetics, 10*, 119–130.

Steffens, M. L., Oller, K., Lynch, M., & Urbano, R. C. (1992). Vocal development in infants with Down syndrome and infants who are developing normally. *American Journal of Mental Retardation, 97*, 235–246.

Sterling, A., & Warren, S. F. (2007). Communication and language development in infants and toddlers with Down syndrome or fragile X syndrome. In Roberts, J.E., Chapman, R.S., & Warren, S.F. (Eds.), *Speech and language development and intervention in Down syndrome and fragile X Syndrome*. Brookes Publishing, pp. 53–76.

Stoel-Gammon, C. (2001). Down syndrome phonology: developmental patterns and intervention strategies. *Downs Syndrome Research and Practice, 7*, 93–100.

Strominger, A. Z., Winkler, M. R., & Cohen, L. T. (1984). Speech and language evaluation. In S. M. Pueschel (Ed.), *The young child with Down syndrome* (pp. 253–261). New York: Human Sciences Press.

Tannock, R. (1988). Mothers' directiveness in their interactions with their children with and without Down syndrome. *American Journal on Mental Retardation, 93*, 154–165.

Thordardottir, E. (November, 2002). Parents' views on language impairment and bilingualism. Presented at the annual meeting of the American Speech-Language-Hearing Association, Atlanta, Georgia.

Thordardottir, E., Chapman, R., & Wagner, L. (2002). Complex sentence production by adolescents with DS. *Applied Psycholinguistics, 24*, 163–183.

Thorndike R., Hagen E., & Sattler J. (1986). *Stanford-Binet Intelligence Scale, Fourth Edition*. Chicago, IL: The Riverside Publishing Company.

Turner, S., & Alborz, A. (2003). Academic attainments of children with Down's syndrome: A longitudinal study. *British Journal of Educational Psychology, 73*, 563–583.

Vallar, G., & Papagno, C. (1993). Preserved vocabulary acquisition in Down's syndrome: The role of phonological short-term memory. *Cortex, 29*, 467–483.

Van Borsel, J. (1996). Articulation in Down's syndrome adolescents and adults. *European Journal of Disorders in Communication, 31*, 415–444.

Vicari, S., Bellucci, S., & Carlesima, G. A. (2006). Evidence from two genetic syndromes for the independence of spatial and visual working memory. *Developmental Medicine and Child Neurology, 48*, 126–131.

Vicari, S., Caselli, M. C., & Tonucci, F. (2000). Asynchrony of lexical and morphosyntactic development in children with DS. *Neuropsychologia, 38*, 634–644.

Vicari, S., Marotta, L., & Carlesima, G. A. (2004). Verbal short-term memory in Down's syndrome: An articulatory loop deficit? *Journal of Intellectual Disabilities Research, 48*, 80–92.

Williams, K. R., Wishart, J. G., Pitcairn, T. K., & Willis, D. S. (2005). Emotion recognition by children with Down syndrome: Investigation of specific impairments and error patterns. *American Journal on Mental Retardation, 110*, 378–392.

Woll, B., & Grove, N. (1996). On language deficits and modality in children with Down syndrome: A case study of twins bilingual in BSL and English. *Journal of Deaf Studies and Deaf Education, 1,* 271–278.

Zelazo, P. D., (2006). The Dimensional Change Card Sort (DCCS): A method of assessing executive function in children. *Nature Protocols, 1,* 297–301.

Zelazo, P. D., Burack, J. A., Benedetto, E., & Frye, D. (1996). Theory of Mind and rule use in individuals with Down's Syndrome: A test of the uniqueness and specificity claims. *Journal of Child Psychology and Psychiatry, 37,* 479–484.

Literacy Development in Childhood, Adolescence, and Young Adulthood in Persons with Down Syndrome

Elizabeth Kay-Raining Bird *and* Robin S. Chapman

Abstract

Literacy enriches and expands opportunities for participation in activities in the home, school, work and community. There are many economic, social, and cultural benefits to being literate (Robinson-Pant, 2005). For example, individuals with more advanced literacy skills are more frequently employed, earn higher wages, and are more likely to be promoted (Johnson, 2000). Furthermore, they tend to have increased self-esteem, greater empowerment, and expanded recreational opportunities. Becoming literate presumably has the same advantages for individuals with Down syndrome (DS) as it would for any other person in a literate society. With changing policies and demographics, the literacy potential of individuals with DS is only now becoming understood and may well be underestimated in the early literature in this area. In this chapter, we review the literature on the literacy abilities of individuals with DS and make recommendations for future research.

Keywords: Down syndrome, literacy, reading, writing, development

Do Individuals with Down Syndrome Learn to Read and Write?

Buckley, Emslie, Haslegrave, & LePrevost (1986) published the first detailed descriptions of literacy development in children with Down syndrome (DS). Their chapter provided case histories of three children with DS and outlined their recommendations for teaching reading and writing to children with DS. In a second edition of this work, Buckley and Bird (1993) claimed that 80% of children with DS have the capacity to learn to read and write. Further, if taught consistently and systematically, they claimed that many children with DS are capable of beginning to read as early as 3 years of age. As well, they stated that word recognition skills in reading would often keep pace with chronological age (CA)-level expectations but would surpass measures of oral language and cognitive skills, at least in the elementary school years. Indeed, some children with DS were reported to begin to read even before they used spoken words spontaneously and most improved their spoken language skills while learning to read,

suggesting to the authors that learning to read can enhance oral language development.

Buckley and Bird (1993) based their argument on extensive experience teaching individuals with DS to read and write, and upon evidence exemplified through three case studies that they presented. In these three cases, the individuals each started reading real words before 4 years of age (2;1, 2;7, and 3;5 years; months). They progressed to functional uses of literacy (i.e., writing stories, playing Scrabble, using the computer for a variety of purposes, using cookbooks, and reading for pleasure) by the time they were 8–13 years of age. Clearly, having DS does not preclude learning to read and write in highly functional ways.

Evidence in subsequent studies is consistent with the notion that most individuals with DS acquire at least some testable reading skills by adulthood. For example, Buckley (2003) reported that approximately 89% of a sample of teenagers who attended special schools in the United Kingdom in both 1987 and 1999 had at least some ability to read and write. Table 13.1 outlines other available studies of DS reading ability. In these studies, the percentage of individuals who have at least some testable reading skill increases with age and varies from a low of 16% of 127 individuals aged 9–14 years in the United Kingdom (Sloper, Cunningham, Turner, & Knussen, 1990) who were scorable on the Spar Reading Test (Young, 1976) to a high of 87% of 30 adults aged 18–36 years also in the United Kingdom (Bochner, Outhred, & Pieterse, 2001) who had "some reading" as tested on the Waddington Diagnostic Reading Test (Waddington, 1988). In the longitudinal studies reviewed in Table 13.1 as well (Casey, Jones, Kugler, & Watkins, 1988; Kay-Raining Bird, Cleave, & McConnell, 2000; Laws & Gunn, 2002), participants were able to demonstrate at least minimal reading skill as they age.

Most studies in Table 13.1 reported measures of reading but not writing achievement. Reading achievement was measured using real-word (word recognition) or nonword (decoding) reading tasks and less often with reading comprehension tasks. Word recognition achievement scores in these studies ranged from a low of 6;2 (years; months) for 12 children with DS between the ages of 6;2 and 11;8 years (Kay-Raining Bird et al., 2000) to a high of 8;6 in a sample of 33 teenagers and adults aged 17–25 years (Fowler, Doherty, & Boynton, 1995). All three studies that included adults with DS (Bochner et al., 2001; Carr, 2000; Fowler et al., 1995) reported very similar mean word recognition age-equivalency scores (range 8;0–8;6). Thus, mean word recognition age-equivalent scores tended to increase with the age of the samples to an average age-equivalent of about 8½ years. The highest reported word recognition age-equivalent score was 11;7, achieved by one child in a relatively young sample (Kay-Raining Bird et al., 2000, Time 3, ages 10.7–16.1). Nonword reading or decoding mean scores tended to be lower than word recognition scores in these studies, ranging from a low of 5;10 (very limited ability) in the first two time periods of the Kay-Raining Bird et al. study, to a high of 7;9 for a sample of teenagers and adults (Fowler et al., 1995). Mean age-equivalent scores for reading comprehension were also lower than word recognition scores, ranging from 5;8 (i.e., virtually no testable comprehension) to a high of 7.1 in the adults (30 years) studied by Carr (2000).

When reported (Table 13.1), measures of writing achievement were more difficult to interpret than were measures of reading achievement because

only one study included a measure that permitted comparison to a standardization sample (Byrne, MacDonald, & Buckley, 2002). In this study, mean age-equivalent scores were available for the spelling subtest of the British Ability Scales, and scores were similar to those obtained on the word reading subtest at all three time periods tested. Participants ranged in age from 4;11 to 12;7 at the onset of the study, and were tested again both 1 and 2 years later.

Across the studies in Table 13.1, several generalizations can be made. One, scores on all reading measures increased with the CA of the participants, both when comparing results across studies and comparing scores longitudinally within studies. Two, when multiple reading measures were completed by the same group, word reading scores were typically higher than either nonword reading (decoding) or reading comprehension scores. Three, age-equivalent scores and CAs diverged, even in the youngest samples, and this divergence increased with increasing CA of samples. Four, age-equivalent scores for real-word reading subtests exceeded full-scale or nonverbal MA scores and/or receptive vocabulary scores for the same samples. Five, much more is known about the reading than the writing abilities of children with DS. These generalizations should be treated with caution as the scoring systems across studies may not be directly comparable, and some authors included and others excluded raw scores of zero in their summary statistics.

Predictors of Writing Ability in Individuals with Down Syndrome

A single study has investigated the written discourse skills of individuals with DS (Kay-Raining Bird, Cleave, White, Pike, & Helmkay, 2008). In this study, regression analyses revealed that the best predictor of written narrative skills for a group of school-aged children with DS was vocabulary comprehension, reflecting the important link between vocabulary and literacy skills. Other predictors of writing ability were age, fine motor ability, digit span performance, and phoneme awareness. Word processed and handwritten narratives for a child with DS are provided in Figure 13.1.

Predictors of Reading in Individuals with Down Syndrome

A variety of factors have been shown to influence reading and writing achievement in individuals with DS.

Table 13.1 A sampling of developmental studies of reading and writing abilities in individuals with Down syndrome

Authors	Sample size	Age/Mental Age (MA)	Reading scores	% Readers
Boudreau (2002) US	20 Nonverbal MA-matched typically developed comparison group	Age 11.3 (3.3), 5;06–17;3 MA (Stanford-Binet, 3 subtests) 4.1 (0.7), 3.1–5.8	Wd ID (raw) 17.2 (18.0), 0–50 6;7 (6;7), 5;9–7;11[1] Wd Atr (raw) 1.7 (3.5), 0–12 6;1 (6;2), 5;7–7;0[1] Passage Comprehension (raw) 2.1 (3.4), 0–13 5;8 (6;0), 5;0–6;10[1]	Not reported
Bochner et al. (2001) Australia	30 No comparison group	Age 18–36 years	Waddington Diagnostic Reading Test (a–e) 8;1 (1;1) (n = 28) Mainstream > separate	26/30 some reading, 87% 4/30 no reading = 13% 6/30 "poor readers" = 20% 14/30 "very good" readers, 47%
Byrne et al. (2002) UK	24 Chronological age (CA)-matched, average reader typically developed comparison group CA and word-level reading matched "slow" reader comparison group	Age T1: 8;2, 4;11–12;7 T2: 1 year later T3: 2 years later (from baseline) BPVS T1: 4;5 T2: 4;5 T3: 5;4	British Ability Scales (a–e) Word Reading T1: 6;3 T2: 6;6 T3: 6;8 Spelling T1: 6;4 T2: 6;4 T3: 6;7 WORD Reading Comprehension T1: 6;0 T2: 6;0 T3: 6;0	Not reported

Study	N	Participant details	Measures	Results
Carr (2000) UK	38	Age T1: 21 years T2: 30 years MA (Leiter, 1980) T1: 5;7 (2;0) T2: 5;6 (2;3) Women > Men Home reared > not SES positively related	Neale Analysis of Reading Test (a-e) Word ID T1: 7.8 (1.6) T2: 8.0 (1.5) Reading Comprehension T1: 6.8 (0.9) T2: 7.1 (1.3)	Able to score on the reading test Word reading: 14/38 = 37% Reading comprehension: 12/38 = 32%
Casey et al. (1988) UK	36 No comparison group	Age T1: 6.2, 3.7–9.9 years T2: 1 year later T3: 2 years later (from baseline) MA (Stanford-Binet, Full scale, 1960) 3.7, 2.3–6.7	Neale Analysis of Reading Ability Wd ID Reading Comprehension Girls > Boys Mainstream > separate	Able to obtain a reading score on Neale WdID T1:9/36 = 25% T2:20/36 = 55% T3: 25/36 = 69% Reading Comprehension T1: 6/36 = 17% T2: 10/36 = 28% T3: 21/36 = 58%
Fletcher & Buckley (2002) UK	17 No comparison group	12;2 (1;4), 9;2–14;5	BAS word reading (a-e) 7;2 (1;10), 5;5–9;0 BAS spelling (a-e) 7;2 (0;3), 6;0–9;11 Wechsler Reading Comprehension subtest (a-e) 6;3 (0;6), 6;0–7;9 Nonword spelling 10/17 scored 0/10	Included if reading scores were ≥ 7 years

(Continued)

Table 13.1 A sampling of developmental studies of reading and writing abilities in individuals with Down syndrome (*Continued*)

Study	N	Age	Measures / Scores	Reading outcome
Fowler et al. (1995) US	33 No comparison group	17–25 years	Word Identification (a-e) 8.5 (2.3) Word Attack (a-e) 7.9 (3.8) Comprehension 6.9 (1.3)	Read ≥1 real-word 100% (recruited adults with DS who could read)
Kay-Raining Bird et al. (2000) Canada	12 No comparison group	Age T1: 9.7 (1.7), 6.2–11.6 years T2: 12.9 (1.7), 9.3–14.8 T3: 14.3 (1.7), 10.7–16.1 MA (Stanford-Binet, 2 subtests)	Word Identification (Gr-e) T1: 1.1 (1.1) < K–2.9 6;2 (6;2), 5;9–8;0 [1] T2: 1.7 (1.2), < K–4 6;11 (6;4), 5;9–9;1 [1] T3: 1.9 (1.6) 0–5.2 7;2 (6;9), 5;9–10;7 [1] Word Attack (Gr-e) T1: 0.5 (0.8), 0–2 5;10 (6;1), 5;7–7;4 [1] T2: 0.7 (0.9), 0–2.5 5;10 (6;1), 5;7–7;10 [1] T3: 0.9 (1.1), 0–3.4 6;1 (6;2), 5;7–8;10 [1]	Read ≥1 real-word: 7/12 = 58% 10/12 = 83% 9/12 = 75%
Laws & Gunn (2002) UK	30 No comparison group	Age T1: 11;3 (4;0) T2: 16;6 (4;0), 10–24 years	Scores reported for readers only K-ABC decoding (a-e) T1: 6;0 T2: 6;9, 5;3–11;3 K-ABC Comprehension (a-e) T1: 6;6 T2: 6;9	Decode ≥1 nonword T1: 11/30 = 37% T2: 16/30 = 53%

Sloper et al. (1990) UK	127 No comparison group	Age 9.2, 6–14 years MA (McCarthy [122] or Bayley-[6]) 3.6 (1.1), 0.7–7.5 years Best predictors of academic achievement: MA, Type of school (mainstream > separate), gender (F>M), father's "locus of control," age	Reading checklist (max = 51) 28.2 (8.0), 17–50 Writing checklist (max = 57) 29.9 (6.5), 19–52	Spar Reading Test 20/127 scored = 15.7%
Turner & Alborz (2003) UK	T1: 102 T2: 101 T3: 79	Age T1: 9.1 (1.7) T2: 13.7 (1.6) T3: 21.1 (1.3) IQ T1: 40.3 (11.0) Reading and writing: T1<T2<T3	Academic achievement Index scores (DS specific scale) Reading (M scores) T1: 4.83 (3.67) T2: 7.38 (4.53) T3: 9.14 (4.82) Writing T1: 4.62 (2.92) T2: 7.76 (4.06) T3: 10.08 (4.70)	NA

[1] Converted from raw scores for the purposes of comparison in this table. Not reported by the authors. TD, typically developing children.

Adolescent with Down Syndrome
Chronological Age: 18 years 4 months
Nonverbal MA, *Stanford Binet, 4^(th) edition*: 5 years
6 months
PPVT-R: 8 years 11 months
Word Identification, WRMT-R: 8 years 11 months
Word Attack, WRMT-R: 7 years 3 months
AAT(PA): 16/40

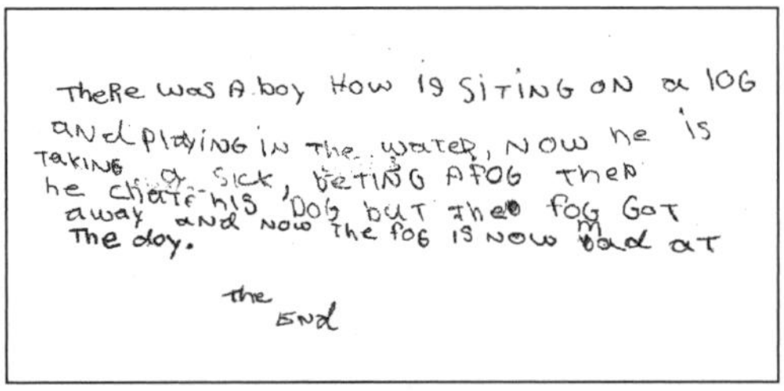

There was A boy how is siting on a log
and playing in the water, now he is
taking o... sick, geting afog then
he chate his Dog but the fog got
away and now the fog is now bad at
the doy.
the
End

A little boy who is frishin
with is dog and then he felt a
taug at the end of his frishing
word but then he went in but
his hand went in frist then the
dog went after him then the
frg went in to and that is then
end

Fig. 13.1 Two writing samples: Handwritten and word-processed.

Chronological Age

Age has a strong influence on literacy achievement in individuals with DS. Significant improvement in reading and writing abilities can be seen across participants of increasing age in different studies and within subjects in longitudinal analyses of children with DS (Byrne et al., 2002; Kay-Raining Bird et al., 2000; Laws & Gunn, 2002; Turner & Alborz, 2003). Furthermore, age is correlated with reading and writing performance (Boudreau, 2002; Kennedy & Flynn, 2003a; Sloper, Cunningham, Turner, & Knussen, 1990). In some studies, growth in literacy skill appears to slow or even plateau with age. For example, Turner and Alborz (2003) reported a plateauing in the growth of reading and writing achievement scores after 16 years of age, using a cross-sectional analysis of participants between the ages of 8 and 22 years. The plateau occurred even though the top ends of the scales were not reached and continued growth would have been expected. Plateauing in numeracy and IQ were also observed. The authors interpreted these findings as suggesting that some of the older individuals in their study were reaching "the limits of their 'academic potential'" (p. 573). Similarly, few significant changes were observed in measures of cognition, language, or reading between 21 and 30 years in the cohort studied by Carr (2000). A reduction in opportunities for literacy instruction in secondary school

(Trenholm & Mirenda, 2006) and beyond may account, at least in part, for the observed plateau in literacy skills. The onset of early effects of Alzheimer disease may also play a role (see Chapman & Kay-Raining Bird, 2011, Chapter 12, this volume).

Cognition

Cognitive abilities are also related to reading and writing acquisition in individuals with DS. For example, in a study of the effects of a large number of intrinsic and extrinsic factors on academic performance by Sloper et al. (1990), stepwise regression revealed that MA (measured using the McCarthy Scales, McCarthy, 1972) or the Bayley Scale (Bayley, 1969) was the strongest predictor of reading and writing achievement. Even so, general measures of nonverbal cognition tend to underestimate word reading abilities in children with DS (Buckley, 2003; Fowler et al., 1995; Kay-Raining Bird et al., 2000), such that matching on reading abilities leads to lower MAs relative to comparison groups (e.g., Fowler et al., 1995; Kay-Raining Bird et al., 2008). Memory measures may also be related to literacy skills in individuals with DS. Verbal short-term memory, measured using a digit span task, was found to be positively related to reading ability in some (Fowler et al., 1995; Kay-Raining Bird et al., 2000) but not all (Boudreau, 2002) studies. Furthermore, phonological memory measured with a nonsense word repetition task has been found to predict later reading abilities in this population (Laws & Gunn, 2002).

Home Environment

The impact of institutionalization on literacy development in individuals with DS seems to be long-lasting. At both 21 and 30 years of age, Carr (2000) reported that home-reared individuals with DS outperformed institutionally reared individuals on all measures of reading. Similarly, Bochner et al. (2001) found that the oldest participants in their study (>24 years) had the lowest reading scores, a finding that the authors attributed to the fact that four of these five individuals lived in institutions most of their lives.

An enriched home literacy environment fosters emergent literacy skills and predicts later reading, writing, and academic success in typically developing children (Justice, 2006). Emergent literacy skills and early literacy experiences have been understudied in individuals with DS. Fitzgerald, Roberts, Pierce, and Schuele (1995) described the availability of literacy-related materials and literacy activities in the homes of three children with DS (aged 33, 37, and 46 months), as well as the interaction styles of mothers during joint storybook reading. They found that the three children were being raised in environments that contained many literacy materials but were experiencing a limited number of different literacy activities. Two of the three mothers used an interactive style during storybook reading with their children that has been shown to support language and cognitive development in typically developing children. The generalizability of these findings is limited. Trenholm and Mirenda (2006) also reported on home literacy issues in their survey study of parents and guardians of 418 individuals with DS aged 0–41 years. Like Fitzgerald et al. (1995), they found that individuals with DS were reported to engage in only a few different reading and writing activities at home. Nonetheless, three-quarters of the respondents reported that the individuals with DS used literacy materials at least once a day, 71% reported the individuals with DS visited the library, while only 37% reported discussing what their children read for more than 15 minutes per day. Thus, it appears that home-raised children with DS generally have higher literacy achievements than institutionally raised children with DS. However, it is possible that more severely impaired individuals were also more likely to be institutionalized, confounding this finding. It is also important to recognize that there may be considerable variability in the quality of both the informal literacy experiences and the formal literacy training of individuals with DS in institutional and home settings alike. The finding that children with DS seem to engage in a limited number of different literacy activities should be explored further.

Schooling

Integrated school settings are found to favorably impact the development of literacy skills in individuals with DS in some studies. For example, Sloper et al. (1990) found that enrollment in mainstream schools was a positive indicator of academic achievement, relative to schools for the moderately or severely intellectually disabled. Similarly, Bochner et al. (2001) reported more advanced reading skills in adults who had attended integrated as opposed to segregated schools. They attributed the higher scores in individuals who had attended integrated schools to "more effective reading instruction and greater opportunity to learn to read" (p.79) in integrated classrooms, although they did not document the learning opportunities in each school setting

provided to their participants. In contrast, Casey et al. (1988) reported that similar percentages of children with DS were scorable on a standardized reading test in either mainstreamed or special education for children with moderate intellectual disabilities settings.

The variability in findings across studies can be explained, at least in part, by the lack of a one-to-one correspondence between the school setting label and the experiences of students in that setting. For example, Kliewer (1998) documented in his ethnographic study that, six of ten school-age children with DS enrolled in "integrated" school settings did not participate at all or participated minimally in the literacy experiences of the regular classroom.

Gender and Socioeconomic Status

Consistent with the evidence that typically developing girls enter literacy earlier, develop literacy more quickly (e.g., Chatterji, 2006), and read more often recreationally (Nippold, Duthie, & Larsen, 2005), gender is an important predictor of literacy skills in individuals with DS as well (Carr, 2000; Sloper et al., 1990), with females outperforming males.

Also similar to findings obtained for typically developing children (e.g., Chatterji, 2006), children with DS from higher socioeconomic backgrounds, as measured by either employment or parent education, perform better on literacy measures (Buckley & Sacks, 1987; Carr, 2000; Sloper et al., 1990). However, parental education ceases to have an impact on reading or writing ability in adults with DS (Carr, 2000).

Expressive and Receptive Spoken Language

Individuals with DS who read have better language abilities than those who are nonreaders (e.g., Buckley, 1995, 2003; Laws & Gunn, 2002). Also, real-word and nonword reading abilities are predicted by measures of receptive vocabulary (Carr, 2000, Fowler et al., 1995), syntax comprehension (Fowler et al., 1995), and general language ability (Reynell Language Test, Shepperdson, 1988) in individuals with DS. Reading comprehension, on the other hand, is predicted by syntax comprehension (TACL-R, Fowler et al., 1995; TROG, Laws & Gunn, 2002). Boudreau (2002) reported that receptive language measures only (vocabulary and syntax comprehension) predicted real-word reading scores, whereas both expressive and receptive language measures predicted reading comprehension scores in 20 children and adolescents with DS that she studied. However, when age was controlled, only the relationship between mean length of utterance (MLU) and reading comprehension remained, suggesting that age was a mediating factor for many observed language–literacy relationships. (Reading comprehension was measured using the Passage Comprehension subtest of the Woodcock Reading Mastery Test-Revised, WRMT-R; Woodcock, 1987.) A bidirectional causal relationship between language and literacy was supported in a study by Laws and Gunn (2002), who demonstrated that reading ability (real-word reading and reading comprehension) positively predicted expressive (i.e., MLU) but not receptive (i.e., syntax comprehension) language abilities 5 years later. Similarly, receptive vocabulary and syntax measures positively predicted later real-word reading skills in the same individuals.

Phonological Awareness

One language component of particular interest in terms of its relationship to reading decoding ability is phonological awareness. Phonological awareness refers to the metalinguistic ability to consciously analyze and manipulate the sounds of a language. Common tasks used to measure phonological awareness include rhyming, segmentation (e.g., tap and say each sound in "pat"), elision (say "pat" without the /p/), and blending (the sounds /p/ /æ/ /t/ combine to make the word "pat"). In typically developing individuals, phonological awareness is a strong predictor of the development of reading decoding, and the two components seem to be related in a bidirectional causal manner (e.g., Blachman, 1994).

The relationship between phonological awareness and reading decoding ability in individuals with DS has received considerable attention in the last decade and a half. Indeed, a special issue of *Reading and Writing* was devoted to this topic in 2002. Interest was initially sparked by an influential article published by Cossu, Rossini, and Marshall (1993), who argued that phonological awareness could not be an "essential prerequisite" (p. 129) for the development of reading decoding skills since children with DS showed decoding ability despite a "failure" on phonological awareness tasks. Cossu et al. (1993) based their conclusions on the finding that the phonological awareness skills of a group of children with DS were impaired relative to that of a typically developed comparison group, matched on reading ability. Subsequent studies have supported this finding of impaired phonological awareness abilities in children with DS (Boudreau, 2002; Evans, 1994; Kay-Raining Bird et al., 2000; Verucci, Menghini, & Vicari, 2006), but not Cossu et al.'s (1993) conclusions.

Despite having lower than expected phonological awareness skills relative to word-level reading ability, many individuals with DS do develop phonological awareness (Boudreau, 2002; Cupples & Iacono, 2000; Kay-Raining Bird et al., 2000; Kennedy & Flynn, 2003a; Laws & Gunn, 2002). Therefore, there is not a general failure to acquire phonological awareness in the DS population. Further, phoneme-level phonological awareness in particular is positively correlated with measures of real-word reading (Boudreau, 2002; Fletcher & Buckley, 2002; Kennedy & Flynn, 2003a), nonword reading (Cupples & Iacono, 2000; Fletcher & Buckley, 2002; Fowler et al., 1995; Kay-Raining Bird et al., 2000; Kennedy & Flynn, 2003a), prose reading (Gombert, 2002), reading comprehension (Fletcher & Buckley, 2002), and spelling (Fletcher & Buckley, 2002) in both children and adults with DS. Phoneme awareness predicts later reading abilities in this population as well (Laws & Gunn, 2002). For example, Fowler et al. (1995) found that phonological awareness accounted for 36% of the variance in Word Identification scores and 49% of the variance in Word Attack scores on the WRMT-R (Woodcock, 1987) among adults with DS. In addition, they reported that no participant showed evidence of decoding (Word Attack) skill without also achieving a raw score of at least 10 on an elision task of phonological awareness (Auditory Analysis Test, Rosner & Simon, 1971). This suggested that a criterion level of phoneme awareness may be required to develop decoding abilities.

Some researchers suggest that individuals with DS may have particular difficulty with one aspect of phonological awareness: rhyming or rhyme awareness (Cardosa-Martins, Michalick, & Pollo, 2002; Gombert, 2002; Snowling, Hulme, & Mercer, 2002). Not all researchers report rhyming to be deficient in this population (Kay-Raining Bird et al., 2000), however. Also, certain rhyming tasks seem to be performed better than others by individuals with DS. For example, rhyme detection and rhyme matching tasks seem to elicit group differences (Cardosa-Martins et al., 2002, Gombert, 2002; Snowling et al., 2002), whereas rhyme generation (Kay-Raining Bird et al., 2008) and nursery rhyme completion tasks (Snowling et al., 2002) do not. Explanations of specific difficulty with rhyming include the suggestion that children with DS are more sensitive to the beginnings than the endings of words (Snowling et al., 2002).

The ability to detect beginning sounds rather than rimes may reflect the instructional focus of early reading efforts. For example, Snowling et al. (2002) reported that typically developing as well as DS groups performed better on an alliteration than a rhyme judgment task when the two tasks were carefully equated in terms of task demands and both groups were in the early stages of reading. This view is similar to one discussed by Gombert (2002), who hypothesized that reading instruction "precipitates the development" (p. 406) of explicit phonological awareness and, consequently, rhyming ability might be outdistanced by phoneme awareness as reading ability progresses because phoneme awareness is more practiced than rhyming during reading instruction. Gombert (2002) suggested that a deficit in meta-representational ability in children with DS might be more explanatory. A specific difficulty with rhyming also seems contrary to the findings of Bourassa, Cleave, and Kay-Raining Bird (2005) and Cupples and Iacono (2002). In these studies, rhyme-based methods were found to be particularly efficacious during reading instruction with children with DS (see intervention section), suggesting that rhymes are indeed accessible to children with DS.

The Profile of Reading and Writing Abilities in Individuals with Down Syndrome

Individuals with DS have an identifiable profile of reading strengths and weaknesses that appears to change somewhat with age. First, word-level reading ability is a strength for this population, and this ability is often in advance of general developmental measures. For example, in studies in which groups were matched on real-word reading ability (Buckley, 2003; Kay-Raining Bird et al., 2008; Snowling et al., 2002; Verucci et al., 2006), cognition, general language, and/or receptive vocabulary scores were consistently reported to be significantly lower in groups with DS. Similarly, when groups were matched on nonverbal cognition, real-word reading ability was reported to be more advanced in individuals with DS (Boudreau, 2002).

A second component of the profile of reading abilities of individuals with DS is that they are typically better at reading real words than nonwords. That is, decoding skills are delayed relative to real-word reading skills in the same individuals (Fowler et al., 1995; Kay-Raining Bird et al., 2000; Verucci et al., 2006). The phonological awareness difficulties experienced by individuals with DS are likely to account for at least some of the decoding problems that they experience, given the consistent relationship found between these two variables.

Gombert (2002) has shown that individuals with DS but not a reading matched comparison group experience particular difficulty reading nonwords with few orthographic neighbors (i.e., few real words that are visually similar to the nonword). This suggested that, when reading nonwords, individuals with DS are more dependent upon a visual strategy of drawing an analogy between unknown and known words, rather than an auditory strategy of sounding out words. Word identification scores are also significantly correlated with visual perception scores for individuals with DS but not for those with developmental disabilities of mixed etiology matched on nonverbal IQ and ranging in age from 7 to 21 years (Fidler, Most, & Guiberson, 2005). Together, these findings are consistent with the view expressed by a number of authors (Buckley, 1995; Kay-Raining Bird et al., 2000; Oelwein, 1995) that individuals with DS show a greater dependence upon the memorization of visual wholes than do typically developing children when learning to read. The phonological route to reading seems to be particularly impaired in the DS population.

Three, real-word reading skills are more advanced than reading comprehension skills in the same individuals (Boudreau, 2002; Fowler et al., 1995; Roch & Levorato, 2009; Verucci et al., 2006). When Gombert (2002) matched DS and typically developing groups on a measure of reading prose (Gombert, 2002), he found that they were also matched on nonword reading ability. This suggests that the difficulties this population experiences with nonword reading and reading comprehension may be comparable in degree, at least for French-speaking children and adolescents between the ages of 10 and 20 years. Fowler et al. (1995) also reported comparable nonword reading and reading comprehension scores in their adults with DS, except for those who were classified as "skilled readers." For the skilled readers, decoding ability outstripped real-word reading scores which, in turn, outstripped reading comprehension. This pattern of findings suggests that reading comprehension is particularly problematic for individuals with DS. It also suggests that decoding ability will be delayed, but can be mastered by some.

The profile of writing abilities in children with DS has not been studied as extensively as that of reading. Nonetheless, writing abilities seem to develop simultaneous to and in lock-step with reading in this population. For example, when groups of school-aged children with DS or typical development were matched on real-word reading ability, Kay-Raining Bird et al. (2008) reported that their written narrative abilities were quite similar. Written narratives of the groups did not differ on MLU, number of different words, story grammar complexity, or spelling. Indeed, only narrative length and handwriting legibility differed significantly, with the group with DS producing longer but less legible written narratives. This is consistent with other evidence (Byrne et al., 2002; Sloper et al., 1990; Turner & Alborz, 2003). For example, Byrne et al. (2002) reported that children with DS achieved very similar age-equivalent scores in word reading and spelling tests at approximately 5–13 years of age and that this comparability remained when the children were tested 1 and 2 years later. Similarly, Sloper et al. (1990) reported comparable achievements in reading and writing on checklists of abilities of a group of 6- to 14-year-old children with DS, and Turner and Alborz (2003) reported almost identical reading and writing index scores in each of three time periods tested over a span of 12 years, starting at a mean age of 9 years.

Although speculative in nature, the described profile of strengths and weaknesses is illustrated in Figure 13.2A and B. Two developmental patterns are presented. The intent is to suggest that the relationship between illustrated components will change as knowledge and skill in each component advances. Distances between components should be considered very rough indicators of relative developmental progress. Figure 13.2A shows a hypothesized developmental relationship between major components of literacy and general development in children with DS who are beginning the literacy learning process. In this figure, whole-word reading is developmentally close to CA and in advance of any other illustrated component. Figure 13.2B shows the hypothesized relationship between literacy and general developmental indicators later in development, once more literacy knowledge and skill has been accumulated. Perhaps the most contentious aspect of Figure 13.2B is where MA and receptive vocabulary skills fall relative to literacy components in later development. Their low position on the time line is supported by evidence presented in Table 13.1, but could be an artifact of comparing age-equivalent scores across different standardization samples or floor effects on standardized tests of comprehension and decoding. An additional component to Figure 13.2 could potentially have been included to illustrate how relationships between components change in skilled readers with DS. In these cases, decoding

ability would be expected to equal or surpass word reading skill (Fowler et al., 1995).

Literacy Intervention

Sue Buckley and her colleagues in Portsmouth, United Kingdom (e.g., Bird & Buckley, 1994; Buckley, 2003, 2005; Buckley & Bird, 1993) and Oelwein in the United States (Oelwein, 1995) have both developed systematic intervention programs to teach reading to children with DS. Using the extant literature, they advocate a process of errorless learning (i.e., programmed to experience success rather than failure) in which initial intervention builds on the word recognition reading strengths of individuals with DS and later incorporates direct work on phonics and comprehension. Buckley and colleagues and Oelwein also support the simultaneous teaching of reading and writing abilities and the use of literacy in functional contexts. Controlled intervention studies of the efficacy of these interventions are currently lacking, although detailed case reports have been published (e.g., Buckley & Bird (1993).

Studies of interventions with a more limited scope have been reported. One investigated the impact of parent implemented print referencing on emergent literacy skills of young children with DS (van Bysterveldt, Gillon, & Moran, 2006). Pre- and post-treatment measures of letter naming, letter sound knowledge, print concepts, and initial phoneme identification were collected. Seven parents of children with DS were trained to use print-referencing techniques (i.e., point to and name beginning letter, identify sound letter makes, identify letter as first sound in word) while engaging in joint book reading of familiar books with their 4-year-old children. Intervention involved four 10-minute sessions per week for 6 weeks. Performance of the seven children with DS was compared to that of seven typically developing children matched for age.

The children with DS performed more poorly on all measures at both pre- and post-testing, relative to the comparison group. Nonetheless, as a group, the children with DS improved significantly from pre- to post-testing on all measures except letter naming, which approached significance. Gain scores for five of the children with DS fell within or above a 1 standard deviation range of the typically developing group on all measures. Thus, parents were shown to be effective teachers of emergent literacy skills, including beginning sound knowledge or phoneme awareness.

Several additional studies have investigated the efficacy of phonological awareness interventions as

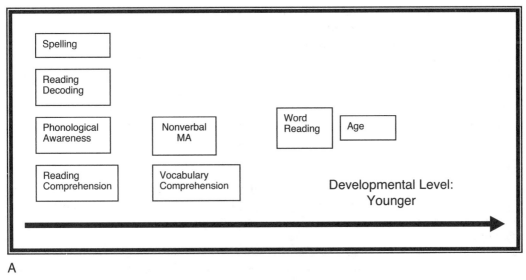

A

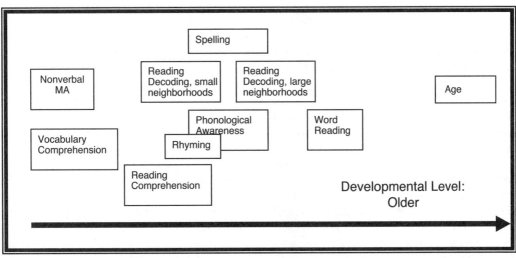

B

Fig. 13.2 (A) Hypothesized profile of literacy strengths and weaknesses for beginning readers with Down syndrome (DS). (B) Hypothesized profile of literacy strengths and weaknesses for more advanced readers with DS.

their sole focus. Kennedy and Flynn (2003b) studied the efficacy of a phonological awareness intervention using a multiple baseline across behaviors study of three 7- or 8-year-olds with DS. The children participated in eight 1-hour sessions in a 4-week period. The intervention focused upon alliteration, initial sound identification, spelling of orthographically consistent one-syllable words, and rhyming recognition. Results provided evidence for improvement in phoneme level phonological awareness abilities and spelling for all three children and improvement in rhyming for two of the three children. Generalization to phoneme segmentation (not trained) was not demonstrated, and the intervention had minimal effects on speech intelligibility.

The authors attributed these latter findings to the short period of intervention. No follow-up data were provided.

Cleave, Kay-Raining Bird, & Bourassa (in press) reported on the efficacy of a phonological awareness intervention for eight school-aged children with DS with a mean age of 11.7 years. Half-hour sessions were conducted twice weekly for a period of 22 weeks. Rhyming was taught in the first 4 weeks, and the subsequent 18 weeks focused upon beginning, then ending sound activities. A comparison group received a narrative intervention hypothesized to be independent in effect of the phonological awareness intervention. Analyses revealed that more participants in the phonological awareness group made phonological awareness gains than in the narrative comparison group, although the gains were typically modest. Gains were most notable in the identification of ending sounds. Teachers reported that initial, more often than final, sound identification was an intervention target in the classroom for both groups, but especially for the children in the comparison group, a fact that may have reduced the effect size of the intervention, at least for initial sound identification.

In terms of reading interventions, both Cupples and Iacono (2002) and Bourassa et al. (2005) compared the effectiveness of a rime-based versus a whole-word approach to teaching word-level reading. Rime-based approaches teach phonics directly by having children segment words into onset and rime during instruction. For example, when teaching the word "cat," the instructor would ask the child to read "c" (onset) then "at" (rime) and then the two together "cat." A rime-based approach would also teach several members of a rime family at the same time (e.g., cat, fat, hat), so that the child's attention is drawn to the relationships between the spellings of words in the family. In contrast, whole-word approaches teach children to read individual words without drawing attention to the relationship between words. Rime-based approaches have been shown to result in faster learning and greater generalization to untrained words than whole-word approaches for typically developing children (Haskell, Foorman, & Swank, 1992; Levy & Lysynchuk, 1997). Using a replicated single-subject design, Cupples and Iacono (2002) compared the performance of four children trained with a rime-based approach to that of three children trained with a whole-word approach. Children were instructed individually once a week for 6 weeks, with parents supervising homework. Although both instructional approaches led to equivalent gains on trained words, the analytic approach resulted in greater generalization to untrained words in the same rime families. Since only 30 words were being trained in this study, it is possible that ceiling effects masked differences in learning trained words for the two instructional programs.

Bourassa et al. (2005) studied 30 school-aged children with DS in an intervention conducted twice a week for 18 weeks. The participants were trained on 90 words, again using either a rime-based or whole-word training strategy. Analyses of pre- and post-test data revealed that the group receiving rime training improved significantly on reading trained words and on a standardized test, whereas the group receiving whole-word training improved

less than the rime-trained group on the word probes and showed no significant change on standardized test scores. As well, only the group receiving the rime-based instruction generalized reading performance to new words in the same rime families that were used in intervention and maintained generalization gains in a follow-up session. Thus, rime-based training advantages can be demonstrated in the DS population as well as in typically developing children. As well, the work of both Cupples and Iacono (2002) and Bourassa et al. (2005) provide further evidence for the importance of phonological awareness to decoding acquisition in the DS population.

There is preliminary evidence that training orthographic conventions (spelling rules) can be efficacious in individuals with DS. This is of some importance, as knowledge of orthography is necessary for skilled decoding and, as has been discussed previously in this review, decoding is an area of deficit in individuals with DS. Two unpublished studies have investigated the efficacy of teaching orthographic conventions to participants with DS using a single-subject A-B-A multiple baseline design. In the first (Spidel & Vogan, 2004), a 15-year-old boy with DS (MA = 5;3, WRMT, Word Identification age-equivalent = 7;4) was taught successive targets in two half-hour sessions per week for 6.5 weeks. Targets included digraphs (two letters spelling one sound, such as sh-, th-, or ea-), clusters (two or more letters spelling two or more sounds, such as br- and sl-), and long (ea̲t) and short (me̲t) vowels. Direct intervention was followed by a home program. Pre-, post- and follow-up measures showed improvement for many targets as well as maintenance of some of those gains 13 weeks later. Improvement was greatest for targets that received more intensive intervention and those for which the participant had demonstrated some knowledge prior to the intervention. Gains were demonstrated on trained targets as well as on the Word Attack subtest of the WRMT. Phoneme awareness skills also improved without direct intervention over the period studied.

Using the same experimental design (St. Pierre, Cleave, & Kay-Raining Bird, 2007), progress in a young adult woman with DS (CA = 21;6, MA = 5;7, WRMT, Word Identification age-equivalent = 6;6) who had experienced difficulties learning to read throughout her public schooling was studied. She received intervention twice a week for 14 weeks, again followed by a home program. The targeted orthographic conventions were digraphs, clusters, and rime families (e.g., -at, -ope). The results were less dramatic for this individual than for the participant in Spidel & Vogan, despite the increased intensity and length of the intervention and the reduced number of targets. Nonetheless, modest gains were made in the ability to accurately read several orthographic targets, and some of these gains were maintained 20 weeks post-intervention. Improvement on an independent measure of word-level reading was also found. Once again, behaviors that were targeted for longer periods of time showed greater changes in performance.

Moni, Jobling, and colleagues (Gallaher, van Kraayenoord, Jobling, & Moni, 2002; Moni & Jobling, 2001; Morgan, Moni, & Jobling, 2004) studied the impact of a broad-based sociocultural form of reading and writing instruction that was operationalized as the postsecondary school Latch-On ™ program. The program involves use of a variety of strategies and technology to teach the comprehension and reproduction of written texts. Thus, communication about texts and functional uses of literacy are emphasized. The program is ongoing, and publications vary in the length of time studied. Moni and Jobling (2001) report on the results of intervention with 17 students, each in one of three cohorts, over an intervention period of 1 year 10 months. Results from these case studies suggest that the Latch-On ™ program had a beneficial effect on the decoding, reading fluency and, to a lesser extent, reading comprehension skills of young adults with DS. The authors argued that comprehension gains in particular required "sustained support and effort" (p. 391; Moni & Jobling, 2001) and the use of a variety of scaffolding strategies.

Conclusion

Although individual differences are large, our review of the literature suggests that individuals with DS have considerable potential to develop literacy skills. Many individuals with DS achieve some level of functional reading skill. Many children with DS appear to have the potential to begin to read in the preschool years and evidence suggests that they continue to develop reading and writing skills at least through early adulthood, although there may be a plateauing of reading development at this point. Word recognition in reading is a literacy strength for many individuals with DS, and studies often report word recognition abilities that are in advance of cognitive and language measures. In contrast, word decoding and reading comprehension skills

are areas of deficit in this population. Although decoding can be mastered in skilled readers with DS, reading comprehension appears to be a deficit for all, a finding that is apparently related to the expressive language difficulties of this population. The profile of reading strengths and weaknesses appears to change as individuals with DS age. Individuals with DS also have difficulty acquiring phoneme-level phonological awareness skills and, perhaps, rhyming ability.

Not surprisingly, many factors have been shown to influence literacy development in individuals with DS, including intrinsic factors such as age, cognition, gender, expressive and receptive language ability, and phonological awareness (particularly phoneme awareness), and extrinsic factors such as home environment, schooling, and socioeconomic status (parental education, social class). Reading and writing abilities also positively influence each other. In general, better readers with DS are older, female, more cognitively and/or linguistically advanced, raised in the home, attend inclusive educational settings, and have been recipients of intensive training in reading and writing.

Emerging evidence suggests that interventions can improve emergent literacy, word recognition and decoding skills, orthographic knowledge, and phonological awareness. Of particular note is the finding that rime-based approaches to word-level reading instruction result in larger gains and more generalization than do whole-word approaches. We may be just beginning to understand the true capabilities of individuals with DS with regards to literacy development. More studies that focus upon underlying mechanisms of reading and writing, the profile of writing abilities, and specific intervention strategies are critical to extending our knowledge base.

Acknowledgments

The preparation of this chapter was supported by grants to the first author from the Social Sciences and Humanities Research Council of Canada (#410-2000-1409 and #410-2003-1875).

References

Bayley, N. (1969). *Manual for Bayley scales of infant development.* New York: Psychological Corporation.

Bird, G., & Buckley, S. (1994). *Meeting the educational needs of children with Down's syndrome.* Portsmouth, UK: Sarah Duffen Centre, University of Portsmouth.

Blachman, B. (1994). Early literacy acquisition: The role of phonological awareness. In G. P. Wallach, & K. G. Butler (Eds.), *Language learning disabilities in school-age children and adolescents* (pp. 253–274). Toronto: Maxwell MacMillan.

Bochner, S., Outhred, L., & Pieterse, M. (2001). A study of functional literacy skills in young adults with Down syndrome. *International Journal of Disability, Development and Education, 48*, 67–90.

Boudreau, D. (2002). Literacy skills in children and adolescents with Down syndrome. *Reading and Writing: An Interdisciplinary Journal, 15*, 497–525.

Bourassa, D. C., Cleave, P., & Kay-Raining Bird, E. (June, 2005). *Teaching children with Down syndrome to read: An update.* Paper presented at the annual meeting of Canadian Language and Literacy Research Network Centre of Excellence, Toronto, Canada.

Buckley, S. (1995). Teaching children with Down's syndrome to read and write. In L. Nadel, & D. Rosenthal (Eds.), *Down syndrome: Living and learning.* New York: Wiley-Liss.

Buckley, S. (2003). Literacy and language. In J. A. Rondal, & S. Buckley (Eds.), *Speech and language intervention in Down syndrome.* London: Whurr Publishers.

Buckley, S., & Bird, G. (1993). Teaching children with Down syndrome to read. *Down's Syndrome Research and Practice, 1*, 34–39.

Buckley, S., & Bird, G. (1993). In S. Buckley, M. Emslie, G. Haslegrave, P. LePrevost, & G. Bird (Eds.), *The development of language and reading skills in children with Down's syndrome* (2nd ed, pp. 38–51). Southsea, Hants, UK: Sarah Duffen Centre, University of Portsmouth.

Buckley, S., Emslie, M., Haslegrave, G., & LePrevost, P. (Eds.), *The development of language and reading skills in children with Down's syndrome.* Southsea, Hants, UK: Sarah Duffen Centre, University of Portsmouth.

Buckley, S., & Sacks, B. (1987). *The adolescent with Down syndrome: Life for the teenager and for the family.* Portsmouth, UK: University of Portsmouth.

Byrne, A., MacDonald, J., & Buckley, S. (2002). Reading, language, and memory skills: A comparative longitudinal study of children with Down syndrome and their mainstream peers. *British Journal of Educational Psychology, 72*, 513–529.

Cardosa-Martins, C., Michalick, M. F., & Pollo, T. C. (2002). Is sensitivity to rhyme a developmental precursor to sensitivity to phoneme?: Evidence from individuals with Down syndrome. *Reading and Writing: An Interdisciplinary Journal, 15*, 439–454.

Carr, J. (1995). *Down's syndrome: Children growing up.* New York: Cambridge University Press.

Carr, J. (2000). Intellectual and daily living skills of 30-year-olds with Down's syndrome: Continuation of a longitudinal study. *Journal of Applied Research in Intellectual Disabilities, 13*, 1–16.

Casey, W., Jones, D., Kugler, B., & Watkins, B. (1988). Integration of Down's syndrome children in the primary school: Longitudinal study of cognitive development and academic attainments. *British Journal of Educational Psychology, 58*, 279–286.

Chapman, R. S., & Kay-Raining Bird, E. (2011). Language development in childhood, adolescence, and young adulthood in persons with Down syndrome. In J. A. Burack, R. M. Hodapp, G. Iarocci, & E. Zigler (Eds.), *The Oxford handbook of intellectual disability and development*, 2nd ed. New York: Oxford University Press.

Chatterji, M. (2006). Reading achievement gaps, correlates, and moderators of early reading achievement: Evidence from the Early Childhood Longitudinal Study (ECLS) kindergarten to first grade sample. *Journal of Educational Psychology, 98*(3), 489–507.

Cleave, P. L., Kay-Raining Bird, E., & Bourassa, D. (in press). Developing phonological awareness skills in children with Down syndrome. *Canadian Journal of Speech-Language Pathology and Audiology.*

Cossu, G., Rossini, F., & Marshall, J. C. (1993). When reading is acquired but phonemic awareness is not: A study of literacy in Down's syndrome. *Cognition, 46*, 129–138.

Cupples, L., & Iacono, T. (2000). Phonological awareness and oral reading skill in children with Down syndrome. *Journal of Speech, Language and Hearing Research, 43*, 595–608.

Cupples, L., & Iacono, T. (2002). The efficacy of "whole word" versus "analytic" reading instruction for children with Down syndrome. *Reading and Writing: An Interdisciplinary Journal, 15*, 549–574.

Evans, R. (1994). Phonological awareness in children with Down's syndrome. *Down's Syndrome Research and Practice, 2*, 102–105.

Fidler, D. J., Most, D. D., & Guiberson, M. M. (2005). Neuropsychological correlates of word identification in Down syndrome. *Research in Developmental Disabilities, 26*, 487–501.

Fitzgerald, J., Roberts, J., Pierce, P., & Schuele, M. (1995). Evaluation of home literacy environment: An illustration with preschool children with Down syndrome. *Reading and Writing Quarterly: Overcoming Learning Difficulties, 11*, 311–334.

Fletcher, H., & Buckley, S. (2002). Phonological awareness in children with Down syndrome. *Down Syndrome Research and Practice, 8*, 11–18.

Fowler, A., Doherty, B., & Boynton, L. (1995). The basis of reading skill in young adults with Down syndrome. In L. Nadel, & D. Rosenthal (Eds.), *Down syndrome: Living and learning in the community.* New York: John Wiley & Sons.

Gallaher, K. M., van Kraayenoord, C. E., Jobling, A., & Moni, K. B. (2002). Reading with Abby: A case study of individual tutoring with a young adult with Down syndrome. *Down Syndrome Research and Practice, 8*, 59–66.

Gombert, J.-E. (2002). Children with Down syndrome use phonological knowledge in reading. *Reading and Writing: An Interdisciplinary Journal, 15*, 455–409.

Haskell, D. W., Foorman, B. R., & Swank, P. R. (1992). Effects of three orthographic/phonological units on first-grade reading. *Remedial and Special Education, 13*, 40–49.

Johnson, A. H. (2000). *Changing skills for a changing world. Recommendations for adult literacy policy in Aoteareo/New Zealand.* A report for the Department of Labour, New Zealand.

Justice, L. (2006). *Clinical approaches to emergent literacy intervention.* San Diego: Plural Publishing.

Kay-Raining Bird, E., Cleave, P., & McConnell, L. (2000). Reading and phonological awareness in children with Down syndrome: A longitudinal study. *American Journal of Speech-Language Pathology, 9*, 319–330.

Kay-Raining Bird, E., Cleave, P. L., White, D., Pike, H., & Helmkay, A. (2008). Written and oral narratives of children and adolescents with Down syndrome. *Journal of Speech, Language, and Hearing Research, 51*, 436–450.

Kennedy, E. J., & Flynn, M. C. (2003a). Early phonological awareness and reading skills in children with Down syndrome. *Down Syndrome Research and Practice, 8*, 100–109.

Kennedy, E. J., & Flynn, M. C. (2003b). Training phonological awareness skills in children with Down syndrome. *Research in Developmental Disabilities, 24*, 44–57.

Kliewer, C. (1998). Citizenship in the literate community: An ethnography of children with Down syndrome and the written word. *Exceptional Children, 64,* 167–180.

Laws, G., & Gunn, D. (2002). Relationship between reading, phonological skills, and language development in individuals with Down syndrome: A five year follow-up study. *Reading and Writing: An Interdisciplinary Journal, 15,* 527–548.

Levy, B. A., & Lysynchuk, L. (1997). Beginning word recognition: Benefits of training by segmentation and whole word methods. *Scientific Studies of Reading, 1,* 359–387.

McCarthy, D. (1972). *McCarthy scales of children's abilities.* San Antonio, TX: The Psychological Corporation.

Moni, K. B., & Jobling, A. (2001). Reading-related literacy learning of young adults with Down syndrome: Findings from a three year teaching and research program. *International Journal of Disability, Development and Education, 48,* 377–394.

Morgan, M., Moni, K. B., & Jobling, A. (2004). What's it all about? Investigating reading comprehension strategies in young adults with Down syndrome. *Down Syndrome Research and Practice, 9,* 37–44.

Nippold, M., Duthie, J., & Larsen, J. (2005). Literacy as a leisure activity: Free-time preferences of older children and young adolescents. *Language, Speech, and Hearing Services in Schools, 36*(2), 93–102.

Oelwein, P. L. (1995). *Teaching reading to children with Down syndrome.* Bethesda, MD: Woodbine House.

Robinson-Pant, A. (2005). *Cross-cultural perspectives in educational research (Conducting educational research).* NY, NY: Open University Press.

Roch, M., & Levorato, M. C. (2009). Simple View of Reading in Down's syndrome: the role of listening comprehension and reading skills. *International Journal of Language and Communication Disorders, 44,* 206–223.

Rosner, J. & Simon, D. P. (1971). The auditory analysis test: An initial report. *Journal of Learning Disabilities, 4,* 384–392.

Shepperdson, P. (1988). *Growing up with Down's syndrome.* London: Cassell.

Sloper, P., Cunningham, C., Turner, S., & Knussen, C. (1990). Factors related to the academic attainments of children with Down syndrome. *British Journal of Educational Psychology, 60,* 284–298.

Snowling, M. J., Hulme, C., & Mercer, R. C. (2002). A deficit in rime awareness in children with Down syndrome. *Reading and Writing: An Interdisciplinary Journal, 15,* 471–495.

Spidel, M., & Vogan, S. (2004). *A reading intervention program for a child with Down syndrome.* Unpublished master's project, Dalhousie University, Halifax, Nova Scotia, Canada.

St. Pierre, J., Cleave, P., & Kay-Raining Bird, E. (November, 2007). *Down syndrome & decoding skills training: A case study.* Poster to be presented at the annual American Speech-Language-Hearing Association Convention, Boston, MA.

Turner, S., & Alborz, A. (2003). Academic attainments of children with Down's syndrome: A longitudinal study. *British Journal of Educational Psychology, 73,* 563–583.

Trenholm, B., & Mirenda, P. (2006). Home and community literacy experiences of individuals with Down syndrome. *Down Syndrome Research and Practice, 10,* 30–40.

van Bysterveldt, A. K., Gillon, G. T., & Moran, C. (2006). *International Journal of Disability, Development and Education, 53*(3), 301–329.

Verucci, L., Menghini, D., & Vicari, S. (2006). Reading skills and phonological awareness acquisition in Down syndrome. *Journal of Intellectual Disability Research, 50,* 477–491.

Waddington, N. J. (1988). *Waddington diagnostic reading and spelling tests: A book of tests and diagnostic procedures for children with learning disabilities.* Ingle Farm, South Australia: Waddington Educational Resources.

Woodcock, R. W. (1987). *Woodcock Reading Mastery Tests-Revised.* Circle Pines, MN: American Guidance Services.

Young, D. (1976). *Spar Reading Test.* London: Hodder Stoughton Educational.

Language Development in Fragile X Syndrome: Syndrome-specific Features, Within-syndrome Variation, and Contributing Factors

Leonard Abbeduto, Andrea McDuffie, Nancy Brady, *and* Sara T. Kover

Abstract

This chapter reviews what is known about the language problems of individuals with fragile X syndrome (FXS). The chapter is organized into four major sections. The first section provides a comprehensive characterization of the language problems typically associated with FXS, describing the extent and profile of delays and impairments and, where possible, the syndrome-specific features of the linguistic profile. The second section describes within-syndrome variation in the linguistic profile, emphasizing the relationship between language and gender and autism status. The third section considers the genetic and environmental factors that lead to the syndrome-specific features of, and within-syndrome variation in, the linguistic phenotype of FXS. The final section identifies important gaps in our knowledge of the language problems of FXS and suggests some directions for future research.

Keywords: Fragile X syndrome, language problems, language ability, linguistic profile, autism

In this chapter, we review what is known about the language problems of individuals with fragile Xsyndrome (FXS). We focus largely on individuals with the full mutation (i.e., 200 or more repetitions of the CGG sequence of nucleotides comprising *FMR1*), only briefly considering individuals with the *FMR1* premutation (i.e., between 55 and 200 CGG repeats). We have organized the review into four major sections. In the first, we provide a comprehensive characterization of the language problems typically associated with FXS, describing the extent and profile of delays and impairments and, where possible, the syndrome-specific features of the linguistic profile. In the second section, we describe within-syndrome variation in the linguistic profile, emphasizing the relationship between language and gender and autism status. In the third section, we consider the genetic and environmental factors that lead to the syndrome-specific features of, and within-syndrome variation in, the linguistic phenotype of FXS. In the final section, we identify important gaps in our knowledge of the language

problems of FXS and suggest some directions for future research. Before launching the review, we describe some principles and assumptions that we believe should guide the design and interpretation of research on FXS.

Guiding Principles and Assumptions

We assume that FXS, like Down syndrome (DS), autism, and other neurodevelopmental disorders, is best understood within a developmental framework, using the course, nature, and explanatory mechanisms of typical development to describe and understand the behavioral sequelae of FXS. A developmental framework leads us to adopt the following more specific principles.

Language and cognition are intimately linked over the course of development. Despite early claims about the modularity, or independence, of language and cognitive development, compelling empirical evidence demonstrates that certain cognitive achievements (e.g., a concept of object permanence) are prerequisites for specific linguistic achievements (e.g., the use of words marking disappearance and recurrence; Tomasello & Farrar, 1984, 1986) and that developments in various components of the information processing system (e.g., short-term auditory memory) have pervasive effects on language development (e.g., vocabulary size; Baddeley, Gathercole, & Papagano, 1998). Although there may be language-specific learning mechanisms, there is no denying that nonlinguistic cognitive development sets the stage and provides critical support for language leaning and use (Abbeduto, Keller-Bell, Richmond, & Murphy, 2006). In light of the fact that virtually all males with FXS and as many as one-half of all females with FXS have IQs low enough to meet criteria for intellectual disability (Hagerman, 1999), there is no doubt that many individuals with FXS will have language skills below those of their age-matched typically developing peers. The question of interest from both a research and a clinical perspective is whether language delays are more or less severe relative to cognitive impairments (Abbeduto, Evans, & Dolan, 2001). In the present review, we focus largely on research designed to address this question.

Language learning is embedded in, and influenced by, social interaction. Typically developing children acquire language by participation in recurring events that are meaningful and interesting to them, such as "reading" the same book with a parent (Chapman, 2000). Moreover, typically developing children use their knowledge of the social world to crack the linguistic code; for example, they search for the meanings of new words by attending to the gaze, emotions, knowledge, and interests of the speaker (Baldwin, Markman, Bill, Desjardins, & Irwin, 1996; Hollich, Hirsh-Pasek, & Golinkoff, 2000; Moore, Angelopoulos, & Bennett, 1999; Tomasello, 2003). Consequently, children who have impairments or characteristics that disrupt participation in social interaction or limit the information that they can glean from social interaction are likely to have language difficulties. In fact, individuals with FXS often have comorbid conditions that adversely affect social interaction. These conditions include hyperarousal (Wisbeck et al., 2000), hyperactivity (Baumgardner et al., 1995; Bregman et al., 1987; Dykens, Hodapp, Ort, & Finucane, 1989; Freund, Reiss, & Abrams, 1993; Mazzocco, Pennington, & Hagerman, 1993), and social anxiety (Bregman et al., 1988; Mazzocco et al., 1998). There is also a relatively high comorbidity between FXS and autism, with more than 90% of this population displaying autistic-like behaviors (e.g., Hagerman,

1999) and 25%–35% meeting criteria for autism (Bailey et al., 2004). These comorbid conditions all but ensure delays and impairments in language in FXS. The question of interest for researchers and clinicians is whether these comorbid conditions contribute something to language problems over and above cognitive contributions. We also consider research designed to address this question, especially research focused on autism.

Language is not a unitary ability. By this we mean that different domains of language, such as vocabulary and morphosyntax (i.e., grammar), appear to be influenced by different factors in the case of typically developing children. For example, a maternal responsive style, defined by, among other things, a tendency to follow rather than redirect the child's focus of attention, has been shown to be more strongly related to the subsequent development of vocabulary than of syntax (Gleitman, Newport & Gleitman, 1984; Pine, 1994; Tomasello & Farrar, 1984). Research on individual differences and neurodevelopmental disorders also supports this view. For example, vocabulary is less impaired than morphosyntax in individuals with DS, and the predictors of progress in the two domains are different for this population as well (Chapman, 2003). The question implied by this view of language is whether some domains of language, or achievements within a domain, are more delayed or impaired relative to other domains or achievements in individuals with FXS. Again, we consider research that addresses this question.

Language development is shaped by the environment and biology. Despite claims about the innateness of language and the minimal role of the environment emanating from the nativist position of Chomsky (1965) and others, there is considerable evidence that the environment plays a critical role in the language development of typically developing children. In general, adult caregivers interact with young children in ways that support language learning by talking about the objects and events that are the focus of the child's attention, using language that is at least roughly matched to the child's level of competence, repeatedly engaging the child in routines that minimize information processing demands, and guiding the child's participation to ensure success and meaningful participation in the interaction (Chapman, 2003). Variations along these caregiving dimensions are associated with variations in language outcomes, even among typically developing children. For example, Hart and Risely (1995) documented substantial differences in the amount of talk directed to children in more and less economically advantaged families and important consequences of these differences for children's linguistic outcomes.

Although the environment is important, genetics also contributes to language learning in important ways. Infants are endowed with predispositions that facilitate language learning, such as an affinity for the human face and voice (DeCasper & Fifer, 1980; Farroni, Menon, & Johnson, 2006; Legerstee, Anderson, & Shaffer, 1998), as well as a surprisingly sophisticated ability to extract patterns from the world around them, including patterns of co-occurrence in acoustic input, thereby enabling segmentation into linguistically relevant units, such as syllables, words, and morphemes (Jusczyk, 1999; Saffran, 2002; Saffran, Aslin, & Newport, 1996). Moreover, maturation of the brain systems and peripheral mechanisms underlying language is a gradual process associated with concomitant advances in language (Mills et al., 2004; Mills, Plunkett, Prat, & Shafer, 2005; Ramscar & Gitcho, 2007). Together, such evidence suggests the need to consider the ways in which the *FMR1* mutation (and variations in the mutation) and the environment contribute to the syndrome-specific features of, and within-syndrome variation in, the linguistic phenotype of FXS. We review the research designed to address these contributing factors.

Language development can be disrupted by any of several factors. As discussed, cognitive impairments, comorbid conditions, biological anomalies, and less than optimal environments can lead, either individually or in combination, to a language delay or impairment. Not surprisingly, many children without FXS can have language problems, and there will be variation across children in the severity and profile of linguistic impairments, reflecting differences in their cognitive impairments, comorbid conditions, genetic make-up, and learning environments. Such observations raise the question of whether the constellation of cognitive impairments, comorbid conditions, biological anomalies, and environmental contexts associated with FXS lead to a unique linguistic signature—a profile that distinguishes FXS from other conditions associated with language problems. Addressing this question requires comparisons of FXS to samples displaying other conditions. We review syndrome-comparison studies, which have been surprisingly rare.

Language Learning and Use in Individuals with Fragile X Syndrome

In the following sections, we review research on language learning and use in FXS. We begin by describing the characteristic linguistic profile of relative strengths and weaknesses in FXS. This description is organized in terms of the transition into language and then into the major components of language: vocabulary, morphosyntax, and pragmatics. Where relevant evidence exists, we also indicated the extent to which the profile described is specific to FXS. We then review research on within-syndrome variation in the phenotype, before moving to a consideration of individual biological and environmental factors in language learning and use.

The Linguistic Phenotype of Fragile X Syndrome

THE TRANSITION INTO LANGUAGE

Typically developing children begin to communicate intentionally with gestures and vocalizations by 9 months of age, which is 3–4 months before they produce their first words (Bates et al., 1987; Volterra et al., 2005). The onset of intentional communication is often substantially delayed in children with intellectual disabilities, and many remain in the prelinguistic stage for years, and, in some cases, even into adulthood (Brady et al., 2004). A delay in the transition from prelinguistic to linguistic communication was documented for FXS in a study by Brady et al. (2006). These investigators interviewed the biological mothers of young boys (*n* = 44) and girls (*n* = 11) with FXS ranging in age from 18 to 36 months about their children's communicative development. Three-fourths of the mothers reported that their children communicated through nonverbal means, such as gestures, or produced only a few words, despite the fact that the children were many months past the age at which typically developing children begin to say words.

The transition to linguistic communication is delayed in children with FXS regardless of the language being learned. In a study of 21 9- to 13-year-old boys with FXS who were learning Hebrew as their native language, Levy, Gottesman, Borochowitz, Frydman, and Sagi (2006) found that one-third of the sample was communicating prelinguistically or produced only single words or syllables. Thus, the transition into language may be delayed by many years (and may not occur at all) for some individuals with FXS.

VOCABULARY

After children with FXS begin to talk, they gradually learn new words, albeit at a slower rate than do their typically developing peers (Roberts, Mirrett, & Burchinal, 2001). In fact, the development of vocabulary is delayed throughout childhood and at least into adolescence and early adulthood in FXS (Abbeduto & Hagerman, 1997). Delays occur in both receptive vocabulary (i.e., in how well, or how many, words are understood when heard) and expressive vocabulary (i.e., in the number of different words spoken by the language learner; Abbeduto, Brady, & Kover, 2007). Nevertheless, there is some unevenness in vocabulary development, with some aspects of this development being more delayed than other aspects, and with vocabulary being less problematic, on average, than other aspects of language for those with FXS (Abbeduto et al., 2007; Rice, Warren, & Betz, 2005).

The unevenness of vocabulary development is illustrated by a study conducted by Roberts, Mirrett, Anderson, Burchinal, & Neebe (2002). These investigators administered the Communication and Symbolic Behavior Scales (CSBS; Wetherby & Prizant, 2003) to 21- to 77-month-old boys with FXS who were functioning between 12 and 28 months in terms of their developmental ages. The CSBS is a standardized assessment of early communication development that consists of structured episodes or prompts designed to elicit particular types of communicative behaviors. The boys with FXS achieved their highest scores for the *use of different words* and *use of different word combinations*. Scaled scores for language comprehension, especially vocabulary comprehension, were lower than were the corresponding expressive scores, suggesting that receptive skills lag behind expressive skills, including those involved in word learning, at least early in development.

In contrast to the results of Roberts et al. (2002), other evidence suggests that vocabulary comprehension is not especially problematic for individuals with FXS. In particular, Abbeduto et al. (2003) administered the Test for Auditory Comprehension of Language-Revised (TACL-R; Carrow-Woolfolk, 1985), a standardized test of receptive language, to adolescents and young adults with FXS. The TACL-R includes subtests that distinguish between the lexical and grammatical aspects of language. The mean age of the participants with FXS, who included both males and females who had intellectual disabilities, was 16 years. Abbeduto et al. also included a comparison group of typically developing children who were matched to the participants with FXS on a measure of nonverbal mental age (NVMA). Abbeduto et al. found that scores on the Word Classes and Relations subtest of the TACL-R, which is a measure of vocabulary knowledge, did not differ

between the two groups of participants. Moreover, these scores were significantly correlated with NVMA. In other words, receptive vocabulary was below chronological age (CA) expectations, but similar to expectations based on level of nonverbal cognitive development and thus, not an area of special challenge.

The differing results of the Abbeduto et al. (2003) and Roberts et al. (2002) studies may be due to differences in the age of the participants, which would suggest that the rate of receptive vocabulary development increases between early childhood and adolescence for those with FXS. Additionally, Abbeduto et al. (2003) observed gender differences in receptive vocabulary ability in their FXS sample, suggesting another possible source of difference between their study and that of Roberts et al., who included only males.

Although comparisons of vocabulary in FXS and other developmental disorders have been rare, the evidence to date does not suggest anything unique in terms of the extent or nature of delays in vocabulary in individuals with FXS relative to individuals with other neurodevelopmental disorders. In particular, Abbeduto et al. (2003) included a group of adolescents and young adults with DS, who were matched to the FXS participants groupwise in terms of CA and nonverbal measures of IQ and mental age (MA). These investigators found that, although group differences existed in the extent of delay in receptive syntax, none existed in receptive vocabulary. Clearly, there is a need for considerably more research in this area, with a wider range of assessments, larger samples of individuals with FXS, and multiple diagnostic comparison groups, before we can conclude that there are no syndrome-specific features of vocabulary development in FXS.

MORPHOSYNTAX

Morphosyntax refers to the characteristic ways in which linguistic units, such as words, are combined into phrases, clauses, and sentences by the speakers of a language. Word-order constraints are an important part of the morphosyntax of English; for example, articles and adjectives precede nouns in noun phrases (e.g., "the red hat," not "hat the red"). The morphosyntax of English also includes regular (as well as idiosyncratic, or irregular) means of modifying the meanings of words and phrases through the use of elements called grammatical morphemes (e.g., the grammatical morpheme "-s" to convey plurality).

In general, morphosyntactic abilities are significantly delayed compared to CA-matched typically developing peers in males with FXS and in females with FXS who also have an intellectual disability (Abbeduto & Hagerman, 1997). Morphosyntax, however, like other dimensions of language, improves with age in FXS (Roberts et al., 2001). Nevertheless, age accounts for relatively little variance in morphosyntactic maturity among individuals with FXS (Fisch et al., 1999)—far less than is accounted for by nonverbal cognitive ability (Abbeduto et al., 2003; Roberts et al., 2001).

However, even the relationship between morphosyntactic and cognitive development in FXS is far from perfect and changes over the course of development (Abbeduto et al., 2007). In a study of receptive morphosyntax, Price, Roberts, Vandergrift, and Martin (2007) administered the TACL-3 to boys with FXS, all of whom were under the age of 16 years (mean age near 10 years). They found that the boys with FXS scored more poorly on the morphosyntactic subtests of the TACL-3, one of which focused on combinational word-order rules and the other on grammatical morphemes, than did typically developing children matched to them on NVMA. In contrast, Abbeduto et al. (2003) found that adolescent and young adult males and females with FXS, most of whom were older than 16, did not differ from NVMA-matched typically developing 3- to 6- year-olds in their age-equivalent scores on the morphosyntactically focused subtests of the TACL-R. In studies of adult males, Paul and colleagues (Paul, Cohen, Breg, Watson, & Herman, 1984; Paul, Dykens, Leckman, Watson, Breg, & Cohen, 1987), like Abbeduto et al. (2003) found that receptive morphosyntactic performance on several standardized tests was generally consistent with NVMA expectations. Together, these studies suggest that the development of receptive morphosyntax in individuals with FXS lags behind nonverbal cognitive development during childhood, but "catches up" in adolescence and young adulthood. It is not clear at this point if this profile emerges because of a relative slowing of cognitive development or a relative speeding up of morphosyntactic development, or both.

There have been few studies of expressive morphosyntax in FXS, and the resulting data are less consistent, especially as regards its relationship to nonverbal cognitive development. Madison, George, and Moeschler (1986) analyzed language samples collected in conversational activities from males with FXS, including children and adults. Madison et al. found that mean length of utterance (MLU)—a gross measure of morphosyntactic maturity—was at

or, even in advance of, NVMA-expectations for each of the male participants with FXS. It should be noted that the Madison et al. study included as participants only members of a single extended family and, thus, the generalizability of the findings is not clear. Nevertheless, it is interesting to note that more recent studies with larger samples have found few differences between individuals with FXS and typically developing children matched on nonverbal cognitive level on gross measures of expressive syntax (Finestack & Abbeduto, 2010; Keller-Bell & Abbeduto, 2007). In contrast, Paul et al. (1984) found that expressive morphosyntax measured in a conversational context was more delayed than expected based on NVMA for adult males with FXS. More research on expressive morphosyntax in this population is clearly needed.

Most of the studies in this area have relied on very gross measures of competence, such as MLU, that average over many different aspects of morphosyntax. Such measures may obscure relative strengths and weaknesses in different aspects of morphosyntax that could provide insight into the nature of the learning impairments that give rise to the morphosyntactic deficits of affected individuals (Rice et al., 2005). A recent study by Levy et al. (2006) is noteworthy, therefore, because it involved a more fine-grained analysis of expressive morphosyntax than any study to date. Levy, et al.'s sample was comprised of 15 boys with FXS, ages 9 to 13 years. The study was conducted in Israel, and the boys were all learning Hebrew as their first language. Hebrew has a more complex system of grammatical morphology and fewer word-order constraints than does English. As noted previously, seven of the boys were largely prelinguistic communicators, and they were not included in the morphosyntactic analyses. Language samples collected in conversational and narrative, or storytelling, contexts were compared to those produced by typically developing children (n = 20) who were matched to the FXS sample on MLU and the percentage of utterances of five or more morphemes in length. Levy et al. found that the boys with FXS were more delayed than were the typically developing matches on several measures of expressive morphosyntax; for example, the former produced fewer complex clauses than did the latter. The boys with FXS, however, also scored at a more advanced level than did the comparison children on many other morphosyntactic measures; for example, the former made fewer errors in number agreement (e.g., "the boys is"), particularly in narrative language samples.

Thus, the Levy et al. findings suggest that expressive morphosyntax in FXS is more advanced in some respects, and less advanced in other respects, than expected based on MLU, at least in a narrative context associated with a high degree of visual support. These findings raise the possibility that morphosyntactic development is not simply delayed, but also different in FXS, in the sense that their morphosyntactic development appears to consist of different "strands" that are delayed to varying degrees. There is a need, however, for replication of these findings because of the small sample and the focus on children with FXS learning Hebrew, a morphologically complex language. In fact, Finestack and Abbeduto (2010) analyzed the narratives of American English-speaking adolescents and young adults with FXS on a number of specific syntactic features and found few differences, with a tendency for poorer performance, relative to typically developing children matched on nonverbal MA.

Although little is known about the syndrome specificity of the profile of morphosyntactic impairments associated with FXS, the studies to date suggest areas of strength relative to individuals with some other syndromes. Ferrier, Bashir, Meryash, Johnston, and Wolff (1991) examined expressive language skills in a conversational context for adult males with FXS, autism, or DS. These investigators did not find differences between the groups in expressive morphosyntax. In a study of narratives, however, Keller-Bell and Abbeduto (2007) found that adolescents and young adults with FXS were more likely to produce grammatical (than ungrammatical) utterances than were age- and nonverbal MA-matched individuals with DS. In another cross-syndrome study, Abbeduto et al. (2003) found that adolescent and young adult males and females with FXS scored significantly higher on the Grammatical Morphemes and Elaborated Sentences subtests of the TACL-R, which reflect morphosyntax-related comprehension, than did participants with DS matched on age and nonverbal measures of IQ and MA. Thus, adolescents with FXS differ from those with DS in that morphosyntax does not seem to be a particular weakness in FXS, although there may be specific morphosyntactic features that are quite challenging for them. Further comparisons among these and other populations are necessary, however, before firm conclusions are possible. It would be particularly important to make syndrome comparisons using more fine-grained analyses, such as those conducted by Levy et al. (2006) and Finestack and Abbeduto (2010).

PRAGMATICS

Pragmatics refers to the use of language to accomplish social goals (i.e., to express one's needs, interests, and intentions), to discern the social goals of other speakers, and to do so in a way that conforms to various cultural constraints on informativeness, social appropriateness, and mutual expectations regarding conduct (Levinson, 1983). Pragmatic skills are at work in the decision to use a pronoun, such as "it" or "he," only if the referent can be assumed to be clear to the listener because of, for example, what has already been stated explicitly in the discourse. Deciding to express a request to a waiter at a restaurant by using the impolite, "Get me my check," rather than by the polite, "Can I have the check when you get a chance?" would be another example of pragmatic skills in action. Studies of pragmatics in individuals with FXS have either (a) relied on broad-based summary measures of pragmatic performance, which yield a single score reflecting an "average" performance across numerous domains of pragmatic skill, such as the Communication domain score on the informant-report Vineland Adaptive Behavior Scales (VABS; Sparrow, Balla, & Cicchetti, 1984); (b) involved a more narrowly focused assessment in a domain of skill that could be seen as foundational for successful communication, such as the ability to make clear the objects or events to which the speaker intends to refer; or (c) focused on documenting the occurrence of inappropriate or maladaptive pragmatic behaviors, such as verbal perseveration. Together, these studies suggest that pragmatics may be the most problematic domain of language for individuals with FXS.

Studies in which broad-based measures of pragmatic skills have been administered (Bailey, Hatton, & Skinner, 1998; Dykens et al., 1989; Fisch et al., 1999) have documented that the pragmatic development of males with FXS and females with FXS who have intellectual disabilities is delayed relative to CA expectations (Murphy & Abbeduto, 2003). For example, Dykens et al. (1989) administered the VABS, which was completed by caregivers of the participants, who were males with FXS. Dykens et al. found that the Communication domain scores of their male participants with FXS suggested that they had a level of skill closer to their MAs than to their CAs. There is also evidence that VABS Communication scores and other similar summary measures lag behind scores in other adaptive skill domains (e.g., the Daily Living domain), which suggests that pragmatics may be an area of relative weakness for males with FXS (Bailey et al., 1998; Dykens et al., 1989; Fisch et al., 1999).

There are important limitations of the VABS Communication scores, as well as of many other summary measures derived from adaptive behavior scales, however, which limit their utility for addressing pragmatics in FXS. First, such broad-based summary scores do not allow for determining whether some facets of pragmatics are more delayed or impaired than other facets (Murphy & Abbeduto, 2003). Second, informant reports, such as the VABS, may not always accurately represent the behavior of the individual with disabilities, especially for contexts that do not include the informant (e.g., parents may not know how the individual behaves in school). The use of observational or experimental measures of specific, well-defined aspects of pragmatic skill avoids such limitations and offers the additional advantage of providing a more nuanced characterization of the pragmatic profile associated with the syndrome.

Studies of more narrowly defined domains of pragmatic skill have demonstrated that the degree of delay in FXS varies across different aspects of pragmatic competence. In one such study, Abbeduto et al. (2006) examined the ability to formulate utterances in such a way as to make clear to others the intended referents. Lack of clarity in establishing shared reference leads to discourse that is difficult, if not impossible, to understand. These investigators administered a non–face-to-face laboratory-based task, which required that only the verbal channel of communication be used, to examine the referential skills of adolescents and young adults with FXS. In the Abbeduto et al. task, the participant was the speaker and a researcher served as listener. The speaker's task was to describe a novel target shape, so that the listener could select the corresponding shape from a set of potential referents. There were multiple shapes, and each recurred on multiple trials, so as to resemble natural conversation, which entails both introducing new topics and returning to old topics.

Abbeduto et al. (2006) found that the adolescents and young adults with FXS were less likely than NVMA-matched typically developing children to create unique (i.e., one-to-one) mappings between their descriptions and the target shapes; instead, they often extended the same description to multiple shapes (e.g., using "the muffin" to refer to two or more different shapes). The latter descriptions are technically ambiguous, and thus, uninformative from the perspective of the listener. The participants

with FXS were also less likely than either the NVMA-matched typically developing children or age- and nonverbal IQ- and MA-matched participants with DS to continue to use their previously successful descriptions on subsequent trials (e.g., using "muffin" to refer to a shape on one trial, but "house" to refer to the same shape on subsequent trials). Such inconsistency also decreased the utility of their descriptions for the listener. The participants with FXS were also more likely than those with DS to scaffold their listener's understanding linguistically (e.g., by saying "It looks kind of like a house" rather than simply "It's a house"). These findings suggest variable delay across the different aspects of the referential domain in FXS, with some differences relative to individuals with DS.

In another experimental study, Abbeduto et al. (2008) examined the ability to recognize and take steps to correct misunderstandings when listening to the messages of others. Failure to engage in such noncomprehension signaling will make it difficult to discern the intentions of others or to create a coherent representation of the discourse, as misunderstandings are likely to be compounded as the conversation progresses. The investigators used a laboratory-based task to examine this aspect of pragmatic ability for adolescents and young adults with FXS. In this task, the participant took the role of the listener, and a researcher served as speaker. The listener's task was to respond to simple directions from the speaker, such as "Place the brown duck in the pond," by selecting from two or four drawings, the one that the speaker intended and placing it in a scene in a book. In some cases, the speaker's direction was fully informative. In other cases, however, the direction was inadequate by design, referring to a drawing that the participant did not have (the *incompatible* condition), referring equally well to multiple drawings (the *ambiguous* condition), or containing a word that was novel for the participant (the *unfamiliar* condition). The correct response for the inadequate directions was to signal noncomprehension in some way (e.g., "I don't have a red one") rather than trying to carry out the direction.

Abbeduto et al. (2008) found that the participants with FXS were less likely to signal noncomprehension than were typically developing children matched to them on NVMA. The difference between groups emerged only for the ambiguous and unfamiliar directions; the groups did not differ on the more salient and easier to recognize and resolve incompatible directions. It also was found that the participants with FXS displayed a pattern of performance that did not differ markedly from that of age-, IQ-, and NVMA-matched participants with DS, and that the below-NVMA performance of the FXS groups was due largely to males rather than females. These findings suggest that the development of noncomprehension signaling is delayed (relative to cognitive development) in males with FXS, but that the pattern of development is neither syndrome-specific nor qualitatively different from that of typically developing children.

An experimental study by Simon, Keenan, Pennington, Taylor, and Hagerman (2001) is notable for its focus on females with FXS and for suggesting that pragmatic impairments extend across the full range of affectedness. Simon et al. employed a task in which women with FXS were asked to select humorous endings for brief stories they had read. It was found that the women with FXS had difficulty selecting the correct endings compared to IQ-matched women without FXS. Simon et al. suggested that the women with FXS did poorly because they were unable to follow the connections between the elements and propositions of a discourse (i.e., establish coherence). Although the generalizability of the Simon et al. results to more everyday pragmatic tasks is not clear (Murphy & Abbeduto, 2003), it is important that the women with FXS displayed pragmatic problems despite having normal-range IQs. Thus, the Simon et al. findings suggest that the skills involved in establishing discourse coherence may be especially impaired in FXS. Problems in discourse coherence have also been documented for males with FXS (Roberts et al., 2007).

In addition to examining the degree and profile of competence in pragmatics, researchers have focused on the occurrence of atypical communicative behaviors for individuals with FXS that are either absent or occur infrequently in the language of intellectually typical speakers. Most studied in this regard has been *verbal perseveration*, which is defined as an unusual self-repetition of words, phrases, and topics (Belser & Sudhalter, 2001; Ferrier et al., 1991; Sudhalter, Cohen, Silverman, & Wolf-Schein, 1990). Several studies have demonstrated that males with FXS produce more perseverative language than do linguistic level-matched typically developing children (Levy et al., 2006) or developmental level-matched males with autism, DS, or other forms of intellectual disability (Belser & Sudhalter, 2001; Ferrier et al., 1991; Roberts et al., 2007; Sudhalter et al., 1990; Sudhalter, Maranion, & Brooks, 1992; Sudhalter, Scarborough,

& Cohen, 1991, but see Paul et al., 1987, for an exception).

Although several hypotheses about the causes of perseveration in FXS have been advanced, only two have received any empirical support. In one hypothesis, frontal lobe abnormalities are thought to result in a failure to inhibit personally salient or previously activated responses, leading to the intrusion of idiosyncratic or previously produced content (Abbeduto & Hagerman, 1997). This hypothesis is supported by the well-documented finding that individuals with FXS, particularly males, have problems with sustained and directed attention as well as impulsive responding (Baumgardner et al., 1995; Cohen, 1995; Hagerman, 1996; Hatton et al., 1999; Lachiewicz et al., 1994; Miller et al., 1999). The second hypothesis is that a problem in regulating the autonomic nervous system, which results in hyperarousal, may exacerbate problems in inhibitory control, particularly in anxiety-provoking situations (Belser & Sudhalter, 1995; Cohen, 1995). This latter hypothesis is supported by the finding that, compared to typically developing controls, youth with FXS (again, particularly males) display higher levels of cortisol, as well as physiological and behavioral signs of an inability to adapt to stressful situations (Belser & Sudhalter, 1995; Hessl et al., 2006; Miller et al., 1999; Wisbeck et al., 2000).

Perseveration, however, may be a more complex problem than previously recognized. In particular, Murphy and Abbeduto (2007) found that the rates of perseveration of different types of verbal units (i.e., topics, rote conversational phrases, or within-utterance syllables, words, or phrases) by adolescent males and females with FXS were influenced by different variables. In particular, the rates of some types of perseveration varied with gender, whereas the rates of other types varied with the contexts in which speaking took place (i.e., conversation and narration). Murphy and Abbeduto suggest that multiple, interacting factors account for perseveration in FXS.

Within-syndrome Variation in the Linguistic Phenotype of Fragile X Syndrome
GENDER DIFFERENCES

As expected for an X-linked disorder, FXS differentially affects the sexes. This difference reflects in large measure differences in fragile X mental retardation protein (FMRP) levels, with females having higher levels due to the presence of a second X chromosome carrying a healthy *FMR1* allele. Thus, the prevalence of affected individuals is 1 in

2,500-4,000 males and 1 in 4,000-6,000 females (Crawford, Acuna, & Sherman et al., 2001; Hagerman, 2008). In terms of broad measures of functioning, such as IQ, males with FXS are more severely delayed in their development and more likely to display psychopathology, on average, than are females with FXS (Keysor & Mazzocco, 2002). Despite the difference in the severity of affectedness, the profile of relative cognitive strengths and weaknesses and the pattern of development associated with FXS are not thought to vary according to gender (Dykens, Hodapp, & Finucane, 2000; Kau, Meyer, & Kaufmann, 2002; Keysor & Mazzocco, 2002). For example, sequential processing is more impaired than simultaneous processing in both males and females with the syndrome (Hagerman, 1999). For the most part, recent data on studies of language and communication involving direct comparisons of males and females under comparable measurement conditions also support this conclusion for all stages of development and components of language investigated to date.

The transition from prelinguistic to linguistic communication is more delayed in males than in females with FXS. In the Brady et al. (2006) study, 35 (80%) of 44 boys with FXS boys and seven (64%) of 11 girls with FXS were reported by their parents to communicate only nonverbally. The mean CA of the prelinguistic girls was reported to be 18.5 months compared to 26.4 months for the prelinguistic boys. More studies of the prelinguistic period in FXS are needed, particularly those employing direct observation and longitudinal designs, so as to determine if the sequence of prelinguistic achievements is similar in males and females, which would yield insights into whether gender differences during this period of development are only quantitative in nature.

Gender differences in the extent of delay in vocabulary development in FXS have also been documented. Among the adolescents and young adults studied by Abbeduto et al. (2003), males achieved lower age-equivalent scores on the TACL-R compared to females, including on the subtest measuring vocabulary; however, receptive vocabulary scores on the TACL-R were appropriate for the participants' NVMAs for both males and females, suggesting a global delay that is greater in males than females. Unfortunately, other studies of vocabulary have purposely excluded females with FXS (Philofsky, Hepburn, Hays, & Hagerman, 2004; Roberts et al., 2001, 2002) and thus, little else is known about the vocabulary development of girls.

The evidence on morphosyntactic development also indicates that females with FXS are less impaired, on average, than same-aged males with FXS, but with no evidence of qualitative differences (Fisch et al., 1999). In one such study, Abbeduto et al. (2003) found that, although the female adolescents and young adults with FXS had higher age-equivalent scores, on average, than did the similarly aged male participants with FXS on all of the TACL-R subtests, the magnitude of the difference was constant across subtests. Moreover, both males and females achieved scores on all subtests that were appropriate for their NVMAs. These results suggest a profile of delayed, but synchronous, development across the different strands of receptive morphosyntax and between receptive morphosyntax and nonverbal cognition for males and females with FXS—a profile of quantitative, not qualitative, differences. However, this study included only 13 males and six females; thus, there is a need for additional comparisons of males and females with larger samples of participants, as well as for studies of different segments of the life course before firm conclusions are possible.

Problems in pragmatics also appear to be more severe for males than for females with FXS, and this appears true for both the development of pragmatic competencies and the occurrence of atypical pragmatic behaviors; however, there is no evidence of qualitative differences. In their study of noncomprehension signaling ability, Abbeduto et al. (2008) found that, among the adolescents and young adults with FXS in their sample, the females were significantly more likely to recognize and take steps to solicit more information when faced with inadequate messages than were the males. Moreover, this difference was found even after controlling for differences in NVMA, reflecting the fact that the females signaled noncomprehension at a NVMA-appropriate rate, whereas the males signaled at a rate below NVMA expectations. Importantly, the difference in rate of noncomprehension signaling was constant across the different types of inadequate directions, again suggesting that the differences between males and females were quantitative, not qualitative, in nature.

In their study of the maladaptive pragmatic behaviors, Murphy and Abbeduto (2007) examined the relationship between different types of perseverative language and both gender and sampling context in adolescents and young adults with FXS. Murphy and Abbeduto found that the males produced more conversational device repetitions (i.e., repetition of rote phrases typically used to manage an interaction, such as "that's it" and "that's a wrap") than did the females. Additionally, it was found that more topic repetitions were produced by both males and females in conversation than in the more structured context of narration, which suggests that similar mechanisms may underlie the occurrence of perseveration in both genders. Again, these findings support the conclusion that only quantitative gender differences exist for those with FXS in the pragmatic domain.

DIFFERENCES RELATED TO AUTISM STATUS

Individuals with FXS and comorbid autism (or autism spectrum disorders, ASD) have been found to have lower IQs, on average, than individuals with only one of these disorders (Bailey et al., 1998; Bailey, Hatton, Skinner, & Mesibov, 2001a; Kaufmann et al., 2004; Lewis et al., 2006; McDuffie, Abbeduto, Lewis, Kover, Kim, & Brown, 2010). This observation, together with the social impairments inherent in the diagnosis of autism, lead to the hypothesis that language should also be especially impaired in the comorbid group relative to individuals with only FXS. In fact, the evidence suggests a more nuanced picture of the linguistic profile associated with comorbid FXS and autism.

There is evidence that language development in individuals with comorbid FXS and autism is delayed to a greater extent than is true in individuals with FXS without autism (but see Price et al., 2007, for an exception). For example, Philofsky and colleagues (2004) found that toddlers and preschoolers with both FXS and autism performed worse on both the expressive and receptive scales of the Mullen Scales of Early Learning (Mullen, 1995) compared to children with only FXS or only autism. In a study of older children, Roberts et al. (2001) found that the presence of autism was associated with an increased degree of language impairment, as measured by the Reynell scales, in children with FXS. Similar results have been reported by Bailey et al. (2001a).

Although these studies are important in demonstrating an impact of autism status on language, their reliance on broad summary measures of language that do not distinguish between different language domains makes it impossible to discern the precise impact of this comorbid condition. The importance of making finer distinctions is highlighted by the finding that receptive language is more of a problem than expressive language for individuals with comorbid FXS and autism, at least when very broad summary measures of these different modalities are employed; however, a similar receptive–expressive difference has been reported for individuals with only FXS (Lewis et al., 2006; Philofsky et al., 2004).

Further evidence of the unique linguistic profile of individuals with comorbid FXS and autism is provided by several recent studies. Using the TACL-R, Lewis et al. (2006) found that receptive language was more impaired relative to nonverbal cognition in adolescents and young adults with FXS who had comorbid autism compared to those with FXS only. Moreover, the magnitude of the difference between these two groups was similar for grammatical morphology, multiword combinatorial rules, and vocabulary, suggesting that receptive language in general is negatively affected by autism status. Receptive language is an area of special challenge for individuals with idiopathic autism as well (Tager-Flusberg, Paul, Lord, 2005), which suggests that receptive language impairments may be central to autism regardless of the co-occurring condition. Replications are needed, however, with larger samples of varying ages and with a more comprehensive battery of measures of various language domains.

In contrast to Lewis et al. (2006), Roberts et al. (2007) focused on the pragmatic aspects of the speaker role. The sample included boys with FXS with and without a comorbid ASD between the ages of 3 and 14 years, all of whom produced at least some word combinations in their spontaneous language samples. Roberts et al. also included NVMA-matched comparison groups of typically developing boys and boys with DS. Conversations between each boy and an examiner during standardized testing were coded to assess a number of pragmatic skills and atypical pragmatic behaviors. Among other things, Roberts et al. found that the boys with FXS and comorbid ASD were the most impaired of the groups, being more likely to maintain old or initiate new topics by producing turns with no conceptual relation to the immediately prior discourse. Although the rate of perseveration was higher among boys with FXS only than among the typically developing boys or those with DS, the boys with comorbid FXS and ASD produced the highest rates of perseveration of any group. Thus, comorbid ASDs in FXS, as in idiopathic cases (Tager-Flusberg et al., 2005), are associated not only with unusually severe impairments in understanding the more formal aspects of language, but also in dealing with the more social elements of language when speaking.

Kover and Abbeduto (2010) examined the conversations and narratives of adolescents and young adults with FXS in relation to autism status. These investigators found that after controlling for IQ, participants with comorbid FXS and autism produced speech that was less intelligible than those with only FXS. Whether this reflects a motor difference or a higher-level language or cognitive difference remains to be determined.

Factors Contributing to Language Development and Impairments in Fragile X Syndrome

In this section, we consider the factors that lead to the emergence of the FXS linguistic phenotype and variation in the phenotype across individuals. We consider the contributions to language learning from both genetic and environmental factors. Although there is no doubt that other genes affect and are affected by the FMR1 gene and that individuals may have different alleles of these "background" genes (Belmonte & Bourgeron, 2006), these genes have yet to be identified and thus, we leave this topic for the future.

CONTRIBUTIONS FROM THE *FMR1* MUTATION

Variations in many dimensions of the FXS behavioral phenotype have been shown to be related to variation in the *FMR1* mutation (Brown, 2002). Among males with the full mutation, there is variation in terms of the size of the CGG expansion, the extent to which there is methylation (i.e., a silencing) of the genes, and whether some cells contain the premutation rather than the full mutation (Nolin et al., 1994). Among females, there is similar variation, but also variation in the relative proportion of cells in which the affected X chromosome, rather than the healthy allele, is active or functioning (Tassone, Hagerman, Chamberlain, & Hagerman, 2000). Such variations among males and females with the full mutation are important because they are associated with variations in levels of FMRP, the protein normally produced by the gene and that has been found to play a critical role in synapse maturation and functioning (Koukoui & Chaudhuri, 2007). In light of the involvement of FMRP in neural development, correlations of FMRP with language would be expected.

In studies of the relation of measures of *FMR1* variation to language development, the focus has been on gross measures of language learning products. For example, Bailey et al. (2001b) found that FMRP levels of young boys with FXS were positively correlated with their VABS Communication domain scores.

Kuo et al. (2002) found that activation ratios of young girls with FXS predicted verbal IQ. In a study of adult females with FXS, most with IQs in the normal range, Simon et al. (2001) found a positive correlation between activation ratio and story comprehension ability. Together, these studies suggest that FMRP is involved in the development of those brain systems involved in language. However, given the numerous brain systems engaged by complex language tasks, identifying the neural mediators of the FMRP–language relationship in FXS remains a formidable task. Because FMRP (and related biological measures) may be more closely related to some dimensions of behavior than to others (Cornish, Munir & Cross, 2001), mapping the involvement of FMRP in language at a neural level will require that researchers move away from a reliance on broad summary measures of language and toward more fine-grained measures. Moreover, FMRP is correlated with many dimensions of the FXS phenotype, including a range of cognitive skills and symptoms of comorbid conditions (Bailey et al., 2001a, b; Cohen et al., 1996; Kwon et al., 2001; Loesch et al., 2002, 2007; Loesch, Huggins, & Hagerman, 2004; Menon, Kwon, Eliez, Taylor, & Reiss, 2000; Reiss et al., 1995; Riddle et al., 1998; Tassone et al., 1999; Willemsen, Olmer, De Diego Otero, & Oostra, 2000), which raises the possibility that the relationship between *FMR1* and language may be mediated, not only by intervening neural systems, but by other domains of competence and behavior.

Although significant correlations between FMRP (and related measures) and language have emerged, the correlations have generally been modest, accounting for a relatively small proportion of variance in language outcomes. These less than impressive correlations may reflect, in part, limitations of the biological markers themselves. In particular, estimates of FMRP from lymphocytes can be assumed to be virtually identical to FMRP in brain tissue for males with the full mutation, but may not be in females and mosaic males (Brown, 2002). Moreover, these studies relied on a measure of FMRP that is not truly quantitative, as it reflects the proportion of cells expressing FMRP rather than the amount of FMRP expressed in each cell – new, truly quantitative, measures are beginning to be used. Caution in interpreting findings, particularly null findings, is necessary, therefore, for these latter groups.

CONTRIBUTIONS FROM THE ENVIRONMENT

Variations in the environment, especially in interactions with parents and other adults, shape the trajectory of language development for typically developing children (Hart & Risely, 1995; Hoff-Ginsberg, 1991. For example, maternal responsivity has been found to be a particularly important determinant of variations in vocabulary and pragmatic development in typically developing children (Bornstein & Tamis-LeMonda, 1989; Gleitman, Newport & Gleitman, 1984; Masur, 1982; Pine, 1994; Tomasello & Farrar, 1984; Tamis-LeMonda et al., 1996) as well as in children with various developmental disabilities (Hauser-Cram et al., 2001; Mahoney, 1988; Siller & Sigman, 2002; Yoder & Warren, 1999). This maternal style of interaction is characterized by high rates of positive, contingent responding to child initiations, while not being overly directive in attempting to change the child's focus of attention (Girolametto, Greenberg, & Manolson, 1986; Spiker et al., 2002). Maternal responsivity and other aspects of the environment have been hypothesized to account for some dimensions of the characteristic phenotype and of individual differences in the phenotype (Murphy & Abbeduto, 2005). Data supporting this hypothesis have recently come from a study by Warren and colleagues of parents interacting with their young children with FXS (Warren, Brady, Sterling, Fleming, & Marquis, 2010); however, replications and extension to different age periods are needed.

Studies of maternal responsivity in FXS should be an especially high priority as there are reasons to believe that, as a group, mothers of individuals with FXS may find it difficult to engage successfully in reciprocal interactions with their children. First, biological mothers who carry the *FMR1* full mutation may have cognitive deficits, increased social anxiety, and depression (Abbeduto, Seltzer, Krauss, Orsmond, & Murphy, 2004), which could impact their responsivity. In addition, some reports indicate increased rates of affective disorders or at least stress among women who carry the premutation (Hagerman & Hagerman, 2002; Roberts, Bailey, & Mankowsky); for example, Abbeduto and colleagues (2004) found that mothers of adolescents with FXS were more pessimistic about their son's and daughter's future and had more depressive symptoms than did mothers of adolescents with DS. Lower levels of maternal psychological well-being may interfere with maternal responsivity (Murphy & Abbeduto, 2005). Second, the behaviors characteristic of children with FXS are likely to affect the ways in which mothers interact with their sons and daughters, limiting the extent to which mothers can provide responsive language input (Murphy & Abbeduto, 2005). Gaze avoidance; hypersensitivity to sensory input; social anxiety; perseveration; stereotypical and challenging behaviors; delays in speech, language, and prelinguistic social communication skills; and autistic-like behaviors may provide mothers with fewer opportunities to be responsive to their children, even when they are motivated to do so (Abbeduto et al., 2007; Bailey et al., 1998). In short, characteristics of mothers and of their children with FXS may lead to less responsive interactions with the child, thereby leading to poorer linguistic outcomes in the children.

Conclusion

In general, individuals with FXS display delays in all domains of language learning and use that have been examined to date; however, more serious delays and impairments occur in some areas. Most notably, pragmatics appears to be an area of especially great challenge, with below-MA performance being the norm; development of the form and content of language (i.e., vocabulary and morphosyntax) tends to more or less keep pace with nonverbal cognitive development, although there may be aspects of morphosyntactic that are unusually challenging. Aspects of the linguistic profile described for FXS, including perseveration and referential communication, are different from those of other neurodevelopmental disorders, although comparisons with a larger number of such disorders are necessary before we can confidently accept this conclusion. Substantial within-syndrome variation also occurs, in the extent of delays and in conformity to the phenotype. Males with FXS do more poorly in language than do females with FXS, with such differences being best conceptualized in terms of degree of impairment rather than qualitatively distinct profiles. Autism status is also associated with fairly substantial differences in language profiles. In particular, receptive vocabulary and morphosyntax appear to be especially impaired in those individuals with FXS who also have an autism diagnosis compared to those with FXS and no comorbid autism diagnosis. Individual biological variation, especially in FMRP levels, is also associated with differences in language, with less FMRP in lymphocytes being associated with lower levels of language, at least at a gross level. The environment also contributes to individual differences in language in FXS; however, those characteristics of the environment that are responsible for language differences are only beginning to be understood.

There remains much that we do not know, however, about the typical course of language learning and use in FXS. There is a pressing need for more data on the early developmental period for children with FXS, including data on the period of prelinguistic intentional communication. Although vocabulary does not appear to be an area of special concern for FXS, studies to date have focused largely on the mastery of concrete vocabulary and thus, there is a need to gather data on the learning of more abstract types of words. We also need to know more about the processes by which individuals with FXS learn new words, using paradigms created to study online word learning in typically developing children. Because studies of morphosyntactic development have relied almost exclusively on broad, summary measures, such as MLU, we know little about the profile of impairments in FXS or their causes. Data on the sequence of morphosyntactic acquisitions and on the types of errors made prior to mastery would be useful in this regard. There is also a need for more data on the relationship between pragmatic development and other dimensions of the FXS behavioral phenotype, including executive function (Cornish et al., 2004) and attention (Mirrett et al., 2003). These gaps in our understanding limit our ability to develop effective interventions for this population.

There is also a need for more research on within-syndrome variation for virtually all domains of language. Additional data are needed on gender differences in language for individuals with FXS. This will require designs in which males and females with FXS are compared under similar measurement conditions. Such studies are necessary to determine whether gender differences in language are quantitative or qualitative in nature (Murphy & Abbeduto, 2003). Further, there is a need for more data regarding the linguistic profiles of those with FXS who do and do not have a comorbid diagnosis of autism. Studies of the relationship between autism status and pragmatics are especially important given the deficits in social reciprocity that are requisite for a diagnosis of autism.

We also require more data on parent–child interactions and the ways in which those interactions affect children's subsequent learning and use of language. It is reasonable to hypothesize that the lower levels of psychological well-being characteristic of some mothers who carry the full or premutation of the *FMR1* gene, together with the many challenging behaviors of their children, might make it difficult for these dyads to engage in the responsive interactions that have been shown to facilitate language

learning for both typically developing children and children who face challenges in acquiring language and communication skills. Such data are critical for determining the need for, and nature of, parent-focused interventions.

There is need for researchers to take more of a developmental approach to the study of language learning and use in FXS. It is clear that the FXS phenotype, including its linguistic characteristics, emerges and changes over the life course; however, there is much that we do not understand about the course of development. Thus, more studies employing developmental, and preferably longitudinal, designs are needed, so that the development of well-defined dimensions of language learning and use can be identified, especially in relation to developments in other domains (e.g., nonverbal cognition). Additionally, there is a need to apply developmental models to understanding the causes of the developmental trajectories observed. Minimally, such models will need to take into account the dynamic relationships among genes, environments, and individual characteristics and profiles (Murphy & Abbeduto, 2005). A developmental approach would allow us to provide more complete information to families and professionals about likely outcomes for individuals with FXS in the language domain. In addition, identifying the predictors of language development, especially the early predictors, and targeting these predictors within the context of intervention studies will allow us, ultimately, to design interventions that will optimize language outcomes for individuals with FXS.

Acknowledgments
Preparation of this manuscript was supported by NIH grants R01 HD024356, R01 HD054764, R03 HD048884, P30 HD003352, P30 HD002528, and P30 HD003110, and by a fellowship awarded to S. T. Kover by the Graduate School of the University of Wisconsin-Madison.

References
Abbeduto, L., Brady, N., & Kover, S. (2007). Language development and fragile X syndrome: Profiles, syndrome-specificity, and within-syndrome differences. *Mental Retardation and Developmental Disabilities Research Reviews, 13*, 36–46.

Abbeduto, L., Evans, J., & Dolan, T. (2001). Theoretical perspectives on language and communication problems in mental retardation and developmental disabilities. *Mental Retardation and Developmental Disabilities Research Reviews, 7*, 45–55.

Abbeduto, L., & Hagerman, R. (1997). Language and communication in fragile X syndrome. *Mental Retardation and Developmental Disabilities Research Reviews, 3*, 313–322.

Abbeduto, L., & Murphy, M. M. (2004). Language, social cognition, maladaptive behavior, and communication in Down syndrome and fragile X syndrome. In M. Rice, and S. F. Warren (Eds.), *Developmental language disorders: From phenotypes to etiologies.* Mahwah, NJ: Erlbaum.

Abbeduto, L., Murphy, M., Cawthon, S., Richmond, E., Amman, A., Beth, P., et al. (2006). Collaboration in referential communication: Comparison of youth with Down syndrome or fragile X syndrome. *American Journal on Mental Retardation, 3,* 170–183.

Abbeduto, L., Murphy, M., Cawthon, S., Richmond, E., Weissman, M., Karadottir, S., & O'Brien, A. (2003). Receptive language skills of adolescents and young adults with mental retardation: A comparison of DS and fragile X syndrome. *American Journal on Mental Retardation, 108,* 149–160.

Abbeduto, L., Seltzer, M. M., Krauss, M., Orsmond, G., & Murphy, M. (2004). Psychological well-being and coping in mothers of youths with autism, Down syndrome, or fragile X syndrome. *American Journal on Mental Retardation, 109*(3), 237–254.

Baddeley, A., Gathercole, S., & Papagno, C. (1998). The phonological loop as a language learning device. *Psychological Review, 105*(1), 158–173.

Bailey, D. B., Jr., Hatton, D. D., & Skinner, M. (1998). Early developmental trajectories of males with fragile X syndrome. *American Journal on Mental Retardation, 103,* 29–39.

Bailey, D. B., Jr., Hatton, D. D., Skinner, M., & Mesibov, G. (2001a). Autistic behavior, FMR1 protein, and developmental trajectories in young males with fragile X syndrome. *Journal of Autism and Developmental Disorders, 31,* 165–174.

Bailey, D. B., Hatton, D. D., Tassone, F., Skinner, M., & Taylor, A. K. (2001b). Variability in FMRP and early development in males with fragile X syndrome. *American Journal on Mental Retardation, 106,* 16–27.

Bailey, D., Mesibov, G. B., Hatton, D. D., Clark, R. D., Roberts, J. E., & Mayhew, L. (1998). Autistic behavior in young boys with fragile X syndrome. *Journal of Autism and Developmental Disorders, 28,* 499–508.

Bailey, D. B., Roberts, J. E., Hooper, S. R., Mirrett, P. L., Roberts, J. E., & Schaaf, J. M. (2004). Research on fragile X syndrome and autism. Implications for the study of genes, environments, and developmental language disorders. In M. Rice, & S. F. Warren (Eds.), *Genes, environments, and language disorders.* Mahwah, NJ: Lawrence Erlbaum.

Baldwin, D. A., Markman, E. M., Bill, B., Desjardins, R. N., & Irwin, J. M. (1996). Infants' reliance on a social criterion for establishing word-object relations. *Child Development, 67,* 3135–3153.

Bates, E., O'Connell, B., & Shore, C. (1987). Language and communication in infancy. In J. D. Osofsky (Ed.), *Handbook of infant development* (pp. 149–203). New York: John-Wiley & Sons.

Baumgardner, T. L., Reiss, A. L., Freund, L. S., & Abrams, M. T. (1995). Specification of the neurobehavioral phenotype in males with fragile X syndrome. *Pediatrics, 95,* 744–752.

Belmonte, M. K., & Bourgeron, T. (2006). Fragile X syndrome and autism at the intersection of genetic and neural networks. *Nature Neuroscience, 9,* 1221–1225.

Belser, R., & Sudhalter, V. (1995). Arousal difficulties in males with fragile X syndrome: A preliminary report. *Developmental Brain Dysfunction, 8,* 270–279.

Belser, R., & Sudhalter, V. (2001). Conversational characteristics of children with fragile X syndrome: Repetitive speech. *American Journal on Mental Retardation, 106,* 28–38.

Bornstein, M. H., & Tamis-LeMonda, C. S. (1989). Maternal responsiveness and cognitive development in children. In M. H. Bornstein (Ed.), *Maternal responsiveness: Characteristics and consequences: New directions for child development.* (pp. 49–61). San Francisco: Jossey-Bass.

Brady, N., Marquis, J., Fleming, K., & McLean, L. (2004). Prelinguistic predictors of language growth in children with developmental disabilities. *Journal of Speech, Language and Hearing Research, 47,* 663–667.

Brady, N., Skinner, M., Roberts, J., & Hennon, E. (2006). Communication in young children with fragile X syndrome: A qualitative study of mothers' perspectives. *American Journal of Speech-Language Pathology, 15,* 353–64.

Bregman, J. D., Dykens, E., Watson, M., Ort, S. I., & Leckman, J. F. (1987). Fragile-X syndrome: Variability of phenotypic expression. *Journal of the American Academy of Adolescent Psychiatry, 26,* 463–471.

Bregman, J. D., Leckman, J. F., & Ort, S. I. (1988b). Fragile X syndrome: Genetic predisposition to psychopathology. *Journal of Autism & Developmental Disorders, 18*(3), 343–354.

Brown, W. T. (2002). The molecular biology of the fragile X mutation. In R. Hagerman, & P. J. Hagerman (Eds.), *Fragile X syndrome: Diagnosis, treatment and research* (3rd ed., pp 110–135). Baltimore: Johns Hopkins University Press.

Carrow-Woolfolk, E. (1985). *Test for Auditory Comprehension of Language-Revised.* Allen, TX: DLM Teaching Resources.

Chapman, R. (2000). Children's language learning: An interactionist perspective. *Journal of Child Psychology and Psychiatry, and Allied Disciplines, 41,* 33–54.

Chapman, R. (2003). Language and communication in individuals with Down syndrome. In L. Abbeduto (Ed.), *International review of research in mental retardation, Vol. 26,* (1–34). New York: Academic Press.

Chomsky, N. (1965). *Aspects of the theory of syntax.* Cambridge, MA: M.I.T. Press.

Cohen, I. L. (1995). A theoretical analysis of the role of hyperarousal in the learning and behavior of fragile X males. *Mental Retardation and Developmental Disabilities Research Reviews, 1,* 286–291.

Cohen, A. L., Nolin, S. L., Sudhalter, V., Ding, X., Dobkin, C. S., & Brown, W. T. (1996). Mosaicism for the FMR1 gene influences adaptive skills development in fragile X-affected males. *American Journal of Medical Genetics, 64,* 365–369.

Cornish, K. M., Munir, F., & Cross, G. (2001). Differential impact of the FMR-1 full mutation on memory and attention functioning: A Neuropsychological perspective. *Journal of Cognitive Neuroscience, 13,* 144–150.

Cornish, K., Sudhalter, V., & Turk, J. (2004). Attention and language in fragile X. *Mental Retardation and Developmental Disabilities Research Reviews, 10,* 11–16.

Crawford, D. C., Acuna, J. M., & Sherman, S. L. (2001). FMR1 and the fragile X syndrome: Human genome epidemiology review. *Genetics in Medicine, 3,* 359–371.

DeCasper, A. J., & Fifer, W. P. (1980). Of human bonding: Newborns prefer their mothers' voices. *Science, 208,* 1174–1176.

Dyer-Friedman, J., Glaser, B., Hessl, D., Johnston, C., Huffman, L. C., Taylor, A., et al. (2002). Genetic and environmental influences on the cognitive outcomes of children with fragile X syndrome. *Journal of the American Academy of Child and Adolescent Psychiatry, 41,* 237–244.

Dykens, E., Hodapp, R., & Finucane, B. (2000). *Genetics and mental retardation syndromes: A new look at behavior and interventions.* Baltimore: Brookes.

Dykens, E., Hodapp, R., Ort, S., & Finucane, B. (1989). The trajectory of cognitive development in males with fragile X syndrome. *Journal of the American Academy of Child and Adolescent Psychiatry, 28,* 422–426.

Farroni, T., Menon, E., & Johnson, M. H. (2006). Factors influencing newborns' preference for faces with eye contact. *Journal of Experimental Child Psychology, 95,* 298–308.

Ferrier, L., Bashir, A., Meryash, D., Johnston, J., & Wolff, P. (1991). Conversational skill of individuals with fragile X syndrome: A comparison with autism and DS. *Developmental Medicine and Child Neurology, 33,* 776–788.

Finestack, L.H., & Abbeduto, L. (2010). Expressive language profiles of verbally expressive adolescents and young adults with Down syndrome or fragile X syndrome. *Journal of Speech, Language, and Hearing Research, 53,* 1334–1348.

Fisch, G. S., Holden, J. J. A., Carpenter, N. J., Howard-Peebles, P. N., Maddalena, A., Pandya, A., & Nance, W. (1999). Age-related language characteristics of children and adolescents with fragile X syndrome. *American Journal of Medical genetics, 83,* 253–256.

Freund, L. S., Reiss, A. L., & Abrams, M. T. (1993). Psychiatric disorders associated with fragile X in the young female. *Pediatrics, 91*(2), 321–329.

Girolametto, L., Verbey, M., & Tannock, R. (1994). Improving joint engagement in parent-child interaction: An intervention study. *Journal of Early Intervention, 18*(2), 155–167.

Gleitman, L. R., Newport, E. L., & Gleitman, H. (1984). The current status of the motherese hypothesis. *Journal of Child Language, 11,* 43–79.

Hagerman, P. (2008). The fragile X prevalence paradox. *Journal of Medical Genetics, 45,* 498–499.

Hagerman, R. (1999). *Neurodevelopmental disorders.* Oxford: Oxford University Press.

Hagerman, R. (1996). Physical and behavioral phenotype. In R. J. Hagerman, & A. Cronister (Eds.), *Fragile X Syndrome: Diagnosis, treatment, and research* (pp. 3–87). Baltimore: The Johns Hopkins University Press.

Hagerman, R. J., & Hagerman, P. J. (2002). Fragile X Syndrome: Diagnosis, treatment, and research. Baltimore: Johns Hopkins University Press.

Hart, B., & Risley, T. R. (1995). *Meaningful differences in the everyday experience of young American children*: Baltimore: Paul H. Brookes Publishing.

Hatton, D. D., Bailey, D. B., Jr., Hargett-Beck, M. Q., Skinner, M., & Clark, R. D. (1999). Behavioral style of young boys with fragile X syndrome. *Developmental Medicine & Child Neurology, 41*(9), 625–632.

Hauser-Cram, P., Warfield, M. E., Shonkoff, J. P., Krauss, M. N., Upshur, C. C., & Sayer, A. (2001). Children with disabilities: A longitudinal study of child development and parent well-being. *Monographs of the Society for Research in Child Development, 66*(3), 1–131.

Hessl, D., Glaser, B., Dyer-Friedman, J., & Reiss, A. L. (2006). Social behavior and cortisol reactivity in children with fragile X syndrome. *Journal of Child Psychology and Psychiatry, and Allied Disciplines, 47*(6), 602–610.

Hoff-Ginsberg, E. (1991). Mother-child conversations in different social classes and communicative settings. *Child Development, 62,* 782–796.

Hollich, G. J., Hirsh-Pasek, K., Golinkoff, R. M., Brand, R. J., Brown, E., Chung, H. L., et al. (2000). Breaking the language barrier: An emergentist coalition model for the origins of word learning. *Monographs of the Society for Research in Child Development, 65,* 1–123.

Jusczyk, P. W., Houston, D. M., & Newsome, M. (1999). The beginnings of word segmentation in English-learning infants. *Cognitive Psychology, 39,* 159–207.

Kau, A. S. M., Meyer, W. M., & Kaufmann, W. E. (2002). Early development in males with fragile X syndrome: A review of the literature. *Microscopy Research and Technique, 57,* 174–178.

Kaufmann, W. E., Cortell, R., Kau, A. S. M., Bukelis, I., Tierney, E., Gray, R. M., et al. (2004). Autism Spectrum Disorder in fragile X syndrome: Communication, social interaction, and specific behaviors. *American Journal of Medical Genetics, 129A,* 225–234.

Keller-Bell, Y. D., & Abbeduto, L. (2007). Narrative development in adolescents and young adults with fragile X syndrome. *American Journal on Mental Retardation, 112,* 289–299.

Keysor, C., & Mazzocco, M. (2002). Physiological arousal in females with fragile X or Turner syndrome. *Developmental Psychobiology, 41,* 133–146.

Kover, S.T., & Abbeduto, L. (2010). Expressive language in male adolescents with fragile X syndrome with and without comorbid autism. *Journal of Intellectual Disability Research, 54,* 246–265.

Kuo, A. Y., Reiss, A. L., Freund, L. S., & Huffman, L. C. (2002). Family environment and cognitive abilities in girls with fragile-X syndrome. *Journal of Intellectual Disability Research, 46,* 328–340.

Koukoui, S.D., & Chaudhuri, A. (2007). Neuroanatomical, molecular genetic, and behavioral correlates of fragile X syndrome. *Brain Research Reviews, 53,* 27–38.

Kwon, H., Menon, V., Eliez, S., Warsofsky, I. S., White, C. D., Dyer-Friedman, J., et al. (2001). Functional neuroanatomy of visuospatial working memory in fragile X syndrome: Relation to behavioral and molecular measures. *American Journal of Psychiatry, 158,* 1040–1051.

Lachiewicz, A. M., Spiridigliozzi, G. A., Gullion, C. M., Ransford, S. N., & Rao, K. (1994). Aberrant behaviors of young boys with fragile X syndrome. *American Journal of Mental Retardation, 98*(5), 567–579.

Legerstee, M., Anderson, D., & Schaffer, A. (1998). Five- and eight-month-old infants recognize their faces and voices as familiar and social stimuli. *Child Development, 69,* 37–50.

Levinson, S.C. (1983). *Pragmatics.* Cambridge: Cambridge University Press.

Levy, Y., Gottesman, R., Borochowitz, Z., Frydman, M., & Sagi, M. (2006). Language in boys with fragile X syndrome. *Journal of Child Language, 33,* 125–144.

Lewis, P., Abbeduto, L., Murphy, M., Richmond, E., Giles, N., Bruno, L., & Schroeder, S. (2006). Cognitive language and social-cognitive skills of individuals with fragile X syndrome with and without autism. *Journal of Intellectual Disability Research, 50,* 532–545.

Loesch, D. Z., Huggins, R. M., Bui, Q. M., Epstein, R. M., Taylor, A. K., & Hagerman, R. J. (2002). Effects of the deficits of fragile X mental retardation protein on cognitive status of fragile X males and females assessed by robust pedigree analysis. *Developmental and Behavioral Pediatrics, 23,* 416–423.

Loesch, D. Z., Huggins, R. M., & Hagerman, R. J. (2004). Phenotypic variation and FMRP levels in fragile X. *Mental Retardation and Developmental Disabilities Research Reviews, 10*(1), 31–41.

Loesch, D. Z., Bui, Q. M., Dissanyake, C., Clifford, S., Gould, E., Bulhak-Paterson, D., et al. (2007). Molecular and cognitive predictors of the continuum of autistic behaviors in fragile X. *Neuroscience and Biobehavioral Reviews, 31,* 315–326.

Madison, L., George, C., & Moeschler, J. (1986). Cognitive functioning in the fragile X syndrome: A study of intellectual, memory, and communication skills. *Journal of Mental Deficiency Research, 30,* 129–148.

Mahoney, G. (1988). Maternal communication style with mentally retarded children. *American Journal on Mental Retardation, 92,* 352–359.

Masur, E. F. (1982). Mothers' responses to infants' object-related gestures: Influences on lexical development. *Journal of Child Language, 9,* 23–30.

Mazzocco, M. M. M., Pennington, B., & Hagerman, R. J. (1993). The neurocognitive phenotype of female carriers of fragile X: Further evidence for specificity. *Journal of Development and Behavioral Pediatrics, 14,* 328–335.

McDuffie, A., Abbeduto, L., Lewis, P., Kover, S.T., Kim, J.-S., & Brown, W.T. (2010). Autism spectrum disorder in children and adolescents with fragile X syndrome: Within-syndrome differences and age-related changes. *American Journal on Intellectual and Developmental Disabilities, 115,* 307–326.

McLean, J., McLean, L., Brady, N., & Etter, R. (1991). Communication profiles of two types of gesture using nonverbal persons with severe to profound mental retardation. *Journal of Speech and Hearing Research, 34,* 294–308.

McLean, L., Brady, N., McLean, J., & Behrens, G. (1998). Communication forms and functions of children and adults with severe mental retardation in community and institutional settings. *Journal of Speech and Hearing Research, 42,* 231–240.

Menon, V., Kwon, H., Eliez, S., Taylor, A. K., & Reiss, A. L. (2000). Functional brain activation during cognition is related to FMR1 gene expression. *Brain Research, 877,* 367–370.

Miller, L. J., McIntosh, D. N., et al (1999). Electrodermal responses to sensory stimuli in individuals with fragile X syndrome: A preliminary report. *American Journal of Medical Genetics, 83,* 268–279.

Mills, D. L., Plunkett, K., Prat, C., & Schafer, G. (2005). Watching the infant brain learn words: Effects of vocabulary size and experience. *Cognitive Development, 20,* 19–31.

Mills, D. L., Prat, C., Zangl, R., Stager, C. L., Neville, H. J., & Werker, J. F. (2004). Language experience and the organization of brain activity to phonetically similar words: ERP evidence from 14- and 20-month-olds. *Journal of Cognitive Neuroscience, 16,* 1452–1464.

Mirrett, P. L., Roberts, J. E., & Price, J. (2003). Early intervention practices and communication intervention strategies for young males with fragile X syndrome. *Language, Speech, and Hearing Services in Schools, 34,* 320–331.

Moore, C., Angelopoulos, M., & Bennett, P. (1999). Word learning in the context of referential and salience cues. *Developmental Psychology, 35*(1), 60–68.

Mullen, E. (1995). *Mullen scales of early learning.* Circle Pines, MN: AGS.

Murphy, M., & Abbeduto, L. (2003). Language and communication in fragile X syndrome. In L. Abbeduto (Ed.), *International review of research in mental retardation* Vol. 26 (pp. 83–119). New York: Academic Press.

Murphy, M. M., & Abbeduto, L. (2005). Indirect genetic effects and the early language development of children with genetic mental retardation syndromes: The role of joint attention. *Infants and Young Children, 18,* 47–59.

Murphy, M. M., & Abbeduto, L. (2007). Gender differences in repetitive language in fragile X syndrome. *Journal of Intellectual Disability Research, 51,* 387–390.

Nolin, S. L., Glicksman, A., Houck, G. E., Jr., Brown, W. T., & Dobkin, C. S. (1994). Mosaicism in fragile X affected males. *American Journal of Medical Genetics, 51*(4), 509–512.

Paul, R., Cohen, D., Breg, R., Watson, M., & Herman, S. (1984). Fragile X syndrome: Its relations to speech and language disorders. *Journal of Speech and Hearing Disorders, 49,* 326–336.

Paul, R., Dykens, E., Leckman, F., Watson, M., Breg, W., & Cohen, D. (1987). A comparison of language characteristics of mentally retarded adults with fragile X syndrome and those with nonspecific mental retardation and autism. *Journal of Autism and Developmental Disorders, 17,* 457–468.

Paul, R., Dykens, E., Leckman, F., Watson, M., Breg, W. R., & Cohen, D. (1987). A comparison of language characteristics of mentally retarded adults with fragile X syndrome and those with nonspecific mental retardation and autism. *Journal of Autism and Developmental Disorders, 17,* 457–468.

Philofsky, A., Hepburn, S., Hayes, A., Hagerman, R., & Rogers, S. (2004). Linguistic and cognitive functioning and autism symptoms in young children with Fragile X syndrome. *American Journal on Mental Retardation, 109,* 208–218.

Pine, J. M. (1994). The language of primary caregivers. In C. Gallaway and B. J. Richards (Eds.), *Input and interaction in language acquisition* (pp. 15–37): Cambridge: Cambridge University Press.

Price, J., Roberts, J., Vandergrift, N., & Martin, G. (2007). Language comprehension in boys with fragile X syndrome and boys with Down syndrome. *Journal of Intellectual Disability Research, 51,* 318–326.

Ramscar, M., & Gitcho, N. (2007). Developmental change and the nature of learning in childhood. *Trends in Cognitive Sciences, 11,* 274–279.

Reiss, A. L., Freund, L. S., Baumgardner, T. L., Abrams, M. T., & Denckla, M. B. (1995). Contribution of the FMR1 gene mutation to human intellectual dysfunction. *Nature Genetics, 11,* 331–334.

Rice, M., Warren, S. F., & Betz, S. (2005). Language symptoms of developmental language disorders: An overview of autism, Down syndrome, fragile X, specific language impairment, and Williams syndrome. *Applied Psycholinguistics, 26,* 7–27.

Riddle, J. E., Cheema, A., Sobesky, W. E., Gardner, S. C., Taylor, A. K., Pennington, B. F., et al. (1998). Phenotypic involvement in females with the FMR1 gene mutation. *American Journal on Mental Retardation, 102,* 590–601.

Roberts, J., Martin, G. E., Moskowitz, L., Harris, A. A., Foreman, J., & Nelson, L. (2007). Discourse skills of boys with fragile X syndrome in comparison to boys with Down syndrome. *Journal of Speech, Language, and Hearing Research, 50,* 475–492.

Roberts, J. E., Mirrett, P., Anderson, K., Burchinal, M., & Neebe, E. (2002). Early communication, symbolic behavior, and social profiles of young males with fragile X syndrome. *American Journal of Speech-Language Pathology, 11,* 295–304.

Roberts, J., Mirrett, P., & Burchinal, M. (2001). Receptive and expressive communication development of young males with fragile X syndrome. *American Journal on Mental Retardation, 106,* 216–230.

Roberts, J.E., Bailey, D., & Mankowsky, J. (2008). Mood and anxiety disorders in females with the FMR1 premutation. *American Journal of Medical Genetics, 150B,* 130–139.

Saffran, J. R. (2002). Constraints on statistical language learning. *Journal of Memory and Language, 47,* 172–196.

Saffran, J., Newport, A., & Aslin, R. (1996). Statistical learning by 8-month-old infants. *Science, 274*, 1926–1928.

Simon, J., Keenan, J., Pennington, B., Taylor, A., & Hagerman, R. (2001). Discourse processing in women with fragile X syndrome: Evidence for a deficit establishing coherence. *Cognitive Neuropsychology, 18*, 1–18.

Siller, M., & Sigman, M. (2002). The behaviors of parents of children with autism predict the subsequent development of their children's communication. *Journal of Autism and Developmental Disorders, 32*(2), 77–89.

Sparrow, S., Balla, D., & Cicchetti, D. (1984). *Vineland adaptive behavior scales.* Circle Pines, MN: American Guidance Co.

Spiker, D., Boyce, G. C., & Boyce, L. K. (2002). Parent-child interactions when young children have disabilities. *International Review of Research in Mental Retardation, 25*, 35–70.

Sudhalter, V., Cohen, I., Silverman, W., & Wolf-Schein, E. (1990). Conversational analysis of males with fragile X, Down syndrome, and autism: Comparison of the emergence of deviant language. *American Journal on Mental Retardation, 94*, 431–441.

Sudhalter, V., Maranion, M., & Brooks, P. (1992). Expressive semantic deficit in the productive language of males with fragile X syndrome. *American Journal of Medical Genetics, 43*, 65–71.

Tager-Flusberg, H., Paul, R., & Lord, C. (2005). Language and communication in autism. In F. R. Volkman, R. Paul, A. Klin, & D. Cohen (Eds.), *Handbook of autism and pervasive developmental disorders, Volume 1: Diagnosis, development, neurobiology, and behavior.* (pp. 335–364). Hoboken, NJ: Wiley.

Tamis-LeMonda, C. S., Bornstein, M. H., Baumwell, L., & Damast, A. M. (1996). Responsive parenting in the second year: Specific influences on children's language and play. *Early Development & Parenting, 5*(4), 173–183.

Tassone, F., Hagerman, R. J., Ikle, D., Dyer, P. N., Lampe, M. N., Willemson, R., et al. (1999). FMRP expressions as a potential prognostic indicator in fragile X syndrome. *American Journal of Medical Genetics, 84*, 250–261.

Tassone, F., Hagerman, R. J., Chamberlain, W. D., & Hagerman, P. J (2000). Transcription of the FMR1 gene in individuals with fragile X syndrome. *American Journal of Medical Genetics, 97*, 195–203.

Tomasello, M. (2003). Constructing a language: A usage-based theory of language acquisition. Cambridge: Harvard University Press.

Tomasello, M., & Farrar, M. J. (1986). Object permanence and relational words: A lexical training study. *Journal of Child Language, 13*, 495–505.

Tomasello, M., & Farrar, M. J. (1984). Cognitive bases of lexical development: Object permanence and relational words. *Journal of Child Language, 11*, 477–493.

Volterra, V., Caselli, M. C., Capirci, O., & Pizzuto, E. (2005). Gesture and the emergence and development of language. In M. Tomasello, & D. Slobin (Eds.), *Beyond nature-nurture: Essays in honor of Elizabeth Bates* (pp 3–41). Mahwah, NJ: Lawrence Erlbaum Associates.

Warren, S., Brady, N., Sterling, A., Fleming, K., & Marquis, J. (2010). Maternal responsivity predicts language in young children with fragile X syndrome. *American Journal of Intellectual and Developmental Disabilities, 115*, 54–75.

Wetherby, A. M., Prizant, B. M., & Hutchinson, T. A. (1998). Communicative, social/affective, and symbolic profiles of young children with autism and pervasive developmental disorders. *American Journal of Speech-Language Pathology, 7*(2), 79–91.

Willemsen, R., Olmer, R., Otero, Y. D., & Oostra, B. A. (2000). Twin sisters, monozygotic with the fragile X mutation, but with a different phenotype. *Journal of Medical Genetics, 37*, 603–604.

Wisbeck, J., Huffman, L., Freund, L., Gunnar, M., Davis, E., & Reiss, A. (2000). Cortisol and social stressors in children with fragile X: A pilot study. *Journal of Developmental and Behavioral Pediatrics, 21*, 278–282.

Yoder, P., Warren, S. F. (1999). Maternal responsivity mediates the relationship between prelinguistic intentional communication and later language. *Journal of Early Intervention, 22*(2), 126–136.

Language Development in Williams Syndrome

Carolyn B. Mervis

Abstract

This chapter begins with a brief description of Williams syndrome (WS). It then summarizes the findings from research on intellectual ability as measured by intelligence tests and considers research on early language acquisition, followed by findings from research on the language abilities of school-aged children and adolescents with WS. A central theme will be that, far from demonstrating the independence of language from cognition, WS provides strong evidence for their interdependence throughout development. The chapter ends with a short section on implications of these findings for future research and for intervention.

Keywords: Williams syndrome, language development, intellectual ability, language acquisition, cognition

Research on the language development of children with developmental disabilities was initially approached from two different perspectives. One group of researchers chose to study children with certain types of developmental disabilities to address theoretical questions that could not be examined in research on typically developing children because the variables of interest could not be manipulated experimentally. A second group of researchers chose to study children with developmental disabilities for practical reasons; this group was concerned with remediating the children's language and educational difficulties. *Language Development in Exceptional Circumstances*, edited by Dorothy Bishop and Kay Mogford and published in 1988, was intended to address the interests of both types of researchers. This book included a chapter on Williams syndrome (WS) by Ursula Bellugi and her colleagues (Bellugi, Marks, Bihrle, & Sabo, 1988) that used data from a small sample of adolescents with WS, a very rare syndrome for which there were only three other published studies of language abilities, to address the theoretical question of whether language was

modular—that is, independent of cognition. This chapter, combined with conference presentations regarding Bellugi's research (e.g., Bates, 1990), brought WS to the attention of researchers concerned with the relation between language and cognition.

The three original studies of the language abilities of children with WS were intended to provide information for practitioners such as speech–language therapists and special education teachers. The findings from these studies did not suggest anything noteworthy about the language abilities of individuals with WS. Both Kataria, Goldstein, and Kushnick (1984) and Meyerson and Frank (1987) reported that the language abilities of children with WS were well below chronological age (CA) expectations. MacDonald and Roy (1988) found that the language abilities of children with WS were at the same level as those of children with other types of developmental disabilities matched for CA and standard score on the Peabody Picture Vocabulary Test-Revised (PPVT-R; Dunn & Dunn, 1981). However, in one of the earliest reports on the general psychological characteristics associated with WS, children with this syndrome were described as having an "unusual command of language," despite severe intellectual disability (von Armin & Engel, 1964, p. 367). Not surprisingly for studies of a syndrome whose estimated prevalence at the time was 1/50,000, all four of these articles were based on very small samples. [For further historical discussion, see Mervis and John (2010b).]

Bellugi et al. (1988) argued that, although the adolescents with WS they studied had severe intellectual disability and were still in Piaget's preoperational period, they nevertheless had excellent language abilities. In particular, although they were unable to conserve either number or quantity, they nevertheless could comprehend and produce complex linguistic constructions such as reversible passives, conditionals, and tag questions. In addition, they had excellent vocabularies, including a variety of unusual words. The combination of the ability to comprehend and produce reversible passives with the inability to conserve led Bellugi et al. to argue that WS provided strong evidence of the independence of language from cognition.

This message quickly attracted the attention of researchers and pundits interested in the relation between language and cognition. Comparisons of the language and cognitive abilities of individuals with WS by authors who had not studied WS directly were considerably more strident than those offered by Bellugi and her colleagues, culminating in Piattelli-Palmarini's statement, "For instance, children with Williams syndrome have barely measurable general intelligence and require constant parental care, yet they have an exquisite mastery of syntax and vocabulary. They are, however, unable to understand even the most immediate implications of their admirably constructed sentences" (2001, p. 887).

The cumulative body of research on language and cognition in WS offers clear evidence that Piattelli-Palmarini's position is untenable and provides a more tempered set of findings than might have been expected from Bellugi et al.'s original report. In the next paragraph, I provide a brief description of WS. In the remainder of the chapter, I briefly summarize the findings from research on intellectual ability as measured by intelligence tests. I then consider research on early language acquisition, followed by research on the language abilities of school-aged children and adolescents with WS. A central theme will be that, far from demonstrating the independence of language from cognition, WS

provides strong evidence for their interdependence throughout development. The chapter ends with a short section on implications of these findings for future research and for intervention.

Williams syndrome is a neurodevelopmental disorder caused by a hemizygous microdeletion of approximately 26 genes on chromosome 7q11.23 (Hillier et al., 2003; Osborne, 2006). This syndrome, which is now considered to have a prevalence of 1/7,500 live births (Strømme, Bjørnstad, & Ramstad, 2003), is associated with a recognizable pattern of physical characteristics, including a specific set of facial features, heart disease (most commonly supravalvar aortic stenosis), connective tissue abnormalities, failure to thrive, and growth deficiency (Morris, 2006; Mervis & Morris, 2007). Individuals with WS have developmental delay that typically leads to mild to moderate intellectual disability or learning difficulties, although some individuals have low average to average intelligence and a smaller proportion have severe intellectual disability. Williams syndrome is characterized by a specific cognitive profile, including relative strengths in verbal short-term memory and language (primarily concrete vocabulary), extreme weakness in visuospatial construction (Mervis et al., 2000), and a specific personality profile, including overfriendliness, gregariousness, and anxiety (Klein-Tasman & Mervis, 2003).

General Intellectual Ability

In this section, I present findings from large-sample studies of the performance of individuals with WS on a variety of standardized assessments of general intellectual ability. These results directly address the claim that individuals with WS have severe intellectual disability or "barely measurable general intelligence."

The most commonly used assessments of the intellectual ability of persons with below-average IQ, including individuals with WS, are the Wechsler tests. Most assessment reports completed by school psychologists and most assessments for vocational placement report IQs derived from these tests. Bellugi, Lichtenberger, Jones, Lai, and St. George (2000) assessed 82 school-aged children and adults with WS on the age-appropriate Wechsler IQ measure (WISC-R; Wechsler, 1974 or WAIS-R; Wechsler, 1981). Mean overall IQ was 55, with a range of 40 to 90. Separate verbal and performance IQs were not reported. Howlin, Davies, and Udwin (1998) reported a mean WAIS-R IQ of 60.85 (range: <40–76) with a mean verbal IQ of 64.55

and a mean performance IQ of 60.77 for 62 adults with WS. Searcy et al. (2004), describing results from a sample of 80 adults with WS, reported slightly higher IQs; mean overall IQ was 67.4, mean verbal IQ was 71.5, and mean performance IQ was 66.0. Of the 80 participants, 19 (24%) had a significantly higher verbal IQ than performance IQ, and one had a significantly higher performance IQ than verbal IQ. Overall, the Wechsler test findings indicate a mean IQ in the mild intellectual disability range, with a range from severe intellectual disability to average intelligence. For most individuals, verbal IQ did not differ significantly from performance IQ.

My laboratory has used the Differential Ability Scales (DAS; Elliott, 1990 or DAS-II; Elliott, 2007) to assess the intellectual abilities of children with WS. These measures provide separate Verbal, Nonverbal Reasoning, and Spatial cluster standard scores as well as an overall General Conceptual Ability standard score (GCA; similar to IQ). Results from 120 children with WS aged 4.01–17.71 years tested with the DAS-II indicated a mean GCA of 64.56 (range: 31–96); mean cluster standard scores were 74.06 for Verbal, 78.89 for Nonverbal Reasoning, and 54.82 for Spatial (Mervis & John, 2010a; see Mervis & Morris, 2007 and Meyer-Lindenberg, Mervis, & Berman, 2006 for findings from the first edition of the DAS). For 86% of the children, Verbal cluster standard score, Nonverbal Reasoning cluster standard score, or both were significantly higher than Spatial cluster standard score. For 2% of the children, Spatial cluster standard score was significantly higher than Verbal cluster standard score (Mervis & John, 2010a). Overall, mean DAS-II GCA is in the mild intellectual disability range, similar to mean overall Wechsler IQ. However, a much higher proportion of children showed significant discrepancies between cluster standard scores than showed a significant difference between verbal and performance IQ. Thus, for individuals with WS, performance on the DAS and DAS-II provides a better indication of the pattern of intellectual strengths and weaknesses associated with WS than does performance on the Wechsler tests.

The same pattern of considerably better performance on verbal and nonverbal reasoning than on visuospatial construction is apparent even in younger children. On the Mullen Scales of Early Learning (Mullen, 1995), mean Early Learning Composite standard score [ELC; similar to developmental quotient (DQ)] for 144 children with WS aged 2.01–4.96 years was 61.45 [range = 49 (floor)–96]. Mean T scores for the scales were 29.51 for Visual Reception (nonverbal reasoning), 21.18 (floor = 20) for Fine Motor (measuring primarily visuospatial construction), 29.45 for Receptive Language, and 32.60 for Expressive Language (Mervis & John, 2010a).

The Kaufman Brief Intelligence Test (KBIT; Kaufman & Kaufman, 1990 or KBIT-2; Kaufman & Kaufman, 2004) is the most commonly used measure of general intellectual ability in research on English-speaking individuals with WS. The KBIT and KBIT-2 assess verbal and nonverbal reasoning abilities but not spatial ability. On the KBIT, mean Composite IQ for 306 4- to 17-year-olds was 69.32 (range: 40 [floor]–112); mean verbal IQ was 71.35, and mean nonverbal IQ was 72.47 (Mervis & Becerra, 2007). On the KBIT-2, mean Composite IQ for 99 4- to 16-year-olds was 72.34 (range: 40 [floor]–105); mean verbal IQ was 74.99 and mean nonverbal IQ was 76.52 (Mervis & Morris, 2007).

In summary, across a variety of measures of intelligence, children with WS score on average in the mild intellectual disability to borderline range for verbal ability and nonverbal reasoning ability and in the moderate intellectual disability range on visuospatial construction ability. It is clearly inappropriate to state that they have "barely measurable general intelligence." On the other hand, a clear pattern of strengths and weaknesses reliably emerges when intellectual ability is assessed with the DAS, DAS-II, or Mullen test instruments. Thus, the possibility remains that language ability is independent of cognitive ability. This possibility has been addressed by examining the correlations among performance on a series of standardized assessments measuring vocabulary (PPVT-R, KBIT-Verbal), grammar (Test for Reception of Grammar, Bishop, 1989), nonverbal reasoning (KBIT-Matrices), visuospatial construction (DAS Pattern Construction), and verbal memory (forward and backward digit recall). All correlations were significant. Partial correlations indicated that the significant correlations between the language measures and the visuospatial construction measures were mediated primarily by nonverbal reasoning and verbal working memory (Mervis, 1999; Mervis, Robinson, Rowe, Becerra, & Klein-Tasman, 2004). As discussed later in this chapter, verbal memory has been found to be more closely related to grammatical development for children with WS than for typically developing children (Robinson, Mervis, & Robinson, 2003). These findings indicate that the language abilities of individuals with WS are, in fact, not independent of their cognitive abilities.

Early Language Acquisition

Despite the importance of early language acquisition, this topic has not been a focus for research on WS. There have been a few studies, however, on speech production and perception, early vocabulary acquisition, and early communicative/pragmatic development. These studies are reviewed below. For a more in-depth discussion, see Mervis and John (in press).

Early Speech Production and Perception

The onset of language acquisition by children with WS is almost always delayed (Mervis & Klein-Tasman, 2000; Mervis & Becerra, 2007). This delay has been attributed to delays in the onset of both nonlinguistic and linguistic rhythmic productions (Masataka, 2001) and the ability to segment words out of the speech stream (Nazzi, Paterson, & Karmiloff-Smith, 2003), as well as to overall developmental delay.

To examine the relations among early language and motor milestones, Masataka (2001) conducted a longitudinal study of eight children with WS from ages 6 to 30 months. All motor and language milestones were delayed. The only motor milestone related to language milestones was the onset of rhythmic hand banging, which was significantly correlated with the onset of canonical babble and the attainment of a 25-word expressive vocabulary. The correlation between the two language measures also was significant. In addition, when children with WS first began to produce canonical babble, their production was facilitated by the simultaneous production of rhythmic hand banging. Mervis and Bertrand (1997) reported that, for the two children in their longitudinal study who had not started to produce canonical babble prior to entry into the study, the onsets of rhythmic hand banging and canonical babble occurred in the same month. Masataka argued that rhythmic hand banging provides the motor substrate for canonical babble and that without canonical babble, word production is for the most part impossible. Thus, a delay in rhythmic hand banging would be expected to lead to delays in both canonical babble and word production.

The results of one study of the phonological development of children with WS have been reported (Mervis & Becerra, 2007; Velleman, Currier, Caron, Curley, & Mervis, 2006). In this study, the phonological repertoires of six 18-month-olds with WS were compared to those of CA-matched groups of children who were developing typically or who had Down syndrome (DS). Although the three groups produced about the same mean proportion of canonical syllables, the syndrome groups showed considerably more variability than did the typically developing group. One child in each of the syndrome groups had not yet begun to produce canonical babble. On several other measures, including proportion of vowel-only syllables, number of syllables per babble, number of different consonants, and mean babble level (as defined by Stoel-Gammon, 1989), the babble of the typically developing children was more complex than that of the children with WS or DS. Consistent with Masataka's (2001) argument that production of canonical babble is critical for word production, the two children with WS whose language development was most advanced also had the most "normal" babble histories, and the child whose language was the most delayed had not met the criterion for attainment of canonical babble even at age 36 months.

The speech perception abilities of young children with WS have been addressed in two studies. In the first, Nazzi, Paterson, and Karmiloff-Smith (2003) considered the ability of 17 children aged 17–47 months (mean CA = 33 months, mean mental age [MA] = 19 months) to segment words with a strong–weak stress pattern (the predominant pattern in English) and words with a weak–strong stress pattern from ongoing speech. The paradigm established by Jusczyk, Houston, and Newsome (1999) was used. The children were successful at segmenting the strong–weak words, but not the weak–strong words, from the speech stream. Nazzi et al. argued that this pattern indicated that children with WS relied on prosodic cues (which are adequate to identify strong–weak words) rather than distributional information (which is needed to identify weak–strong words) to segment words from the speech stream, and that difficulty attending to distributional information may be an important contributor to the language delay associated with WS. Mervis and Becerra (2007) noted that the difficulty Nazzi et al. identified in segmenting weak–strong words from the speech stream may have a relatively limited effect on language development in WS, for two reasons. First, weak–strong words are rare in the vocabularies of typically developing toddlers, accounting for only eight of 396 words on the Words and Gestures form of the MacArthur-Bates Communicative Development Inventory (CDI;

Fenson et al., 1993, 2007). Second, young children with WS clearly are able to learn these words, perhaps because they are used in isolation in conjunction with their referents; parents of 13 of the 17 participants in Nazzi et al. (2003) reported that their child already understood "balloon," one of the possible target weak–strong words.

Cashon et al. (2009) used Saffran, Aslin, and Newport's (1996) paradigm to study the speech segmentation abilities of ten 9- to 20-month-olds (mean CA = 14 months) with WS. The participants were exposed to a 2-minute segment of speech from an artificial language in which all syllables received equal stress. Three-syllable sequences were considered "words" if they co-occurred statistically more often during familiarization than did other syllable sequences; "part-words" consisted of three-syllable sequences in which the syllables occurred equally often during familiarization, but did not occur together. Looking times during test trials were significantly longer for "part-words" than for "words," indicating that the children had succeeded in segmenting the "words" from the speech stream even when there were no prosodic cues available, thus providing them with an important foundational ability for word learning. These findings do not address the question of whether the onset of the ability to segment words from the speech stream is delayed in children with WS, as the youngest child in the study was 9 months old, and Saffran et al. (1996) found that typically developing 8-month-olds are able to segment words from the speech stream.

Early Vocabulary Acquisition

Early vocabulary acquisition is almost always delayed. Mervis, Robinson, Rowe, Becerra, and Klein-Tasman (2003) followed the early vocabulary development of 13 children with WS longitudinally, using the CDI Words and Sentences form. Age of acquisition of a ten-word expressive vocabulary was below the 5th percentile (the lowest percentile provided) for all 13 children; for 12 of these children, age of acquisition of 50- and 100-word expressive vocabularies also was below the 5th percentile. Median age of acquisition of a 100-word expressive vocabulary was 37 months for the children with WS, but only 18 months for typically developing children (Fenson et al., 1993).

Two cross-sectional studies comparing the expressive vocabulary sizes of young children with WS to those of young children with DS have been conducted. Mervis and Robinson (2000) compared 30-month-olds with the two syndromes and found that the children with WS (mean = 132 words, range: 3–391) had significantly larger expressive vocabularies than did the children with DS (mean = 79 words, range: 0–324 words). Both spoken and signed words were included in the expressive vocabulary counts. Vicari, Caselli, Gagliardi, Tonucci, and Volterra (2002) found that MA-matched groups of children with WS and DS had similar expressive vocabulary sizes, although the WS group had significantly more advanced grammatical ability and verbal memory skills (see also Volterra, Caselli, Capirci, Tonucci, & Vicari, 2003).

Studies of typically developing children and children with DS have identified several links between early cognitive development and early language development that hold for both groups (see summary in Mervis & Bertrand, 1993). Mervis and Bertrand (1993; see also Mervis, 2006) have shown that some of these links also obtain for children with WS. First, the extension of children's early object labels corresponded to their play patterns; both were at the child-basic level. For example, the children rolled a wide variety of approximately spherical objects, whether or not they were balls; they also comprehended and produced "ball" in relation to these objects. Second, the onset of spontaneous sorting of objects and the onset of fast-mapping of object labels was demonstrated in the same session for all but one child, for whom fast mapping preceded spontaneous exhaustive sorting by 2 weeks. In contrast, the well-established link between referential pointing and the onset of referential language does not hold for children with WS. For typically developing children and children with DS, the onset of referential pointing precedes the onset of referential language. In sharp contrast, the reverse relation holds for children with WS; the onset of referential language precedes the onset of referential pointing by an average of 6 months. Because joint attention to the referent is necessary for the child to acquire labels, alternative methods must be used. Mervis and Bertrand (1993) identified three such methods, all of which are also used successfully by parents of typically developing children and children with DS.

Early Communicative/Pragmatic Development

The delay in onset of comprehension and production of pointing gestures even beyond the delay in onset of referential language presages significant communicative/pragmatic difficulties for toddlers and preschoolers with WS. Laing et al. (2001) compared the performance of a group of young children with WS (aged 17–55 months, mean age 31 months) to a MA-matched group of typically developing infants and toddlers on the Early Social Communication Scales (Mundy & Hogan, 1996). Although the children with WS had significantly larger expressive vocabularies, they were significantly less likely to comprehend or produce pointing gestures or to engage in triadic joint attention.

Rowe, Peregrine, and Mervis (2005) used a similar measure, the Behavior Sample of the Communication and Symbolic Behavior Scales, Developmental Profile (Wetherby & Prizant, 2002) to compare the communicative abilities of toddlers with WS to those of toddlers with DS individually matched for CA, MA, and expressive vocabulary size. The children with WS produced significantly fewer gaze shifts, engaged in significantly fewer episodes of triadic joint attention, and used significantly fewer distal gestures (including points) and significantly fewer conventional gestures. The nonverbal communicative abilities of the children with WS were strongly related to their language, nonverbal reasoning, and visuospatial constructive abilities, as measured by the Mullen Scales of Early Learning (Mullen, 1995).

John and Mervis (2010) used the hiding game developed by Behne, Carpenter, and Tomasello (2005) to determine if CA-matched groups of preschoolers with WS or DS were able to infer communicative intent as expressed through pointing gestures or eye gaze. Despite having a significantly lower mean DQ, the DS group was significantly better at inferring communicative intent than was the WS group; 60% of the children with DS, but only 27% of the children with WS, found the toy at a rate significantly above that expected by chance.

The types of communicative problems identified by Laing et al. (2002) and Rowe et al. (2005) overlap with the difficulties associated with autism spectrum disorders (ASD). To provide a more in-depth examination of the sociocommunicative abilities of young children with WS, Klein-Tasman, Mervis, Lord, and Phillips (2007) administered the Autism Diagnostic Observation Schedule (ADOS; Lord et al., 2000) Module 1 to 29 children with WS aged 30–63 months (mean CA = 42 months) who had very limited or no expressive language. The results confirmed and extended those of previous studies: More than half of the children evidenced difficulties with pointing, giving, showing, and appropriate use of eye contact. Many children also showed difficulties

with initiation of joint attention or response to the examiner's bids for joint attention and with integration of eye gaze with other behaviors. Fourteen children (48%) met or exceeded the ADOS algorithm cut-off for "autism spectrum disorder"; three of these children met or exceeded the ADOS algorithm cut-off for "autism." By itself, ADOS performance is not sufficient to make a diagnosis of autism or ASD. However, the three children who met the ADOS algorithm for autism were later clinically diagnosed with autism. Klein-Tasman, Phillips, Lord, Mervis, and Gallo (2009) have compared the ADOS data for the children with WS who participated in the Klein-Tasman et al. (2007) study to data for three groups of CA- and Mullen performance-matched children: a group clinically diagnosed with autism, a group clinically diagnosed with pervasive developmental disorders–not otherwise specified (PDD-NOS), and a mixed-etiology group who did not have an autism or PDD-NOS diagnosis. Klein-Tasman et al. (2009) found that, although the sociocommunicative abilities of the WS group were better than those of the autism group, they were at about the same level as those of the PDD-NOS group. The social reciprocity skills of the WS group were more limited than those of the mixed-etiology group.

Klein-Tasman et al. (2007, 2009) argue that difficulties with pointing, showing, and giving are characteristic of WS and should not be considered diagnostic for ASD in children with this syndrome. However, when these gestural difficulties are combined with difficulties directing vocalization or facial expressions to other people, and the quality of social overtures is generally poor, Klein-Tasman et al. (2007, 2009) suggest that consideration of a comorbid ASD is warranted.

Language Abilities of School-aged Children and Adolescents

Most of the research on the language abilities of school-aged children and adolescents with WS has focused on semantics and grammar, with a smaller number of studies of pragmatic abilities and literacy. In this section, these studies are briefly reviewed.

Semantics
CONCRETE VOCABULARY
Studies of the receptive vocabularies of English-speaking children with WS almost always include a version of the Peabody Picture Vocabulary Test (PPVT-R, Dunn & Dunn, 1981; PPVT-III, Dunn & Dunn, 1997; PPVT-4; Dunn & Dunn, 2007) as

part of their protocol. From the early studies of WS (e.g., Bellugi et al., 1988) to recent ones (e.g., Brock, Jarrold, Farran, Laws, & Riby, 2007; Mervis & Becerra, 2007; Mervis & John, 2010a, 2010b; Mervis & Morris, 2007), performance on the PPVT has consistently yielded the highest mean standard score for any standardized assessment. Mervis and John (2010a) reported a mean PPVT-4 standard score of 81.84 (range: 20–124) for 129 children aged 4.01–17.71 years, with 83% scoring at least 70 and 8% scoring at least 100. Nevertheless, performance on the PPVT-4 clearly was not above the level expected for children in the general population and was not consistent with "exquisite" mastery of vocabulary. Furthermore, the finding that mean level of performance is higher on the PPVT than on any other standardized assessment is not unique to WS. Glenn and Cunningham (2005) documented this pattern for individuals with DS, and Facon, Bollengier, and Grubar (1993), in a meta-analysis of studies that reported performance on both the PPVT and a full-scale IQ measure, found that for most studies in which participants' mean IQ was less than 70, mean PPVT standard score was higher than mean IQ. The participants in the studies included in the meta-analysis had a wide range of etiologies.

The expressive concrete vocabulary of individuals with WS is often measured with a version of the Expressive Vocabulary Test (EVT; Williams, 1997, or EVT-2: Williams, 2007). Most items on the EVT-2 (which was co-normed with the PPVT-4) require the child to name a picture or the action depicted in the picture; for a small proportion of items the child is asked to provide a synonym for a word produced by the examiner. Mervis and John (2010a) reported a mean EVT-2 standard score of 79.43 (range: 20–120) for the same 129 children whose performance on the PPVT-4 was described above, with 83% earning a standard score of at least 70 and 6% earning a standard score of at least 100. These findings suggest that, when measured in a parallel manner, the concrete receptive and expressive vocabulary abilities of individuals with WS typically are at about the same level relative to the general population.

RELATIONAL/CONCEPTUAL VOCABULARY

Relational/conceptual vocabulary includes both terms for basic relational concepts (e.g., spatial, quantitative, temporal, and dimensional terms) and more advanced relational concepts such as conjunctions and disjunctions (e.g., and, or, although,

nevertheless, neither. . . . nor). In striking contrast to their performance on concrete vocabulary measures, the performance of children with WS on relational vocabulary measures is very low, approximating the level of their performance on measures of visuospatial construction such as DAS Pattern Construction (Mervis & John, 2008), the signature weakness for individuals with WS (Mervis et al., 2000). Mervis and John (2008), reporting on 92 5- to 7-year-olds with WS, found that, in contrast to their mean PPVT-III standard score of 86.73 (range: 59–118), the children's mean standard score on an assessment of receptive knowledge of simple relational concepts (Test of Relational Concepts; TRC; Edmonston & Litchfield Thane, 1988) was 55.79 (range: 25–104). The pattern of errors indicated that children with WS have difficulty with relational language in general, rather than specifically with spatial language.

Lukács (2005) tested the spatial language of Hungarian children and adolescents with WS and found that, although they made significantly more errors than did typically developing children matched for Hungarian PPVT raw score, the pattern of spatial language errors was the same for both groups. Landau and Zukowski (2003) and Lukács, Pléh, and Racsmány (2004) have argued that the difficulty children with WS have in describing more complex spatial relations such as bounded-from and via paths, which require memory for two spatial locations, is due to problems with spatial memory, which is considerably weaker than verbal memory (Rowe & Mervis, 2006).

Not surprisingly given the difficulty that children with WS have with simple relational concepts, individuals with WS also evidence considerable weakness with regard to more complex relational concepts. Mervis and John (2008) administered the Clinical Evaluation of Language Fundamentals-IV (CELF-IV; Semel, Wiig, & Secord, 2003) Formulated Sentences subtest, which includes both simple and advanced relational concepts, to 29 9- to 11-year-olds with WS. Twelve children earned a scaled score of 1, the lowest possible. Stojanovik, Perkins, and Howard (2006), who administered the CELF-R Formulated Sentences subtest to five 7- to 12-year-olds, also reported very poor performance.

SEMANTIC ORGANIZATION

Semantic organization (how a person cognitively relates the members of a category) is usually measured by word fluency tests in which the participant is asked to list as many category members as possible.

Bellugi, Wang, and Jernigan (1994) compared the semantic organization of the "animal" category for six adolescents with WS, six CA- and IQ-matched adolescents with DS, and a group of typically developing second-graders. Based on the finding that the WS group was more likely than the other groups to name unusual (defined as low word-frequency) animals, Bellugi et al. concluded that the semantic organization of individuals with WS was deviant.

The results of more recent studies suggest that the semantic organization of individuals with WS is appropriate. Mervis, Morris, Bertrand, and Robinson (1999) found that the semantic organization of 8- to 10-year-olds with WS was comparable to that of a CA- and IQ-matched group of children with DS and a MA-matched group of typically developing children on all but one measure. On that measure, the WS and DS groups performed similarly to a CA-matched group of typically developing children; all three groups performed significantly differently than the MA-matched group of typically developing children. Jarrold, Hartley, Phillips, and Baddeley (2000) found no differences between a group of 7- to 27-year-olds (mean CA = 16.75 years) with WS and a group of individuals with moderate learning difficulties matched for raw score on the British version of the PPVT on the usual measures of semantic fluency. Levy and Bechar (2003) compared a group of 6- to 17-year-olds (mean CA = 12 years) with WS to a CA- and IQ-matched group of individuals with intellectual disability of unknown etiology and a MA-matched group of typically developing children and found no differences between groups. Volterra, Capirci, Pezzini, Sabbadini, and Vicari (1996), Temple, Almazan, and Sherwood (2002), and Lukács (2005) found that the semantic organization of children and adolescents with WS was similar to that of MA-matched typically developing children. Thus, at least within the semantic fluency paradigm, individuals with WS are not more likely than matched groups to use unusual vocabulary.

Stojanovik and van Ewijk (2008) addressed the question of whether children with WS used unusual vocabulary by comparing the vocabulary used by a group of 7- to 13-year-olds with WS to that of three groups of typically developing children: one matched for CA, one matched for receptive grammatical ability, and one matched for nonverbal reasoning ability. The children's task was to relate the story in the wordless picture book, *Frog, Where Are You?* (Mayer, 1969) while looking at the pictures. The WS group did not differ from the other groups

on either the number of different word roots used or mean word frequency for the roots. The WS group was significantly less likely to use especially infrequent words than any of the comparison groups. For the WS group, but not the typically developing groups, the correlation between the number of low-frequency words produced and nonverbal reasoning ability was significant.

Grammar

Bellugi and her colleagues (e.g., 1988, 1994, 2000) have argued that grammatical ability is a strength for individuals with WS. In particular, the fact that adolescents with WS were able to comprehend and produce complex grammatical constructions even though they were still in Piaget's preoperational period of cognitive development was considered to provide strong evidence for the independence of language and cognition. This position is based on Beilin's (1975) argument that comprehension and production of reversible passive utterances requires reversible thought (the hallmark of the concrete operational period), as evidenced by success on conservation tasks. However, studies of typically developing children have provided evidence that preschoolers learning English (e.g., Brooks & Tomasello, 1999; Maratsos, Kuczaj, Fox, & Chalkley, 1979) and 2-year-olds learning non-European languages in which passive constructions are common (Allen & Crago, 1996) are able to comprehend and produce reversible passives, indicating that attainment of concrete operational thought is not necessary for knowledge of passive constructions.

As a second part of their argument, Bellugi and her colleagues (1988, 1994, 2000) provided a series of demonstrations that adolescents with WS had considerably more advanced grammatical abilities than CA- and IQ-matched adolescents with DS. These results have been replicated for both children acquiring English as their native language (Joffe & Varlokosta, 2007a, b; Mervis et al., 2003) and children acquiring Italian (Vicari et al., 2004). However, these findings probably reflect the inordinate difficulties that individuals with DS have with grammar rather than that individuals with WS have usually good grammatical abilities. In fact, comparisons of the grammatical ability of individuals with WS relative to that of CA- and IQ-matched individuals with forms of intellectual disability other than DS or MA-matched typically developing children consistently indicate that the WS group is at or below the level of the contrast group. This finding has been reported for English (e.g., Grant et al., 1997; Grant, Valian, & Smith, 2002; Joffe & Varlokosta, 2007a, b; Mervis & Becerra, 2007; Perovic & Wexler, 2007; Udwin & Yule, 1990; Zukowski, 2004), German (Gosch, Städing, & Pankau, 1994), Hungarian (Lukács, 2005), and Italian (Volterra, Capirci, Pezzini, Sabbadini, & Vicari, 1996; Volterra et al., 2003). For a discussion of potential difficulties in interpreting the results of studies in which individuals with intellectual disabilities are compared to much younger typically developing children, see Mervis and Klein-Tasman (2004) and Mervis and Robinson (2005).

Studies of the morphological abilities of English-speaking individuals with WS have focused primarily on the acquisition of the past tense. Researchers agree that, by late childhood, most individuals with WS correctly mark the past tense on regular verbs but often overregularize the past tense of irregular verbs (e.g., "runned"). Interpretation of these results led to a vigorous debate between researchers favoring a dual-mechanism model of language acquisition (Clahsen & Almazan, 1998; Clahsen, Ring, & Temple, 2003; Clahsen & Temple, 2003; Marshall & van der Lely, 2006) and those arguing for a single-mechanism model (Thomas et al., 2001; Thomas & Karmiloff-Smith, 2003). Studies of the morphological abilities of individuals with WS acquiring languages with more complex morphology than English indicate that morphological abilities are at or slightly below those of MA-matched typically developing children (for French: e.g., Boloh, Ibernon, Royer, Escudier, & Danillon, 2009; Karmiloff-Smith et al., 1997; for Hebrew: Levy & Hermon, 2003; for Hungarian: Lukács, 2005; Lukács et al., 2004). A more detailed summary of grammatical development, including both syntax and morphology, is provided in Mervis (2006).

Many researchers concerned with the receptive grammatical abilities of individuals with WS have included the Test for Reception of Grammar (TROG; Bishop, 1989 or TROG-2; Bishop, 2003) in their protocols. The constructions tested by these measures range from simple positive statements through complex sentences such as those containing center-embedded clauses. Mervis and Becerra (2007) reported a mean TROG-2 standard score of 70.25 (range: 55 [lowest possible]–111) for 110 5- to 18-year-olds with WS. The modal score was 55 (floor), indicating that many individuals with WS have considerable difficulty with grammatical comprehension, especially of complex constructions. Karmiloff-Smith et al. (1997) reported similar

findings for a smaller sample. Translations of the TROG into Italian and Hungarian have been used to compare the receptive grammatical abilities of individuals with WS acquiring these languages to those of MA-matched typically developing children. The findings indicated that the children with WS performed significantly worse than the contrast group, but that the pattern of performance was the same (Lukács, 2005; Volterra et al., 1996). Thus, the order of difficulty of various types of grammatical constructions is similar for children with WS and children in the general population. The receptive grammatical ability of children with WS is strongly related to verbal working memory ability. Robinson et al. (2003) found that backward digit recall ability accounted for the largest amount of variance in the TROG performance of a sample of 39 4- to 16-year-olds. The correlation between backward digit recall ability and TROG performance was significantly higher for the WS group than for a group of typically developing children matched for number of blocks correct on the TROG, suggesting that children with WS may rely more heavily on verbal working memory when parsing complex grammatical constructions than do typically developing children.

Pragmatics

As indicated earlier, the sociocommunicative abilities of young children with WS are quite limited. These difficulties continue into the school-aged and adult years, and are of considerable concern to parents. Most children and adolescents with WS have Individualized Educational Program (IEP) goals targeting aspects of pragmatics such as turn-taking, conversational and topic maintenance, and appropriate use of eye gaze (Mervis, 2006). Studies of pragmatics have focused on general assessment of sociocommunicative abilities by parental or caregiver responses to standardized questionnaires, analyses of children's conversation skills, and examination of their comprehension monitoring skills.

QUESTIONNAIRE-BASED STUDIES

To assess the general pragmatic abilities of individuals with WS, three studies using a version of the Children's Communication Checklist (CCC; Bishop, 1998 or CCC-2; Bishop, 2002) have been conducted. Laws and Bishop (2004) asked parents of 19 6- to 25-year-olds with WS (mean CA = 14.83 years) to complete the CCC. Based on the parents' responses, 15 of the 19 participants met the CCC cut-off for pragmatic language impairment. The WS group evidenced significant difficulties in all areas of pragmatics measured by the CCC, with particular difficulty in the use of stereotyped conversations, inappropriate initiation of conversations, and overdependence on context to interpret what was said to them. Peregrine, Rowe, and Mervis (2005) found that 6- to 12-year-olds with WS received significantly lower scaled scores than their 6- to 12-year-old typically developing siblings on all 10 CCC-2 scales. The areas of greatest difficulty for the WS group were the same as those identified by Laws and Bishop. Philofsky, Fidler, and Hepburn (2007) compared the CCC-2 scaled scores for a group of 6- to 12-year-old children with WS (mean CA = 9.1 years) to those of a CA-matched group of children with autism and a younger group of typically developing children. All children spoke in complete sentences. The scaled scores for the WS group were significantly below those of the typically developing group for all ten scales. The performance of the WS group was significantly better than that of the autism group on two of the four pragmatics scales (Stereotyped Language and Nonverbal Communication) and at the same level as the autism group's on the other two pragmatics scales (Inappropriate Initiation and Use of Context).

CONVERSATIONAL SKILLS

To address the claim that children with WS use "cocktail party speech," Udwin and Yule (1990) engaged 43 6- to 15-year-olds (mean CA = 11.1 years) in 30-minute one-on-one conversations with a researcher. Sixteen of the children (37%) met the authors' criteria for hyperverbal speech (fluent speech including an excessive number of stereotyped phrases or idioms, overfamiliarity, introduction of irrelevant personal experiences, and perseverative responding). Jones et al. (2000) compared the conversational abilities of ten adolescents and adults with WS (mean CA = 15.8 years), ten CA- and IQ-matched adolescents and adults with DS, and ten MA-matched typically developing children during a biographical interview. Although all three groups answered equivalent numbers of questions, the WS group used significantly more evaluative devices (including descriptions of affective states, evaluative comments, character speech, and emphatic markers) than did either comparison group. The WS group also displayed the overfamiliarity described by Udwin and Yule, asking the researcher personal questions and often perseverating on these types of questions even after the researcher attempted to redirect the participant. These types of behaviors were not exhibited by

individuals in the comparison groups. The types of problems identified in these two studies are consistent with parental and caregiver reports on the CCC and CCC-2.

Stojanovik and her colleagues have analyzed the conversational abilities of a small sample of 7- to 12-year-olds (mean CA = 9.2 years) with WS. The findings from the initial analyses (Stojanovik, 2006) indicated that the children with WS were considerably more likely than slightly older children with specific language impairment matched for receptive grammatical ability as measured by the TROG to provide too little information in response to the researcher's questions. Results of later analyses (Stojanovik, Perkins, & Howard, 2006), which included an additional comparison group of slightly younger typically developing children, again indicated that, regardless of whether the researcher asked for new information or for clarification, the responses of the children with WS were more likely than the responses of the other groups to be inadequate. In particular, the children with WS were more likely to provide too little information or to misinterpret what their conversational partner had meant and were considerably less likely to produce a response that continued the conversation.

COMPREHENSION MONITORING

Successful comprehension monitoring requires the child to attend to whether he or she understands what the speaker has said and to request clarification if needed. Only one study of the comprehension monitoring abilities of children with WS has been reported. John, Rowe, and Mervis (2009) considered the performance of 57 6- to 12-year-olds with WS in the listener role of a referential communication task modeled after Abbeduto et al. (2008). Children were asked to place one of several pictures into a scene based on the researcher's instructions. Although the children performed very well when they understood the instructions and the required picture was available, they had considerable difficulty when the researcher's instruction was inadequate (the requested picture was not among the available choices, the researcher's instruction was ambiguous, or the researcher's instruction contained vocabulary that the child did not understand). In particular, the children verbally indicated that there was a problem only 45% of the time; 55% of the time, the child placed a picture into the scene even though the correct picture was not available or more information was needed to identify the picture that had been requested. Even when the child indicated that there was a problem, he or she often did not identify the correct problem. Performance was related to CA and first-order theory of mind.

Literacy

The first studies of the reading abilities of individuals with WS were published in the late 1980s. Pagon, Bennett, LaVeck, Stewart, and Johnson (1987) tested nine individuals aged 10–20 years and found that all but one was able to read at least at the mid-first grade level. The person with the best reading skills scored at her grade level (ninth grade) on both decoding and reading comprehension. Median reading grade level was mid-second grade. In contrast, Udwin, Yule, and Martin (1987), in a study of 44 children aged 6–16 years, found that only 50% could read at all. For the children who could read (mean CA = 12.0 years), mean reading age equivalent (AE) was 7.75 years for decoding and 7.83 years for reading comprehension. Udwin, Davies, and Howlin (1996) retested 23 of the 44 participants in Udwin et al.'s study (1987) an average of approximately 9 years later. This group included 14 individuals who had been originally classified as "readers." Thirteen of the 14, plus four additional participants, were able to read at least a few words at the time of the follow-up study. The grade-equivalent scores were almost identical to those at the original assessment. Howlin, Davies, and Udwin (1998) tested the reading abilities of 62 adults (including the 23 in Udwin et al., 1996) and found that 47 (62%) could read at least a few words. Once again, mean reading AEs for the individuals who could read at all were quite low (8.65 years for decoding and 7.16 years for comprehension). IQ was related to reading ability; although no individual with IQ less than 50 was able to read, 78% of individuals with IQs 50–69 and 100% of individuals with IQs 70 or higher could read. Levy, Smith, and Tager-Flusberg (2003) also found a significant relation between IQ and reading ability for a group of 12- to 20-year-olds (mean CA = 12.42 years).

Phonological awareness is strongly related to both single-word reading and nonword reading ability for typically developing children (see reviews in Ehri, 2004, and McCardle, Chhabra, & Kapinus, 2008). This relation has also been studied for individuals with WS. Laing, Hulme, Grant, and Karmiloff-Smith (2001), studying individuals aged 9–27 years (mean CA = 15.08 years) learning to read English, found significant correlations between all the phonological awareness measures used and single-word reading. However, once CA and IQ were controlled, these correlations were no longer significant. Levy et al. (2003), also studying individuals who were learning to read English, administered the Comprehensive Test of Phonological Processing (CTOPP; Wagner, Torgesen, & Rashotte, 1999) as well as a test of single-word reading. The participants performed relatively well on the CTOPP, with mean standard score for Elision (deletion of specified syllables or phonemes) in the borderline range and mean standard scores for Segmenting Words and Segmenting Nonwords (dividing words and nonwords into syllables or individual phonemes) in the low average range. Elision ability was significantly correlated with both word reading ability and nonword reading ability, and word segmentation was significantly correlated with nonword reading even after nonverbal reasoning ability was controlled. Menghini, Verucci, and Vicari (2004), studying individuals learning to read Italian (mean CA = 17.58 years, range: 10–30 years), found that syllable deletion (elision) was significantly correlated with both single-word reading and nonword reading. Levy and Antebi (2004) studied 17 11- to 22-year-olds (mean CA = 16.2 years) learning to read Hebrew, a language that is likely to be more challenging to learn to read because reading requires integrating visuospatial information along several different axes (in Hebrew, vowels are indicated above or below the consonants rather than on the same axis). For the 11 participants who could read both words and nonwords, median word-reading grade level was third grade. One participant (aged 19 years) read at the level expected for her age. For the participants who could read, phoneme deletion was significantly correlated with single-word reading and phoneme identification, and single-word reading was significantly correlated with nonword reading. Based on these findings, Levy and colleagues (Levy & Antebi, 2004; Levy et al., 2003) recommended that children with WS be taught to read using a phonics approach.

Becerra, John, Peregrine, and Mervis (2008) considered the relation between primary method of reading instruction and reading ability. Initial analyses treated the 44 participants (mean CA = 12.49 years, range: 8.93–17.71 years) as a single group, to provide information about the reading ability of children with WS relative to general population peers of the same CA. The children completed the Reading section of the Wechsler Individual Achievement Test-II (WIAT-II, Wechsler, 2005). Standard scores indicated considerable variability, with SDs >15 for all measures. Mean standard scores were 73.00 (range: 40 [floor]–112) for Word Reading, 78.75 (range: 0 correct–113 [standard score]) for Pseudoword Decoding, and 64.61 (range: 40 [floor]–102] for Reading Comprehension. All the children were able to read at least a few real words, but 8 (18%) could not read any of the non-words. Several participants, including one in 11th grade, read and comprehended at grade level. As would be expected given previous studies, the mean standard score was significantly higher for Word Reading than for Reading Comprehension.

The 44 participants were divided into two groups according to primary method of reading instruction: phonics (*n* = 24) and whole (sight) word (*n* = 20). Although there was a wide range of DAS-II GCAs for both groups (for Phonics: 49–98; for Whole Word: 39–80), mean GCA was significantly higher for the Phonics group (67.42) than for the Whole Word group (58.00). To compare the reading abilities of the two groups relative to their GCAs, predicated WIAT-II reading scores were determined for each child based on his or her GCA, using the tables in the DAS-II manual. Discrepancy scores (obtained reading standard score minus predicted reading standard score) were calculated for each child. Results indicated large and significant differences as a function of group both for Reading Composite and for each of the reading subtests. All of the children who could not read any nonwords were in the Whole Word group. Most children in the Phonics group read at or above the level expected for their GCA. In contrast, most children in the Whole Word group read below the level expected for their GCA. These findings are consistent with those of the meta-analyses conducted by the National Reading Panel (see summaries in Ehri, 2004 and McCardle et al., 2008), which stressed the importance of early, explicit, and systematic instruction in phonemic awareness and phonics for all children.

Conclusion

In this section, I briefly summarize the findings reported in this chapter. I then consider how one might address the question of whether the pattern of language strengths and weaknesses found for individuals with WS is likely to be specific to that syndrome. Finally, I address future directions for research and implications of the findings reported for intervention.

As Bishop and Mogford (1988) noted about research on language disorders in general, in the late 1980s studies of the language abilities of individuals with WS focused on either theoretical questions (in this case, about the relation between language and cognition) or practical concerns about language remediation, but did not simultaneously address both. In contrast, many of the more recent studies have attempted to address both theoretical and practical questions. Despite the original arguments that WS demonstrated the independence of language from cognition—in particular that excellent language abilities coexisted with severe intellectual disability—and the more extreme claims by academicians who had never conducted research on WS, subsequent research has shown that, although the overall language ability of individuals with WS is considerably stronger than overall visuospatial construction ability (the signature weakness for this syndrome), overall language ability is not at the average level for the general population. Furthermore, very few individuals with WS have severe intellectual disability; overall IQ typically is in the mild intellectual disability range, with language and nonverbal reasoning abilities in the borderline to mild intellectual disability range and spatial abilities in the moderate intellectual disability range. Language abilities and cognitive abilities are strongly related. For example, verbal working memory is more important for grammatical comprehension for children with WS than for children in the general population, spatial memory limitations have been hypothesized to be related to difficulties in relational language, and the relations of both concrete vocabulary ability and grammatical ability to visuospatial construction ability are mediated by nonverbal reasoning and verbal working memory.

Just as there is a pattern of general intellectual strengths and weaknesses associated with WS, there is also a pattern of strengths and weaknesses within the language domain that characterizes most individuals with WS, beginning during early childhood and extending through adulthood. In particular, the strongest area of language ability is typically concrete vocabulary. For example, the majority of individuals with WS score in the normal range on the PPVT-4 (measuring receptive concrete vocabulary) and the EVT-2 (measuring expressive concrete vocabulary). Grammatical ability is more limited; most individuals with WS have difficulty with comprehension of complex grammatical constructions (as measured both by the TROG and by related CCC items), and expressive grammatical ability appears to be at about the same level as for individuals with other forms of intellectual disability (excluding DS) matched for CA and IQ. Conceptual/relational vocabulary ability is much more limited, with performance only slightly above that for visuospatial construction.

The pragmatics abilities of most individuals with WS are also very limited. For young children, both comprehension and use of communicative gestures are more limited than expected for vocabulary ability, and sociocommunicative abilities are about at the level of CA- and DQ-matched children with PDD-NOS. Furthermore, the early pragmatic abilities of preschoolers with WS are significantly weaker than those of CA-matched children with DS, even though the children in the DS group had a significantly lower mean Mullen DQ than did the children in the WS group. For older children and adolescents with WS, pragmatics skills typically remain very weak, with data from both transcript analyses and performance on the CCC suggesting that conversational skills are especially weak.

Reading ability is greatly affected by method of instruction; children with WS who are taught to read with systematic phonics methods read at or above the level expected for their GCA, whereas children taught primarily with whole-word (sight-word) methods read below the level expected for their GCA. The single-word reading abilities of both groups are considerably better than their reading comprehension abilities, reflecting in part the difficulties with complex grammar, conceptual/relational language, and pragmatics associated with WS.

Determination of the Specificity of the Williams Syndrome Language Profile

The specificity of this language profile to WS has not been addressed directly. However, as mentioned earlier, receptive concrete vocabulary has been identified as a strength for individuals with a variety of etiologies of intellectual disability. To address the specificity question directly, studies that compare CA- and IQ-matched individuals with different etiologies of intellectual disability would be particularly valuable. Such studies are often impractical, however. For example, if mean IQ is considerably different for two syndromes, then comparing CA- and IQ-matched samples will likely result in a comparison of children in the top part of the IQ distribution for Syndrome A to children in the bottom part of the IQ distribution for Syndrome B, yielding non-representative samples for both groups. To avoid this problem, many researchers have compared groups of individuals with a particular syndrome to much younger typically developing children matched for AE score on a control variable. This method is fraught with difficulties, both with the use of AE scores and with acceptance of the often-incorrect assumption that everyone who has earned a particular AE score on the control variable should be expected to earn the same AE score on the target variable, even when there are large differences in CA. These problems are addressed in Mervis and Robinson (2005) and Mervis and Klein-Tasman (2004).

Another approach is to compare profiles based on standard scores. Mervis and Robinson (2005) have provided guidelines for when comparison of standard scores across assessments normed on different samples is appropriate. However, for this approach to be effective, the norms for the assessment must extend low enough to capture the variability present within a syndrome. This has historically been difficult for many syndromes. For example, the subtests on the Wechsler IQ tests are normed to only 3 SDs below the population mean, with the result that a large proportion of individuals with many syndromes (e.g., DS, males with fragile X syndrome) score at floor. However, the norms for some of the most recent assessments extend considerably lower. For example, the DAS-II subtests are normed to 4 SDs below the mean and the PPVT-4 and EVT-2 are normed to >5 SDs below the mean. In a promising approach, Hessl et al. (2009) obtained the WISC-III raw norms data from Psychological Corporation and used these data to calculate normalized scores based on participants' raw scores, using a z-score transformation. Hessl et al. demonstrated that subtest z-scores actually fit a normal distribution for individuals with fragile X syndrome, a finding that had been obscured when the published norms were used, as between 65% and 94% of the scaled scores for each subtest were at floor for the males in their sample. This method could be applied to the standardization sample data from any assessment for which the publisher was willing to make these data available. Alternatively, the publishers could implement this approach themselves to provide extended norms for use with individuals with intellectual disabilities.

Directions for Future Research

Most of the research that has been conducted on the language abilities of individuals with WS has focused on semantics and grammar. Although much has been learned about both, considerably more research is needed in these areas; especially important is research that takes a developmental approach. The two remaining major components of language, phonology and pragmatics, have hardly been studied at all. Almost nothing is known about either speech perception or speech production by individuals with WS. The recent finding that WS is associated with sensorineural hearing loss that typically begins during childhood (e.g., Marler, Elfenbein, Ryals, Urban, & Netzloff, 2005; Marler, Sitcovsky, Mervis, Kistler, & Wightman, 2010) makes a developmental approach to the study of speech perception and the potential impact of speech perception on other aspects of language acquisition especially important. Although pragmatics is known to be an area of considerable difficulty for individuals with WS, much more research is needed to carefully characterize the pragmatics abilities of school-aged children with WS. Additional studies of literacy are needed, especially studies focused on reading comprehension, spelling, and written composition. Although individuals with WS show a relative strength in concrete vocabulary, very little is known about the strategies that children with WS use to acquire words and how these strategies may change with age. The impact of the home environment on language acquisition has not been studied at all, although findings from studies of typically developing children and children with DS have implicated factors such as parental responsiveness and the amount of language addressed to the child in rate of language development (e.g., Hart & Risley, 1995; Mervis & Becerra, 2003). These findings suggest that characteristics of the home environment are likely to play a role in variability in language ability across children with WS. Characteristics of the school environment also are likely to be important, although the only characteristic that has been studied so far is type of reading instruction.

Although approximately 95% of individuals with WS have the same genes deleted, there are also a few individuals with shorter or longer deletions (Mervis & Morris, 2007). Comparisons of these individuals to individuals with classic deletions may allow for the identification of genes that, in transaction with other genes and the environment, are involved in language development. Recently, individuals who have duplications of the WS region have been identified. Most of these individuals have intelligence in the normal range, although during early childhood most have significant speech delay, with many showing symptoms of childhood apraxia of speech and some meeting full criteria for this disorder (Osborne & Mervis, 2007). Studies of children with duplications of this region may lead to identification of genes in the WS region that, once again in transaction with other genes and the environment, are important for speech development.

Implications for Intervention

Almost all children with WS have delayed onset of language, and most continue to have significant delays or difficulties with at least some aspects of language throughout the school years. Thus, language therapy is critical for older infants, toddlers, and preschoolers, and continues to be important throughout the school years, although the focus will change with development. Children who are very young or who have moderate or severe intellectual or language disability would benefit from intensive language therapy focused on all aspects of language. For older children and adolescents who have intellectual ability in the mild disability to low average range, language intervention is also important, especially with regard to conceptual/relational language and pragmatics, but this often is not provided.

The pattern evidenced by young children with WS of starting to produce referential language prior to using (or even comprehending) referential gestures often leads to significant delays in the onset of language therapy, as many therapists use the onset of referential communicative gestures as the indicator that children are ready for language therapy aimed at the acquisition of vocabulary. Similarly, if children do not come to the attention of early-intervention programs until after they have begun to talk, the presumption is often made that they have mastered the referential gesture system. Both these presumptions are incorrect. Children with WS are ready to begin therapy aimed at vocabulary acquisition well before they begin to produce referential pointing gestures, and children with WS who talk well almost always still have difficulty with pragmatic aspects of language, including referential gesture comprehension and production. Thus, a full assessment of all aspects of language and communication, including extensive observation of the child's linguistic interactions with teachers and peers, both in the classroom and on the playground, is critical to determining if an individual child would benefit from language intervention. All too often, language intervention ends once the child's speech is clear and he or she is no longer making significant grammatical errors, even though the child continues to have difficulty with conceptual/relational language and with pragmatics. These difficulties have a serious impact not only on the child's academic performance but also on his or her social interactions with other children, limiting the child's ability to make and keep friends. These types of difficulties are best addressed by a coordinated multidisciplinary approach including the language therapist, classroom teachers, special educators, and aides, as well as the child's parents; as the child gets older and more aware of these difficulties, he or she should also be included in goal selection and implementation. Intervention also should target both reading comprehension, which is considerably weaker than decoding for almost all children with WS, and prose composition, which is reported by parents and teachers to be an area of great difficulty for most children with WS. Strategies recommended by the National Reading Panel for both good readers and children who are having difficulty learning to read are summarized in McCardle et al. (2008). Recommendations regarding both reading intervention and language intervention for children with WS are provided in Mervis (2009) and Mervis and John (2010a).

Unfortunately, research addressing the impact of intervention on the language abilities of children with WS has been extremely limited. One study has considered the effect of type of reading instruction method on children's performance on standardized reading assessments (Becerra et al., 2008; Mervis, 2009). Results indicated the importance of using a systematic phonics approach, which had previously been endorsed by the National Reading Panel for all children, rather than a whole-word or whole-language approach. Data from this study suggest that only about half of the children with WS are being taught reading using a systematic phonics approach. There have been no studies targeting the efficacy of particular methods of language intervention (including, among other methods, either music therapy or the use of music within more traditional language therapy) for children and adolescents with WS, the relative advantages and disadvantages of individual or group therapy for improving the language skills of individuals with WS, or more generally the impact of language intervention on their language and communicative abilities. Carefully conceived and implemented intervention studies would provide crucial input for the design of an educational environment that would allow children and adolescents with WS the opportunity to reach their full academic and social potential.

Acknowledgments

Preparation of this manuscript was supported by the National Institute of Child Health and Human Development grant R37 HD29957 and by the National Institute of Neurological Disorders and Stroke grant R01 NS35102. I thank the individuals with WS and their families for participating so enthusiastically in the research reported in this manuscript. Their commitment has made progress in understanding the development of individuals with WS possible.

References

Abbeduto, L., Murphy, M. M., Kover, S. T., Giles, N. D., Karadottir, S., Amman, A., et al. (2008). Signaling noncomprehension of language: A comparison of fragile X syndrome and Down syndrome. *American Journal on Mental Retardation, 113*, 214–230.

Allen, S. E. M., & Crago, M. B. (1996). Early passive acquisition in Inuktitut. *Journal of Child Language, 23*, 129–155.

Bates, E. (1990, April). *Early language development: How things come together and how they come apart.* Invited address presented at the International Conference on Infant Studies, Montreal, Quebec.

Becerra, A. M., John, A. E., Peregrine, E., & Mervis, C. B. (2008, June). *Reading abilities of 9–17-year-olds with Williams syndrome: Impact of reading method.* Poster presented at the Symposium on Research in Child Language Disorders, Madison, WI.

Beilin, H. (1975). *Studies in the cognitive basis of language development.* New York: Academic Press.

Bellugi, U., Marks, S., Bihrle, A., & Sabo, H. (1988). Dissociation between language and cognitive functions in Williams syndrome. In D. Bishop, & K. Mogford (Eds.), *Language development in exceptional circumstances* (pp. 177–189). London: Churchill Livingstone.

Bellugi, U., Lichtenberger, L., Jones, W., Lai, Z., & St. George, M. (2000). The neurocognitive profile of Williams syndrome: A complex pattern of strengths and weaknesses. *Journal of Cognitive Neuroscience, 12*(Supplement 1), 7–29.

Bellugi, U., Wang, P., & Jernigan, T. L. (1994). Williams syndrome: An unusual neuropsychological profile. In S. H. Broman, & J. Grafman (Eds.), *Atypical cognitive deficits in developmental disorders: Implications for brain function* (pp. 23–56). Hillsdale, NJ: Erlbaum.

Behne, T., Carpenter, M., & Tomasello, M. (2005). One-year-olds comprehend the communicative intentions behind gestures in a hiding game. *Developmental Science, 8*, 492–499.

Bishop, D. V. M. (1989). *Test for the Reception of Grammar.* Manchester, UK: Chapel Press.

Bishop, D. V. M. (1998). Development of the Children's Communication Checklist (CCC): A method for assessing the qualitative aspects of communication impairment in children. *Journal of Child Psychology and Psychiatry, 39*, 879–891.

Bishop, D. V. M. (2002). *The Children's Communication Checklist, 2nd ed.* London: Psychological Corporation.

Bishop, D. V. M. (2003). *Test for Reception of Grammar, Version 2.* London: Psychological Corporation.

Bishop, D., & Mogford, K. (Eds.). (1988). *Language development in exceptional circumstances.* London: Churchill Livingstone.

Boloh, Y., Ibernon, L., Royer, S., Escudier, F., & Danillon, A. (2009). Gender attribution and gender agreement in French Williams syndrome. *Research in Developmental Disabilities, 30*, 1523–1540.

Brock, J., Jarrold, C., Farran, E. K., Laws, G., & Riby, D. M. (2007). Do children with Williams syndrome really have good vocabulary knowledge? Methods for comparing cognitive and linguistic abilities in developmental disorders. *Clinical Linguistics & Phonetics, 21*, 673–688.

Brooks, P. J., & Tomasello, M. (1999). Young children learn to produce passives with nonce verbs. *Developmental Psychology, 35*, 29–44.

Cashon, C. H., Ha, O.-R., Allen, C. L., Graf, K. M., Saffran, J. R., & Mervis, C. B. (2009, April). *9- to 20-month-olds with Williams syndrome are linguistic statistical learners.* Poster presented at the biennial meeting of the Society for Research in Child Development, Denver, CO.

Clahsen, H., & Almazan, M. (1998). Syntax and morphology in children with Williams syndrome. *Cognition, 68*, 167–198.

Clahsen, H., Ring, M., & Temple, C. (2003). Lexical and morphological skills in English-speaking children with Williams syndrome. *Essex Research Reports in Linguistics, 43*, 1–27.

Clahsen, H., & Temple, C. (2003). Words and rules in children with Williams syndrome. In Y. Levy, & J. Schaeffer (Eds.), *Language competence across populations: Toward a definition of specific language impairment* (pp. 323–352). Mahwah, NJ: Erlbaum.

Dunn, L. E., & Dunn, L. E. (1981). *Peabody Picture Vocabulary Test-Revised.* Circle Pines, MN: American Guidance Service.

Dunn, L. E., & Dunn, L. E. (1997). *Peabody Picture Vocabulary Test (3rd ed.).* Circle Pines, MN: American Guidance Service.

Dunn, L. E., & Dunn, D. M. (2007). *Peabody Picture Vocabulary Test (4th ed.).* Minneapolis, MN: Pearson Assessments.

Edmonston, N. K., & Litchfield Thane, N. (1988). *TRC: Test of Relational Concepts.* Austin, TX: PRO-ED.

Ehri, L. C. (2004). Teaching phonemic awareness and phonics: An explanation of the National Reading Panel meta-analyses. In P. McCardle, & V. Chhabra (Eds.), *The voice of evidence in reading research* (pp. 153–186). Baltimore: Brookes.

Elliott, C. D. (1990). *Differential Ability Scales.* San Antonio, TX: Psychological Corporation.

Elliott, C. D. (2007). *Differential Ability Scales* (2nd ed.). San Antonio, TX: Psychological Corporation.

Facon, B., Bollengier, T., & Grubar, J.-C. (1993). Overestimation of mental retarded persons' IQ using the PPVT: A re-analysis and some implications for future research. *Journal of Intellectual Disability Research, 37*, 373–379.

Fenson, L., Dale, P. S., Reznick, J. S., Thal, D., Bates, E., Hartung, J. P., et al. (1993). *MacArthur communicative development inventories: User's guide and technical manual.* San Diego: Singular.

Fenson, L., Marchman, V. A., Thal, D. J., Dale, P. S., Reznick, J. S., & Bates, E. (2007). *MacArthur-Bates communicative development inventories: User's guide and technical manual* (2nd ed.). Baltimore: Brookes.

Glenn, S., & Cunningham, C. (2005). Performance of young people with Down syndrome on the Leiter-R and British Picture Vocabulary Scales. *Journal of Intellectual Disability Research, 49*, 239–244.

Gosch, A., Städing, G., & Pankau, R. (1994). Linguistic abilities in children with Williams-Beuren syndrome. *American Journal of Medical Genetics, 52*, 291–296.

Grant, J., Karmiloff-Smith, A., Gathercole, S. A., Paterson, S., Howlin, P., Davies, M., & Udwin, O. (1997). Phonological short-term memory and its relationship to language in Williams syndrome. *Cognitive Neuropsychiatry, 2*, 81–99.

Grant, J., Valian, V., & Karmiloff-Smith, A. (2002). A study of relative clauses in Williams syndrome. *Journal of Child Language, 29*, 403–416.

Hart, B., & Risley, T. R. (1995). *Meaningful differences in the everyday experience of young American children.* Baltimore: Brookes.

Hessl, D., Nguyen, D. V., Green, C., Chavez, A., Fassone, F., Hagerman, R. J., et al. (2009). A solution to limitations of cognitive testing in children with intellectual disabilities: The case of fragile X syndrome. *Journal of Neurodevelopmental Disorders, 1*, 33–45.

Howlin, P., Davies, M., & Udwin, O. (1998). Cognitive functioning in adults with Williams syndrome. *Journal of Child Psychology and Psychiatry, 39*, 183–189.

Jarrold, C., Hartley, S. J., Phillips, C., & Baddeley, A. D. (2000). Word fluency in Williams syndrome: Evidence for unusual semantic organization? *Cognitive Neuropsychiatry, 5*, 293–319.

Joffe, V., & Varlokosta, S. (2007a). Language abilities in Williams syndrome: Exploring comprehension, production, and repetition skills. *Advances in Speech Language Pathology, 9*, 213–225.

Joffe, V., & Varlokosta, S. (2007b). Patterns of syntactic development in children with Williams syndrome and Down's syndrome: Evidence from passives and wh-questions. *Clinical Linguistics & Phonetics, 21*, 705–727.

John, A. E., & Mervis, C. B. (2010). Comprehension of the communicative intent behind pointing and gazing gestures by young children with Williams syndrome or Down syndrome. *Journal of Speech, Language, and Hearing Research, 53*, 950–960.

John, A. E., Rowe, M. L., & Mervis, C. B. (2009). Referential communication skills of children with Williams syndrome: Understanding when messages are not adequate. *American Journal on Intellectual and Developmental Disabilities, 114*, 85–99.

Jones, W., Bellugi, U., Lai, Z., Chiles, M., Reilly, J., Lincoln, A., & Adolphs, R. (2000). Hypersociability in Williams syndrome. *Journal of Cognitive Neuroscience, 12*(Supplement 1), 30–46.

Jusczyk, P. W., Houston, D. M., & Newsome, M. (1999). The beginnings of word segmentation in English-learning infants. *Cognitive Psychology, 39*, 159–207.

Karmiloff-Smith, A., Grant, J., Berthoud, I., Davies, M., Howlin, P., & Udwin, O. (1997). Language and Williams syndrome: How intact is "intact"? *Child Development, 68*, 274–290.

Kataria, S., Goldstein, D. J., & Kushnick, T. (1984). Developmental delays in Williams ("Elfin facies") syndrome. *Applied Research in Mental Retardation, 5*, 419–423.

Kaufman, A. S., & Kaufman, N. L. (1990). *Kaufman Brief Intelligence Test.* Circle Pines, MN: American Guidance Services.

Kaufman, A. S., & Kaufman, N. L. (2004). *Kaufman Brief Intelligence Test, 2nd ed.* Circle Pines, MN: American Guidance Services.

Klein-Tasman, B. P., & Mervis, C. B. (2003). Distinctive personality characteristics of 8-, 9-, and 10-year-olds with Williams syndrome. *Developmental Neuropsychology, 23*, 269–290.

Klein-Tasman, B. P., Mervis, C. B., Lord, C. E., & Phillips, K. D. (2007). Socio-communicative deficits in young children with Williams syndrome: Performance on the Autism Diagnostic Observation Schedule. *Child Neuropsychology, 13*, 444–467.

Klein-Tasman, B. P., Phillips, K. D., Lord, C., Mervis, C. B., & Gallo, F. (2009). Overlap with the autism spectrum in young children with Williams syndrome. *Journal of Developmental and Behavioral Pediatrics, 30*, 289–299.

Laing, E., Butterworth, G., Ansari, D., Gsödl, M., Longhi, E., Panagiotaki, G., et al. (2002). Atypical development of language and social communication in toddlers with Williams syndrome. *Developmental Science, 5*, 233–246.

Laing, E., Hulme, C., Grant, J., & Karmiloff-Smith, A. (2001). Learning to read in Williams syndrome: Looking beneath the surface of atypical reading development. *Journal of Child Psychology and Psychiatry, 42*, 729–739.

Landau, B., & Zukowski, A. (2003). Objects, motions, and paths: Spatial language in children with Williams syndrome. *Developmental Neuropsychology, 23*, 107–139.

Laws, G., & Bishop, D. V. M. (2004). Pragmatic language impairment and social impairment in Williams syndrome: A comparison with Down's syndrome and specific language impairment. *International Journal of Language and Communication Disorders, 39*, 45–64.

Levy, Y., & Antebi, V. (2004). Word reading and reading-related skills in Hebrew-speaking adolescents with Williams syndrome. *Neurocase, 10*, 444–451.

Levy, Y., & Bechar, T. 2003). Cognitive, lexical, and morphosyntactic profiles of Israeli children with Williams syndrome. *Cortex, 39*, 255–271.

Levy, Y., & Hermon, S. (2003). Morphological abilities of Hebrew-speaking adolescents. *Developmental Neuropsychology, 23*, 61–85.

Levy, Y., Smith, J., & Tager-Flusberg, H. (2003). Word reading and reading-related skills in adolescents with Williams syndrome. *Journal of Child Psychology and Psychiatry, 44*, 576–587.

Lord, C., Risi, S., Lambrecht, L., Cook, E. H., Jr., Leventhal, B. L., DiLavore, P. C., et al. (2000). The Autism Diagnostic Observation Schedule-Generic: A standard measure of social and communication deficits associated with the spectrum of autism. *Journal of Autism and Developmental Disorders, 30*, 205–223.

Lukács, A. (2005). *Language abilities in Williams syndrome.* Budapest, Hungary: Akadémiai Kiadó.

Lukács, A., Pléh, C., & Racsmány, M. (2004). Language in Hungarian children with Williams syndrome. In S. Bartke, & J. Siegmüller (Eds.), *Williams syndrome across languages* (pp. 187–220). Amsterdam, The Netherlands: John Benjamins Publishing.

MacDonald, G. W., & Roy, D. L. (1988). Williams syndrome: A neuropsychological profile. *Journal of Clinical and Experimental Neuropsychology, 10*, 125–131.

Maratsos, M., Kuczaj, S. A., Fox, D. E. C., & Chalkley, M. A. (1979). Some empirical studies in the acquisition of transformational relations: Passives, negatives, and the past tense. In W. A. Collins (Ed.), *The Minnesota Symposia on Child Psychology,* Vol. 12 (pp. 1–46). Hillsdale, NJ: Erlbaum.

Marler, J. A., Elfenbein, J. L., Ryals, B. M., Urban, Z., & Netzloff, M. L. (2005). Sensorineural hearing loss in children and adults with Williams syndrome. *American Journal of Medical Genetics. Part A, 138*, 318–327.

Marler, J. A., Sitcovsky, J. L., Mervis, C. B., Kistler, D. J., & Wightman, F. L. (2010). Auditory function and hearing loss in children and adults with Williams syndrome: Cochlear impairment in individuals with otherwise normal hearing. *American Journal of Medical Genetics Part C, 154C*, 249–265.

Marshall, C. R., & van der Lely, H. K. J. (2006). A challenge to current models of past tense inflection: The impact of phonotactics. *Cognition, 100*, 302–320.

Masataka, N. (2001). Why early linguistic milestones are delayed in children with Williams syndrome: Late onset of hand banging as a possible rate-limiting constraint on the emergence of canonical babbling. *Developmental Science, 4*, 158–164.

Mayer, M. (1969). *Frog, where are you?* New York: Dial Press.

McCardle, P., Chhabra, V., & Kapinus, B. (2008). *Reading research in action: A teacher's guide for student success.* Baltimore: Brookes.

Menghini, D., Verucci, L., & Vicari, S. (2004). Reading and phonological awareness in Williams syndrome. *Neuropsychology, 18*, 29–37.

Mervis, C. B. (1999). The Williams syndrome cognitive profile: Strengths, weaknesses, and interrelations among auditory short term memory, language, and visuospatial constructive cognition. In E. Winograd, R. Fivush, & W. Hirst (Eds.), *Ecological approaches to cognition: Essays in honor of Ulric Neisser* (pp. 193–227). Mahwah, NJ: Erlbaum.

Mervis, C. B. (2006). Language abilities in Williams-Beuren syndrome. In C. A. Morris, H. M. Lenhoff, & P. P. Wang (Eds.), *Williams-Beuren syndrome: Research, evaluation, and treatment* (pp. 159–206). Baltimore: Johns Hopkins University Press.

Mervis, C. B. (2009). Language and literacy development of children with Williams syndrome. *Topics in Language Disorders, 29*, 149–169.

Mervis, C. B., & Becerra, A. M. (2003). Lexical development and intervention. In J. A. Rondal, & S. Buckley (Eds.), *Speech and language intervention in Down syndrome* (pp. 63–85). London: Whurr.

Mervis, C. B., & Becerra, A. M. (2007). Language and communicative development in Williams syndrome. *Mental Retardation and Developmental Disabilities Research Reviews, 13*, 3–15.

Mervis, C. B., & Bertrand, J. (1993). Acquisition of early object labels: The roles of operating principles and input. In A. P. Kaiser, & D. B. Gray (Eds.), *Enhancing children's communication: Research foundations for intervention* (pp. 281–316). Baltimore: Brookes.

Mervis, C. B., & Bertrand, J. (1997). Developmental relations between cognition and language: Evidence from Williams syndrome. In L. B. Adamson, & M. A. Romski (Eds.), *Communication and language acquisition: Discoveries from atypical development* (pp. 75–106). New York: Brookes.

Mervis, C. B., & John, A. E. (2008). Vocabulary abilities of children with Williams syndrome: Strengths, weaknesses, and relation to visuospatial construction ability. *Journal of Speech, Language, and Hearing Research, 51*, 967–982.

Mervis, C. B., & John, A. E. (2010a). Cognitive and behavioral characteristics of children with Williams syndrome: Implications for intervention approaches. *American Journal of Medical Genetics Part C, 154C*, 229–248.

Mervis, C. B., & John, A. E. (2010b). Williams syndrome: Psychological characteristics. In B. Shapiro, & P. Accardo (Eds.), *Neurogenetic syndromes: Behavioral issues and their treatment* (pp. 81–98). Baltimore: Brookes.

Mervis, C. B., & John, A. E. (in press). Precursors to language and early language development in Williams syndrome. In E. K. Farran & A. Karmiloff-Smith (Eds.), *Neuroconstructivism: The multidisciplinary study of genetic syndromes from infancy to adulthood.* Oxford, UK: Oxford University Press.

Mervis, C. B., & Klein-Tasman, B. P. (2000). Williams syndrome: Cognition, personality, and adaptive behavior. *Mental Retardation and Developmental Disabilities Research Reviews, 6*, 148–158.

Mervis, C. B., & Klein-Tasman, B. P. (2004). Methodological issues in group-matching designs: Alpha levels for control variable comparisons and measurement characteristics of control and target variables. *Journal of Autism and Developmental Disorders, 34*, 7–17.

Mervis, C. B., & Morris, C. A. (2007). Williams syndrome. In M. M. M. Mazzocco, & J. L. Ross, *Neurogenetic developmental disorders: Variation of manifestation in childhood* (pp. 199–262). Cambridge, MA: MIT Press.

Mervis, C. B., & Robinson, B. F. (2000). Expressive vocabulary of toddlers with Williams syndrome or Down syndrome: A comparison. *Developmental Neuropsychology, 17*, 111–126.

Mervis, C. B., & Robinson, B. F. (2005). Designing measures for profiling and genotype/phenotype studies of individuals with genetic syndromes or developmental language disorders. *Applied Psycholinguistics, 26*, 41–64.

Mervis, C. B., Robinson, B. F., Bertrand, J., Morris, C. A., Klein-Tasman, B. P., & Armstrong, S. C. (2000). The Williams Syndrome Cognitive Profile. *Brain and Cognition, 44*, 604–628.

Mervis, C. B., Robinson, B. F., Rowe, M. L., Becerra, A. M., & Klein-Tasman, B. P. (2003). Language abilities of individuals who have Williams syndrome. In L. Abbeduto (Ed.), *International review of research in mental retardation* Vol. 27 (pp. 35–81). Orlando, FL: Academic Press.

Mervis, C. B., Robinson, B. F., Rowe, M. L., Becerra, A. M., & Klein-Tasman, B. P. (2004). Relations between language and cognition in Williams syndrome. In S. Bartke, & J. Siegmüller (Eds.), *Williams syndrome across languages* (pp. 63–92). Amsterdam, The Netherlands: John Benjamins Publishing.

Meyer-Lindenberg, A., Mervis, C. B., & Berman, K. F. (2006). Neural mechanisms in Williams syndrome: A unique window to genetic influences on cognition and behavior. *Nature Reviews Neuroscience, 7*, 380–393.

Meyerson, M. D., & Frank, R. A. (1987). Language, speech, and hearing in Williams syndrome: Intervention approaches and research needs. *Developmental Medicine and Child Neurology, 29*, 258–262.

Morris, C. A. (2006). The dysmorphology, genetics, and natural history of Williams-Beuren syndrome. In C. A. Morris, H. M. Lenhoff, & P. P. Wang (Eds.), *Williams-Beuren syndrome: Research, evaluation, and treatment* (pp. 3–17). Baltimore: Johns Hopkins University Press.

Mullen, E. M. (1995). *Mullen Scales of Early Learning.* Circle Pines, MN: American Guidance Service.

Mundy, P., & Hogan, A. (1996). *A preliminary manual for the abridged Early Social Communication Scales (ESCS).* Coral Gables, FL: University of Miami Psychology Department. http://www.psy.miami.edu/faculty/pmundy/ESCS.pdf

Nazzi, T., Paterson, S., & Karmiloff-Smith, A. (2003). Early word segmentation by infants and toddlers with Williams syndrome. *Infancy, 4*, 251–271.

Osborne, L. R. (2006). The molecular basis of a multisystem disorder. In C. A. Morris, H. M. Lenhoff, & P. P. Wang (Eds.), *Williams-Beuren syndrome: Research, evaluation, and treatment* (pp. 18–58). Baltimore: Johns Hopkins University Press.

Osborne, L. R., & Mervis, C. B. (2007). Rearrangements of the Williams-Beuren syndrome locus: Molecular basis and implications for speech and language development. *Expert Reviews in Molecular Medicine, 9*(15), 1–16.

Pagon, R. A., Bennett, F. C., LaVeck, B., Stewart, K. B., & Johnson, J. (1987). Williams syndrome: Features in late childhood and adolescence. *Pediatrics, 80*, 85–91.

Peregrine, E., Rowe, M. L., & Mervis, C. B. (2005). *Pragmatic language difficulties in children with Williams syndrome.* Poster presented at the biennial meeting of the Society for Research in Child Development, Atlanta, GA.

Perovic, A., & Wexler, K. (2007). Complex grammar in Williams syndrome. *Clinical Linguistics & Phonetics, 21*, 729–745.

Philofsky, A., Fidler, D. J., & Hepburn, S. (2007). Pragmatic language profiles of school-age children with autism spectrum disorders and Williams syndrome. *American Journal of Speech-Language Pathology, 16*, 368–380.

Robinson, B. F., Mervis, C. B., & Robinson, B. W. (2003). Roles of verbal short-term memory and working memory in the acquisition of grammar by children with Williams syndrome. *Developmental Neuropsychology, 23*, 13–31.

Rowe, M. L., & Mervis, C. B. (2006). Working memory in Williams syndrome. In T. P. Alloway, & S. E. Gathercole (Eds.), *Working memory and neurodevelopmental conditions* (pp. 267–293). Hove, UK: Psychology Press.

Rowe, M. L., Peregrine, E., & Mervis, C. B. (2005, April). *Communicative development in toddlers with Williams syndrome.* Poster presented at the biennial meeting of the Society for Research in Child Development, Atlanta, GA.

Saffran, J. R., Aslin, R. N., & Newport, E. L. (1996). Statistical learning by 8-month-old infants. *Science, 274*, 1926–1928.

Searcy, Y. M., Lincoln, A. J., Rose, F. E., Klima, E. S., & Bavar, N. (2004). The relationship between age and IQ in adults with Williams syndrome. *American Journal on Mental Retardation, 109*, 231–236.

Semel, E., Wiig, E. H., & Secord, W. A. (2003). *Clinical evaluation of language fundamentals–4th Edition.* San Antonio, TX: Harcourt Assessment.

Stoel-Gammon, C. (1989). Prespeech and early speech development of two late talkers. *First Language, 9*, 207–224.

Stojanovik, V. (2006). Social interaction deficits and conversational inadequacy in Williams syndrome. *Journal of Neurolinguistics, 19*, 157–173.

Stojanovik, V., Perkins, M., & Howard, S. (2006). Language and conversational abilities in Williams syndrome: How good is good? *International Journal of Language and Communication Disorders, 36*(Supplement), 234–239.

Stojanovik, V., Perkins, M., & Howard, S. (2006). Linguistic heterogeneity in Williams syndrome. *Clinical Linguistics & Phonetics, 20*, 547–552.

Stojanovik, V., & van Ewijk, L. (2008). Do children with Williams syndrome have unusual vocabularies? *Journal of Neurolinguistics, 21*, 18–34.

Strømme, P., Bjørnstad, P. G., & Ramstad, K. (2002). Prevalence estimation of Williams syndrome. *Journal of Child Neurology, 17*, 269–271.

Temple, C. M. (2006). Developmental and acquired dyslexias. *Cortex, 42*, 898–910.

Temple, C. M., Almazan, M., & Sherwood, S. (2002). Lexical skills in Williams syndrome: A cognitive neuropsychological analysis. *Journal of Neurolinguistics, 15*, 463–495.

Thomas, M. S. C., Grant, J., Barham, Z., Gsödl, M., Laing, E., Lakusta, L., et al. (2001). Past tense formation in Williams syndrome. *Language & Cognitive Processes, 16*, 143–176.

Udwin, O., Davies, M., & Howlin, P. (1996). A longitudinal study of cognitive abilities and educational attainment in Williams syndrome. *Developmental Medicine and Child Neurology, 38*, 1020–1029.

Udwin, O., & Yule, W. (1990). Expressive language of children with Williams syndrome. *American Journal of Medical Genetics Supplement, 6*, 108–114.

Udwin, O., Yule, W., & Martin, N. (1987). Cognitive and behavioral characteristics of children with idiopathic infantile hypercalcaemia. *Journal of Child Psychology and Psychiatry, 28*, 297–309.

Velleman, S. L., Currier, A., Caron, T., Curley, A., & Mervis, C. B. (2006, May). *Phonological development in Williams syndrome.* Paper presented at the annual meeting of the International Clinical Phonetics and Linguistics Association, Dubrovnik, Croatia.

Vicari, S., Bates, E., Caselli, M. C., Pasqualetti, P., Gagliardi, C., Tonucci, F., & Volterra, V. (2004). Neuropsychological profile of Italians with Williams syndrome: An example of a dissociation between language and cognition? *Journal of the International Neuropsychological Society, 10*, 862–876.

Vicari, S., Caselli, M. C., Gagliardi, C., Tonucci, F., & Volterra, V. (2002). Language acquisition in special populations: A comparison between Down and Williams syndromes. *Neuropsychologia, 40*, 2461–2460.

Volterra, V., Capirci, O., Pezzini, G., Sabbadini, L., & Vicari, S. (1996). Linguistic abilities in Italian children with Williams syndrome. *Cortex, 32*, 663–677.

Volterra, V., Caselli, M. C., Capirci, O., Tonucci, F., & Vicari, S. (2003). Early linguistic abilities of Italian children with Williams syndrome. *Developmental Neuropsychology, 23*, 33–59.

von Arnim, G., & Engel, P. (1964). Mental retardation related to hypercalcaemia. *Developmental Medicine and Child Neurology, 6*, 366–377.

Wagner, R. K., Torgesen, J. K., & Rashotte, C. A. (1999). *Comprehensive Test of Phonological Processing.* Austin, TX: PRO-ED.

Wechsler, D. (1974). *Wechsler Intelligence Scale for Children-Revised.* New York: Psychological Corporation.

Wechsler, D. (1981). Wechsler Adult Intelligence Scale-Revised. New York: Psychological Corporation.

Wechsler, D. (2005). *Wechsler Individual Achievement Test-II Update 2005.* San Antonio, TX: Harcourt Assessment.

Wetherby, A. M., & Prizant, B. M. (2002). *CSBS DP manual: Communication and Symbolic Behavior Scales: Developmental Profile, 1st normed ed.* Baltimore: Brookes.

Williams, K. T. (1997). *Expressive Vocabulary Test.* Circle Pines, MN: American Guidance Service.

Williams, K. T. (2007). *Expressive Vocabulary Test (2nd ed.).* Minneapolis, MN: Pearson Assessments.

Zukowski, A. (2004). Investigating knowledge of complex syntax: Insights from experimental studies of Williams syndrome. In M. L. Rice & S. F. Warren (Eds.), *Developmental language disorders: From phenotypes to etiologies* (pp. 99–119). Cambridge, MA: MIT Press.

PART 5

Social-Emotional Development

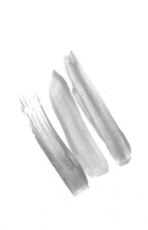

Emotional Development in Children with Developmental Disabilities

Connie L. Kasari, Laudan B. Jahromi, *and* Amanda C. Gulsrud

Abstract

Research into the emotional development of children with developmental disabilities has dramatically increased over the past decade. Studies investigating the development of children with an autism spectrum disorder (ASD) account for the largest increase in the field, but progress has also been made in better understanding emotional development in children with Down syndrome (DS). This chapter reviews the evidence on emotional strengths and weaknesses in children with autism, DS, and other developmental disorders. It identifies continuing gaps in our knowledge of emotional development and suggests some promising lines of research for the future.

Keywords: Emotional development, developmental disabilities, children, Down syndrome, autism

Research into the emotional development of children with developmental disabilities has exploded over the past decade. Studies investigating the development of children with an autism spectrum disorder (ASD) account for the largest increase in the field, but progress has also been made in better understanding emotional development in children with Down syndrome (DS). In this chapter, we will review the evidence on emotional strengths and weaknesses in children with autism, DS, and other developmental disorders. We will identify continuing gaps in our knowledge of emotional development and suggest some promising lines of research for the future.

Any consideration of the development of children with developmental disabilities is often couched in terms of a typical child developmental trajectory. By contrasting the development of children with developmental disabilities with typical development, both similarities and differences can be better understood. In this chapter, we will highlight important developmental milestones for typical child development and use this model as a framework for considering the extent to which children with

developmental disabilities are delayed or different in their emotional development. We address several areas of emotional development, including emotion recognition and understanding, emotional expressions, emotion responsiveness, and emotion regulation.

Emotion Recognition and Understanding *social aspect*

Important to children's social functioning is the ability to recognize emotions and understand their meaning in self and others. In typical children, the ability to discriminate and label simple emotions such as happiness, sadness, anger, and fear, emerges in the first 2 years of life, whereas the recognition and understanding of complex emotions such as embarrassment, guilt, pride, and empathy emerge later (Cohn, Campbell, Matias, & Hopkins, 1990; Huebner & Izard, 1988). These complex emotions are thought to develop simultaneously with more sophisticated cognitive skills, as they require the capacity for self-evaluation, perspective-taking, and social comparison. In typical young children, emotion recognition and understanding are positively related to social competence. Children who are more adept at identifying and understanding the emotions of others are rated as more socially competent by their teachers, are more liked by peers, and display more prosocial behaviors (Denham, 1986; Denham et al., 2003).

Less is known about the development of emotion recognition and understanding in atypical children, but in the last few decades, researchers have become increasingly aware of its importance. These studies have focused largely on distinct groups of children with disabilities, including children with DS, autism, and fragile X syndrome (FXS).

Down Syndrome

Children with DS provide one of the clearest examples of specific impairment in emotion recognition. Kasari and Freeman (2001) found that recognition of simple emotions was significantly more impaired for children with DS compared to mental age (MA)-matched children with mental retardation and typical controls. Specifically, the emotions of fear and anger were particularly difficult for these children to expressively label and identify. This discrepancy was evident in children matched at 4 years MA but not 3 years, suggesting that children with DS may not progress at the same rate as typical peers in their emotion recognition ability between the third and fourth year of life. It appears that the emotion recognition abilities of children with DS fail to keep pace with their cognitive advancements (Kasari, Freeman, & Bass, 2003; Kasari, Freeman, & Hughes, 2001).

Other researchers find similar weakness in emotion recognition of children with DS. Wishart and Pitcairn (2000) found that children with DS were significantly worse at identifying emotions during a photo-matching expression task than were typical control children. In this paradigm, the emotions of fear and surprise emerged as particularly difficult for children with DS, thus confirming the particular difficulty children with DS have in recognizing the emotion of fear. In a more recent study by the same group, Williams et al. (2005) continued to investigate this emerging profile of impairment. To provide greater confidence in research findings, an increased number of trials were employed, as well as the elimination of any task that required expressive language demands. Consistent with previous research, children with DS had significant difficulties in nonverbal identification of expressed emotion, especially fearful expressions. In a 2007 study by the same group (Wishart, Cebula, Willis, & Pitcairn, 2007) children with DS were compared to

matched samples of children with FXS, nonspecific developmental delays, and typical control children. Again, children with DS performed significantly worse but only compared to the typical children, with fear recognition being particularly impaired. Children with FXS and nonspecific developmental delays performed similarly to developmentally matched typical children. Thus, research has confirmed that children with DS present with a specific impairment in emotion recognition particularly in the domain of fear when compared to typical children and children with other developmental delays.

Autism Spectrum Disorder

In contrast to the specific and consistently found deficits in the area of emotion recognition for children with DS, there is considerable debate in the field of autism research about both the presence and origin of emotion-related deficits. Due to contradictory findings, researchers have been unable to agree on whether a specific deficit in emotion recognition exists in this population.

Some research suggests that children with autism have a specific deficit in emotion recognition stemming from a broader deficit in facial processing. More specifically, these studies have found that children with autism are impaired in their ability to attend to and draw meaning from others' faces and this, in turn, impedes their ability to recognize and understand emotions in others. Hobson (1986) found that children with autism were more proficient when matching non–emotion-related items and less proficient when matching emotion-related items. However, these differences for the most part diminished when the children were matched for verbal abilities. Hobson et al. (1989) also found that children with autism were significantly more impaired in coordinating emotionally expressive sounds and faces than in coordinating the sounds and appearances of non–emotion-related objects. Both of these findings support Hobson's notion that perceptual difficulties in children with autism are specific to other people's faces. This suggests that children with autism may have a specific deficit in processing emotion-related stimuli due to their difficulty in processing facial features.

This finding has been independently supported in the work of Gross (2004). When looking at error patterns for identifying emotions in humans and other animals, he found that children with autism more often attended to the lower region and not the whole face, compared to typical and MR controls. In this study, nonautistic children performed better on the emotion recognition task when they saw the whole face as opposed to partial features. Conversely, this had no effect on the accuracy of response for children with autism. Again, these findings point to a specific deficit in facial processing that impedes the development of emotion recognition.

Downs and Smith (2004) examined emotion recognition and understanding in a group of children with high-functioning autism (HFA). Compared with children with attention deficit hyperactivity disorder (ADHD) and typical controls, the children with autism performed significantly worse when asked to identify emotion expressions in photographs. Surprisingly, when subjects were probed for more detailed understanding of emotions and the causes of emotions, the ADHD children were the most impaired. The children with autism did not differ from typical controls in overall emotional understanding, including understanding belief-based emotions. In another sample of HFA children, Bailey (unpublished dissertation) found similar specific deficits when she probed for emotion recognition from videotaped vignettes. This finding was robust despite each child undergoing intensive behavioral therapy that incorporated emotion recognition training. In addition, some research suggests that compared to typical children, children with autism are slower in identifying emotions and make more errors in identifying specific emotions in faces (Bal et al, 2010). Within the ASD group, severity of autism symptoms and decreased gaze to the eye region were both related to more difficulties in emotion recognition.

Age-related differences in emotion recognition may also exist in this population. A study by Kuusikko et al. (2009) found that older children with autism (over 12 years of age) performed better than younger children with autism on identifying blended emotions. While improvements may be evident with increasing age, children with ASD continued to score lower than controls on emotion recognition tasks. They also tended to attribute ambiguous stimuli to a negative emotion, and were particularly impaired in identifying expressions of anger relative to age matched controls (Wright et al, 2008).

Not all emotion recognition studies find differences between children with and without autism. Heery et al. (2003) compared children with HFA to typical controls and found no significant differences in the ability to recognize simple emotions from photos, but did find that children with HFA performed significantly worse when asked to recognize complex emotions, such as embarrassment and shame. Hobson, Chidambi, Lee & Meyer (2006) also find that children with HFA often can recognize simpler emotions, but have mixed findings with respect to the social emotions of pride, guilt and embarrassment. While several studies find particular difficulty in recognizing social and complex emotions, there are exceptions. Hillier and Allinson (2002) failed to find significant difficulties for children with HFA in the recognition and understanding of the complex emotion of embarrassment. Williams and Happe (2010) failed to find any differences between a sample of children with autism and a matched sample of children with learning disabilities. Both groups had more difficulty identifying the social as compared to non-social emotions. This difficulty was related to individual differences in the ability to recognize social emotions in others and was independent of group, age or verbal ability. In another study, children and adolescents with ASD showed no greater impairment in the speed or accuracy of identifying simple and complex emotions compared to typical controls (Tracy, Robins, Schriber & Solomon, 2011). These contradictory results raise some important issues in the study of emotion recognition and understanding in children with autism, and suggest the need for additional studies that tease apart issues related to individual differences, task and context.

For example, as autism is a spectrum disorder composed of a heterogeneous population, emotion recognition and understanding deficits may be present in some, but not all children with the disorder. For children with autism who are lower functioning, emotion-related difficulties appear to be widespread and span both emotion recognition and understanding domains (Hobson, 1986; Kasari & Sigman, 1996; Ozonoff, Pennington, & Rogers, 1990). For children on the spectrum who are higher functioning, the presence of emotion recognition and understanding deficits are less clearly defined. It appears that these children may have more specific difficulties in self-evaluative or complex emotions, and their knowledge of simple emotions may be relatively intact (Heery, Keltner, & Capps, 2003; Hobson et al, 2006). Further research into the nature of emotion-related deficits is needed in order to conclude for whom and what types of emotions (simple vs. complex) are affected.

Other Disabilities

Emotion recognition and understanding has had limited study in children with other specific disabilities.

Some information is available for children with FXS, the most common inherited intellectual disability. In contrast to children with DS and some children with autism, children with FXS do not appear to have specific deficits in emotion recognition. Turk and Cornish (1998) compared both the facial and vocal identification of emotional expressions in differing contexts in boys with FXS, children with DS, and typical peers matched on chronological age. Results showed that FXS children did not differ significantly from a typical sample matched on chronological age for facial recognition, but did differ from the DS sample, with the DS sample performing significantly worse. There were no group differences in the ability to recognize emotion from facial expressions or emotion from vocalization, but children with DS performed significantly worse than typical controls when the emotions were presented in varying contexts. These results illustrate that the ability to recognize emotion may be relatively unaffected for children with FXS. Although social impairments are very clearly present in children with FXS, the origin may not be in the domain of emotion recognition or understanding.

Some additional work has examined children with Williams syndrome. This group of children presents as highly social and expressive and hypotheses about whether this presentation is linked to better recognition of emotions have been tested. Plesa-Skewerer and colleagues (2006) found that compared to a group of children with intellectual disabilities (ID) and typically developing children, children with Williams perform similarly to the ID group and both perform significantly worse than typical matched controls. Both the Williams and ID groups had more difficulty identifying negative emotions, such as sadness, fear, and anger. All three groups identified positive emotions with similar accuracy. In this study, the children with Williams syndrome showed deficits in recognizing negative emotions but these deficits do not appear unique to Williams syndrome as children with ID showed similar deficits. In a more recent study, children with Williams syndrome were compared to a group of children with autism and results showed that children with autism were more adept at identifying emotions (Lacriox, Guidette, Roge, & Reilly, 2009). These studies suggest that children with Williams syndrome, similar to other children with intellectual disabilities, show deficits in their abilities to identify emotions. However, the deficits for children with Williams syndrome may be greater than for children with ASD.

The literature to date on emotion recognition and understanding provides a relatively clear profile for some disabilities, such as DS and FXS, and a less clear profile for other disabilities, such as autism. In the case of autism, more research is needed to draw conclusions about the nature of emotion-related deficits and to profile which types of children are most greatly affected. More research is needed on other disabilities, including FXS and Williams, and across more diverse tasks, to have greater confidence in the findings from the current limited database.

Emotional Expression

An important element of children's healthy social functioning can be explained by their appropriate expression of emotions (Eisenberg, Cumberland, & Spinrad, 1998; Halberstadt, Crisp, & Eaton, 1999), which is often considered to be a function of children's temperaments. In infancy, facial expressions serve the purpose of communicating emotions. Children who express more positive and less negative affect are generally viewed more favorably by parents and teachers, and have better relationships with peers (e.g., Denham & Bruger, 1991; Denham & Grout, 1992). Similarly, positive temperament styles are associated with increased peer interactions for children with disabilities, whereas negative temperament is associated with higher levels of negative teacher–child interactions (Keogh & Burstein, 1988). It is important, therefore, to understand the emotional expressions and responses of infants and young children with developmental delays and other developmental disabilities. A good deal of work in this area has focused on children with DS, who display different patterns of affect expression than do other children with and without delay. Most of the research in this area has examined children's facial and vocal affective responses to social interactions and to various emotion-eliciting situations. Although in previous years the emphasis has been on positive affect and smiling, more recent work has revealed interesting findings concerning negative affect and frustration, particularly in older children.

Down Syndrome

Early work on infants with DS suggested that they show decreased emotionality and responsiveness to their environment. For example, Emde, Katz, and Thorpe (1978) found that infants with DS showed dampened smiles with little or no bodily activity, such as a waving arm or leg, which is common in typical infants. They also displayed shorter and less frequent affective expressions, and longer latencies to express affect than did typically developing infants and young children (Cicchetti & Sroufe, 1976; Emde & Brown, 1978; Kasari, Mundy, Yirmiya, & Sigman, 1990). Delays in smiling and laughing have been shown to be greatest in infants with the most pronounced hypertonia and hypotonia (Gallagher, Jens, & O'Donnell, 1983). Finally, although studies indicate that infants with DS do show distress upon separation from their mothers in the Strange Situation (Berry, Gunn, & Andrews, 1980), those who have compared them to typically developing infants have found that infants with DS display significantly less negative emotional intensity and a longer latency to distress than do matched typical infants (Thompson et al., 1985).

Work on toddlers and children with DS indicate mixed findings concerning their expressions of positive affect. Some studies show that, in contrast to their behaviors in infancy, these children show greater positive expressions than MA-matched children, and commonly pair smiles with looks to the social partner (Capps, Kasari, Yirmiya, & Sigman, 1993; Kasari, Mundy, Yirmiya, & Sigman, 1990; Kasari & Sigman, 1996; Landry & Chapieski, 1990). More specifically, Kasari et al.'s (1990) findings indicate that, although the frequency of positive affect appears to increase post-infancy, the intensity of these expressions may remain somewhat stable during childhood. Others have found *less* positive affect in children with DS compared to children with developmental delay, physical impairments, or typical development (Bieberich & Morgan, 2004; Brooks-Gunn & Lewis, 1982).

With respect to negative affect post-infancy, researchers have found more variability in the temperamental ratings of children with DS, similar to that among typical children (Bridges & Cicchetti, 1982), and even signs of a "difficult" temperament among children with DS (Gunn & Berry, 1985). In a recent study by Jahromi, Gulsrud, and Kasari (2008), which examined negative affective expressions during a challenging task in a sample of children with DS, children with DS displayed significantly more frustration than matched samples of typical children and children with nonspecific developmental delays.

Fidler and colleagues (Fidler, Most, Booth-LaForce, & Kelly, 2006; Fidler, Barret, & Most, 2005) found an interesting pattern of change in temperamental style with age in the DS population. Fidler et al.'s (2006) longitudinal study of temperament and behavioral problems in children with DS

and those with mixed etiologies at 12, 30, and 45 months of age reveals that, although 12-month-olds with DS did not differ from the comparison sample in the measure of "difficult temperament" (including negative mood) at 12 months, they did show a significant increase in problem behaviors from 30 to 45 months. Moreover, although temperament ratings at 12 months predicted problem behaviors in the mixed-etiology sample, early temperament did not predict later problem behaviors for the children with DS, indicating a lack of stability, or discontinuity, in these processes for children with DS (Fidler et al., 2006).

Yet another pattern seems to appear when even older children, adolescents, and young adults with DS are studied. In a sample of individuals aged 5 through 20, the older individuals with DS showed significantly fewer and shorter durations of smiles than did the younger children with DS. Individuals with developmental delays of mixed etiology, in contrast, showed longer smile durations with increasing age (Fidler et al., 2005). Smiling behavior was inversely related to social problems, such that individuals who displayed more smiling had fewer social problems. This finding is in line with research that suggests changes in psychopathology and maladjustment in adolescents with DS (Dykens, Shah, Sagun, Beck, & King, 2002). Although the study utilized a cross-sectional design, it highlights an important developmental shift in emotional development for adolescents and young adults with DS.

Autism Spectrum Disorders

Children with autism offer an interesting comparison to those with DS. The emotional expressions of children with autism are often more negative (Kasari & Sigman, 1997) or ambiguous (Yirmiya, Kasari, Sigman, & Mundy, 1989). Studies of parents' perceptions and those involving observation indicate that children with autism display more negative and less positive affect than do comparison children (Capps et al., 1993; Joseph & Tager-Flusberg, 1997). Recent physiological work has explored autonomic reactivity and the subjective experience of emotion in children with autism. For example, in a study of high functioning children with autism and Asperger syndrome, Shalmon et al. (2006) found that children with autism or Asperger syndrome were similar to typical controls in their autonomic emotional response (i.e., skin conductance) to viewing positive, negative, and neutral pictures. Children with autism were, however, different in their affective self-reports of the three pictures, such that they failed to differentiate among pictures of positive, negative, and neutral expressions. In another study of physiological emotional expressions, Bolte, Feineis-Matthews, and Poustka (2008) induced specific emotional states (e.g., fear, anger, disgust, happiness, and sadness) in adults with autism and typical controls. The authors examined both physiological emotional expressions and affective self-reports in response to the stimuli and found that individuals with autism showed a different physiological trajectory in response to the stimuli as compared to typical adults. With respect to affective reports, individuals with autism indicated less emotional arousal in response to the sad pictures but higher arousal in response to the neutral stimuli. Together, the early findings concerning physiological emotional reactivity in individuals with autism suggest a possible mismatch between emotional experiences and subjective reports of affective expressions.

Other Disabilities

In the area of emotional expression, there is again limited research in populations of children other than FXS. Similar to the work on emotion recognition and understanding, studies find that children with FXS do not show clear delays in emotion expressiveness, but they do show a tendency toward more negative temperamental characteristics. Although these children show frequent smiling and enjoyment of social interactions in familiar settings, they also display clear signs of a negative temperament and increased irritability, particular as they get older and enter more demanding situations (Hagerman, 1996; Kau, Reider, Payne, Meyer, & Greund, 2000). Temper tantrums and aggressive outbursts are a consequence of this increasing irritability. Research suggests that, in comparison to typical matched controls, children with FXS are significantly slower to adapt, less persistent, more withdrawing, and more active (Bailey, Hatton, Mesibov, & Ament, 2000; Kau et al., 2000; Roberts, Boccia, Hatton, Skinner, & Sideris, 2006). In comparison to children with autism, children with FXS were also found to be more active, more intense, more distractible, and to have a lower threshold for change along with more negative moods (Bailey et al., 2000). It is thought that heightened physiological arousal may explain this behavioral style.

Together, research suggests that children with different etiologies show varying patterns of emotional expressions across childhood. Development also explains some of this variability, as affective expressions and the associated behaviors also appear to change from infancy through childhood within specific syndromes. Future research is needed to further understand the contextual factors that may explain change in affective expressions, for example the role of parents and peers. In addition, it will be important to further explore the consequences of varying affective styles on these children's functioning.

Emotion Responsiveness

The ability to respond appropriately to other's emotional expressions is another important developmental milestone. In typical children, this emerges simultaneously with the ability to recognize and understand the meaning of expressed emotion in self and others. The ability to respond to others' expressed emotion in a prosocial manner is important to the successful emotional development of any child. Children who can read the emotions of another and respond contingently have more positive relationships with peers and adults (Denham, 1986; Denham et al., 2003).

Children with atypical development do not always fit the same profile of emotion responsiveness as typical children. For example, responses to negative emotions in others have been examined in children with autism compared to typical controls. Many independent accounts have confirmed that children with autism gaze less at a experimenter or parent who is displaying distress (e.g., Bauminger et al., 2008; Bacon, Fein, Morris, Waterhous, & Allen, 1998; Corona et al., 1998; Dawson et al., 2004; Dissanyake, Sigman, & Kasari, 1996; Sigman, Kasari, Kwon, & Yirmiya, 1992) and show less empathic concern (e.g., Bacon et al., 1998; Charman et al., 1998; Dawson et al., 2004; Sigman et al., 1992). More recent work in this area suggests that the empathic difficulties of children with ASD could be related to their delays with cognitive perspective-taking (Jones, Happe, Gilbert, Burnett, & Viding, 2010) or emotional processing (Clark, Winkielman, & McIntosh, 2008). Moreover, work by Hudry and Slaughter (2009) suggests that while children with ASD have been described by parents as less responsive (e.g., to show less comforting acts) overall than typical controls, the familiarity of and type of emotion expressed by the agent appear to moderate these children's empathic expressions. Like their typical peers, children with ASD in Hudrey and Slaughter's (2009) study showed the most empathy toward familiar individuals and the least responsiveness toward unknown individuals. However, children with ASD differed from comparison peers in the variability of their responses, with stronger, more negative, personal distress responses to others' fear and anger, and more sympathetic responses to others' pain, illness and frustration (Hudry & Slaughter, 2009).

Responses to emotions have also been examined as they relate to other emotional outcomes in these children. Bauminger et al. (2008) found that this ability to respond to others distress is related to the ability to express the outward emotion of jealousy in children with autism. Children with autism who engaged in more emotional responsiveness such as hugging the adult also displayed more jealous behaviors, as indicated by the child's gaze and higher ratings on a jealousy index.

In contrast, children with DS have been found to show greater empathic responses when compared to children with nonspecific developmental delays and typical children. In a 2003 study, Kasari et al. found that children with DS showed little positive or negative expressed emotion during a distress paradigm but did orient to the experimenter more and display more prosocial comforting behaviors than did children with nonspecific mental retardation and typical children. Although these children showed greater concern, they had difficulty understanding the abstract concept of empathy in a hypothetical testing situation.

From the limited work in this area, an interesting profile of emotional responsiveness emerges. It appears that although children with DS have limited emotional expressions when faced with another's distress, they do provide more comfort seeking and prosocial behaviors than do those with nonspecific mental retardation and typical children. Children with autism are perhaps the most impaired in this area, as these children gaze less at others in distress and display less concern

Emotion Regulation

In typically developing children, the earliest forms of emotion regulation appear in infancy (Mangelsdorf, Shapiro, & Marzolf, 1995; Stifter, 2002). Infants have been shown to use a range of regulatory behaviors in response to negativity, including attentional strategies (orienting, distraction, and gaze aversion), avoidance, non-negative communication, and self-comforting behaviors (Buss & Goldsmith, 1998; Crockenberg & Leerkes, 2004; Diener & Mangelsdorf, 1999; Stifter & Braungart, 1995). Across the first few years of development, the behavioral repertoire of toddlers and young children also includes coping strategies that reflect their increasing cognitive capacity. Young children begin to use more constructive strategies, including cognitive reappraisals and mental re-evaluations (Calkins & Johnson, 1998; Diener & Mangelsdorf, 1999; Grolnick, Bridges, & Connell, 1996; Spinrad, Stifter, Donelan-McCall, & Turner, 2004; Stansbury & Sigman). The association between specific strategies (e.g., distraction, instrumental coping, and goal-directed behaviors) and decreased negativity has been documented with typical samples in the context of delay of gratification and other tasks involving negativity or frustration (e.g., Calkins & Johnson, 1998; Eisenberg et al., 1995; Jahromi & Stifter, 2007). Children's ability to appropriately self-regulate their emotions is important for their social competence, including the ability to avoid aggressive behavior (Eisenberg & Fabes, 1992).

Given the importance of emotion regulation for typical children's social outcomes, it is not surprising that, in the past decade, there has been increasing interest in understanding the development of emotion regulation in children with developmental disability. Although this area of research is in its early stages, recent work on children with DS and FXS indicate interesting etiological differences in this developmental skill and point to the importance of future work on this topic.

Down Syndrome

The earliest work on infants with DS revealed an interesting pattern of affective reactivity and regulation in this population. Cicchetti and Sroufe (1978) noted a general dampening of negative reactivity in these infants during a visual cliff, but also found that the infants who did show fear had greater difficulty calming themselves than did typical infants. One interpretation of this behavioral pattern is that of an inadequate affect modulation system.

A few studies have addressed affect modulation in toddlers and children with DS. In the context of a challenging task, children with DS have been shown to use social distraction behaviors (i.e., orienting to an experimenter, establishing eye-contact, comfort-seeking) and off-task behaviors that focus their attention away from completing a task, whereas typical children use more goal-directed strategies, such as assistance-seeking and cognitive self-soothing (Jahromi, Gulsrud, & Kasari, 2008; Kasari & Freeman, 2001; Pitcairn & Wishart, 1994). Given that children with DS also show heightened frustration in these contexts, it appears that they are limited in the use of strategies that are effective for coping with their negativity (Jahromi, Gulsrud, & Kasari, 2008). These findings are consistent with those of Baker et al. (2007), who found greater evidence of observed dysregulation in frustrating laboratory tasks in a sample of children classified as intellectually delayed based on Bayley Mental Development Index (MDI) scores, as compared to a comparison sample of children with normal intellectual development.

Although there is limited work addressing emotion regulation behaviors in children with mental retardation, work on other forms of behavior regulation may offer some insight on the topic. Children with an inability to regulate heightened emotions are also likely to show problems with situations requiring compliance to others' demands and in situations that involve a delay of gratification. In recent years, there has been increased attention to such behaviors in children with developmental and intellectual delays, including those with DS. Early work by Mischel and Ebbesen (1970) revealed that children with DS use significantly fewer strategies to regulate their emotion while waiting in a delay-of-gratification task (Kopp, Krakow, & Johnson, 1983) and they are less able to delay gratification than are typical matched subjects (Cuskelly, Zhang, & Hayes, 2003; Kopp et al., 1983). Bieberich and Morgan (1998, 2004) have found that children with DS, in comparison to those with autism, showed *higher* self-regulation and fewer ratings of deviant behavior. However, a comparison to typically developing children was not available in their study. More recently, McIntyre, Blacher, and Baker (2006) compared a sample of children with intellectual disability and typical development at 3 and 5 years of age and found that at both ages, those with intellectual disability were less likely to delay gratification and showed significantly shorter latencies to delay. Together, these studies provide further evidence that children with DS may be limited in their use of regulatory strategies to modulate the negative affect that is associated with behavioral control.

What are some hypotheses about the possible developmental shift toward greater dysregulation in children with DS? One suggestion is that a consequence of the early dampened emotional expressions seen in this population is that it compromises their caregiver's ability to effectively recognize and respond to their affective states (Cicchetti, Ganiban, & Barnett, 1991; Kasari & Sigman, 1996). Caregivers serve as a source of external regulation for young infants, and early experience with external regulation is thought to facilitate infants' development of self-regulatory skills (Kopp, 1989; Thompson, 1994). It may be that, with age, children with DS are faced with more challenging contexts that elicit negative arousal, but have little experience coping with such situations. A decline in cognitive ability offers another explanation for the increasing difficulty with affect modulation. Children with DS often decline cognitively across late childhood (Hodapp, Evans, & Gray, 1999; Wishart, 1993), and this cognitive deceleration may result in greater failure and frustration in these children over time. Moreover, as cognitive skills facilitate higher-order emotion regulation strategies (e.g., constructive coping, mental re-evaluation), failures to self-regulate may be a function of decreases in cognitive development.

Autism and Fragile X Syndrome

The development of emotion regulation has also been addressed in both children with FXS and autism, with evidence of poor behavioral and emotional self-regulation in both populations. Children with FXS often exhibit heightened physiological arousal and inadequate arousal modulation. Differences have been documented between children with FXS and typically developing children in the physiological process thought to underlie behavioral regulation. One such physiological measure is cardiac vagal tone, which is a component of the parasympathetic activity of the autonomic nervous system that reflects the system's ability to maintain a regulated state of homeostasis (Porges, 2003). Compared to typical children, children with FXS show both elevated reactivity measures of physiological arousal and reduced baseline vagal tone and vagal reactivity, which indicate a pattern of high arousal and poor arousal modulation (Belser & Sudhalter, 1995; Keysor & Mazzocco, 2002; Roberts et al., 2006).

Individuals with autism also appear to be impaired in their ability to regulate emotional arousal or reactivity (Loveland, 2005; Wetherby, Prizant, & Schuler, 2000). Similar to children with FXS, they show increased emotional reactivity (Hirstein, Iversen, & Ramachandran, 2001), the consequence of which appears to be a decreased capacity to properly engage in self-regulatory strategies that require input from cognitive, attentional, and motor processes (Whitman, 2004). Konstantareas and Stewart (2006) found evidence of less adaptive affective regulation strategies in a laboratory situation that involved frustration among children with ASD than typical matched controls. Moreover, children with autism differed significantly from typical controls in the temperament factor of effortful control, which is comprised of scales that are highly connected to emotion self-regulation (i.e., measures of inhibitory control, attentional focusing, low intensity pleasure, smiling and laughter, and soothability) (Konstantareas & Stewart, 2006). Evidence from clinical measures of self-regulation such as the Temperament and Atypical Behavior Scale (TABS) have shown that 80 percent of children with autism were reported as having "self-regulatory difficulties" at 1 year of age (Gomez & Baird, 2005), and that children with autism were significantly more impaired in all but one TABS scale than a comparison sample of developmental delayed children with 22q13 Deletion Syndrome (Glaser & Shaw, 2011). Even high functioning children with ASD, including those with average range IQs, have been reported by mainstream teachers as exhibiting behavioral and emotional difficulties that affect classroom performance, including difficulty maintaining their attention and regulating their emotions (Ashburner, Zivaniani, & Rodger, 2010). Taken together, research indicates that children with developmental disability may have compromised self-regulatory processes. Further research addressing the antecedents and consequences of emotion regulation in delayed populations will enable us to better understand the source of this deficit and the degree to which dysregulation predicts these children's overall functioning. In the case of ASD, it may be that several core features of the disorder, including difficulties with joint attention and associated hyperactivity symptoms, may be related to the challenges noted in emotion regulation. For example, in typically-developing children, Morales, et al. (2005) found that joint attention skills, particularly the ability to follow the direction of a mother's gaze at 6 months, were related to children's use of effective emotion regulation strategies at 2 years of age, and that coordination of joint attention and emotion regulation were related concurrently at 2 years of age. Similarly, Raver (1996) found that typical children who were able to engage in more joint attention during free-play with their mothers were more likely to engage in distraction self-regulation techniques during a delay of gratification task. Interestingly, in a study of a caregiver-driven intervention targeting joint engagement in children with autism, Gulsrud, Jahromi, and Kasari (2010) found that both caregivers' and their children with autism employed significantly more emotion co-regulation behaviors during distress episodes over the course of

the intervention, and that children decreased their expression of negativity across the intervention, lending further support of a link between the development of joint attention and emotion self-regulation abilities. In another study targeting the hyperactivity behaviors of children with Pervasive Developmental Disorder and symptoms associated with ADHD (i.e., hyperactivity, distractibility, and impulsivity), a significant, positive clinical effect of the psychostimulant medication methylphenidate was found on these children's emotion self-regulation and affective behaviors in addition to positive effects on those behaviors directly targeted by the medication (Jahromi, Kasari, McCracken, et al., 2009). These findings suggest that not only do children with ASD have difficulties with emotion self-regulation, but that such difficulties may be associated with other core dimensions of the disorder and that treatments targeting the core deficits may have cumulative positive effects on children's emotion regulation.

Implications for Intervention

Intervention is always an important area for discussion when studying children with developmental disabilities. Specific interventions for emotional development, however, have only recently begun to emerge. Most interventions to date focus on parent training and/or child-directed interventions. Within this framework, various theoretical approaches are employed, including social-cognitive, behavioral, cognitive-behavioral, and psychoeducational, and most are commonly adapted from existing interventions with typical or at-risk children.

Several intervention programs have been developed to target emotional development in children using a child-directed approach. Some of these programs utilize a universal intervention model, thus providing program- or school-wide interventions to all children regardless of developmental level or disability. Two well-validated programs include a universal childcare intervention program, the Social Emotional Intervention (Denham & Burton, 1996) and an elementary school-aged intervention, Promoting Alternative Thinking Strategies (PATHS) program (Greenberg, Kusche, Cook, & Quamma, 1995). Specific outcomes for developmentally disabled, at-risk, and typical children have been reported.

In the Social Emotional Intervention, teachers were trained to build a relationship with the child, improve children's understanding and regulation of emotions, and improve children's social problem solving abilities in the childcare setting (Denham & Burton, 1996). After 32 weeks of individualized instruction, children showed decreased negative emotion, greater involvement with peers, and more initiative in positive peer play compared to children who did not receive the intervention. Similar positive results were found in the PATHS program, where second- and third-grade classrooms received treatment targeting self-control, emotion knowledge, and problem solving abilities in a randomized control study design (Greenberg et al., 1995). Teachers carried out the curriculum over an entire school year, with results including improvement in children's range of emotion vocabulary, fluency in discussing emotion experiences, and overall improved in emotion understanding. In this study, special education students made particularly large gains, partly because of their lower levels of understanding when the program started. These two studies provide evidence for the effectiveness of a universal treatment approach on the emotional development of children and suggest it may even by more powerful for children with developmental disabilities.

More recently, efforts have been made to evaluate several emotion-related interventions specifically designed for children with autism. The Social Communication, Emotion Regulation, and Transactional Supports (SCERTS) program is an autism-specific intervention designed to specifically target social communication and emotion regulation outcomes (Prizant, Wetherby, Rubin, Laurent, & Rydell, 2006). In this program, the child's use of more effective and socially appropriate self-regulation strategies are assessed, then targeted by intervening directly with the child to encourage the use of behavioral strategies (removing self from overstimulation) and language (metacognitive self-talk) to regulate levels of arousal. This program is the first of its kind to specifically target emotion regulation in children with autism, and studies are under way to test its efficacy.

Interventions specifically targeting emotion recognition in children with autism have also been studied. Ryan and Charragain (2010) implemented a training to help children identify the components of facial expressions through the use of verbal labels, repeated opportunity for mastery, role-play, homework and parent involvement. Compared to a wait-list control group, children who received the immediate training improved in their emotion recognition with a large effect size (d=1.42).

Several social-cognitive interventions for high-functioning children with autism have also been tested in the field. Some of the most effective have utilized the principles of cognitive-behavior therapy and adapted the curriculum to target the specific social-emotional deficits in children with autism. For example, Bauminger (2002) tested an adapted school-based intervention (Margalit & Weisel, 1990; Spivack & Shure, 1974) and showed positive outcomes in preadolescent children with HFA (Bauminger, 2002). The 7-month intervention consisted of teaching problem solving, emotional knowledge, and social skills to 15 children with HFA. In addition to these child-directed intervention sessions, teacher and peers were trained to implement strategies at school, and parents were educated on the treatment goals at home. After intervention, significant gains were noted in several areas, including social interaction, problem solving, and emotional knowledge, thus suggesting that a relatively intense and global intervention can produce positive social-emotional outcomes for children with HFA.

In 2007, Bauminger again found improved social-cognitive and emotional outcomes for children with HFA who underwent a cognitive-behavioral intervention. Children increased social behaviors compared to typical children during blindly rated observations and maintained these behaviors for 4 months after treatment. Children also improved in their social problem solving strategies and their understanding of complex emotions. In another social-cognitive intervention designed for children with HFA, Solomon et al. (2004) evaluated emotion recognition and understanding, theory of mind, and executive function (problem solving) in 18 boys with HFA, Asperger syndrome, or pervasive developmental disorder-NOS (PDD-NOS). Child-directed group intervention sessions were held 1.5 hours weekly for 20 weeks. Parent training sessions were concurrently conducted. A wait-list control versus active intervention design was implemented, and results revealed that children assigned to the intervention group made significant gains in emotion recognition and problem solving.

Recently, Stichter and colleagues (2010) implemented an intervention in a group-design again utilizing cognitive-behavioral principles. This intervention targeted theory of mind, emotion recognition and executive functioning and found positive results on parent report of social skills, child emotion recognition and theory of mind and problem solving. These studies provide evidence of the potential effectiveness of a global cognitive-behavioral intervention for children with autism, but future work is necessary to determine the efficacy of these principles compared to other potential interventions. Comparing treatments through the use of randomized controlled trials will provide more information on the active ingredients of intervention for children with autism.

Another promising approach for teaching emotions concerns the implementation of computer-based interventions. Silver and Oakes (2001) utilized computer-based emotion recognition software to teach 11- to 18-year-old children with autism. In this study, 22 children were matched for age, gender, and school, and then randomly assigned to treatment or control. The 11 children who received the computer intervention made significant gains in the identification of facial expressions of emotions and understanding of social situations. Positive results were also noted by Lacava et al. (2007), who recorded increases in facial and vocal emotion recognition as a result of their computer-based emotion software. They also noted some generalization of the identification of complex emotions not included in the computer program. Again using media, Golan and colleagues (2010) found positive results of an animated series that used vehicles with emotional expressions. Children who used the software everyday for 4 weeks outperformed a clinical sample of children with autism who did not receive the intervention and scored equivalently to typical controls at the end of treatment. In general, the small sample size and exclusion of lower-functioning individuals with autism require more studies using computer-based programs and media.

Most of the intervention studies designed for children with disabilities focus on children on the autism spectrum, largely ignoring children with other disabilities. Children with DS and FXS show significant delays and differences in emotion development and thus also are in need of targeted interventions. However, at this point, we have little knowledge about how these children might respond to treatment and which treatments might provide the most optimal outcomes. The next steps for intervention research should include the development of innovative and targeted interventions to improve emotional outcomes in children with these disabilities.

Conclusion

At this junction, we know much more about the emotional development of children with disabilities than we did a decade ago, yet there are still many gaps in our knowledge. These gaps are most apparent in our understanding of the relations between emotions and other developmental abilities, and in our understanding of change in emotional knowledge over different ages. We also have much more knowledge of some disorders than we do of others. For example, although we have many new studies on children with autism, we have a lack of consistency in results. Because autism is a spectrum disorder, there is much more variability in presentation of children's abilities. Thus, future studies are needed to further explore the variability in findings for children with autism.

For children with DS, we are beginning to see a consistent picture in the emotional development of these children at the earliest stages and the youngest ages. However, we still lack a consistent developmental picture in terms of the changes and importance of emotional understandings to overall functioning. Finally, for children with other developmental disabilities, we have little to no information in some cases, and limited, but consistent findings in others (e.g., children with FXS). For all children, we need to pay more attention to the development of interventions aimed at improving emotional development across different ages and contexts. We hope that future efforts may find the "active ingredients" of interventions, so that we can target effective interventions for particular children at different ages.

References

Ashburner, J., Ziviani, J., & Rodger, S. (2010). Surviving in the mainstream: Capacity of children with autism spectrum disorders to perform academically and regulate their emotions and behavior at school. *Research in Autism Spectrum Disorders, 4*, 18–27.

Bacon, A. L., Fein, D., Morris, R., Waterhouse, L., & Allen, D. (1998). The responses of autistic children to the distress of others. *Journal of Autism and Developmental Disorders, 28*, 129–142.

Bailey, K. J. (2001). Social competence of children with autism classified as best-outcome following behavior analytic treatment. *Dissertation Abstracts International: Section B: The Sciences and Engineering, 61*, 6696.

Bailey, D. B., Hatton, D. D., Mesibov, G., & Ament, N. (2000). Early development, temperament, and functional impairment in autism and Fragile X syndrome. *Journal of Autism and Developmental Disorders, 30*, 49–59.

Baker, J. K., Fenning, R. M., Crnic, K. A., Baker, B. L., & Blacher, J. (2007). Prediction of social skills in 6-year-old children with and without developmental delays: Contributions of early regulation and maternal scaffolding. *American Journal on Mental Retardation, 112*, 375–391.

Bal, E., Harden, E., Lamb, D., Van Hecke, A., Denver, J.W., & Porges, S.W. (2010). Emotion recognition in children with autism spectrum disorders: Relations to eye gaze and autonomic state. *Journal of Autism and Developmental Disorders, 40*, 358–370.

Bauminger, N. (2007). Brief Report: Individual social-multi-modal intervention for HFASD. *Journal of Autism and Developmental Disorders, 37*, 1593–1604.

Bauminger, N. (2002). The facilitation of social-emotional understanding and social interaction in high-functioning children with autism: Intervention outcomes. *Journal of Autism and Developmental Disorders, 32*, 283–298.

Bauminger, N., Chomsky-Smolkin, L., Orbach-Caspi, E., Zachor, D., & Levy-Shiff, R. (2008). Jealousy and emotional responsiveness in young children with ASD. *Cognition and Emotion, 22*, 595–619.

Belser, R. C., & Sudhalter, V. (1995). Arousal difficulties in males with fragile X syndrome: A preliminary report. *Developmental Brain Dysfunction, 8*, 270–279.

Ben Shalmon, D., Mostofsky, S. H., Hazlett, R. L., Goldberg, M. C., Landa, R. J., Faran, Y., et al. (2006). Normal physiological emotions but differences in expression of conscious feelings in children with high-functioning autism. *Journal of Autism and Developmental Disorders, 36*, 395–400.

Berry, P., Gunn, P., & Andrews, R. (1980). Behavior of Down syndrome infants in a strange situation. *American Journal of Mental Deficiency, 85*, 213–218.

Bieberich, A. A., & Morgan, S. B. (1998). Affective expression in children with autism or Down syndrome. *Journal of Autism and Developmental Disorders, 28*, 333–338.

Bieberich, A. A., & Morgan, S. B. (2004). Self-regulation and affective expression during play in children with autism or down syndrome: A short-term longitudinal study. *Journal of Autism and Developmental Disorders, 34*, 439–448.

Bolte, S., Feineis-Matthews, S., & Poustka, F. (2008). Brief Report: Emotional processing in high-function autism: Physiological reactivity and affective report. *Journal of Autism and Developmental Disorders, 38*, 776–781.

Bridges, F. A., & Cicchetti, D. (1982). Mothers' ratings of the temperament characteristics of Down syndrome infants. *Developmental Psychology, 18*, 238–244.

Brooks-Gunn, J., & Lewis, M. (1982). Affective exchanges between normal and handicapped infants and their mothers. In T. Field, & A. Fogel (Eds.), *Emotion and early interaction* (pp. 161–212). Hillsdale, NJ: Erlbaum.

Buss, K. A., & Goldsmith, H. H. (1998). Fear and anger regulation in infancy: Effects on the temporal dynamics of affective expression. *Child Development, 69*, 359–374.

Calkins, S. D., & Johnson, M. C. (1998). Toddler regulation of distress to frustrating events: Temperamental and maternal correlates. *Infant Behavior & Development, 21*, 379–395.

Capps, L., Kasari, C., Yirmiya, N., & Sigman, M. (1993). Parental perception of emotional expressiveness in children with autism. *Journal of Consulting and Clinical Psychology, 61*, 475–484.

Charman, T., Swettenham, J., Baron-Cohen, S., Cox, A., Baird, G., & Drew, A. (1998). An experimental investigation of social-cognitive abilities in infants with autism: Clinical implications. *Infant Mental Health. Special Issue: 6th World Congress, World Association of Infant Mental Health, 19*, 260–275.

Cicchetti, D., Ganiban, J., & Barnett, D. (1991). Contributions from the study of high-risk populations to understanding the development of emotion regulation. In J. Garber, & K. A. Dodge (Eds.), *The development of emotion regulation and dysregulation* (pp. 15–48). New York: Cambridge University Press.

Cicchetti, D., & Sroufe, L. A. (1976). The relationship between affective and cognitive development in Down's syndrome infants. *Child Development, 47*, 920–929.

Cicchetti, D., & Sroufe, L. A. (1978). An organizational view of affect: Illustration from the study of Down syndrome infants. In M. Lewis, & L. A. Rosenblum (Eds.), *The development of affect* (pp. 309–350). New York: Plenum.

Clark, T. F., Winkielman, P., & McIntosh, D. N. (2008). Autism and the extraction of emotion from briefly presented facial expressions: Stumbling at the first step of empathy. *Emotion, 8*, 803–809.

Cohn, J. F., Campbell, S. B., Matias, R., & Hopkins, J. (1990). Face-to-face interactions of postpartum depressed and non-depressed mother-infant pairs at 2 months. *Developmental Psychology, 26*, 15–23.

Corona, R., Dissanayake, C., Arbelle, S., Wellinton, P., & Sigman, M. (1998). Is affect aversive to young children with autism? Behavioral and cardiac responses to experimenter distress. *Child Development, 69*, 1494–1502.

Crockenberg, S. C., & Leerkes, E. M. (2004). Infant and maternal behaviors regulate infant reactivity to novelty at 6 months. *Developmental Psychology, 40*, 1123–1132.

Cuskelly, M., Zhang, A., & Hayes, A. (2003). A mental age-matched comparison study of delay of gratification in children with Down syndrome. *International Journal of Disability, Development & Education, 50*, 239–251.

Dawson, G., Toth, K., Abbott, R., Osterling, J., Munson, J., Estes, A., & Liaw, J. (2004). Early social attention impairments in Autism: Social orienting, joint attention, and attention to distress. *Developmental Psychology, 40*, 271–283.

Denham, S. A. (1986). Social cognition, prosocial behaviors, and emotion in preschoolers: Contextual validation. *Child Development, 57*, 194–201.

Denham, S. A., Blair, K. A., DeMulder, E., Levitas, J., Sawyer, K., Auerbach-Major, S., & Queenan, P. (2003). Preschool emotional competence: Pathway to social competence? *Child Development, 74*, 238–256.

Denham, S. A., & Bruger, C. (1991). Observational validation of teacher rating scales. *Child Study Journal, 21*, 185–202.

Denham, S. A., & Burton, R. (1996). A social-emotional intervention for at-risk 4-year olds. *Journal of School Psychology, 34*, 225–245.

Denham, S. A., & Grout, L. (1992). Socialization of emotion: Pathways to preschoolers' emotional and social competence. *Journal of Nonverbal Behavior, 17*, 205–227.

Diener, M. L., & Manglesdorf, S. C. (1999). Behavioral strategies for emotion regulation in toddlers: Associations with maternal involvement and emotional expressions. *Infant Behavior & Development, 22*, 569–583.

Dissanayake, C., Sigman, M., & Kasari, C. (1996). Long-term stability of individual difference in the emotional responsiveness of children with autism. *Journal of Child Psychology and Psychiatry, 37*, 461–467.

Downs, A., & Smith, T. (2004). Emotional understanding, cooperation, and social behavior in high-functioning children with autism. *Journal of Autism and Developmental Disorders, 34*, 625–635.

Dykens, E. M., Shah, B., Sagun, J., Beck, T., & King, B. H. (2002). Maladaptive behavior in children and adolescents with Down syndrome. *Journal of Intellectual Disability Research, 46*, 484–492.

Eisenberg, N., Cumberland, A., & Spinrad, T. L. (1998). Parental socialization of emotion. *Psychological Inquiry, 9*, 241–273.

Eisenberg, N., & Fabes, R. (1992). Emotion, regulation, and the development of social competence. In M. S. Clark (Ed.), *Emotion social behavior: Review of personality social psychology* (pp. 119–150). Newbury Park, CA: Sage.

Eisenberg, N., Fabes, R., Murphy, B., Maszk, P., Smith, M., & Karbon, M. (1995). The role of emotionality and regulation in children's social functioning: A longitudinal study. *Child Development, 66,* 1360–1384.

Emde, R. N., & Brown, C. (1978). Adaptation after birth of Down's syndrome infant. *Journal of American Academy Child Psychiatry, 17,* 299–323.

Fidler, D. J., Most, D. E., Booth-LaForce, C., & Kelly, J. F. (2006). Temperament and behavior problems in young children with Down syndrome at 12, 30, and 45 months. *Down Syndrome Research and Practice, 10,* 23–29.

Fidler, D. J., Barret, K. C., & Most, D. E. (2005). Age-related differences in smiling and personality in Down syndrome. *Journal of Developmental and Physical Disabilities, 17,* 263–280.

Gallagher, R. J., Jens, K. G., & O'Donnell, K. J. (1983). The effect of physical status on the affective expression of handicapped infants. *Infant Behavior and Development, 6,* 73–77.

Glaser, S. E., Shaw, S. R. (2011). Emotion regulation and development in children with autism and 22q13 deletion syndrome: Evidence for group differences. *Research in Autism Spectrum Disorder, 5,* 926–934.

Golan, O., Ashwin, E., Grander, Y., McClintock, S., Day, K., Leggett, V., & Baron-Cohen, S. (2010). Enhancing emotion recognition in children with autism spectrum conditions: An intervention using animated vehicles with real emotional faces. *Journal of Autism and Developmental Disorders, 30,* 269–279.

Gomez, C. R. & Baird, S. (2005). Identifying early indicators for autism in self-regulation difficulties. *Focus on Autism and Other Developmental Disabilities, 20,* 106–116.

Greenberg, M., Kusche, C., Cook, E., & Quamma, J. P. (1995). Promoting emotional competence in school-aged children: The effects of the PATHS curriculum. *Development and Psychopathology, 7,* 117–136.

Grolnick, W. S., Bridges, L. J., & Connell, J. P. (1996). Emotion regulation in two-year-olds: Strategies and emotional expression in four contexts. *Child Development, 67,* 928–941.

Gross, T. F. (2004). The perception of four basic emotions in human and nonhuman faces by children with autism and other developmental delays. *Journal of Abnormal Child Psychology, 32,* 469–480.

Gulsrud, A. C., Jahromi, L. B., & Kasari, C. (2010). The co-regulation of emotions between mothers and their children with autism. *Journal of Autism and Developmental Disorders, 40,* 227–237. doi: 10.1007/s10803-009-0861-x.

Gunn, P., & Berry, P. (1985). The temperament of Down's syndrome toddlers and their siblings. *Journal of Child Psychology & Psychiatry, 26,* 973–979.

Hagerman, R. J. (1996). Fragile X syndrome. *Child and Adolescent Psychiatric Clinics of North America, 5,* 895–911.

Halberstadt, A. G., Crisp, V. W., & Eaton, K. L. (1999). A retrospective and new directions for research. In P. Philippot, R. S. Feldman, & E. J. Coats (Eds.), *The social context of nonverbal behavior: Studies in emotion and social interaction* (pp. 109–155). New York: Cambridge University Press.

Heery, E. A., Keltner, D., & Capps, L. M. (2003). Making sense of self-conscious emotion: Linking theory of mind and emotion in children with autism. *Emotion, 3,* 394–400.

Hillier, A., & Allinson, L. (2002). Understanding embarrassment among those with autism: Breaking down the complex emotion of embarrassment among those with autism. *Journal of Autism and Developmental Disorders, 32,* 583–592.

Hirstein, W., Iversen, P., & Ramachandran, V. S. (2001). Autonomic responses of autistic children to people and objects. *Proceedings of the Royal Society of London Series B, 268,* 1883–1888.

Hobson, R. P. (1986). The autistic child's appraisal of expressions of emotion. *Journal of Child Psychology and Psychiatry, 27,* 321–342.

Hobson, R. P., Chidambi, G., Lee, A., Meyer, J. (2006). Foundations for self-awareness: An exploration through Autism. *Monographs of the Society for Research in Child Development, vol. 71,* serial number 284.

Hobson, R. P., Ouston, J., & Lee, A. (1989). Naming emotion in faces and voices: Abilities and disabilities in autism and mental retardation. *British Journal of Developmental Psychology, 7,* 237–250.

Hodapp, R. M., Evans, D., & Gray, F. L. (1999). Intellectual development in children with Down syndrome. In J. A. Rondal, J. Perera, & L. Nadel (Eds.), *Down's syndrome: A review of current knowledge* (pp. 124–132). London: Whurr Publishers.

Hudry, K., & Slaughter, V. (2009). Agent familiarity and emotional context influence the everyday empathic responding of Young childrne with autism. *Research in Autism Spectrum Disorders, 3,* 74–85.

Huebner, R. R., & Izard, C. E. (1988). Mothers' responses to infants' facial expressions of sadness, anger, and physical distress. *Motivation and Emotion, 12,* 185–196.

Jahromi, L. B., Gulsrud, A., & Kasari, C. (2008). Emotional competence in children with Down syndrome: Negativity and regulation. *American Journal on Mental Retardation, 113,* 32–43.

Jahromi, L. B., Kasari, C. L., McCracken, J., T., Lee, L. S-Y., Aman, M. G., McDougle, C. J., Scahil, L., Tierney, E., Arnold, E., Vitiello, B., Ritz, L., Witwer, A., Kustan, E., Ghuman, J., & Posey, D. J. (2009). Positive effects of methylphenidate on social communication and self-regulation in children with pervasive developmental disorders and hyperactivity. *Journal of Autism and Developmental Disorder, 39,* 395–404. doi: 10.1007/s10803-008-0636-9.

Jahromi, L. B., & Stifter, C. A. (2007). Individual differences in preschoolers' self-regulation and theory of mind. *Infancy, 11,* 255–269.

Jones, A., Happe, F. G., Gilbert, F., Burnett, S., & Viding, E. (2010). Feeling, caring, knowing: Different types of empathy deficit in boys with psychopathic tendencies and autism spectrum disorder. *Journal of Child Psychology and Psychiatry, 51,* 1188–1197.

Joseph, R. M., & Tager-Flusberg, H. (1997). An investigation of attention and affect in children with autism and Down syndrome. *Journal of Autism and Developmental Disorders, 27,* 385–396.

Kasari, C., Freeman, S., & Bass, W. (2003). Empathy and response to distress in children with Down syndrome. *Journal of Child Psychology and Psychiatry, 44,* 424–431.

Kasari, C., Freeman, S., & Hughes, M. (2001). Emotion recognition of children with Down syndrome. *American Journal on Mental Retardation, 106,* 59–72.

Kasari, C., Mundy, P., Yirmiya, N., & Sigman, M. (1990). Affect and attention in children with Down syndrome. *American Journal on Mental Retardation, 95,* 55–67.

Kasari, C., & Sigman, M. (1996). Expression and understanding of emotion in atypical development: Autism and Down syndrome. In M. Lewis, & M. Sullivan (Eds.), *Emotions in atypical development* (pp 109–130). Hillsdale, NJ: Erlbaum.

Kau, A. S., Reider, E. E., Payne, L., Meyer, W. A., & Greund, L. (2000). Early behavior signs of psychiatric phenotypes in fragile X syndrome. *American Journal of Mental Retardation, 105,* 286–299.

Keogh, B. K., & Burstein, N. D. (1988). Relationship of temperament to preschoolers' interactions with peers and teachers. *Exceptional Children, 54,* 456–461.

Keysor, C. S., & Mazzocco, M. M. (2002). A developmental approach to understanding fragile X syndrome in females. *Microscopy Research and Technique, 57,* 179–186.

Konstantareas, M. M., & Stewart, K. (2006). Affect regulation and temperament in children with autism spectrum disorder. *Journal of Autism and Developmental Disorders, 36,* 143–154.

Kopp, C. B. (1989). Regulation of distress and negative emotions: A developmental view. *Developmental Psychology, 25,* 343–354.

Kopp, C. B., Krakow, J. B., & Johnson, K. L. (1983). Strategy production by young Down syndrome children. *American Journal of Mental Deficiency, 88,* 164–169.

Kuusikko, S., Haapsamo, H., Jansson-Verkasalo, E., Hurtig, T., Mattila, M., Ebeling, H., Jussila, K., Bölte, S., & Moilanen, I. (2009). Emotion recognition in children and adolescents with autism spectrum disorders. *Journal of Autism and Developmental Disorders, 39,* 938–945.

Lacroix, A., Guidetti, M., Rogé, B., & Reilly, J. (2009). Recognition of emotional and nonemotional facial expressions: A comparison between Williams syndrome and autism. *Research in Developmental Disabilities, 30,* 976–985.

Landry, S. H., & Chapieski, M. L. (1990). Joint attention of six-month-old Down syndrome and preterm infants: 1. Attention to toys and mothers. *American Journal of Mental Retardation, 94,* 488–498.

Loveland, K. A. (2005). Social-emotional impairment and self-regulation in autism spectrum disorder. In J. Nadel, & D. Muir (Eds.), *Emotional development: Recent research advance* (pp. 365–382). New York: Oxford University Press.

Mangelsdorf, S. C., Shapiro, J. R., & Marzolf, D. (1995). Developmental and temperamental differences in emotion regulation in infancy. *Child Development, 66,* 1817–1828.

Margalit, M., & Weisel, A. (1990). Computer-assisted social skills learning for adolescents with mild disabilities and social difficulties. *Educational Psychology, 10,* 343–354.

McIntyre, L. L., Blacher, J., & Baker, B. L. (2006). The transition to school: Adaptation in young children with and without intellectual disability. *Journal of Intellectual Disability Research, 50,* 349–361.

Mischel, W., & Ebbesen, E. B. (1970). Attention in delay of gratification. *Journal of Personality & Social Psychology, 16,* 329–337.

Ozonoff, S., Pennington, B. F., & Rogers, S. (1990). Are there emotion perception deficits in young autistic children? *Journal of Child Psychology and Psychiatry, 31,* 343–361.

Pitcairn, T. K., & Wishart, J. G. (1994). Reactions of young children with Down's syndrome to an impossible task. *British Journal of Developmental Psychology, 12,* 485–489.

Porges, S. W. (2003). The polyvagal theory: Phylogenetic contributions to social behavior. *Physiology & Behavior, 79,* 503–513.

Prizant, B. M., Wetherby, A. M., Rubin, E., Laurent, A. C., & Rydell, P. J. (2006). *The SCERTS model: A comprehensive educational approach for children with autism spectrum disorders* Vol. 1. Baltimore: Paul H. Brookes Publishing.

Prizant, B. M., Wetherby, A. M., Rubin, E., Laurent, A. C., & Rydell, P. J. (2006). *The SCERTS model: A comprehensive educational approach for children with autism spectrum disorders* Vol. 2. Baltimore: Paul H. Brookes Publishing.

Roberts, J. E., Boccia, M. L., Hatton, D. D., Skinner, M. L., & Sideris, J. (2006). Temperament and vagal tone in boys with fragile X syndrome. *Developmental and Behavioral Pediatrics, 27,* 193–201.

Ryan, C., & Charragáin, C.N. (2010). Teaching Emotion Recognition Skills to Children with Autism. *Journal of Autism and Developmental Disorders, 40,* 1505–1511.

Sigman, M. D., Kasari, C., Kwon, J., & Yirmiya, N. (1992). Responses to negative emotions of others by autistic, mentally retarded, and normal children. *Child Development, 63,* 796–807.

Silver, M., & Oakes, P. (2001). Evaluations of a new computer intervention to teach people with autism or Asperger syndrome to recognize and predict emotions in others. *Autism, 5,* 299–316.

Solomon, M., Goodlin-Jones, B. L., & Anders, T. F. (2004). A social adjustment enhancement intervention for high functioning autism, Asperger's syndrome, and pervasive developmental disorder NOS. *Journal of Autism and Developmental Disorders, 34,* 649–668.

Spinrad, T. L., Stifter, C. A., Donelan-McCall, N., & Turner, L. (2004). Mothers' regulation strategies in response to toddlers' affect: Links to later emotion self-regulation. *Social Development, 13,* 40–55.

Spivack, G., & Shure, M. B. (1974). *Social adjustment of young children. A cognitive approach to solving real-life problems.* San Francisco: Jossey-Bass.

Stichter, J.P., Herzog, M.J., Visovsky, K., Schmidt, C., Randolph, J., Schultz, T., & Gage, N. (2010). Social Competence Intervention for Youth with Asperger Syndrome and High-functioning Autism: An Initial Investigation. *Journal of Autism and Developmental Disorders, 40,* 1067–1079.

Stifter, C. A. (2002). Individual differences in emotion regulation in infancy: A thematic collection. *Infancy, 3,* 129–132.

Stifter, C. A., & Braungart, J. M. (1995). The regulation of negative reactivity in infancy: Function and development. *Developmental Psychology, 31,* 448–455.

Thompson, R. (1994). Emotion regulation: A theme in search of definition. *Monographs of the Society for Research in Child Development, 59*(2–3, Serial No. 240), 25–52.

Thompson, R. A., Cicchetti, D., Lamb, M. E., & Malkin, C. (1985). Emotional responses of Down syndrome and normal infants in the strange situation: The organization of affective behavior in infants. *Developmental Psychology, 21,* 828–841.

Tracy, J.L., Robins, R.W., Schriber, R.A., & Solomon, M. (2011). Is Emotion Recognition Impaired in Individuals with Autism Spectrum Disorders? *Journal of Autism and Developmental Disorders, 41,* 102–109.

Turk, J., & Cornish, K. (1998). Face recognition and emotion perception in boys with fragile-X syndrome. *Journal of Intellectual Disability Research, 42,* 490–499.

Wetherby, A. M., Prizant, B. M., & Schuler, A. L. (2000). Understanding the nature of communication and language impairments. In A. M. Wetherby, & B. M. Prizant (Eds.), *Autism spectrum disorders: A transactional developmental perspective* (pp. 109–141). Baltimore: Paul H. Brookes.

Whitman, T. (2004). *The development of autism: A self-regulatory perspective.* London: Jessica Kingsley Publishers.

Williams, D., & Happé, F. (2010). Recognising 'social' and 'non-social' emotions in self and others: A study of autism. *Autism, 14*, 285–304.

Williams, K. R., Wishart, J. G., Pitcairn, T. K., & Willis, D. S. (2005). Emotion recognition by children with Down syndrome: Investigation of specific impairments and error patterns. *American Journal on Mental Retardation, 110*, 378–392.

Wishart, J. G. (1993). The development of learning difficulties in children with Down's syndrome. *Journal of Intellectual Disability Research, 37*, 389–403.

Wishart, J. G., Cebula, K. R., Willis, D. S., & Pitcairn, T. K. (2007). Understanding of facial expressions of emotion by children with intellectual disabilities of different etiology. *Journal of Intellectual Disability Research, 51*, 551–563.

Wishart, J. G., & Pitcairn, T. K. (2000). Recognition of identity and expression in faces by children with Down syndrome. *American Journal on Mental Retardation, 105*, 466–479.

Wright, B., Clarke, N., Jordan, J., Young, A.W., Clarke, P., Miles, J., Nation, K., Clarke, L., & Williams, C. (2008). Emotion recognition in faces and the use of visual context in young people with high-functioning autism spectrum disorders. *Autism, 12*, 607–626.

Yirmiya, N., Kasari, C., Sigman, M., & Mundy, P. (1989). Facial expressions of affect in autistic, mentally retarded and normal children. *Journal of Child Psychology & Psychiatry & Allied Disciplines, 30*, 725–735.

Zaja, R.H., & Rojahn, J. (2008). Facial emotion recognition in intellectual disabilities. *Current Opinion in Psychiatry, 21*, 441–444.

Socioemotional and Brain Development in Children with Genetic Syndromes Associated with Developmental Delay

Alison Niccols, Karen Thomas, *and* Louis A. Schmidt

Abstract

This chapter reviews studies of social and behavioral development, emotional development and temperament, and brain development and psychophysiology in children with the six most common genetic syndromes associated with developmental delay (Down syndrome, fragile X syndrome, 22q11.2 deletion syndrome, Williams syndrome, Prader-Willi syndrome, and Angelman syndrome). We review recent research on relations among brain, psychophysiological, and socioemotional development in these children, placing particular emphasis on how each of these genetic disorders provides researchers with evidence and a model to understand the links among gene-, brain-, and behavior relations.

Keywords: Socioemotional, brain, children, genetic syndromes, developmental delay

Over the past several decades, descriptions of the psychological characteristics of individuals with genetic syndromes associated with developmental delay suggest that these syndromes are associated with unique behavioral phenotypes (Burack, 1990; Burack, Hodapp, & Zigler, 1998; Dykens, 1995). In the decade since the last edition of this volume, theoretical and methodological advances in the field of neuroscience have permitted the application of new theories and methods to further our understanding of genetic syndromes and their impact on brain structure and function. Some researchers took advantage of these advances and conducted rigorous studies involving appropriate comparison groups (Burack, Iarocci, Flanagan, & Bowler, 2004; Mervis & Klein-Tasman, 2004; Mervis & Robinson, 1999), resulting in meaningful evidence of the impact of specific genetic syndromes on certain neuroanatomical areas and socioemotional functions. Yet, the biological basis of neurodevelopmental differences is not yet well delineated, and research efforts currently are being expended to investigate direct effects of genetic variation on brain development and indirect effects through other neurochemical

factors (Campbell et al., 2006). Thus, a primary goal of current research in this area is to inform our knowledge of gene–brain–behavior relations in general and with regard to specific behaviors and psychiatric disorders. As genetic syndromes may involve specific changes in brain anatomy, brain development, and psychophysiology, they are well-suited to these types of investigations.

The study of the impact of childhood genetic disorders on brain and social affective development provides researchers with experiments in nature to address longstanding questions related to the origins of complex behaviors in typical and atypical development. Until recently, much of the work in this area largely was concerned with simple associations between a particular genetic disorder and a particular deficit. What was clearly lacking in a majority of prior studies was consideration of a major level of analysis in the equation: the brain. Today, however, researchers have begun to use genetic disorders in childhood as a model to understand complex brain–behavior relations in normal development and to more fully exploit possible mechanisms underlying complex behaviors than in the past.

Recent theoretical and methodological advances in the field of neuroscience have informed neighboring fields of inquiry, such as developmental neuroscience and clinical child psychology and psychiatry, as to what questions to ask, where to look in the brain, and what tools to use to do it (see Schmidt, 2003, 2007 for reviews). For example, the development of models to understand the neurocircuitry of approach–withdrawal, two fundamental behavioral dimensions that are conserved across animals has provided developmental psychologists with new knowledge to understand complex traits in children and the brain-based origins of these traits. The conceptualization of complex socioemotional behaviors, such as sociability and shyness, along two fundamental dimensions of approach–withdrawal has provided researchers with a heuristic from which to derive testable hypotheses. That is, by anchoring phenomenon to behavior, we can measure social behavior more objectively in children than in the past (Schmidt & Schulkin, 1999). Shyness and sociability are characteristic of two genetic disorders reviewed in this chapter, fragile X syndrome (FXS) and Williams syndrome (WS), respectively. Knowing the brain areas affected by these genetic disorders may shed light on the brain areas involved in shyness and sociability and their possible genetic origins.

Along with conceptual advances, the last several decades have seen dramatic methodological advances in the study of complex brain processes. For example, with the advent of faster computers, traditional electroencephalogram (EEG) studies involving the interpretation of analog signals restricted to neurologists in clinical settings has moved to basic research settings, in which frequency analyses of the EEG signals can be performed by those researchers interested in relations between brain dynamics and complex behaviors. Accordingly, questions related to how typically and atypically developing children regulate emotion and what factors impact socioemotional processes can be addressed using relatively noninvasive methods in basic laboratory settings to index the middle level (i.e., the brain) (Schmidt & Segalowitz, 2008).

The purpose of this chapter is to review studies of social and behavioral development, emotional development and temperament, and brain development and psychophysiology in children with the six most common genetic syndromes associated with developmental delay (Down syndrome [DS], FXS, 22q11.2 deletion syndrome, WS, Prader-Willi syndrome, and Angelman syndrome), as well as recent research on relations among brain, psychophysiological, and socioemotional development in these children. We place a particular emphasis in the review on how each of these genetic disorders provides researchers with evidence and a model to understand the links among gene, brain, and behavior relations.

Down Syndrome

Down syndrome results from trisomy 21, a usually spontaneous chromosomal abnormality in which an extra copy of chromosome 21 is present. Occurring in approximately one in every 600 live births, DS is the most common genetic cause of developmental delay.

Social and Behavioral Development

Infants with DS look at faces and appear socially engaging due to their interest in people (Kasari, Freeman, Mundy, & Sigman, 1995). In interactions with their mothers, infants with DS show patterns of social interaction that are functionally similar to typically developing infants (Carvajal & Iglesias, 2002). For example, within the first 3 months of life, infants with DS display turn taking and reciprocal interactions. However, infants with DS show less predictability, clarity, and frequency in social cueing, as well as dampened responsiveness (i.e., lower frequency, duration, and intensity of expressions such as smiling and waving their limbs; Carvajal & Iglesias, 2002). At 7 months, infants with DS are described as more "difficult to read" than typically developing 7-month-olds (Hyche, Bakeman, & Adamson, 1992). During play, infants with DS show fewer approach behaviors and more passivity (Linn, Goodman, & Lender, 2000).

Toddlers with DS look at their parents less often and for less time and exhibit a different pattern of social referencing than do mental age (MA)-matched toddlers without DS (Knieps, Walden, & Baxter, 1994). They appear to use eye gaze for "game" or "personal" purposes, whereas typically developing children use eye gaze mainly for "referential" purposes to refer to another person or object (Jones, 1980).

Preschool- and school-aged children with DS tend to seek out social interaction and be engaging and affectionate, thus appearing to have a high level of social motivation or interest (Kasari & Freeman, 2001; Moore, Oates, Hobson, & Goodwin, 2002). Children with DS have been described as highly sociable with peers, well-behaved in social situations, and active in joining a peer group (Rosner, Hoddapp,

Fidler, Sagun, & Dykens, 2004). However, most studies of social competence in children with DS are based on parent reports rather than direct observation (Iarocci, Yager, Rombough, & McLaughlin, 2008). Direct observations reveal that, compared to their MA-matched peers, children with DS make fewer bids for social interaction (Guralnick, 2002); are less receptive to the social bids of others (Sigman et al., 1999); exhibit some social deficits in recognizing facial expressions, particularly surprise and fear (Laws & Bishop, 2004); show diminished activity in the classroom and in group play (Sinson & Wetherick, 1981); frequently request adult help (Sigman et al., 1999); and experience social isolation at school (Sigman et al., 1999).

Compared with typically developing children, school-aged children with DS are more apt to exhibit provocative and low-level aggressive behaviors (i.e., disobedience, argumentativeness, demanding attention) and other externalizing behavior, such as inattention and impulsivity, but relatively low rates of extreme aggression (i.e., fighting) (Dykens, 2007). Although externalizing symptoms in DS appear to decline from early childhood to adolescence, internalizing symptoms (anxiety, depression, withdrawal) appear to increase (Dykens, 2007). Internalizing symptoms in children with DS may emerge later in development than among children with developmental delay of nonspecific etiologies (Fidler, 2006).

Considerable variability occurs in social adaptation among individuals with DS that cannot be accounted for by IQ alone (Iarocci et al., 2008). Emerging evidence suggests that the limitations of children with DS, as well as inadequate contextual supports, may compromise their development of social competence (Iarocci et al., 2008).

Emotional Development and Temperament
From 6 to 24 months MA, infants with DS appear to display similar types of emotional reactions as children with developmental delay and typically developing children of the same MA, but lower frequency, duration, and intensity of emotional expression (Carvajal & Iglesias, 2002). At 3 years MA, the emotion recognition abilities of children with DS appear on par with their MA-matched delayed and nondelayed peers; however, by the developmental age of 4, they are less accurate in verbally labeling an emotion or identifying emotions from context-based stories than are MA-matched children (Adams & Markham, 1991; Kasari, Freeman & Hughes, 2001; Williams, Wishart,

Pitcairn, & Willis, 2005; Wishart & Pitcairn, 2000). Children with DS have difficulty recognizing emotions such as fear, anger, and surprise and, at times, confuse positive emotions with negative ones (Kasari et al., 2001; Williams et al., 2005; Wishart & Pitcairn, 2000).

With regard to temperament, infants with DS exhibit lower levels of distress to limitations (i.e., anger/frustration), less negative emotionality, longer duration of orienting, more low-intensity pleasure, and more cuddliness and affiliation than typically developing infants (Gartstein, Marmion, & Swanson, 2006). Unlike other children with developmental delay, temperamental style in infancy does not predict future behavior in children with DS (Fidler, 2006). Although the personality style stereotype for DS is sociable, pleasant, and affectionate, adolescents and adults with DS also exhibit inflexibility, resistance to change, stubbornness, lack of persistence, and passivity (Capone, Goyal, Ares, & Lannigan, 2006; Fidler, 2006).

Brain Development and Psychophysiology
Children with DS have several central nervous system abnormalities. The average brain weight of individuals with DS is 25% less than normal, with disproportionately smaller cerebellum, brainstem, and hippocampus; diminished and malformed growth of the frontal and temporal lobes; and reduced cortical area and thickness (Coyle, Oster-Granite, & Gearhart, 1986; Lubec & Endgidawork, 2002; Pennington & Bennetto, 1998; Reeves, 2006). There are reduced levels of those fetal neurotransmitters (chemicals that relay, amplify, and modulate signals between a neuron and another cell) critical for normal brain development (Whittle, Sartori, Dierssen, Lubec, & Singewald, 2007) and clear evidence of disruption of early brain development, including both prenatal and early postnatal abnormalities (Lubec & Engidawork, 2002; Pennington & Bennetto, 1998).

Although much of the research on the DS brain is focused on explaining cognitive deficits and the connection to the increased rates of Alzheimer disease (e.g., Menendez, 2005), neurotransmitters and neurotransmitter systems (e.g., the noradrenaline system, the adrenaline system) in children with DS also are examined. Compared to typically developing infants of the same chronological age, 3- to 12-month-old infants with DS exhibit decreased neurotransmitter activity in the noradrenergic and adrenergic systems (Gartstein et al., 2006). Because these neurotransmitter systems are associated with bringing the nervous system to "high alert," arousal, and voluntary movement, these findings may explain the dampened responsiveness of young children with DS (Gartstein et al., 2006). Thus, differences in the noradrenaline and adrenaline systems may account for the differences in temperament and social behavior observed between infants with DS and typically developing infants.

In addition to brain structure and neurotransmitter systems, brain-based measures of processing, such as EEG measures of cortical regional brain activation have been used with children with DS to assess neuropsychological (Partanen et al., 1996) and cognitive functioning (Devinsky, Sato, Conwit, & Schapiro, 1990) and brain maturation (McAlaster, 1992). In a pilot study, Conrad et al. (2007) investigated frontal EEG activation models and emotion processing in children with DS. Conrad et al. (2007) examined frontal EEG activity patterns in response to the presentation of popular children's video clips that varied in affective content in three children with DS and three typically developing children matched on reading level. All the children exhibited greater relative left frontal activity in response to the happy video clip, and all children exhibited greater relative right frontal activity in response to the fear and sad video clips. These findings suggest that the differentiation of these emotions in children with DS occurs at the neural level in a manner that is not significantly different from that of typically developing children. Despite these similarities, there were notable group differences in the intensity of emotion and the processing of anger. There was, in addition, a group difference in the magnitude of the asymmetry scores, which appeared larger for the children with DS than for the typically developing children, suggesting that the intensity of the emotion processed may be greater for children with DS than for typically developing children, at least with regard to happy, sad, and fear video clips.

In several behavioral studies, children with DS exhibited differences in the intensity of emotional reactions (e.g., Brooks-Gunn & Lewis, 1982; Carvajal & Iglesias, 1997; Cicchetti & Sroufe, 1976; Kasari, Sigman, Mundy, & Yirmiya, 1990; Serafica & Cicchetti, 1976; Thompson, Cicchetti, Lamb, & Malkin, 1985), although in these cases they were typically less intense than those of the typically developing children. Children with DS may have neuropsychological reactions to emotional stimuli that are more intense than typically developing children, but exhibit dampened behavioral responses, perhaps due to other constraints (e.g., motor tone, motor speed).

The second group difference was that the children with DS displayed, on average, right frontal EEG activity, as compared to the left frontal EEG activity displayed by the typically developing children, during the processing of the anger video clip, suggesting that they may suppress anger and experience anger as an emotion associated with withdrawal tendencies. These results may be clinically relevant as right frontal EEG activity is linked to depression (Henriques & Davidson, 1990). Brain-based measures of affective processing can be used to study the differentiation of emotion on an electrocortical level and may be informative regarding atypical brain–emotion–behavior relations in other genetic syndromes.

Summary

Early research and descriptions of children with DS as having a pleasant, affectionate, and passive personality style have been augmented by more recent, nuanced findings of a more complex emotional–behavioral profile that includes, for example, stubbornness, noncompliance, and adolescent depression (Fidler, 2006). Nevertheless, socioemotional abilities appear to be a relative strength for children with DS. In fact, infants with DS constitute an ideal population for studying the development of emotion, as their cognitive impairments may limit what can develop through social learning; that is, studying children with DS may help us understand which aspects of emotional development are maturational and which are environmental (Carvajal & Iglesias, 2002).

There is considerable variation in outcomes for individuals with DS, with some adults with DS able to function semi-independently in supported employment and housing, whereas others are entirely dependent on caregivers. Additional research on predictors of individual differences in socioemotional and brain development may help explain this heterogeneity. Environmental factors, such as parents and peers, likely influence the development of children with DS, and preliminary studies suggest that environmental influences on these children are not minor (e.g., Dyer-Friedman et al., 2002; Hessl et al., 2001; Niccols, Milligan, Chisholm, & Atkinson, in press). Studies designed to elucidate how socioemotional and brain development is moderated and mediated by environmental factors are vital to understanding and optimizing development in these children (Reiss & Dant, 2003).

Fragile X Syndrome

Fragile X syndrome is a result of a defective gene on the X chromosome, one of the pair of chromosomes that determines gender. It is the most common known inherited cause of developmental delay, occurring in approximately one in every 2,000–5,000 live births (Turner, Webb, Wake, & Robinson, 1996).

Social and Behavioral Development

Fragile X syndrome is the most common known cause of autism, responsible for approximately 5% of all cases. Preschool-aged boys with FXS often exhibit gaze aversion, poor eye contact, social withdrawal, attention deficits, hand flapping, hand biting, anxiety, and emotionality (Baumgardner, Reiss, Freund, & Abrams, 1995; Cornish et al., 2005a, b; Eliez, Blasey, Freund, Hastie, & Reiss, 2001; Farzin et al., 2006; Mazzocco, 2000). Boys with FXS are often shy and anxious, avoid unfamiliar people, and display poor eye contact (Teisl, Reiss, & Mazzocco, 1999;Cohen, Vitze, Sudhalter, Jenkins, & Brown, 1991). Approximately 15%–30% of males with FXS meet criteria for autism, although many more show some symptoms (Baumgardner et al., 1995). Although FXS occurs as frequently in girls as boys, girls tend to be less severely affected and have less pronounced social, emotional, and behavioral problems than do boys with FXS (Mazzocco, Baumgardner, Freund, & Reiss, 1998).

To examine the longitudinal course of behavioral and emotional problems, Einfeld, Tonge, and Turner (1999) assessed children and adolescents with FXS (average age 15 years, standard deviation [SD] = 6.73) and then reassessed these same individuals 7 years later (average age 22 years), using the Developmental Behavior Checklist. Despite the persistence of their overall level of emotional and behavioral problems from childhood to adulthood, individuals with FXS showed a reduction in externalizing behavior and an increase in internalizing behavior over time, much like the individuals with developmental delay in the comparison group (Einfeld et al., 1999a). However, the two individual items that distinguished those with FXS from the comparison group ("shy" and "avoids eye contact") continued to do so 7 years later, indicating that shyness and avoidance of eye contact continue to be particular problems for individuals with FXS in adulthood (Einfeld et al., 1999a).

Emotional Development and Temperament

Some have hypothesized that the social anxiety and gaze avoidance of individuals with FXS are due to classic social perception impairments; however, there is no evidence of difficulties in emotion perception, recognition of facial and emotional expression, or perspective-taking skills in children and adults with FXS (Feinstein & Reiss, 1998; Mazzocco, Pennington, & Hagerman, 1994; Turk & Cornish, 1998). An alternative hypothesis is that the social anxiety and gaze avoidance may be due to impaired modulation of arousal. There is evidence that school-aged children with FXS have a strong propensity for hyperarousal: They are sensitive to auditory, tactile, visual, and olfactory stimuli, and may overreact in highly stimulating environments such as a supermarket or mall (Cohen, 1995; Reiss & Dant, 2003).

Behavior problems are the focus of studies of children with FXS. Studies of temperament are generally focused post-infancy, likely because of the relatively late diagnosis of FXS. In a longitudinal study of 45 young boys (3–8 years old) with FXS and using the Behavioral Style Questionnaire (McDevitt & Carey, 1978), Hatton, Bailey, Hargettt-Beck, Skinner, and Clark (1999) found that they were more active and less adaptable, approachable, persistent, and intense than typically developing children. Similarly, in a study of preschoolers and another with a wider age range (1–11 years), boys with FXS were described as more active and withdrawing and less adaptable and persistent than typically developing boys (Bailey, Hatton, Mesibov, Ament, & Skinner, 2000; Roberts, Boccia, Hatton, Skinner, & Sideris, 2006). The temperamental profile of young children with FXS appears to differ not only from typically developing children but also from children with developmental delay: Hepburn and Rogers (2001) reported that 1- to 3-year-old children with FXS were less adaptable, approachable, and persistent than chronological age-matched children with developmental delay. In an attempt to compare FXS and autism, Bailey et al. (2000) investigated temperament in three groups of preschoolers—boys with FXS alone, boys with FXS and autism, and boys with autism alone—and found no differences in temperament among the three groups.

Brain Development and Psychophysiology

Brain abnormalities (differences in the size of various brain structures, alterations in connections between brain areas, and disruptions in the activation of specific brain areas) may account for the emotional, behavioral, and cognitive difficulties of individuals with FXS. Individuals with FXS have abnormalities in several brain structures. The cerebral, ventricular, and hippocampal areas are larger than expected (Kates, Abrams, Kaufmann, Breiter, & Reiss, 1997; Reiss, Freund, Baumgardner, Abrams, &

Denckla, 1995) and the cerebellar vermis area and superior temporal gyrus are smaller than expected (Mostofsky et al., 1998; Reiss, Lee, & Freund, 1994). Abnormalities in these brain areas are associated with disruptions in memory, language, spatial problem solving, and the detection of novel stimuli (hippocampal area; Kates et al., 1997; Reiss et al., 1994) and with difficulties in processing sensory information and modulating attention, emotion, and movement coordination (cerebellar vermis; Reiss, Patel, Kumar, & Freund, 1988). Individuals with FXS also have abnormalities in more specific brain areas, such as the caudate nucleus, as well as in prefrontal–striatal white matter connectivity and frontoparietal activation, which may be associated with difficulties in attention, social behavior, impulse control, behavioral response to environmental cues, and language and motor behavior (Barnea-Goraly et al., 2003; Cummings, 1993; Kwon et al., 2001; Masterman & Cummings, 1997; Rivera, Menon, White, Glaer, & Reiss, 2002).

Much of the psychophysiological research on FXS is focused on understanding gaze aversion (e.g., Reiss & Dant, 2003). In neuroimaging, electrophysiologic, and neuroendocrine studies, there is evidence of neuronal dysfunction involving the fusiform gyrus, abnormal processing of direct gaze, and associations between face-to-face contact and hyperarousal (Belser, & Sudhalter, 2001; Garrett, Menon, MacKenzie, & Reiss, 2004; Hessl, Glaser, Dyer-Friedman, & Reiss, 2006; Miller et al., 1999). Preliminary evidence suggests that the neural basis of gaze aversion may be related partly to reduced brain activation in individuals with FXS (Reiss & Dant, 2003). Individuals with FXS have deficient activation in brain areas associated with gaze processing, especially the superior temporal sulcus, which is involved in interpreting gaze direction in a social context.

Also, children with FXS may have abnormal hypothalamic-pituitary-adrenal (HPA) axis function, as indicated by reports of endocrine abnormalities (Bregman, Leckman, & Ort, 1990; Butler & Najjar, 1988; Loesch, Huggins, & Hoang, 1995), hippocampal enlargement (Kates et al., 1997; Reiss et al.,1995), and hyperarousal (Cronister & Hagerman, 1989), with higher resting heart rates (Keysor & Mazzocco, 2002; Roberts, Boccia, Bailey, Hatton, & Skinner, 2001), lowered baseline vagal tone and reduced vagal reactivity (Roberts et al., 2001, 2006), greater electrodermal responses to skin stimulation (Miller et al., 1999), and increased cortisol levels and cortisol reactivity (Hessl et al., 2002; 2006; Wisbeck et al., 2000). This disruption of the typical HPA axis function may help to explain the variability in stress-related symptoms among children with FXS, including hyperarousal and social anxiety, as well as behavioral overreactivity.

Summary
Children with FXS typically exhibit characteristic behavior such as gaze aversion, hyperarousal, shyness, anxiety, and other autistic symptoms. As such, research on these children could help identify core deficits in autism, which could lead to improved treatment for both autism and FXS. With their strong propensity for hyperarousal and gaze aversion in particular, study of individuals with FXS may help elucidate the neurological and endocrinological underpinnings of these constructs and their role in socioemotional development. Future FXS research examining psychophysiological measures and socioemotional development in the same study will help us comprehensively understand relations among psychophysiology, hyperarousal, gaze aversion, shyness, anxiety, and autism.

Most studies of socioemotional and brain development in individuals with FXS focus on school-aged children (and older individuals), likely due to, in part, the difficulties inherent in identifying and diagnosing FXS in infancy. It is possible that information from genetic and psychophysiological studies may assist in the development of early identification procedures for FXS. Accurate, early diagnosis is important for early intervention and to longitudinal studies of socioemotional and brain development in FXS.

22q11.2 Deletion Syndrome (22qDS)
Caused by a microdeletion on the long arm of chromosome 22 (specifically chromosome 22q11.2), 22qDS is the most common microdeletion syndrome, occurs in approximately 1 in 4,000 live births, and involves multiple anomalies (du Montcel, Mendizabal, Ayme, Levy, & Philips, 1996). Historically, it also has been called various names including *velocardiofacial syndrome, DeGeorge syndrome, Shprintzen syndrome* and *CATCH 22 syndrome*. This caused considerable confusion, until the underlying cause of all these conditions was determined to be the same 22q microdeletion.

Social and Behavioral Development
Children with 22qDS exhibit social withdrawal, shyness, flat affect, impulsivity, overactive and disinhibited behavior, autistic symptoms, moodiness, and many anxiety symptoms (Feinstein, Eliez, Blasey, &

Reiss, 2002; Niklasson, Rasmussen, Oskarsdottir, & Gillberg, 2002; Papolos et al., 1996; Swillenen et al., 1999; Woodlin et al., 2001). Behavioral presentation can be quite variable, and children with 22qDS appear to demonstrate behavioral extremes (e.g., from withdrawal to disinhibition) (Gerdes et al., 1999; Golding-Kushner et al., 1985; Shprintzen, 2000; Swillen et al., 1999). Cross-sectional research suggests progression from more externalizing behavior to more internalizing behavior with increasing age (Swillen et al., 1999). In childhood, individuals with 22qDS are at high risk of developing attention deficit hyperactivity disorder (ADHD) (35%–55%) and autism (14%) (Fine et al., 2005; Gerdes et al., 1999; Gothelf et al., 2003, 2004). By early adulthood, individuals with 22qDS exhibit high rates of psychiatric disorders, such as bipolar disorder, depression, anxiety, and obsessive-compulsive disorder, and approximately 30% develop schizophrenia (Baker & Skuse, 2005; Feinstein et al., 2002; Gothelf et al., 2005). Because of these high risk rates, investigating the precursors of psychiatric vulnerability in children with 22qDS, including emotional development and temperament, could be informative with regard to the early signs of schizophrenia, ADHD, and autism.

Emotional Development and Temperament

Anecdotal observations of preschoolers with 22qDS reveal their difficulties modulating emotion and their high levels of anxiety and phobias. In a study of temperament in 6- to 15-year-old children with 22qDS, parents rated them as moderately difficult, with most difficulty identified in regularity of daily habits, focusing and sustaining attention, mood, and responding flexibly to changes in the environment (Antshel et al., 2007). There was considerable variation among temperamental ratings for the children with 22qDS, however, as was the case with the two comparison groups (siblings and age-, race-, and gender-matched community control participants). A mismatch between parent and child activity level was predictive of behavior problems in children with 22qDS in this study (Antshel et al., 2007). Given the relatively high risk for psychopathology in this population, future investigations of goodness of fit between parents and children with 22qDS and the potential moderating role of overprotection in these families are important.

Brain Development and Psychophysiology

The brain structure and neurodevelopment of children with 22qDS have been of considerable interest due to the relatively high risk for schizophrenia and other psychiatric disorders. Thus, 22qDS may provide a neurological model for the development of severe psychiatric disorder. As alterations of the prefrontal cortex–temporal lobe circuits are robustly associated with severe psychiatric disorder in the general population, Kates et al. (2006) investigated the association between temporal lobe anatomy and psychiatric symptoms in 9- to 15-year-old children with 22qDS. They found that, as predicted, volumes of mesial temporal lobe structures (hippocampus, amygdala, prefrontal cortex-to-hippocampal ratios, and prefrontal cortex-to-amygdala ratios) were altered in children with 22qDS compared to community controls and siblings. Increased amygdala volume, in particular, was associated with anxiety, aggression, and overall behavior problems in these children (Kates et al., 2006). The amygdala, which is involved in assigning emotional valence to stimuli, may be disproportionately larger in children with 22qDS due to disruptions in neural pruning during brain development in the early years (Kates et al., 2006). Inefficient neural pruning is also evident in the corpus callosum of children with 22qDS. Relative to typically developing children, children with 22qDS have larger corpus callosal areas (Antshel, Conchelos, Lanzetta, Fremont, & Kates, 2005; Bingham et al., 1997; Eliez, Schmitt, White, & Reiss, 2000). Also, the shape of the corpus callosum in children with 22qDS is more bowed than in typically developing children, which is significant because it is one of the most robust findings from neuroimaging studies of individuals with schizophrenia (for a review, see Shenton, Dickey, Frumin, & McCarley, 2001).

Children with 22qDS have a wide range of neuroanatomical abnormalities such as high-frequency developmental midline anomalies, ventricular enlargement, and skull base abnormalities (Chow et al., 1999). There are volumetric alterations in several brain regions. Relative to typically developing children, children with 22qDS exhibit reductions in total brain, posterior fossa, cerebellum, parietal gray matter, and frontal, parietal, and temporal white matter volumes (Eliez et al., 2000, 2001; Kates et al., 2001, 2005). White matter development is more compromised than cortical gray matter development (Kates et al., 2001, 2005). White matter alterations may be due to delays in myelin development, disorganization of axon density within the cerebral cortex, or alterations in the cellular structure of white matter (Antshel et al., 2005; Kates et al., 2001).

In the largest study of brain–behavior relations in this population, Campbell et al. (2006) used volumetric and voxel-based morphometry magnetic resonance imaging (MRI) with 39 children and adolescents with 22qDS. Their results revealed a significant reduction in cerebellar gray matter, and white matter reduction in the frontal lobe, cerebellum, and internal capsule, relative to the sibling control group matched on age and socioeconomic status (Campbell et al., 2006). Although white matter is more reduced than gray matter in the brains of children with 22qDS, it is the gray matter volume in specific brain regions that was associated with scores for schizotypy, and emotional, behavioral, and social problems in the children and adolescents with 22qDS (Bearden et al., 2004; Campbell et al., 2006). Because studies suggest that individuals with 22qDS exhibit differences in both white and gray matter, dysfunction within large-scale neural networks may underpin their behavioral characteristics. At least two higher-order functional networks have been hypothesized to be atypical in the brains of children with 22qDS, including the particular prefrontal–striatal network associated with mood lability, irritability, and impulsivity.

Thus, the brain structure of individuals with 22qDS is characterized by a range of regional increases (e.g., amygdala and corpus callosum) and decreases in both white and gray matter volume. These findings may reflect programmed cell death, which may lead to too few or too many neurons (Campbell et al., 2006). Changes in the catechol-O-methyl transferase (COMT) gene may be the genetic basis of these neurodevelopmental differences (Dunham, Collins, Wadey, & Scambler, 1992; Graf et al., 2001; Lachman et al., 1996). *COMT* gene codes for an enzyme involved in the breakdown of dopamine, adrenaline, and noradrenaline (i.e., neurotransmitters involved in arousal, voluntary movement, motivation, desire, and addiction). In the general population, changes in *COMT* gene are linked to obsessive-compulsive disorder, bipolar disorder, and risk for schizophrenia (Akil et al., 2003; Karayiorgou et al., 1995; Lachman et al., 1996). The deleted region in 22qDS contains *COMT* gene. Further, individuals with 22qDS exhibit significant differences in the anatomy of dopamine-rich brain regions (Campbell et al., 2006). Researchers continue to investigate whether the neurological findings in children with 22qDS are due to a direct effect of *COMT* gene on brain development or if they are secondary to an effect of dopamine.

Summary

Children with 22qDS are at high risk of developing psychiatric disorders, especially ADHD, atypical development, and schizophrenia. Like most studies of socioemotional and brain development in individuals with genetic syndromes associated with developmental delay, studies of 22qDS involve individuals of school-aged and older, likely due, in part, to the difficulties inherent in identifying and diagnosing 22qDS. Although it is possible to diagnose 22qDS with genetic testing at any age, this testing is not routinely performed at birth.

As 22qDS is considered a neurological model for the study of gene–brain–behavior relations in schizophrenia, the hope is that research on neuroanatomical characteristics of individuals with 22qDS will help identify biological markers that predict severe psychiatric illness (Eliez et al., 2001). Examining the neuroanatomic differences between individuals with 22qDS who develop psychotic symptoms and those who do not may be helpful in determining the particular patterns in brain region volumes that are explicitly related to psychosis (Bearden et al., 2004). Research is ongoing regarding the biological basis of the neurodevelopmental characteristics of 22qDS and examining hypotheses regarding the interaction of direct effects of genetic variation on brain development and indirect effects of dopamine metabolism (Campbell et al., 2006).

There is considerable heterogeneity within 22qDS, so research is needed on predictors of individual differences in socioemotional and brain development to help explain this heterogeneity. Environmental factors, such as parents and peers, likely influence the development of these children, as suggested by preliminary studies (Antshel et al., 2007). Studies designed to elucidate how socioemotional and brain development is moderated and mediated by environmental factors are vital to understanding and optimizing development in children with 22qDS (Reiss & Dant, 2003).

Longitudinal studies, beginning early in life, of relatively large groups of individuals with 22qDS and appropriate comparison groups would be informative to help understand relations between socioemotional development and brain development (Reiss & Dant, 2003). There is a need for future longitudinal functional imaging studies of individual differences in brain structure and function, neurochemistry, and behavior changes across the lifespan of individuals with 22qDS (Campbell et al., 2006).

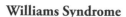

Williams Syndrome

Williams syndrome is a genetic disorder resulting from the deletion of approximately 20 contiguous genes on the long arm of chromosome 7 (7q11.23) (Korenberg et al., 2000). It affects approximately 1 in 7,500–20,000 live births (Duba et al., 2002; Stromme, Bjornstad, & Ramstad, 2002). The deletion is associated with a typical "elfin" facial appearance and a distinctive cognitive profile (low IQ, poor visual–spatial abilities, and surprisingly good verbal abilities and face recognition) (Frigerio et al., 2006).

Social and Behavioral Development

Infants and toddlers with WS are engaging and responsive and demonstrate an extreme form of focused attention and interest in faces (Fidler, Hepburn, Most, Philofsky, & Rogers, 2007; Laing et al., 2002; Mervis et al., 2003). They exhibit unique intensity and duration of attention to people (Mervis et al., 2003). Their intense and prolonged looking at faces leads to a reduction in the ability to monitor the rest of the environment (Mervis et al., 2003). This attentional pattern is adaptive in situations requiring attention to detail, but detrimental in situations that depend upon broad perception of the environment or flexible responding, and reduces the opportunities of individuals with WS to learn about their surrounding environment. Also, despite their interest in faces, children with WS are delayed in their ability to interpret facial expressions of emotion and other subtle social cues (Fidler et al., 2007; Frigerio et al., 2006; Gagliardi et al., 2003). They also exhibit impairment in another important social skill, theory of mind, such that they have difficulty imagining the perspective of others (Sullivan & Tager-Flusberg, 1999).

Children with WS exhibit hypersociability and are excessively friendly, even with strangers (Fidler et al., 2007; Jones et al., 2000). In a study examining their perception of unfamiliar faces, Frigerio et al. (2006) found that they rated some faces as more approachable than others (e.g., happy faces were rated as more approachable than angry faces). Although able to discriminate others in terms of approachability, individuals with WS have difficulty inhibiting their strong compulsion toward social interaction, and may not make use of this approachability knowledge in real-world settings (Frigerio et al., 2006). Thus, an individual with WS may approach an individual even when they think the person looks unapproachable. Frigerio et al. (2006) differentiated between true friendliness (which includes relationship) from what they termed "social stimulus attraction" (which characterizes the social drive or compulsion shown by individuals with WS). Individuals with WS often suffer social problems, including social isolation, anxiety, and depression (Dykens, 2003), possibly because of their social skill deficits, including exhibiting more social stimulus attraction than true friendliness.

Emotional Development and Temperament

Children with WS are empathic and sensitive to the emotional displays of others, perhaps even excessively so (e.g., Fidler et al., 2007). As early as toddlerhood, parents report that their children with WS show awareness of other's distress and offer comfort (Mervis et al., 2003). Although individuals with WS are well known for their tendency to interact with strangers, many (79%) report being scared of them, supporting the notion that the sociability of WS individuals may reflect a form of disinhibition that is characteristic of overly anxious individuals (Dykens, 2003).

Klein-Tasman and Mervis (2003) examined the sensitivity and specificity of the temperamental patterns in children with WS and found that ratings on two scales were particularly unique: Sociability and Empathy. In another study, Tomc, Williamson, and Pauli (1990) found that parents described their children with WS as displaying difficult temperament, and, compared to other children, they display higher activity levels, intensity, negative mood, distractibility, and approachability, and lower rhythmicity, adaptability, persistence, and arousal threshold (Tomc, Williamson, & Pauli, 1990).

Brain Development and Psychophysiology

The unusual characteristics of children with WS may be due to the impact of their particular genetic deletion on brain development. This impact may be direct, in that the missing genes direct early brain cell differentiation and segmentation, or it may be indirect, via the elevated levels of calcium in the blood of individuals with WS. During embryogenesis and postnatal development, elevated calcium levels in brain cells can dysregulate the release of neurotransmitters, potentially leading to aberrant neural organization (Karmiloff-Smith, Klima, Bellugi, Grant, & Baron-Cohen, 1995).

In any case, patterns of brain growth during embryogenesis and ontogenesis result in different brain volume proportions in individuals with WS as compared to typically developing individuals (Karmiloff-Smith et al., 1995). The brains of individuals with WS are only 80%–85% of expected volume. However, there are no obvious left–right symmetry differences and no obvious space-occupying lesions in either the right or left hemisphere (Karmiloff-Smith et al., 1995). The overall brain volume deficit is primarily due to a 15%–21% reduction in white matter and 6%–8% reduction in gray matter (Thompson et al., 2005). In the disproportionately reduced white matter, cortical cells fit over a smaller area, and can pile up and thicken, owing to a crowding effect (Toga, Thompson, & Sowell, 2006).

Thickening is apparent in other cortical areas, particularly across sections of the right frontal cortex and superior temporal sulcus (which are responsible for face and gaze processing) and the perisylvian regions (which are responsible for the processing of language and musical prosody) (Braden & Obrzut, 2002; Frigerio et al., 2006; Thompson et al., 2005). These findings are consistent with the general strengths of individuals with WS in these areas. Cortical complexity also is significantly increased; however, there is no simple relation between thickness and complexity (Thompson et al., 2005; Toga et al., 2006). A thicker cortex is often interpreted as being functionally superior; however, a thicker cortex may instead relate to less efficient neural packing, increased gyrification, and the proportionally greater loss of white than gray matter (Frigerio et al., 2006; Thompson et al., 2005).

Much of the effort expended in examining brain development in individuals with WS has focused on explaining their characteristic hypersociability. There are several hypotheses regarding affected brain regions. Particular abnormalities have been found in the amygdala (an increase in gray matter and of size, taking into account the smaller brains of individuals with WS) and connected areas (Reiss et al., 2004). The amygdala has been linked to the ability to use social information to decide whether to approach, and individuals with WS appear to have strengths in this area (Frigario et al., 2006; Porter, Coltheart, & Langdon, 2007). Other limbic structures of the temporal lobe (uncus, hippocampus, and parahippocampal gyrus) are relatively spared in WS (Galaburda, Wang, Bellugi, & Rossen, 1994), which may account for their ability to process socially relevant information (Karmiloff-Smith et al., 1995). The relatively large size of the cerebellum of infants and toddlers with WS distinguishes them from typically developing individuals and does not vary as a function of age (Jones et al., 2002). The cerebellum also plays a role in language and social–emotional abilities, areas of relative

strength for individuals with WS (Braden & Obrzut, 2002; Jones et al., 2002). Other neurological evidence suggests frontal lobe abnormalities in children with WS and that their abnormal (indiscriminate) social approach is best explained by frontal lobe impairment, particularly poor response inhibition (Frigerio et al., 2006; Porter et al., 2007).

Summary

The hypersociability of children with WS may be explained by neurodevelopmental differences. Research in this area can inform our knowledge of gene–brain–behavior relations, particularly as they pertain to social and emotional development. Williams syndrome involves both widespread and specific changes in brain anatomy, brain development, and psychophysiology. Research is ongoing regarding the biological basis of these neurodevelopmental differences, which may involve interactions between direct effects of the genetic deletion on brain development and indirect effects through elevated calcium levels.

Recent improvements in early identification and diagnosis have allowed for studies of socioemotional and brain development in infants and toddlers with WS. There is a need for future longitudinal imaging studies of individual differences in brain structure, neurochemistry, and brain function (Campbell et al., 2006). Longitudinal studies, beginning early in life, of relatively large groups of individuals with WS and appropriate comparison groups would be informative to help understand relations between socioemotional development and brain development (Reiss & Dant, 2003). Also needed is research on predictors of individual differences in socioemotional and brain development to help explain heterogeneity within WS. Studies designed to elucidate how socioemotional and brain development is moderated and mediated by environmental factors are vital to understanding and optimizing development in these children (Reiss & Dant, 2003).

Prader-Willi Syndrome

Prader-Willi syndrome is a multisystemic genetic disorder caused by deletion or impaired expression of paternal genes in the q11–q13 region of chromosome 15 (Benarroch, Hirsch, Genstil, Landau, & Gross-Tsur, 2007). The incidence ranges from 1 in 10,000–20,000 births (Whittington et al., 2001). It has figured prominently in recent genetic research because of its relation to Angelman syndrome (AS; which has very different clinical features but is caused by deletion of maternal genes in the same area as PWS) and the resulting identification of genomic imprinting in humans (a phenomenon in which gene expression is dictated by the chromosome on which the particular copy of that gene resides) (State & Dykens, 2000).

Social and Behavioral Development

Levels of psychopathology are higher among individuals with PWS than in other syndromes associated with developmental delay (Reddy & Pfieffer, 2007). Intensity and frequency do vary to some extent, but the pattern of behavioral characteristics of children with PWS is quite consistent (Benarroch et al., 2007). Children with PWS characteristically exhibit hyperphagia (excessive eating due to an impaired neural satiety response) and obesity (Akefeldt & Gillberg, 1999; Clarke et al., 2002; Dykens & Kasari, 1997; Einfeld, Smith, Durvasula, Florio, & Tonge, 1999; Greenswag, 1987; Hinton et al., 2006; Holsen et al., 2006; Stein, Keating, Zar, & Hollandar, 1994; Wattendorf & Muenke, 2005). The intense food-seeking related behaviors typically start around the age of 6 years. If unrestricted, children with PWS will eat enormous quantities of food, even frozen, raw, or pet food. The pursuit of food can lead to antisocial behaviors (including lying and stealing to obtain or hoard food) or dangerous behaviors (such as exchanging sex for food). Children with PWS also exhibit obsessive-compulsive behaviors related to food and repeated questioning. Rituals and compulsive behaviors, such as skin picking, hoarding, and ordering, are more common in individuals with PWS than in individuals with other syndromes associated with developmental delay, and cause significant impairment in more than 45% (Dykens, Leckman, & Cassidy, 1996; Greaves, Prince, Evans, & Charman, 2006).

Children with PWS have difficulty recognizing social cues and interpreting social situations (Koenig, Klin, & Shultz, 2004). They show poor social judgment, exhibit social withdrawal, and have poor peer relations (Benarroch et al., 2007). The prevalence of autism among children with PWS is relatively high (Veltman, Craig, & Bolton, 2005).

Emotional Development and Temperament

Parents describe their young children with PWS as rigid, inflexible, stubborn, insisting on sameness, and unable to adjust to changes (Benarroch et al., 2007). Clinicians and researchers have reported impaired affect regulation, mood swings, tantrums, and agitation (Benarroch et al., 2007). Compared to typically developing children, children with PWS are less agreeable, conscientious, open to new experiences, and active, and more irritable and dependent (van Lieshout, De Meyer, Curfs, & Fryns, 1998). In adolescence and adulthood, mood disorders are diagnosed in 15%–17% (Vogels et al., 2004), and 28% have severe affective disorders with psychotic features (Boer et al., 2002).

Brain Development and Psychophysiology

Efforts to elucidate the neural basis for abnormal eating behaviors predominate psychophysiological research on individuals with PWS. Children with PWS have a resting metabolic rate that is lower than expected for their age (Benarroch et al., 2007). Because individuals with PWS exhibit hypothalamic dysregulation, hypothalamic abnormalities have been thought to account for their clinical characteristics. There are several types of evidence in support of this hypothesis, including structural MRI evidence of functional abnormalities in the brain region. However, brain imaging techniques suggest other brain regions also are involved (Kim et al., 2006; Yamada, Matsuzawa, Uchiyama, Kwee, & Nakada, 2006). For example, MRI, magnetic spectroscopy, and positron emission tomography (PET) scans reveal structural, functional, and metabolic abnormalities including enlarged ventricles, cortical atrophy, decreased volume of brain tissue in the parietal-occipital lobe (which also has been associated with obsessive-compulsive behavior), abnormalities in the frontothalamic regions (also associated with psychiatric dysfunction), sylvian fissure polymicrogyria, incomplete insular closure, and a small brainstem (Hashimoto et al., 1998; Hinton et al., 2006; Kim et al., 2006; Miller et al., 2007; State & Dykens, 2000; Yamada et al., 2006).

In a cross-sectional study, Miller et al. (2007) found that the only intracranial abnormality in children with PWS less than 2 years of age was enlarged ventricles. Enlarged ventricles indicate abnormal neuronal development, but it is unclear whether the enlarged ventricles result from a loss or abnormal growth of gray matter, white matter, or both (Miller et al., 2007). Whether the other structural brain abnormalities are present at birth or develop later is unknown; however, Miller et al.'s (2007) findings suggest that they may develop over time. Longitudinal studies are needed to document typical development and the impact of intervention.

Summary

Prader-Willi syndrome involves changes in brain anatomy, development, and metabolism, especially as they relate to the neural basis of an impaired satiety response. Research on the causal gene mechanism for this specific impairment is ongoing, but it likely involves complex interactions between direct effects of genetic variation on brain development and indirect effects through other neurochemical factors. Although there seems to be less heterogeneity in PWS than in other genetic syndromes associated with developmental delay, there is still variation in intensity and frequency of behavior problems that require explanation. Specifically, there is a need for future longitudinal studies, beginning early in life, of relatively large groups of individuals with PWS and appropriate comparison groups to help understand relations between hyperphagia and brain development. It is possible that information from psychophysiological studies may assist in the development of early identification procedures for PWS (e.g., the characteristic metabolic pattern). Early diagnosis is important to early intervention and to longitudinal studies of socioemotional and brain development in PWS. Further, identification of the core deficits, brain structures, and neurochemistry involved might enable the identification of more effective, targeted early intervention strategies (e.g., growth hormone supplementation), and investigation of the impact of intervention on structure and function of the developing brain.

Angelman Syndrome

Angelman syndrome is a genetic disorder caused by a deletion of the maternal genes in the q11–q13 region of chromosome 15. It occurs in 1 in every 10,000–20,000 births (Buckley, Dinno, & Weber, 1998; Petersen, Brondum-Nielsen, Hansen, & Wulff, 1995; Steffenburg, Gillberg, Steffenburg, & Kyllerman, 1996) and is characterized by severe developmental delay, expressive language deficits, and truncal and gait ataxia (tremulous movements) (Walz, 2007). Seizures, microcephaly, and distinctive physical traits are common (Williams et al., 2006).

Social and Behavioral Development

Compared to other children with developmental delay, children with AS (also called the "happy puppet" syndrome) exhibit excessive sociability, laughing, smiling, and initiation of interaction with adults (Clayton-Smith, 2001; Horsler & Oliver, 2006; Oliver et al., 2007). They also exhibit hyperactivity, aggression (grabbing and hair-pulling), noncompliance, sleep disturbance, stereotyped or repetitive behavior (such as hand flapping, tongue thrusting, excessive mouthing), and preference for water play (Clarke & Marston, 2000; Horsler & Oliver, 2006; Ishmael, Begleiter, & Butler, 2002; Miano et al., 2004; Summers & Feldman, 1999; Thompson & Bolton, 2003; Walz & Benson, 2002). Individuals with AS appear to "calm down" as they get older; they exhibit less hyperactivity, noncompliance, and bursts of laughter, with the clinical presentation of AS being most distinct between the ages of 2 and 16 years (Buntinx et al., 1995; Clarke & Marston, 2000; Horsler & Oliver, 2006).

Using the Aberrant Behavior Checklist (Aman & Singh, 1986), a standardized rating scale used to measure maladaptive behavior in individuals with developmental delay, Summers and Feldman (1999) compared children and young adults with AS to matched individuals with developmental delay of mixed etiology. The children and young adults with AS scored significantly lower on scales measuring irritability and lethargy/social withdrawal. These findings are consistent with clinical observations of individuals with AS and with later studies providing empirical evidence in support of a specific behavioral profile for AS.

Recently, Horsler and Oliver (2006) reviewed 64 studies of the behavioral characteristics associated with AS and found that few studies were methodologically rigorous (the majority being case studies), there was a potential bias in studies that did not involve a comparison group, and there was a trend in the literature from a direct gene effect on laughter to a socially mediated effect. Although the laughing and smiling behavior of children with AS is argued to be so characteristic of AS that it is sufficient for the diagnosis (Summers, Allison, Lynch, & Sandler, 1995), there appears to be disagreement as to the cause and function (which have been variously hypothesized as associated with seizure activity, the result of a neurological deficit, a global expressive outlet, a randomly generated motor phenomenon, or simply easily provoked in a social context) and whether it is influenced by the environment or is inappropriate to the context or environment (Horsler & Oliver, 2006).

Emotional Development and Temperament

Infants with AS usually begin smiling and laughing when they are 4 to 6 weeks old (Clayton-Smith, 1993; Clayton-Smith & Laan, 2003), which is concurrent with that of children without developmental delay and in contrast to other children with developmental delay, who typically exhibit a delayed emergence of social smiling and laughing (e.g., Carvajal & Iglesias, 1997). Parents describe their children with AS as having a happy demeanor and easily excitable personality (Walz & Benson, 2002; Williams et al., 1995). Children with AS generally exhibit fewer negative emotion signals (e.g., crying or tearful episodes) (Summers et al., 1995; Summers & Feldman, 1999; Thompson & Bolton, 2003). Parent ratings suggest lower levels of anxiety in children with AS than in other children with developmental delay (Walz & Benson, 2002). However, other characteristics, such as lack of sleep, restlessness, and hyperactivity, may indicate greater anxiety in children with AS (Brown & Consedine, 2004).

Brown and Consedine (2004) assert that the three main affective characteristics of children with AS—namely, high frequency of positive affect signals, low frequency of negative affect expressions, and behaviors indicative of high anxiety in the absence of observable anxiety signaling—comprise a distinctive a distinctive affective phenotype designed to elicit maximal levels of maternal investment and minimize the likelihood of rejection. In a recent observational study of children with AS and a matched control group, Oliver et al. (2007) provided evidence in support of Brown and Consedine's (2004) perspective. They found that the children with AS smiled more than the control group children, their smiling evoked higher levels of adult attention, and smiling by children with AS was frequently preceded by their initiation of contact with an adult. Thus, Oliver et al. (2007) provided evidence to support the perspective that the purpose of heightened sociability and smiling in the context of AS is to significantly increase access to social resources in a competitive setting, specifically the reward of adult contact. This potent social reinforcement from adults, as well as the prolonging of social interaction, also may underpin maladaptive behaviors such as grabbing and hair pulling.

Brain Development and Psychophysiology

Brain MRI or computed tomography (CT) scans of individuals with AS are typically normal but may show nonspecific changes such as mild cortical atrophy, microencephaly, delay in myelination, and ventricular dilation, which are consistent with delayed brain maturation and also observed in individuals with several other chromosomal disorders (Harting et al., 2008; Schumacher, 2001; Williams, 2005). However, more than 80% of individuals with AS have epilepsy and an extremely abnormal and clinically unexpected EEG pattern (Williams, 2005; Williams et al., 1995).

In animal studies, characteristics of AS (unique epileptic patterns and distinctive behavioral features) have been linked to localized central nervous system dysfunction of the ubiquitin ligase gene, UBE3A, located at 15q11.2, and the multiple actions of UBE3A during neuronal development, especially in the hippocampus and cerebellum (Miura et al., 2002; Williams, 2005). UBE3A is thought to play a role in axon guidance (the process by which neurons direct axons towards correct targets), neuronal connectivity, and degradation of potentially harmful proteins (Schumacher, 2001). In Williams' (2005) study of UBE3A-deficient mice, it is also implied that UBE3A disruption can cause mental retardation and seizures that are typical of AS.

Summary

The frequent smiling and laughter exhibited by children with AS may be designed to facilitate social interaction. Brown and Consedine (2004) suggest that perhaps individuals with AS seem to "calm down" as they develop because signals from caregivers indicating successful bonding decrease the frequency of laughing and smiling and other attention-seeking behaviors over time. Further research is needed on the smiling and laughing behavior in children with developmental delay (Burack et al., 1998), particularly its etiology, function, and developmental course in AS, as it is reported to be one of the most salient but least understood features of AS (Horsler & Oliver, 2006). Future research involving larger samples and a variety of comparison groups with relevant diagnoses (e.g., children with autism, PWS, developmental delay, developmental delay and epilepsy, etc.) will enhance our understanding of the pathophysiological overlap between related syndromes (Walz, 2007).

Conclusion

Brain and behavior are clearly affected by genetic syndromes. Genetic syndromes involve both widespread and specific changes in brain anatomy, brain development, and psychophysiology. Some genetic syndromes seem to affect certain neuroanatomical areas and socioemotional functions more than others. In fact, the increased prevalence of some socioemotional difficulties in children with genetic syndromes may be partially explained by neurodevelopmental differences.

For example, infants with DS are socially engaging but show dampened responses and passivity. Their unique temperament and social behavior may be explained by decreased neurotransmitter activity. Children with DS seek out social interaction and are affectionate, but exhibit deficits in emotion recognition.

Frontal EEG activation differences may help explain differences in emotion processing in children with DS. Because of their relative strength in socioemotional abilities, infants with DS constitute an ideal population for studying the development of emotion. Because their cognitive impairments may limit what can develop through social learning, studying children with DS may help us understand which aspects of emotional development are maturational and which are environmental (Carvajal & Iglesias, 2002).

Children with FXS typically exhibit characteristic behavior such as gaze aversion, hyperarousal, shyness, anxiety, and other autistic symptoms. As such, research on these children may help identify the core deficits in autism. With their strong propensity for hyperarousal and gaze aversion in particular, study of individuals with FXS may help elucidate the neurological and endocrinological underpinnings of these constructs and their role in socioemotional development.

Children with 22qDS are at high risk of developing psychiatric disorders, especially ADHD, autism, and schizophrenia. Results of neuroanatomical studies have revealed both widespread and specific changes in brain anatomy in children with 22qDS. Longitudinal research on children with 22qDS may help identify biological markers that predict severe psychiatric illness and 22qDS is considered a neurological model for the study of gene–brain–behavior relations in schizophrenia. (Eliez et al., 2001).

Findings from research on neurodevelopmental differences also may help explain the hypersociability of children with WS. Williams syndrome involves changes in brain anatomy, brain development, and psychophysiology. The biological basis of these neurodevelopmental differences may involve interactions between direct effects of the genetic deletion on brain development and indirect effects through elevated calcium levels.

Prader-Willi syndrome involves neural changes and differences in metabolism that may account for the excessive eating exhibited by individuals with PWS. Information from psychophysiological studies may assist in the development of early identification procedures for PWS (e.g., the characteristic metabolic pattern), and identification of the core deficits, brain structures, and neurochemistry involved might enable the identification of early intervention strategies (e.g., growth hormone supplementation).

Children with AS frequently smile and laugh, infrequently exhibit negative affect, are highly anxious, and have epilepsy. There is disagreement as to the cause and function of the laughing and smiling behavior of children with AS. Various causes have been hypothesized, including seizure activity and a localized neurological deficit. Evidence suggests that the function of the distinctive affective phenotype of AS may be to elicit social interaction and attention from caregivers. Brain scans of individuals with AS show nonspecific changes; however, more than 80% of individuals with AS have an extremely abnormal EEG pattern.

Despite the exciting developments in knowledge of socioemotional and brain development in children with genetic syndromes associated with developmental delay, the field is rife with opportunities for important future research on the link between specific genetic syndromes and psychiatric disorders (Hodapp & Dykens, 2009). For example, findings from research on the overlap of autism characteristics in specific genetic disorders (such as FXS) may improve our understanding of the behavioral phenotypes of these disorders, as well as of the neurobiology of autism (Walz, 2007). That is, findings from research on children with FXS who have some symptoms of autism (i.e., not just those who have been diagnosed with autism) may inform our understanding of the pathophysiology of specific behavioral traits, such as stereotyped behaviors or social interaction difficulties (Dykens, Sutcliffe, & Levitt, 2004; Walz, 2007).

Also needed is more research starting early in life. Most research on socioemotional and brain development in individuals with genetic syndromes associated with developmental delay is focused on school-aged children (and older individuals). This is partly due to the difficulties inherent in identifying and diagnosing some genetic disorders in infancy. Although many disorders can be diagnosed with genetic testing at any age, this testing is not routinely performed at birth. For some genetic syndromes, information from psychophysiological studies may assist in the development of early-identification procedures. For example, noninvasive EEG could be used for early diagnosis of AS if we had more information on the characteristic EEG pattern in AS (including the reliability and validity of this test). Without such research, the difficulties with late diagnosis are likely to continue. Accurate, early diagnosis is important to early intervention and to longitudinal studies of socioemotional and brain development with these populations. Further, identification of the core deficits, brain structures, and neurochemistry involved in genetic syndromes might facilitate the identification of more effective, targeted early intervention strategies (e.g., growth hormone supplementation in PWS), and investigation of the impact of intervention on structure and function of the developing brain.

Research on the biological basis of neurodevelopmental differences in children with genetic syndromes is ongoing, but it likely involves complex interactions between direct effects of genetic variation on brain development and indirect effects through other neurochemical factors (Campbell et al., 2006; Hodapp & Dykens, 2009; for reviews see Schaer & Eliez, 2007; Venkitaramani & Lombroso, 2007). Research on the specific mechanisms underlying neuropathological abnormalities and their relation to socioemotional development would be helpful. Given that the "brain piece" is unfortunately missing in many studies, as are appropriate comparison groups, a multidisciplinary collaboration among geneticists, psychophysiologists, and behavioral researchers likely is needed (Shelley & Robertson, 2005). Longitudinal studies, beginning early in life, of relatively large groups of individuals with specific genetic syndromes and appropriate comparison groups could add to the knowledge base on relations between socioemotional development and brain development (Reiss & Dant, 2003). In addition to informing our knowledge of genetic syndromes, research in this area can inform our knowledge of gene–brain–behavior relations generally (Feinstein & Singh, 2007; Hodapp & Dykens, 2009).

Also needed is research on predictors of individual differences in socioemotional and brain development to help explain heterogeneity within syndromes. Environmental factors, such as parents and peers, likely influence the development of children with genetic syndromes associated with developmental delay, and preliminary studies suggest that environmental influences on these children are not minor (e.g., Dyer-Friedman et al., 2002; Hessl et al., 2001; Niccols et al., in press). Studies designed to elucidate how socioemotional and brain development is moderated and mediated by environmental risk and protective factors are vital to understanding and optimizing development in these children (Hodapp & Dykens, 2009; Reiss & Dant, 2003).

References

Adams, K., & Marham, R. (1991). Recognition of affective facial expressions by children and adolescents with and without mental retardation. *American Journal on Mental Retardation, 96*, 21–28.

Akefeldt, A., & Gillberg, C. (1999). Behavior and personality characteristics of children and young adults with Prader-Willi syndrome: A controlled study. *Journal of the American Academy of Child & Adolescent Psychiatry, 38*, 761–769.

Akil, M., Kolachana, B., Rothmond, D., Hyde, T., Weinberger, D., & Kleinman, J. (2003). Catechol-o-methyl transferase genotype and dopamine regulation in the human brain. *Journal of Neuroscience, 23*, 2008–2013.

Aman, M. G., & Singh, N. N. (1986). *Aberrant behaviour checklist: Manual.* East Aurora, NY: Slosson Educational Publications.

Antshel, K. M., Conchelos, J., Lanzetta, G., Fremont, W., & Kates, W. R. (2005). Behavior and corpus callosum morphology relationships in velocardiofacial syndrome (22q11.2 deletion syndrome). *Psychiatry Research, 138*, 235–245.

Antshel, K. M., Stallone, K., AbdulSabur, N., Shprintzen, R., Roizen, N., Higgins, A. M., et al. (2007). Temperament in velocardiofacial syndrome. *Journal of Intellectual Disability Research, 51*, 3–27.

Bailey, D. B., Hatton, D. D., Mesibov, G., Ament, N., & Skinner, M. (2000). Early development, temperament, and functional impairment in autism and fragile X syndrome. *Journal of Autism and Developmental Disorders, 30*, 49–59.

Baker, K. D., & Skuse, D. H. (2005). Adolescents and young adults with 22q11 deletion syndrome: Psychopathology in an at-risk group. *The British Journal of Psychiatry, 186*, 115–120.

Barnea-Goraly, N., Eliez, S., Hedeus, M., Menon, V., White, C., Moseley, M., & Reiss, A. (2003). White matter tract alterations in fragile X syndrome: Preliminary evidence from diffusion tensor imaging. *American Journal of Medical Genetics. Part B, Neuropsychiatric Genetics, 118*, 81–88.

Baumgardner, T. L., Reiss, A. L., Freund, L. S., & Abrams, M. T. (1995). Specification of the neurobehavioral phenotype in males with fragile X syndrome. *Pediatrics, 95*, 744–752.

Bearden, C. E., van Erp, T. G. M., Monterosso, J. R., Simon, T. J., Glahn, D. C., Saleh, P. A., et al. (2004). Regional brain abnormalities in 22q11.2 deletion syndrome: Association with cognitive abilities and behavioral symptoms. *Neurocase, 10*, 198–206.

Belser, R. C., & Sudhalter, V. (2001). Conversational characteristics of children with fragile X syndrome: repetitive speech. *American Journal of Mental Retardation, 106*, 28–38.

Benarroch, F., Hirsch, H. J., Genstil, L., Landau, Y. E., & Gross-Tsur, V. (2007). Prader-Willi syndrome: Medical prevention and behavioral challenges. *Child and Adolescent Psychiatric Clinics of North America, 16*, 695–708.

Bingham, P. M., Zimmerman, R. A., McDonald-McGinn, D., Driscoll, D., Emanual, B. S., & Zackai, E. (1997). Enlarged Sylvian fissures in infants with interstitial deletion of chromosome 22q11. *American Journal of Medical Genetics (Neuropsychiatric Genetics), 74*, 538–543.

Boer, H., Holland, A., Whittington, J., Butler, J., Webb, T., Clarke, D. (2002). Psychotic illness in people with Prader-Willi syndrome due to chromosome 15 maternal uniparental disomy. *Lancet, 359*, 135–136.

Braden, J., & Obrzut, J. (2002). Williams syndrome: Neuropsychological findings and implications for practice. *Journal of Developmental and Physical Disabilities, 14*, 203–213.

Bregman, J. D., Leckman, J. F., & Ort, S. I. (1990). Thyroid function in fragile-X syndrome males. *The Yale Journal of Biology and Medicine, 63*, 293–299.

Brooks-Gunn, J., & Lewis, M. (1982). Affective exchanges between normal and handicapped infants and their mothers. In T. Field, & A. Fogel (Eds.), *Emotion and early interaction* (pp.161–212). Hillsdale, NJ: Lawrence Erlbaum Associates.

Brown, W. M., & Consedine, N. S. (2004). Just how happy is the happy puppet? An emotion signaling and kinship theory perspective on the behavioral phenotype of children with Angelman syndrome. *Medical Hypotheses, 63*, 377–385.

Buckley, R. H., Dinno, N., & Weber, P. (1998). Angelman syndrome: Are the estimates too low? *American Journal of Medical Genetics, 80*, 385–390.

Buntinx, I. M., Hennekam, R. C., Brouwer, O. F., Stroink, H., Beuten, J., Mangelschots, K., et al. (1995). Clinical profile of Angelman syndrome at different ages. *American Journal of Medical Genetics, 56*, 176–183.

Burack, J. A. (1990). Differentiating mental retardation: The two-group approach and beyond. In R. M. Hodapp, J. A. Burack, & E. Zigler (Eds.), *Issues in the developmental approach to mental retardation* (pp. 27–48). New York: Cambridge University Press.

Burack, J. A., Hodapp, R. M., & Zigler, E. (1998). *Handbook of mental retardation and development*. Cambridge: Cambridge University Press.

Burack, J. A., Iarocci, G., Flanagan, T. D., & Bowler, D. M. (2004). On mosaics and melting pots: Conceptual considerations of comparison and matching strategies. *Journal of Autism and Developmental Disorders, 34*(1), 65–73.

Butler, M. G., & Najjar, J. L. (1988). Do some patients with fragile X syndrome have precocious puberty? *American Journal of Medical Genetics, 31*, 779–781.

Campbell, L. E., Daly, E., Toal, F., Stevens, A., Azuma, R., Catani, M., et al. (2006). Brain and behaviour in children with 22q11.2 deletion syndrome: A volumetric and voxel-based morphometry MRI study. *Brain, 129*, 5–28.

Capone, G., Goyal, P., Ares, W., & Lannigan, E. (2006). Neurobehavioral disorders in children, adolescents, and young adults with Down syndrome. *American Journal of Medical Genetics. Part C, Seminars in Medical Genetics, 142C*, 158–172.

Carvajal, F., & Iglesias, J. (1997). Mother and infant smiling exchanges during face to face interaction in infants with and without Down syndrome. *Developmental Psychobiology, 31*, 277–289.

Carvajal, F., & Iglesias, J. (2002). Face-to-face emotion interaction studies in Down syndrome infants. *International Journal of Behavioral Development, 26*, 104–112.

Chow, E. W., Mikulis, D. J., Zipursky, R. B., Scutt, L. E., Weksberg, R., & Bassett, A. S. (1999). Qualitative MRI findings in adults with 22q11 deletion syndrome and schizophrenia. *Biological Psychiatry, 46*, 1436–1442.

Cicchetti, D., & Sroufe, A. (1976). Relationship between affective and cognitive development in Down's syndrome infants. *Child Development, 47*, 920–929.

Clarke, D. J., Boer, H., Whittington, J., Holland, A., Butler, J., & Webb, T. (2002). Prader-Willi syndrome, compulsive and ritualistic behaviours: The first population-based survey. *British Journal of Psychiatry, 180*, 358–362.

Clarke, D. J., & Marston, G. (2000). Problem behaviors associated with 15q- Angelman syndrome. *American Journal of Mental Retardation, 105*, 25–31.

Clayton-Smith, J. (1993). Clinical research on Angelman syndrome in the United Kingdom: Observations on 82 affected individuals. *American Journal of Medical Genetics, 46*, 12–15.

Clayton-Smith, J. (2001). Angelman syndrome: Evolution of the phenotype in adolescents and adults. *Developmental Medicine and Child Neurology, 43*, 473–480.

Clayton-Smith, J., & Laan, L. (2003). Angelman syndrome: A review of the clinical and genetic aspects. *Journal of Medical Genetics, 40*, 87–95.

Cohen, I. L. (1995). A theoretical analysis of the role of hyperarousal in the learning and behavior of fragile X males. *Mental Retardation and Developmental Disabilities Research Review, 1*, 286–291.

Cohen, I. L., Vietze, P. M., Sudhalter, V., Jenkins, E. C., & Brown, W. T. (1991). Effects of age and communication level on eye contact in fragile X males and in non-fragile X autistic males. *American Journal of Medical Genetics, 38*, 498–502.

Conrad, N. J., Schmidt, L. A., Niccols, A., Polak, C., Riniolo, T., & Burack, J. (2007). Frontal electroencephalogram asymmetry during affective processing in children with Down syndrome: A pilot study. *Journal of Intellectual Disability Research, 51*, 988–995.

Cornish, K., Burack, J., Rahman, A., Munir, F., Russo, N., & Grant, C. (2005a). Theory of mind deficits in children with fragile X syndrome. *Journal of Intellectual Disability Research, 49*, 372–378.

Cornish, K., Kogan, C., Turk, J., Manly, T., James, N., Mills, A., et al. (2005b). The emerging fragile X permutation phenotype: Evidence from the domain of social cognition. *Brain and Cognition, 57*, 53–60.

Coyle, J. T., Oster-Granite, M. L., & Gearhart, J. D. (1986). The neurobiologic consequences of Down syndrome. *Brain Research Bulletin, 16*, 773–787.

Cronister, A. E., & Hagerman, R. J. (1989). Fragile X syndrome. *Journal of Pediatric Health Care, 3*, 9–19.

Cummings, J. L. (1993). Frontal-subcortical circuits and human behavior. *Archives of Neurology, 50*, 873–880.

Devinsky, O., Sato, S., Conwit, R. A., & Schapiro, M. B. (1990). Relation of EEG alpha background to cognitive function, brain atrophy, and cerebral metabolism in Down's syndrome: Age-specific changes. *Archives of Neurology, 47*, 277–281.

Duba, H. C., Doll, A., Neyer, M., Erdel, M., Mann, C., Hammerer, I., et al. (2002). The elastin gene is disrupted in a family with a balanced translocation t(7;16) (q11.23;q13) associated with a variable expression of the Williams-Beuren syndrome. *European Journal of Human Genetics, 10*, 351–361.

du Montcel, S. T., Mendizabal, H., Ayme, S., Levy, A., & Philips, N. (1996). Prevalence of 22q11 microdeletion. *Journal of Medical Genetics, 33*, 719.

Dunham, I., Collins, J., Wadey, R., & Scrambler, P. (1992). Possible role for COMT in psychosis associated with velo-cardial-facial syndrome. *Lancet, 340*, 1361–1362.

Dyer-Friedman, J., Glaser, B., Hessl, D., Johnston, C., Huffman, L.C., Taylor, A., et al. (2002). Genetic and environmental influences on the cognitive outcomes of children with fragile X syndrome. *Journal of the American Academy of Child and Adolescent Psychiatry, 41*, 237–244.

Dykens, E. (1995). Measuring behavioral phenotypes: Provocations from the "new genetics." *American Journal of Mental Retardation, 99*, 522–532.

Dykens, E. (2003). Anxiety, fears, and phobias in persons with Williams syndrome. *Developmental Neuropsychology, 23*, 291–316.

Dykens, E. (2007). Psychiatric and behavioral disorders in persons with Down Syndrome. *Mental Retardation and Developmental Disabilities, 13*, 272–278.

Dykens, E. M., & Kasari, C. (1997). Maladaptive behavior in children with Prader-Willi syndrome, Down syndrome, and nonspecific mental retardation. *American Journal of Mental Retardation, 102*, 228–237.

Dykens, E. M., Leckman, J. F., & Cassidy, S. B. (1996). Obsessions and compulsions in Prader-Willi syndrome. *Journal of Child Psychology & Psychiatry & Allied Disciplines, 37*, 995–1002.

Dykens, E. M., Sutcliffe, J. S., & Levitt, P. (2004). Autism and 15q11-q13 disorders: Behavioral, genetic, and pathophysiological issues. *Mental Retardation and Developmental Disabilities Research Reviews, 10*, 284–291.

Einfeld, S. L., Smith, A., Durvasula, S., Florio, T., & Tonge, B. J. (1999b). Behavior and emotional disturbance in Prader-Willi syndrome. *American Journal of Medical Genetics, 40*, 454–459.

Einfeld, S., Tonge, B., & Turner, G. (1999a). Longitudinal course of behavioral and emotional problems in fragile X syndrome. *American Journal of Medical Genetics, 87*, 436–439.

Eliez, S., Blasey, C. M., Freund, L. S., Hastie, T., & Reiss, A. L. (2001). Brain anatomy, gender and IQ in children and adolescents with fragile X syndrome. *Brain, 124*(Pt. 8), 1610–1618.

Eliez, S., Schmitt, J., White, C., & Reiss, A. (2000). Children and adolescents with velo-cardio-facial syndrome: A volumetric MRI study. *American Journal of Psychiatry, 157*, 409–415.

Farzin, F., Perry, H., Hessl, D., Loesch, D., Cohen, J., Bacalman, S., et al. (2006). Autism spectrum disorders and attention-deficit/hyperactivity disorder in boys with the fragile X premutation. *Journal of Developmental and Behavioral Pediatrics, 27*(Supplement 2), 137–144.

Feinstein, C., Eliez, S., Blasey, C., & Reiss, A. L. (2002). Psychiatric disorders and behavioral problems in children with velocardiofacial syndrome: Usefulness as phenotypic indicators of schizophrenia risk. *Biological Psychiatry, 51*, 312–318.

Feinstein, C., & Reiss, A. L. (1998). Autism: The point of view from fragile X studies. *Journal of Autism and Developmental Disorders, 28*, 393–405.

Feinstein, C., & Singh, S. (2007). Social phenotypes in neurogenetic syndromes. *Child and Adolescent Psychiatric Clinics of North America, 16*, 631–647.

Fidler, D. (2006). The emergence of a syndrome-specific personality profile in young children with Down syndrome. *Down Syndrome Research and Practice, 10*, 53–60.

Fidler, D., Hepburn, S., Most, D., Philofsky, A., & Rogers, S. (2007). Emotional responsivity in young children with Williams syndrome. *American Journal on Mental Retardation, 112*, 194–206.

Fine, S., Weissman, A., Gerdes, M., Pinto-Martin, J., Zackai, E., McDonald-McGinn, D., et al. (2005). Autism spectrum disorders and symptoms in children with molecularly confirmed 22q11.2 deletion syndrome. *Journal of Autism and Developmental Disorders, 35*, 461–470.

Frigerio, E., Burt, D. M., Gagliardi, C., Cioffi, G., Martelli, S., Perrett, D. I., et al. (2006). Is everybody always my friend? Perception of approachability in Williams syndrome. *Neuropsychologia, 44*, 254–259.

Gagliardi, C., Frigerio, E., Burt, D. M., Cazzaniga, I., Perrett, D. I., & Borgatti, R. (2003). Facial expression recognition in Williams syndrome. *Neuropsychologia, 41*, 733–738.

Galaburda, A., Wang, P., Bellugi, U., & Rossen, M. (1994). Cytoarchitectonic findings in a genetically based disorder: Williams syndrome. *NeuroReport, 5*, 758–787.

Garrett, A. S., Menon, V., MacKenzie, K., & Reiss, A. L. (2004). Here's looking at you, kid: Neural systems underlying face and gaze processing in fragile X syndrome. *Archives of General Psychiatry, 61*, 281–288.

Gartstein, M., Marmion, J., & Swanson, H. (2006). Infant temperament: An evaluation of children with Down Syndrome. *Journal of Reproductive and Infant Psychology, 24*, 31–41.

Gerdes, M., Solot, C., Wang, P. P., Moss, E., La Rossa, D., & Randall, P. (1999). Cognitive and behavior profile of preschool children with chromosome 22q11.2 deletion. *American Journal of Medical Genetics, 85*, 127–133.

Golding-Kushner, K. J., Weller, G., & Shprintzen, R. J. (1985). Velo-cardio-facial syndrome: Language and psychological profiles. *Journal of Craniofacial Genetics and Developmental Biology, 5*, 259–266.

Gothelf, D., Eliez, S., Thompson, T., Hinard, C., Penniman, L., Feinstein, C., et al. (2005). COMT genotype predicts longitudinal cognitive decline and psychosis in 22q11.2 deletion syndrome. *Nature Neuroscience, 8*, 1500–1502.

Gothelf, D., Gruber, R., Presburger, G., Dotan, I., Brand-Gothelf, A., Burg, M., et al. (2003). Methylphenidate treatment for attention-deficit/hyperactivity disorder in children and adolescents with velocardiofacial syndrome: An open label study. *Journal of Clinical Psychiatry, 64*, 1163–1169.

Gothelf, D., Presburger, D. L., Nahmani, A., Burg, M., Berant, M., Blieden, L. C., et al. (2004). Genetic, developmental, and physical factors associated with attention deficit hyperactivity disorder in patients with velocardiofacial syndrome. *American Journal of Medical Genetics, 126B*, 116–121.

Graf, W. D., Unis, A. S., Yates, C. M., Sulzbacher, S., Dinulos, M. B., Jack, R. M., et al. (2001). Catecholamines in patients with 22q11.2 deletion syndrome and the low-activity COMT polymorphism. *Neurology, 57*, 410–416.

Greaves, N., Prince, E., Evans, D. W., & Charman, T. (2006). Repetitive and ritualistic behavior in children with Prader-Willi syndrome and children with autism. *Journal of Intellectual Disability Research, 50*, 92–100.

Greenswag, L. R. (1987). Adults with Prader-Willi syndrome: A survey of 232 cases. *Developmental Medicine and Child Neurology, 29*, 145–152.

Guralnick, M. J. (2002). Involvement with peers: Comparisons between young children with and without Down's syndrome. *Journal of Intellectual Disability Research, 46*, 379–393.

Harting, I., Seitz, A., Rating, D., Sartor, K., Zschocke, J., Janssen, B., et al. (2008). Abnormal myelination in Angelman syndrome. *European Journal of Paediatric Neurology* [Epub ahead of print].

Hashimoto, T., Mori, K., Yoneda, Y., Yamaue, T., Miyazaki, M., Harada, M., et al. (1998). Proton magnetic resonance spectroscopy of the brain in patients with Prader-Willi syndrome. *Pediatric Neurology, 18*, 30–35.

Hatton, D. D., Bailey, D. B., Jr., Hargett-Beck, M., Skinner, M., & Clark, R. (1999). Behavioral style of young boys with fragile X syndrome. *Developmental Medicine and Child Neurology, 41*, 625–632.

Henriques, J. B., & Davidson, R. J. (1990). Regional brain electrical asymmetries discriminate between previously depressed and healthy control subjects. *Journal of Abnormal Psychology, 99*, 22–31.

Hepburn, S., & Rogers, S. J. (2001, March). *Temperament in children with fragile X syndrome.* Paper presented at the Gatlinburg Conference on Research in Developmental Disabilities, Charleston, SC.

Hessl, D., Dyer-Friedman, J., Glaser, B., Wisbeck, J., Barajas, R. G., Taylor, A., et al. (2001). The influence of environmental and genetic factors on behavior problems and autistic symptoms in boys and girls with fragile X syndrome. *Pediatrics, 108*, E88.

Hessl, D., Glaser, B., Dyer-Friedman, J., Blasey, C., Hastie, T., Gunnar, M., et al. (2002). Cortisol and behavior in fragile X syndrome. *Psychoneuroendocrinology, 27*, 855–872.

Hessl, D., Glaser, B., Dyer-Friedman, J., & Reiss, A. L. (2006). Social behavior and cortisol reactivity in children with fragile X syndrome. *Journal of Child Psychology and Psychiatry, and Allied Disciplines, 47*, 602–610.

Hinton, E. C., Holland, A. J., Gellatly, M. S. N., Soni, S., Patterson, M., Ghatel, M. A., et al. (2006). Neural representations of hunger and satiety in Prader-Willi syndrome. *International Journal of Obesity, 30*, 313–321.

Hodapp, R. M., & Dykens, E. M. (2009). Intellectual disabilities and child psychiatry: Looking to the future. *Journal of Child Psychology and Psychiatry, 50*(1–2), 99–107.

Holsen, L. M., Zarcone, J. R., Brooks, W. M., Butler, M. G., Thompson, T. I., Ahluwalia, J. S., et al. (2006). Neural mechanisms underlying hyperphagia in Prader-Willi syndrome. *Obesity, 14*, 1028–1037.

Horsler, K., & Oliver, C. (2006). Environmental influences on the behavioral phenotype of Angelman syndrome. *American Journal of Mental Retardation, 111*, 311–321.

Hyche, J. K., Bakeman, R., & Adamson, L. B. (1992). Understanding communicative cues of infants with Down syndrome: Effects of mothers' experience and infants' age. *Journal of Applied Developmental Psychology, 13*(1), 1–16.

Iarocci, G., Yager, J., Rombough, A., & McLaughlin, J. (2008). The development of social competence among persons with Down syndrome: From survival to social inclusion. *International Review of Research in Mental Retardation, 35*, 87–119.

Ishmael, H. A., Begleiter, M. L., & Butler, M. G. (2002). Drowning as a cause of death in Angelman syndrome. *American Journal of Mental Retardation, 107*, 69–70.

Jones, O. H. M. (1980). Prelinguistic communication skills in Down's syndrome and normal infants. In T. F. Field (Ed.), *High-risk infants and children: Adult and peer interactions* (pp. 205–225). New York: Publication Press.

Jones, W., Bellugi, U., Lai, Z., Chiles, M., Reilly, J., Lincoln, A., et al. (2000). II. Hypersociability in Williams syndrome. *Journal of Cognitive Neuroscience, 7*, 196–208.

Jones, W., Hesselink, J., Courchesne, E., Duncan, T., Matsuda, K., & Bellugi, U. (2002). Cerebellar abnormalities in infants and toddlers with Williams syndrome. *Developmental Medicine & Child Neurology, 44*, 688–694.

Karayiorgou, M., Morris, M. A., Morrow, B., Shprintzen, R. J., Goldberg, R., & Borrow, J. (1995). Schizophrenia susceptibility associated with interstitial deletions of chromosome 22q11. *Proceedings of the National Academy of Sciences, 92*, 7612–7616.

Karmiloff-Smith, A., Klima, E., Bellugi, U., Grant, J., & Baron-Cohen, S. (1995). Is there a social module? Language, face processing, and theory of mind in individuals with Williams syndrome. *Journal of Cognitive Neuroscience, 7*, 196–208.

Kasari, C., & Freeman, S. (2001). Task-related social behavior in children with Down syndrome. *American Journal on Mental Retardation, 106*(3), 253–264.

Kasari, C., Freeman, S., & Hughes, M. A. (2001). Emotion recognition by children with Down syndrome. *American Journal on Mental Retardation, 106*, 59–72.

Kasari, C., Freeman, S., Mundy, P., & Sigman, M. (1995). Attention regulation by children with Down syndrome: Coordinated joint attention and social referencing looks. *American Journal on Mental Retardation, 100*(2), 128–136.

Kasari, C., Sigman, M., Mundy, P., & Yirmiya, N. (1990). Affective sharing in the context of joint attention interactions of normal, autistic, and mentally retarded children. *Journal of Autism and Developmental Disorders, 20*, 87–100.

Kates, W. R., Abrams, M. T., Kaufmann, W. E., Breiter, S. N., & Reiss, A. L. (1997). Reliability and validity of MRI measurement of the amygdale and hippocampus in children with fragile X syndrome. *Psychiatry Research, 75*, 31–48.

Kates, W. R., Antshel, K. M., Willhite, R., Bessette, B. A., Abdul-Sabur, N., Higgins, A. M. (2005). Gender moderated dorsolateral prefrontal reductions in 22q11.2 deletion syndrome: Implications for risk for schizophrenia. *Child Neuropsychology, 11*, 73–85.

Kates, W. R., Burnette, C. P., Jabs, E. W., Rutberg, J., Murphy, A. M., Grados, M., et al. (2001). Regional cortical white matter reductions in velocardiofacial syndrome: A volumetric MRI analysis. *Biological Psychiatry, 49*, 677–684.

Kates, W. R., Miller, A. M., Abdulsabur, N., Antshel, K., Conchelos, J., Freemon, W., & Roizen, N. (2006). Temporal lobe anatomy and psychiatric symptoms in velocardiofacial syndrome (22q1.2 deletion syndrome. *Journal of the American Academy of Child and Adolescent Psychiatry, 45*, 587–595.

Keysor, C. S., & Mazzocco, M. M. (2002). A developmental approach to understanding fragile X syndrome in females. *Microscopy Research and Technique, 57*, 179–186.

Kim, S. E., Jin, D. K., Cho, S. S., Kim, J. H., Hong, S. D., Paik, K. H., et al. (2006). Regional cerebral glucose metabolic abnormality in Prader-Willi syndrome: An 18F-FDG PET study under sedation. *Journal of Nuclear Medicine, 47*, 1088–1092.

Klein-Tasman, B. P., & Mervis, C. B. (2003). Distinctive personality characteristics of 8–9 and 10 year olds with Williams syndrome. *Developmental Neuropsychology, 23*, 271–292.

Knieps, L. J., Walden, T. A., & Baxter, A. (1994). Affective expressions of toddlers with and without Down syndrome in a social referencing context. *American Journal on Mental Retardation, 99*, 301–312.

Koenig, K., Klin, A., & Schultz, R. (2004). Deficits in social attribution ability on Prader-Willi syndrome. *Journal of Autism and Developmental Disorders, 34*, 573–582.

Korenberg, J. R., Chen, X., Hirota, H., Lai, Z., Bellugi, U., Burian, D., et al. (2000). Genome structure and cognitive map of Williams syndrome. *Journal of Cognitive Neuroscience, 12*, 89–107.

Kwon, H., Menon, V., Eliez, S., Warsofsky, I. S., White, C. D., Dyer-Friedman, J., et al. (2001). Functional neuroanatomy of visuospatial working memory in fragile X syndrome: Relation to behavioral and molecular measures. *American Journal of Psychiatry, 158*, 1040–1051.

Lachman, H. M., Morrow, B., Shprintzen, R. J., Veit, S., Parsia, S. S., Faedda, G., et al. (1996). Association of codon 108/158 catechol-o-methyl transferase gene polymorphism with the psychiatric manifestations of velo-cardio-facial syndrome. *American Journal of Medical Genetics, 67*, 468–472.

Laing, E., Butterworth, G., Ansari, D., Gsodl, M., Longhi, E., Panagiotaki, G., et al. (2002). Atypical development of language and social communication in toddlers with Williams syndrome. *Developmental Science, 5*, 233–246.

Laws, G., & Bishop, D. (2004). Verbal deficits in Down's syndrome and specific language impairment: a comparison. *International Journal of Language and Communication Disorders, 39*, 423–451.

Linn, M. I., Goodman, J. F., & Lender, W. L. (2000). Played out? Passive behavior by children with Down syndrome during unstructured play. *Journal of Early Intervention, 23*(4), 264–278.

Loesch, D. Z., Huggins, R. M., & Hoang, N. H. (1995). Growth in stature in fragile X families: A mixed longitudinal study. *American Journal of Medical Genetics, 58,* 249–256.

Lubec, G., & Engidawork, E. (2002). The brain in Down syndrome (Trisomy 21). *Journal of Neurology, 249,* 1347–1356.

Masterman, D. L., & Cummings, J. L. (1997). Frontal-subcortical circuits: The anatomic basis of executive, social and motivated behaviors. *Journal of Psychopharmacology, 11,* 107–114.

Mazzocco, M. M. (2000). Advances in research on the fragile X syndrome. *Mental Retardation and Developmental Disabilities Research Reviews, 6,* 96–106.

Mazzocco, M. M., Baumgardner, T., Freund, L. S., & Reiss, A. L. (1998). Social functioning among girls with fragile X or Turner syndrome and their sisters. *Journal of Autism and Developmental Disorders, 28,* 509–517.

Mazzocco, M. M., Pennington, B. F., & Hagerman, R. J. (1994). Social cognition skills among females with fragile X. *Journal of Autism and Developmental Disorders, 24,* 473–485.

McAlaster, R. (1992). Postnatal cerebral maturation in Down's syndrome children: A developmental EEG coherence study. *International Journal of Neuroscience, 65,* 221–237.

McDevitt, S. C., & Carey, W. B. (1978). The measurement of temperament in 3- to 7-year-old children. *Journal of Child Psychology and Psychiatry, and Allied Disciplines, 19,* 245–253.

Menendez, M. (2005). Down syndrome, Alzheimer's disease and seizures. *Brain Development, 27,* 246–252.

Mervis, C. B., & Klein-Tasman, B. P. (2004). Methodological issues in group-matching designs: Alpha levels for control variable comparisons and measurement characteristics of control and target variables. *Journal of Autism and Developmental Disorders, 34,* 7–17.

Mervis, C., Morris, C., Klein-Tasman, B., Bertrand, J., Kwitny, S., Appelbaum, L., et al. (2003). Attentional characteristics of infants and toddlers with Williams syndrome during triadic interactions. *Developmental Neuropsychology, 23,* 243–268.

Mervis, C. B., & Robinson, B. F. (1999). Methodological issues in cross-syndrome comparisons: Matching procedures, sensitivity (Se), and specificity (Sp). Commentary on M. Sigman, & E. Ruskin, Continuity and change in the social competence of children with autism, Down syndrome, and developmental delays. *Monographs of the Society for Research in Child Development, 64*(Serial no. 256), 115–130.

Miano, S., Bruni, O., Leuzzi, V., Elia, M., Verrillo, E., & Ferri, R. (2004). Sleep polygraphy in Angelman syndrome. *Clinical Neurophysiology, 115,* 938–945.

Miller, J. L., Couch, J. A., Schmalfuss, I., He, G., Liu, Y., & Driscoll, D. J. (2007). Intracranial abnormalities detected by three-dimensional magnetic resonance imaging in Prader-Willi syndrome. *American Journal of Medical Genetics. Part A, 143,* 476–483.

Miller, L. J., McIntosh, D. N., McGrath, J., Shyu, V., Lampe, M., Taylor, A. K., et al. (1999). Electrodermal responses to sensory stimuli in individuals with fragile X syndrome: A preliminary report. *American Journal of Medical Genetics, 83,* 268–279.

Miura, K., Kishino, T., Li, E., Webber, H., Dikkes, P., Holmes, G. L., & Wagstaff, J. (2002). Neurobehavioral and electroencephalographic abnormalities in Ube3A maternal-deficient mice. *Neurobiology of Disease, 9,* 149–159.

Moore, D., Oates, J., Hobson, R., & Goodwin, J. (2002). Cognitive and social factors in the development of infants with Down syndrome. *Down Syndrome Research and Practice, 8,* 43–52.

Mostofsky, S. H., Mazzocco, M. M., Aakalu, G., Warsofsky, I. S., Denckla, M. B., & Reiss, A. L. (1998). Decreased cerebellar posterior vermis size in fragile X syndrome: A correlation with neurocognitive performance. *Neurology, 50,* 121–130.

Niccols, A., Milligan, K., Chisholm, V., & Atkinson, L. (in press). Maternal sensitivity and aggression in young children with Down syndrome. *Brain and Cognition, special issue on New Directions in the Study of Aggression.*

Niklasson, L., Rasmussen, P., Oskarsdottir, S., & Gillberg, C. (2002). Chromosome 22q11 deletion syndrome (CATCH 22): Neuropsychiatric and neuropsychological aspects. *Developmental Medicine and Child Neurology, 44,* 44–50.

Oliver, C., Horsler, K., Berg, K., Bellamy, G., Dick, K., & Griffiths, E. (2007). Genomic imprinting and the expression of affect in Angelman syndrome: What's in the smile? *Journal of Child Psychology and Psychiatry, 48,* 571–579.

Papolos, D. F., Faedda, G. L., Veit, S., Goldberg, R., Morrow, V., Kucherlapati, R., et al. (1996). Bipolar spectrum disorders in patients diagnosed with velo-cardio-facial syndrome: Does a hemizygous deletion of chromosome 22q11 result in bipolar affective disorder? *American Journal of Psychiatry, 153,* 1541–1547.

Partanen, J., Soininen, H., Kononen, M., Kilpelainen, R., Helkala, E. L., & Riekkinen, P. (1996). EEG reactivity correlates with neuropsychological test scores in Down's syndrome. *Acta Neurologica Scandinavica, 94,* 242–246.

Pennington, B. F., & Bennetto, L. (1998). A Neuropsychology of mental retardation. In J. Burack, R. Hodapp, & E. Zigler (Eds.), *Handbook of mental retardation and development* (pp. 80–114). New York: Cambridge University Press.

Petersen, M. B., Brodum-Nielsen, K., Hansen, L. K., & Wulff, K. (1995). Clinical, cytogenetic, and molecular diagnosis of Angelman syndrome: Estimated prevalence rate in a Danish county. *American Journal of Medical Genetics, 60,* 261–262.

Porter, M., Coltheart, M., & Langdon, R. (2007). The neuropsychological basis of hypersociability in Williams and Down syndrome. *Neuropsychologia, 45,* 2839–2849.

Reddy, L. A., & Pfeiffer, S. I. (2007). Behavioral and emotional symptoms of children and adolescents with Prader-Willi syndrome. *Journal of Autism and Developmental Disorders, 37,* 830–839.

Reeves, R. H. (2006). Down syndrome mouse models are looking up. *Trends in Molecular Medicine, 12,* 237–240.

Reiss, A. L., & Dant, C. C. (2003). The behavioral neurogenetics of fragile X syndrome: Analyzing gene-brain-behavior relationships in child developmental psychopathologies. *Development and Psychopathology, 15,* 927–968.

Reiss, A. L., Eckert, M. A., Rose, R. E., Karchemskiy, A., Kesler, S., Chang, M., et al. (2004). An experiment of nature: Brain anatomy parallels cognition and behaviour in Williams syndrome. *Journal of Neuroscience, 24,* 5009–5015.

Reiss, A. L., Freund, L. S., Baumgardner, T. L., Abrams, M. T., & Denckla, M. B. (1995). Contribution of the FMR1 gene mutation to human intellectual dysfunction. *Natural Genetics, 11,* 331–334.

Reiss, A. L., Lee, J., & Freund, L. (1994). Neuroanatomy of fragile X syndrome: The temporal lobe. *Neurology, 44,* 1317–1324.

Reiss, A. L., Patel, S., Kumar, A. J., & Freund, L. (1988). Preliminary communication: Neuroanatomical variations of the posterior fossa in men with the fragile X (Martin-Bell) syndrome. *American Journal of Medical Genetics, 31,* 407–414.

Rivera, S. M., Menon, V., White, C. D., Glaser, B., & Reiss, A. L. (2002). Functional brain activation during arithmetic processing in females with fragile X Syndrome is related to FMR1 protein expression. *Human Brain Mapping, 16*, 206–218.

Roberts, J. E., Boccia, M. L., Bailey, D. B., Jr., Hatton, D. D., & Skinner, M. L. (2001). Cardiovascular indices of physiological arousal in boys with fragile X syndrome. *Developmental Psychobiology, 39*, 107–123.

Roberts, J. E., Boccia, M. L., Hatton, D. D., Skinner, M. L., & Sideris, J. (2006). Temperament and vagal tone in boys with fragile X syndrome. *Journal of Developmental and Behavioral Pediatrics, 27*, 193–201.

Rosner, B. A., Hodapp, R. M., Fidler, D. J., Sagun, J. N., & Dykens, E. M. (2004). Social competence in persons with Prader-Willi, Williams and Down's syndrome. *Journal of Applied Research in Intellectual Disabilities, 17*, 209–217.

Schaer, M., & Eliez, S. (2007). From genes to brain: Understanding brain development in neurogenetic disorders using neuroimaging techniques. *Child and Adolescent Psychiatric Clinics of North America, 16*, 557–579.

Schmidt, L. A. (Guest Editor). (2003). Affective neuroscience. [Special Issue]. *Brain and Cognition, 52*(1), 1–133.

Schmidt, L. A. (Guest Editor). (2007). Social cognitive and affective neuroscience: Developmental and clinical perspectives. [Special Issue]. *Brain and Cognition, 65*(1), 1–142.

Schmidt, L. A., & Schulkin, J. (Eds.). (1999). *Extreme fear, shyness, and social phobia: Origins, biological mechanisms, and clinical outcomes* (pp. x–311) (Series in Affective Science). New York: Oxford University Press.

Schmidt, L. A., & Segalowitz, S. J. (Eds.). (2008). *Developmental psychophysiology: Theory, systems, and methods* (pp. xxii–462). New York: Cambridge University Press.

Schumacher, A. (2001). Mechanisms and brain specific consequences of genomic imprinting on Prader-Willi and Angelman syndrome. *Gene Function and Disease, 1*, 1–19.

Serafica, F. C., & Cicchetti, D. (1976). Down's syndrome children in a Strange Situation: Attachment and exploration behaviors. *Merrill-Palmer Quarterly, 22*, 137–150.

Shelley, B. P., & Robertson, M. M. (2005). The neuropsychiatry and multisystem features of the Smith-Magenis syndrome: A review. *The Journal of Neuropsychiatry and Clinical Neurosciences, 17*, 91–97.

Shenton, M. E., Dickey, C. C., Frumin, M., & McCarley, R. W. (2001). A review of MRI findings in schizophrenia. *Schizophrenia Research, 49*, 1–52.

Shprintzen, R. J. (2000). Velo-cardio-facial syndrome: A dinstinctive behavioral phenotype. *Mental Retardation and Developmental Disabilities Research Reviews, 6*(2), 142–147.

Sigman, M., Ruskin, E., Arbeile, S., Corona, R., Dissanayake, C., & Espinosa, M. (1999). Continuity and change in the social competence of children with autism, Down syndrome, and developmental delays. *Monographs of the Society for Research in Child Development, 64*(1), 1–114.

Sinson, J. C., & Wetherick, N. E. (1981). The behaviour of children with Down syndrome in normal playgroups. *Journal of Mental Deficiency Research, 25*(2), 113–120.

State, M. W., & Dykens, E. M. (2000). Genetics of childhood disorders: XV. Prader-Willi syndrome: Genes, brain, and behavior. *Journal of the American Academy of Child and Adolescent Psychiatry, 39*, 797–800.

Steffenburg, S., Gillberg, C. L., Steffenburg, U., Kyllerman, M. (1996). Autism in Angelman syndrome: A population based study. *Pediatric Neurology, 14*, 131–136.

Stein, D. J., Keating, J., Zar, H. J., & Hollander, E. (1994). A survey of the phenomenology and pharmacotherapy of compulsive and impulsive-aggressive symptoms in Prader-Willi syndrome. *The Journal of Neuropsychiatry and Clinical Neuroscience, 6*, 23–29.

Stromme, P., Bjornstad, P. G., & Ramstad, K. (2002). Prevalence estimation of Williams syndrome. *Journal of Child Neurology, 17*, 269–271.

Sullivan, K., & Tager-Flusberg, H. (1999). Second-order belief attribution in Williams syndrome: Intact or impaired? *American Journal of Mental Retardation, 104*, 523–532.

Summers, J. A., Allison, D., Lynch, P., & Sandler, J. A. (1995). Behavioural problems in Angelman syndrome. *Journal of Intellectual Disability Research, 39*, 97–106.

Summers, J. A., & Feldman, M. A. (1999). Distinctive pattern of behavioral functioning in Angelman syndrome. *American Journal of Mental Retardation, 104*, 376–384.

Swillen, A., Devriendt, K., Legius, E., Prinzie, P., Vogels, A., Ghesquiere, P., et al. (1999). The behavioural phenotype in velo-cardio-facial syndrome (VCFS): From infancy to adolescence. *Genetic Counseling, 10*, 79–88.

Teisl, J. T., Reiss, A. L., & Mazzocco, M. M. (1999). Maximizing the sensitivity of a screening questionnaire for determining fragile X at-risk status. *American Journal of Medical Genetics, 83*, 281–285.

Thompson, R. J., & Bolton, P. F. (2003). Case report: Angelman syndrome in an individual with a small SMC(15) and paternal uniparental disomy: A case report with reference to the assessment of cognitive functioning and autistic symptomatology. *Journal of Autism and Developmental Disorders, 33*, 171–176.

Thompson, R. A., Cicchetti, D., Lamb, M. E., & Malkin, C. (1985). Emotional responses of Down syndrome and normal infants in the Strange Situation. *Developmental Psychology, 21*, 828–841.

Thompson, P., Lee, A., Dutto, R., Geaga, J., Hayashi, K., Eckert, M., et al. (2005). Abnormal cortical complexity and thickness profiles mapped in Williams syndrome. *The Journal of Neuroscience, 25*, 4146–4158.

Toga, P., Thompson, P., & Sowell, E. (2006). Mapping brain maturation. *Trends in Neurosciences, 29*, 148–159.

Tomc, S. A., Williamson, N. K., & Pauli, R. M. (1990). Temperament in Williams syndrome. *American Journal of Medical Genetics, 36*, 345–352.

Turk, J., & Cornish, K. (1998). Face recognition and emotion perception in boys with fragile-X syndrome. *Journal of Intellectual Disability Research, 42*, 490–499.

Turner, G., Webb, T., Wake, S., & Robinson, H. (1996). Prevalence of fragile X syndrome. *American Journal of Medical Genetics, 64*, 196–197.

van Lieshout, C. F. M., De Meyer, R. E., Curfs, L. M. G., & Fryns, J. (1998). Family contexts, parental behaviour, and personality profiles of children and adolescents with Prader-Willi, Fragile-X, or Williams Syndrome. *Journal of Child Psychology and Psychiatry, 39*, 699–710.

Vataja, R., & Elomaa, E. (1998). Midline brain anomalies and schizophrenia in people with CATCH 22 syndrome. *The British Journal of Psychiatry, 172*, 518–520.

Veltman, M. W., Craig, E. E., & Bolton, P. F. (2005). Autism spectrum disorders in Prader-Willi and Angelman syndromes: A systematic review. *Psychiatric Genetics, 15*, 243–254.

Venkitaramanie, D. P., & Lomboroso, P. S. (2007). Molecular bases of genetic neuropsychiatric disorders. *Child and Adolescent Psychiatric Clinics of North America, 16*, 541–556.

Vogels, A., De Hert, M., Descheemaeker, M. J., Govers, V., Devriendt, K., Legius, E., et al. (2004). Psychotic disorders in Prader-Willi syndrome. *American Journal of Medical Genetics, 127*, 238–243.

Walz, N. C. (2007). Parent report of stereotyped behaviors, social interaction, and developmental disturbances in individuals with Angelman Syndrome. *Journal of Autism and Developmental Disorders, 37*, 940–947.

Walz, N. C., & Benson, B. A. (2002). Behavioral phenotypes in children with Down syndrome, Prader-Willi syndrome, or Angelman syndrome. *Journal of Developmental and Physical Disabilities, 14*, 307–321.

Wattendorf, D. J., & Muenke, M. (2005). Prader-Willi syndrome. *American Family Physician, 72*, 827–830.

Whittington, J. E., Holland, A. J., Webb, T., Butler, J., Clarke, D., & Boer, H. (2001). Population prevalence and estimated birth incidence and mortality rate for people with Prader-Willi syndrome in one UK Health Region. *Journal of Medical Genetics, 38*(11), 792–798.

Whittle, N., Sartori, S. B., Dierssen, M., Lubec, G., & Singewald, N. (2007). Fetal Down syndrome brains exhibit aberrant levels of neurotransmitters critical for normal brain development. *Pediatrics, 120*, 1465–1471.

Williams, C. A. (2005). Neurological aspects of the Angelman syndrome. *Brain & Development, 27*, 88–94.

Williams, C. A., Angelman, H., Clayton-Smith, J., Driscoll, D. J., Hendrickson, J. E., Knoll, J. H., et al. (1995). Angelman syndrome: consensus for diagnostic criteria. *American Journal of Medical Genetics, 56*, 237–238.

Williams, C. A., Beaudet, A. L., Clayton-Smith, J., Knoll, J. H., Kyllerman, M., Laan, L., et al. (2006). Angelman syndrome 2005: Updated consensus for diagnostic criteria. *American Journal of Medical Genetics, 140*, 413–418.

Williams, K. R., Wishart, J. G., Pitcairn, T. K., & Willis, D. S. (2005). Emotion recognition by children with Down syndrome: Investigation of specific impairments and error patterns. *American Journal on Mental Retardation, 110*(5), 378–392.

Wisbeck, J. M., Huffman, L. C., Freund, L., Gunnar, M. R., Davis, E. P., & Reiss, A. L. (2000). Cortisol and social stressors in children with fragile X: A pilot study. *Journal of Developmental and Behavioral Pediatrics, 21*, 278–282.

Wishart, J. G., & Pitcairn, T. K. (2000). Recognition of identity and expression in faces by children with Down syndrome. *American Journal on Mental Retardation, 105*, 466–479.

Woodlin, M., Wang, P., Aleman, D., McDonald-McGinn, D., Zackai, E., & Moss, E. (2001). Neuropsychological profile of children and adolescents with the 22q11.2 microdeletion. *Genetics in Medicine, 3*, 34–39.

Yamada, K., Matsuzawa, H., Uchiyama, M., Kwee, I. L., & Nakada, T. (2006). Brain developmental abnormalities in Prader-Willi syndrome detected by diffusion tensor imaging. *Pediatrics, 118*, e442–e448.

The Assessment and Presentation of Autism Spectrum Disorder and Associated Characteristics in Individuals with Severe Intellectual Disability and Genetic Syndromes

Joanna Moss, Patricia Howlin, *and* Chris Oliver

Abstract

This chapter considers the prevalence and nature of Autism Spectrum Disorders (ASD) and associated symptomatology in the intellectual disability population, with particular focus on three genetically determined syndromes—Fragile X syndrome, Tuberous Sclerosis Complex, and Rett syndrome—that have received particular attention with respect to their association with ASD. It then considers the importance of accurate assessment and diagnosis of ASD in individuals with genetically determined syndromes. It describes the methods and tools available for assessing ASD in individuals with intellectual disability, and explores the appropriateness of these assessments for identifying ASD in individuals with genetically determined syndromes associated with intellectual disability.

Keywords: Autism Spectrum Disorders, genetic syndromes, behavioural phenotypes, developmental disability, intellectual disability

Autism Spectrum Disorders (ASDs[1]) are classified by the *Diagnostic and Statistical Manual of Mental Disorders, 4th Edition, Text Revision* (DSM-IV-TR; American Psychiatric Association [APA], 2000) and International Classification of Disease (ICD-10; World Health Organization [WHO], 1992) as Pervasive Developmental Disorders (PDD) characterized by the presence of three core features: qualitative impairments in communication and social interaction, the presence of repetitive behavior, and restricted interests. Autism Spectrum Disorders occur in up to 1% of children in the general population (Baird et al., 2006), and in up to 40% of individuals with severe to profound levels of intellectual disability (La Malfa, Lassi, Bertelli, Salvini, & Placidi, 2004).

Advances in the identification of genetic abnormalities have promoted research into the association between ASDs/ASD characteristics and specific genetic abnormalities that are associated with intellectual disability.[2] The presence of ASD or autistic-like characteristics has been reported in a growing list of genetically determined syndromes including Tuberous Sclerosis Complex (TSC), Fragile X syndrome (FXS), Down syndrome (DS), Angelman syndrome (AS), Coffin-Lowry syndrome, Cohen syndrome, Rett syndrome (RS), Cornelia de Lange syndrome (CdLS), and Williams syndrome (WS) (see Fombonne, 1999; Gillberg & Coleman, 2000, for reviews). The study of ASD in these and other genetic syndromes has stimulated interest in a number of different areas.

The apparent association between genetically determined syndromes and ASD symptomatology clearly has important implications. At the level of etiology it has been suggested that the study of genetic syndromes may be influential in identifying and understanding genetic and neural pathways underlying ASD (Abrahams & Gerschwind, 2008; Laumonnier et al., 2004; Persico & Bourgeron, 2006). Alternatively, Skuse (2007) suggests that the association between ASD and genetic syndromes is unlikely to provide us with the answer to the question of etiological pathways underlying ASD. Skuse argues that the associated intellectual disability in these syndrome groups results in a diminished capacity for cognitive compensation of autistic traits, and in this way acts as a risk marker for these characteristics and impairments to be revealed in susceptible individuals. With regard to phenomenology of ASD in individuals with genetic syndromes, atypical or unusual profiles of ASD symptomatology have now been identified in a number of genetic syndromes including Rett, Fragile X, and Cornelia de Lange syndromes (see Cornish, Turk, & Hagerman, 2008; Moss, Oliver, Wilkie, Berg, Kaur, & Cornish, 2008; Mount, Charman, Hastings, Reilly, & Cass, 2003; Mount, Hastings, Reilly, Cass, & Charman, 2003), leading to considerable debate regarding the boundaries of the autism spectrum and the strength of association between ASD and genetically determined syndromes. This more fine-grained approach to ASD symptomatology has stimulated discussion about the suitable methods for identification and assessment of ASD characteristics in individuals with genetic syndromes. Greater awareness and understanding of these conceptual and methodological issues is important to ensure that assessment of ASD in genetic syndromes associated with intellectual disability in both research and clinical settings is conducted carefully and accurately. These areas of debate will be considered in detail throughout this chapter.

In the first section of this chapter, we will consider the prevalence and nature of ASD and associated symptomatology in the intellectual disability population, with particular focus on three genetically determined syndromes—FXS, TSC, and RS—which have received particular attention with respect to their association with ASD. Other syndrome groups that have illustrated particular issues relevant to the syndrome–ASD association and the role of intellectual disability will also be discussed. These include AS, Down, CdLS, and CHARGE syndromes, and phenylketonuria (PKU).[3] In this section, the focus of discussion will be on the role of intellectual disability in understanding the prevalence of ASD in these syndrome groups and the need to carefully consider the presence of atypicalities in the profile of ASD in these populations. In the second section of this chapter, we consider the importance of accurate assessment and diagnosis of ASD in individuals with genetically determined syndromes. We will describe the methods and tools available for assessing ASD in individuals with intellectual disability, and we will critically explore the appropriateness of these assessments for identifying ASD in individuals with genetically determined syndromes associated with intellectual disability.

Prevalence of Autism Spectrum Disorder and Associated Characteristics in Individuals with Intellectual Disability and Genetic Syndromes

Prevalence of Autism Spectrum Disorder in Individuals with Intellectual Disability

Prevalence rates of ASD in individuals with intellectual disability range from 14% to 40% (Deb & Prasad, 1994; La Malfa et al., 2004; Nordin & Gillberg, 1996; Rumeau-Roquette, Grandjean, Cans, Du Mazaubrun, & Verrier, 1997). Specifically, La Malfa et al. (2004) reported a prevalence rate of 60% in individuals with profound intellectual disability and 37%, 24%, and 8% in those with severe, moderate, and mild intellectual disability, respectively. Other studies that have addressed the association from the alternative perspective: That is, the prevalence of intellectual disability in individuals with ASD are consistent with findings in the intellectual disability population. Fombonne (2005) estimated that approximately 30% of individuals with ASD scored in the mild to moderate range and 40% in the severe to profound range.

It is clear that ASD is more prevalent in individuals with intellectual disability, and a strong, positive correlation between severity of ASD and severity of intellectual disability is well established. This association has raised questions regarding the role of intellectual disability in the development or presentation of ASD. The strength of this association has led some researchers to believe that there may be shared genetic and neurobiological pathways leading to the presentation of ASD and intellectual disability (Abrahams & Gerschwind, 2008; Laumonnier et al., 2004). However, in contrast to this, Skuse (2007) suggests that the presence of intellectual disability simply increases the risk that ASD or autistic characteristics will be revealed. Skuse's argument is based around the suggestion that, whereas predisposition to autistic features may be common and independently heritable, level of cognitive ability determines whether or not these characteristics manifest themselves. In this way, lower general intelligence reduces the possibility for cognitive compensation for independently determined ASD traits. Skuse argues that intellectual ability is one of many factors that may influence the expression or manifestation of autistic traits.

Autism Spectrum Disorder in Individuals with Genetic Syndromes Associated with Intellectual Disability

Rapid advances in technologies for the identification of genetic disorders over the last decade have had a significant impact on research into specific genetic syndromes. In particular, genetically linked disorders associated with intellectual disability have received increased attention within the literature. Three syndrome groups that have received a raised profile with regard to their association with ASD are FXS and RS, and TSC (Table 18.1). In particular, the study of ASD in these three syndrome groups has highlighted that, although individuals with a given genetic syndrome may score above diagnostic/clinical cut-off scores on diagnostic assessments for ASD, the specific profile of behaviors, the quality and nature of impairments, and the trajectory of development of these characteristics may not be typical of idiopathic ASD. Rather, a unique, syndrome-specific "signature" of ASD characteristics and impairments may better describe the phenomenology identified in some of these syndrome groups (Cornish et al., 2008). These findings highlight the need for conducting fine-grained investigation of ASD phenomenology in genetic syndrome groups that goes beyond basic clinical diagnostic levels.

Autism Spectrum Disorder in Fragile X Syndrome

Reported prevalence rates of ASD in males with FXS vary widely (see Table 18.1), although estimates from studies conducted since 2001 are more consistent, ranging from 21% to 50% (Bailey et al., 2001; Cohen et al., 1991; Demark, Feldman, & Holden, 2003; Hatton et al., 2006; Kau et al., 2004; Sabaratnam, Turk, & Vroegop, 2003; Turk & Graham, 1997). The variability in prevalence estimates among the earlier studies is likely to be accounted for by the different methodologies, and diagnostic and participant inclusion criteria employed across studies. Recent studies report a strong correlation between degree of disability and

Table 18.1 Reported prevalence estimates of Autism Spectrum Disorder in genetic syndromes

Syndrome	Range of prevalence estimates	Dates of prevalence studies	Notes
FXS	0–60%[1]	1986–2006	Prevalence rate for ASD reported in females are from 1% to 6%[2]
RS	25%–40%[3]	1987–2003	Prevalence reported to be 97% in preserved speech variant of the syndrome[4]
TSC	5%–89%[5]	1994–2006	Suggested association between ASD in TSC and temporal lobe tubers, although evidence is not consistent[6]
AS	50%–81%[7]	2004	Caution required, given associated degree of intellectual ability in this syndrome
CdLS	50%–67%[8]	1999–2008	
DS	5%–39%[9]	1986–2007	
PKU	5%–20%[10]	1986–2003	ASD only identified in late-diagnosis cases or cases in which dietary control is poor[11]
CHARGE syndrome	15%–50%[12]	2005–2006	

[1] Brown et al., 1986; Bailey et al., 2001; Cohen et al.,1991; Demark et al., 2003; Hagerman et al., 1986; Hatton et al., 2006; Kau et al., 2004; Levitas et al., 1983; Reiss & Freund, 1990; Sabaratnam et al., 2003; Turk & Graham, 1997

[2] Mazzocco et al., 1997; Hatton et al., 2006

[3] Mount et al., 2003a; Naidu et al., 1990; Sandberg et al., 2000; Witt-Engerstrom & Gillberg, 1987

[4] Zappella, et al., 1998

[5] Baker et al., 1998; Bolton & Griffiths, 1997; Bolton et al., 2002; Gillberg et al., 1994; Gutierrez et al., 1998; Humphrey et al., 2006; Hunt & Shepherd, 1993; Jambaque et al., 1991; Park & Bolton, 2001; Smalley et al., 1992; Williamson & Bolton, 1995; Webb et al., 1996

[6] Asano et al., 2001; Bolton et al., 2002

[7] Trillingsgaard & Ostergaard, 2004; Peters et al., 2004

[8] Oliver et al., 2008; Basile et al., 2007; Berney, et al., 1999; Bhyuian et al., 2006, Moss et al., 2008

[9] Capone et al., 2005; Gillberg et al., 1986; Ghaziuddin et al., 1992; Kent et al.,1999; Lowenthal et al., 2007; Lund, 1988; Starr et al., 2005; Turk & Graham, 1997

[10] Baieli et al., 2003; Reiss et al., 1986

[11] Baieli et al., 2003

[12] Hartshorne et al., 2005; Johansson et al., 2006; Smith, et al., 2005.

presence of ASD characteristics in FXS (Demark et al., 2003; Kaufmann et al., 2004; Loesch et al., 2007), although ASD has also been identified in individuals with the premutation FXS, who have only mild cognitive impairments or IQ in the normal range (Hagerman, Ono, & Hagerman, 2005).

Severe autism (as measured by the Childhood Autism Rating Scales, CARS; Schopler, Reichller, & Renner, 1988) is relatively rare in FXS (Bailey, Hatton, Skinner, & Mesibov, 2001; Demark et al., 2003) and a milder presentation is more characteristic. However, fine-grained analysis of ASD characteristics has identified specific areas of behavior that may be qualitatively different from those in idiopathic autism. Social anxiety, extreme shyness, and gaze avoidance are highly characteristic of FXS, alongside seemingly preserved emotion sensitivity and willingness to interact (Cornish, Turk, & Levitas, 2007; Hall, de Benardis, & Reiss, 2006; Lesniak-Karpiak, Mazzocco, & Ross, 2003; Roberts, Weisenfeld, Hatton, Heath, & Kaufmann, 2007; Turk & Cornish, 1998). Furthermore, the gaze avoidance and perseverative speech described in FXS are reported to be unrelated to verbal ability or age (in contrast to the autism population), and are more marked than in autism or "nonspecific" intellectual disability (Sudhalter, Cohen, Silverman, & Wolfschein, 1990). The developmental trajectory of ASD symptomatology in FXS is also reported to differ from idiopathic autism. According to some studies, the rate of autism and social avoidance behaviors increases with age in males with full mutation FXS (Hatton et al., 2006; Roberts et al., 2007), whereas improvements in core symptomatology with age are typically identified in individuals with idiopathic ASD (Charman et al., 2005; Moss, Magiati, Charman, & Howlin, 2008).

A similar pattern of findings has emerged with regard to the identification of sociocognitive characteristics, including theory of mind (ToM). Although initial studies of individuals with FXS and ASD described deficits in ToM (Cornish et al., 2008), subsequent research has showed that a general information processing and working memory deficit may account for poor performance in this area rather than a specific ToM deficit (Grant, Apperly, & Oliver, 2007). These findings suggest that the subtle differences between ASD and FXS at the level of behavior may also be reflected at the level of social-cognition.

Autism Spectrum Disorder in Rett Syndrome

Prevalence figures for ASD reported in RS are described in Table 18.1. The overlap between RS and ASD has previously been considered to be so robust that the syndrome is currently classified as a pervasive developmental disorder (PDD) alongside autism in both the DSM-IV-TR (APA, 2000) and ICD-10 (WHO, 1992) classification systems. This inclusion within the PDD category is now considered by many to be inappropriate (Tsai, 1992), largely due to the fact that there are distinct differences in phenomenology between ASD and RS. For example, many (although not all) individuals with RS develop simple speech prior to regression. Despite the marked deterioration in social skills, eye contact is often maintained, and social impairments and autistic characteristics also tend to improve with age after the initial regression (Nomura & Segawa, 2005). Furthermore, the characteristic repetitive hand movements in RS are very different in nature to those observed in individuals with ASD (Howlin, 2002). Even when diagnostic criteria for autism are met, individuals with RS demonstrate an atypical profile of phenomenology, with fewer core features (Mount, Hastings et al., 2003).

Given the difficulties in identifying ASD in individuals with severe intellectual disability, the severity of intellectual disability typically found in RS is likely to further complicate the understanding of its association with ASD. However, studies have identified that the severe degree of intellectual ability cannot solely account for the heightened prevalence of ASD in RS (Mount, Charman et al., 2003, Zappella, Gillberg, & Ehlers, 1998; Zappella, Meloni, Longo, Hayek, & Renieri, 2001).

Autism Spectrum Disorder in Tuberous Sclerosis Complex

Reported prevalence rates of ASD in TSC are described in Table 18.1. Few studies have considered the profile of ASD phenomenology in TSC in detail. Smalley et al. (1992) reported that individuals with TSC had somewhat higher (although nonsignificant) scores than individuals with autism on the social and communication domains of the Autism Diagnostic Interview-Revised (ADI-R; Rutter, LeCouteur, & Lord, 2003), and scored significantly lower on the repetitive behavior domain of this measure. Others have reported a global deficit in play skills in all children with TSC, regardless of ASD status (Jeste, Sahin, Bolton, Ploubidis, & Humphrey, 2008). The male-to-female ratio in TSC is also different to that reported in the ASD population (Smalley, 1998). Such findings suggest that ASD features in TSC may be atypical to those identified in individuals with idiopathic ASD.

Although recent studies have identified a greater risk of autism and ASD with increased degree of disability in TSC (de Vries, Hunt, & Bolton, 2007; Jeste et al., 2008; Wong, 2006), others have suggested that the ASD–TSC association may be independent of intellectual disability, with up to 25% of individuals who meet criteria for autism having an IQ of over 70 (Harrison & Bolton, 1997; Smalley, 1998). This is notably higher than the prevalence of ASD in the general population, suggesting that degree of disability cannot solely account for the raised prevalence of ASD in TSC. Further research is needed to further delineate the profile of ASD phenomenology in TSC. It remains important for any further studies of ASD in TSC to continue to consider what the role of intellectual disability might be in the ASD–TSC association.

In addition to the increasing interest in the association between ASD and FXS, RS, or TSC, there are several other syndrome groups in which identification of ASD characteristics has important clinical and research issues. These are principally AS, Down, CdLS, and CHARGE syndromes, and PKU.

Autism Spectrum Disorder in Angelman Syndrome

Reported prevalence rates of ASD in AS are described in Table 18.1. Peters, Beaudit, Madduri, and Bacino (2004) reported that individuals with AS and autism are significantly more intellectually impaired than are individuals with AS who do not meet criteria for autism. Bonati et al. (2007) also reported that individuals with AS with better expressive language skills did not meet ASD or autism criteria on the Autism Diagnostic Observation Schedule (ADOS; Lord, Rutter, DiLavore, & Risi, 2000) or ADI-R (Rutter, LeCouteur, & Lord, 2003). It is therefore possible that the identification of ASD in AS may be influenced by the profound disability associated with the syndrome and the overlap in phenomenology that profound disability has with ASD. In line with this, Trillingsgaard and Østergaard (2004) found that individuals with AS and autism were significantly less impaired than were individuals with idiopathic autism on items such as social smile, facial expression directed to others, shared enjoyment in interaction, and response to name, and in unusual interests or repetitive behavior, all of which are less reliant on developmental level. These findings suggest that degree of disability in AS may have a significant role to play in the association with ASD, and it is less likely to represent a syndrome-specific association between AS and ASD. Furthermore, syndrome-specific characteristics of AS, such as hand flapping, excessive sociability, excessive motivation for eye contact, and lack of stranger discrimination, may be misrepresented in any autism-specific assessment as inappropriate social behavior. Thus, the core features of the syndrome itself may be interpreted as indicators of ASD even though the etiology of such behaviors may differ. Caution should therefore be taken when assessing and diagnosing ASD in this syndrome group.

With regard to the profile of ASD behaviors in AS, Walz and Benson (2002) and Walz (2007) found that some of the characteristic features of ASD, such as finger/hand flicking, object spinning, lining up objects, looking through people, and lack of affection, were rarely reported in AS. Taken together, these studies suggest that even when individuals with AS meet diagnostic criteria for ASD, the profile of behaviors and the reasons for meeting criteria may be somewhat different to that of idiopathic ASD.

Autism Spectrum Disorder in Cornelia de Lange Syndrome

Cornelia de Lange syndrome is caused by a deletion in *NIPBL* on chromosome 5 (locus 5p13) in 20%–50% of cases (Gillis et al., 2004; Krantz et al., 2004; Miyake et al., 2005; Tonkin, Wang, Lisgo, Bamshad, & Strachan, 2004). Additional mutations on *SMC3*, on chromosome 10 (Deardorff et al., 2007) and on the X-linked *SMC1* (Musio et al., 2006) are reported to account for 5% of cases. Cornelia de Lange syndrome is characterized by developmental delay, delayed growth, distinctive facial features, and limb abnormalities (Jackson, Kline, Barr, & Koch, 1993).

Prevalence rates of autism in CdLS are reported in Table 18.1, and they range from 50% to 67%. Using the CARS (Schopler et al., 1988), Oliver, Arron, Sloneem, and Hall (2008) reported that 32.1% of 54 individuals with CdLS scored within the "severe autism" category of the CARS, compared to only 7.1% of a matched control group of individuals with intellectual disability, suggesting that the relationship between CdLS and ASD is not solely accounted for by associated degree of disability. Oliver et al. (2005) also report that those with CdLS scored significantly higher on the Autism Screening Questionnaire (Berument, Rutter, Lord, Pickles, & Bailey, 1999) did than individuals with Cri du Chat and Prader-Willi syndromes, with a mean score comparable to that of a group with FXS.

Fine-grained investigation has indicated that the presentation of the triad of impairments in CdLS may not be typical of that observed in idiopathic ASD. Specifically, social impairment in CdLS may be characterized by selective mutism, extreme shyness, and social anxiety (Goodban, 1993; Collis, Oliver, & Moss, 2006; Moss, Oliver, Wilkie, Berg, Kaur, & Cornish, 2008; Richards, Moss, O'Farrell, Kaur, & Oliver, 2009). Oliver et al. (2006) also described a high prevalence of socially avoidant behaviors such as "wriggling out of physical contact" and "attempting to move away during an interaction" in 14 out of 16 individuals with CdLS. These studies indicate that social anxiety and social avoidance may be characteristic of individuals with CdLS, and this presentation appears similar to the social anxiety and shyness that is reported in individuals with FXS (see Cornish et al., 2008). Further detailed study of early social interaction skills has demonstrated that poor social relatedness may be highly characteristic of CdLS. Poor eye contact in the first year of life has been found to be predictive of social relatedness in later years (Sarimski, 2007). With regard to repetitive behaviors, individuals with CdLS demonstrate a heightened prevalence of compulsive behaviors relative to matched controls with nonspecific intellectual disability (Hyman, Oliver, & Hall, 2002). Further detailed investigation has revealed that lining up and tidying up behaviors appear to show high levels of specificity in CdLS when compared to six other genetic syndrome groups and individuals with intellectual disability of heterogeneous cause (Moss et al., 2009). As with other areas of the triad of impairments in CdLS, and indeed other genetic syndrome groups, investigation of repetitive behaviors at the subscale level masks these highly specific patterns of behavior, highlighting the need for fine-grained study of behavioral phenomenology. As with FXS, changing profiles of ASD symptom severity and social anxiety in CdLS have been identified as individuals move into late adolescence and adulthood (Collis et al., 2006).

In summary, although prevalence rates of CdLS are reported to be high, a potentially atypical profile of ASD characteristics and impairments has been identified in CdLS, with social anxiety and selective mutism occurring at unusually high rates, and the presence of highly specific repetitive behaviors.

Autism Spectrum Disorder in Down Syndrome

Prevalence rates of ASD in DS are described in Table 18.1. Although not necessarily directly indicative of an association with ASD, difficulties in ToM and emotion perception have also been reported in some children with DS (Barisnikov, Hippolyte, & van der Linden, 2008; Wishart, 2007; Wishart, Cebula, Willis, & Pitcairn, 2007; Zelazo, Burack, Benedetto, & Frye, 1996). According to Wishart (2007), some of these difficulties cannot be solely accounted for by degree of disability. Interestingly, higher rates of impaired social skills have been reported in family members of individuals with DS and ASD, in comparison to individuals with DS without ASD (Lowenthal, Paula, Schwartzman, Brunoni, & Mercadante, 2007). Individuals with DS and ASD are reported to have a greater degree of intellectual disability and higher rates of stereotyped behaviors, hyperactivity, and inappropriate speech, compared to individuals with DS but without ASD (Capone, Grados, Kaufmann, Bernad-Ripoll, & Jewell, 2005). It is not clear how much the increased severity of intellectual disability in this subgroup explains the heightened prevalence of ASD symptomatology.

Autism Spectrum Disorder in Phenylketonuria

Phenylketonuria is an inherited defect in protein metabolism, resulting in an inability to break down the amino acid phenylalanine. Phenylketonuria occurs in approximately 1 in 10,000 live births (Scriver, Eisensmith, Woo, & Kaufmann, 1994). With early diagnosis and a controlled diet, the effects of PKU are minimal. However, late diagnosis and high levels of protein in the diet can produce toxic levels of phenylalanine hydroxylase (PAH), resulting in intellectual disability, seizures, and physical abnormalities. Degree of intellectual disability in PKU can range from mild to severe, particularly in late-diagnosis cases (although this is not inevitable), but many individuals with PKU have an IQ within the normal range (Yalaz, Vanli, Yilmaz, Tokatli, & Anlar, 2006).

With advances in pre- and postnatal screening and early intervention, the effects of PKU, at least in developed countries, have become far less prevalent. As a result, the association between ASD and PKU is difficult to determine, but it is now currently thought that ASD is largely only identified in those individuals with late PKU diagnosis and a poorly controlled diet (Baieli, Pavone, Meli, Fiumara, & Coleman, 2003). This contrasts with the high rates of association reported in earlier studies conducted prior to the introduction of improved screening methods (Reiss, Feinstein, & Rosenbaum, 1986). Overlap in the cognitive profiles of individuals with autism (notably good performance on Block Design and comparatively low scores on Comprehension) and poorly controlled PKU, matched for age and IQ, have been reported (Dennis et al., 1999). Individuals with better-controlled PKU did not demonstrate this profile. The changes in PKU since the introduction of pre- and postnatal screening and early intervention present a natural test of the effects of PAH on cognitive development and more importantly, the development of ASD characteristics.

Autism Spectrum Disorder in CHARGE Syndrome

The prevalence rate of ASD in CHARGE syndrome is described in Table 18.1. Information is limited regarding the role of intellectual disability and sensory deficits in the development of ASD in the syndrome. Two case studies described by Smith, Nichols, Issekutz, and Blake (2005) suggest that ASD is more likely to occur in nonverbal individuals with severe to profound intellectual disability, which might account for their very impaired social skills. However, Hartshorne, Grialou, and Parker (2005) reported that the presence of ASD symptomatology in CHARGE could not be wholly accounted for by the visual and hearing impairments typically associated with the syndrome. Further research is needed to identify the role that the associated intellectual disability and sensory impairments may have on the manifestation of ASD characteristics in this group.

Summary

The number of genetic syndromes reported to show an association with ASD is ever growing. The importance of employing a detailed and fine-grained assessment of ASD characteristics in genetic syndromes is well illustrated in the examples of FXS, CdLS, and RS. Initial descriptions at a superficial behavioral level suggested a significant, even causal, relationship with ASD. However, further detailed investigation of the phenomenology of ASD characteristics within these groups revealed very different developmental, behavioral, and cognitive profiles to those found in individuals with idiopathic ASD. It may be helpful to consider these differences as unique and syndrome-specific "signatures" of ASD phenomenology. Further research to consider other syndrome-specific signatures of ASD will be important in furthering our conceptual understanding of the triad of impairments. The fact that the phenomenology of ASD appears to differ across genetic syndromes has particular implications for the debate concerning the boundaries of the autism spectrum. The main question that is raised from this

issue is: Where does the ever-growing number of syndrome groups identified as showing apparently unusual or atypical profiles of ASD sit, conceptually, within the spectrum of autism characteristics?

The complex and often unusual behavioral and cognitive patterns that are characteristic of many genetic syndromes may result in individuals obtaining scores above the autism cut-off on standard autism-specific assessments even though the underlying neurobiological or cognitive pathways may be different from idiopathic ASD. For example, eye gaze avoidance in FXS and ASD was initially considered to be a shared characteristic in both populations. It is now suggested that, in FXS, eye gaze avoidance occurs in response to hypersensitivity to sensory stimuli, hyperarousal, and social anxiety, whereas in ASD the same behavior is thought to result from a more general impairment of social interaction (Cornish et al., 2007, 2008; Hall et al., 2006). Additionally, syndrome-specific characteristics, such as hand flapping or inappropriate sociability in AS, can easily be misidentified in autism-specific assessments. It is important to avoid accepting superficial similarities between syndrome groups and ASD and to look beyond the diagnostic and clinical cut-off scores that are so often assumed to be definitive.

The study of ASD in genetic syndromes also raises debate regarding the role of intellectual disability in the presentation of ASD characteristics. According to Skuse (2007), associated intellectual disability in these syndrome groups results in diminished capacity for cognitive compensation of autistic traits, and in this way acts as a risk marker for these characteristics and impairments to be revealed in susceptible individuals. It is clear from our review of RS and CdLS that degree of disability cannot always account fully for the presentation of ASD characteristics. However, there is certainly a need to be extremely cautious when assessing ASD in syndrome groups associated with severe and profound intellectual disability. In AS, autism-specific assessments and indeed diagnostic criteria may not be sensitive enough to distinguish between ASD-related characteristics and the effects of the profound intellectual disability.

Identification and Assessment of Autism Spectrum Disorder and Associated Characteristics in Individuals with Intellectual Disability and Genetic Syndromes

Distinguishing between autism spectrum phenomenology and the impairments and behaviors associated with intellectual disability (particularly severe intellectual disability) becomes particularly difficult in individuals with genetic syndromes associated with intellectual disability. These individuals often evidence a range of complex cognitive, communicative, behavioral, emotional, and physical difficulties that may mask or emulate aspects of ASD, or give rise to an atypical presentation of the triad of impairments. From a pragmatic perspective, the etiology of the behavior presentation is, arguably, unimportant. Rather, it is the ability to accurately assess and identify these shared characteristics and impairments in individuals with intellectual disability that is essential (Moss, Oliver, Wilkie, Berg, Kaur, & Cornish et al., 2008). Nevertheless, clinical experience and case studies of individuals with genetic syndromes suggest that often differential diagnoses and recognition of ASD symptomatology is not considered when in fact, it would be beneficial to do so. There is sometimes a tendency to attribute *all* the behaviors and difficulties shown by an individual directly to the specific genetic disorder, rather than considering the possibility of other additional or differential diagnoses. "Diagnostic overshadowing" (Dykens, 2007; Reiss, Levitan, & Szyszko, 1982) of this kind can be a particular problem in the case of rare genetic syndromes, with the result that other causes and, more importantly, possible interventions, may not be considered by parents or professionals. Case studies reported by Howlin, Wing, and Gould (1995) and Moss and Howlin (2009) illustrate how failure to identify ASD characteristics or appropriate recognition of ASD symptomatology in individuals with genetic syndromes can have a significant impact on the individual's behavioral difficulties, mood, and quality of life (see Box 18.1 for example case studies). As a point of caution, although the

---

Box 18.1   Case study examples illustrating the implications of recognizing ASD in genetic syndromes[*]

Jeremy was an 18-year-old with Cornelia de Lange syndrome (CdLS). In his teens, he became progressively more withdrawn and uncommunicative, and was diagnosed as being selectively mute. However, his eye contact had always been poor, and since childhood he had a keen preference for routine and engaged in various repetitive and stereotyped behaviors. The possibility of ASD was not considered until he was 17 years old, despite his parents' previous requests for assessment. The move to college, where the emphasis was on flexibility and student choice rather than the structure and routine he needed, led to significant deterioration in his mood and behavior. The college was unwilling to modify its program, insisting that Jeremy needed to "learn to be more flexible and cope with the changes." Jeremy became increasingly tearful and withdrawn, stopped taking part in his usual daily activities, and refused to go to classes. Although he has since received a formal diagnosis of ASD, Jeremy still remains at home, with no educational provision. His outcome contrasts markedly with that of David, another 18-year-old with CdLS for whom, following a period of regression in his late teens, the recognition that he showed many characteristics of ASD led to his being transferred to specialist autism provision, resulting in significant improvements in his mood and behavior.

Ivan was an 11-year-old boy with Leber's congenital amaurosis, attending a school for visually impaired children. Although he had some very specific areas of skill, especially in music, he showed no interest in other children, had very stereotyped and repetitive language, and very fixed routines. The headmaster did not agree with the possibility that he might have ASD and therefore did not support his parents' request for transfer to a specialist ASD unit. Ivan became increasingly isolated, self-injurious behaviors increased, and his parents found it more and more difficult to cope. He eventually required placement in a residential school.

Jake was an 8-year-old boy with Down syndrome; he showed a typical ASD profile of repetitive, noncommunicative speech, poor eye contact, limited interaction with other people, and a host of repetitive and restricted interests. Although his parents had become increasingly concerned about his lack of progress, school staff interpreted his behaviors as being "difficult" or "naughty" and again rejected the possibility of comorbid ASD. Over time, Jake's behavior became steadily more disruptive and aggressive; diagnostic assessment for ASD indicated that he met all the criteria for this disorder and transfer to a specialist autism unit was recommended.

---

[*] Please note that although each of the case studies reported here are all individual cases that have been observed/ assessed by the authors in clinical or research settings, all cases are reported using pseudonyms.
Case studies reprinted by permission from Moss & Howlin (2009).

impact of accurate ASD diagnosis in individuals with intellectual disability and genetic syndromes is clear from these case examples, it is also important not to be overinclusive of the term ASD (see Box 18.2 for example case study). Careful investigation in both clinical and research settings, taking into account the overlap in phenomenology of ASD, severe and profound intellectual disability, and syndrome-specific characteristics and impairments, is essential in ensuring that individuals receive appropriate support and education.

For example, the behavior management strategies, educational programming, and therapeutic interventions that are effective for individuals with autism and those without may be very different (Howlin, 2000; Jordan, 2001). Identification and recognition of ASD characteristics in individuals with intellectual disability and genetic syndromes may also have implications for the way in which challenging behavior may be perceived by professionals and parents. Thus, the reported "stubbornness" that is frequently identified by parents, teachers, and researchers as a personality trait of individuals with DS may be better understood in individuals with DS and ASD as a strong preference for routine. In other words, this is a *behavioral* challenge that can be managed with behavioral methods and strategies. Thus, the correct identification of ASD or, at the very least, recognition that the individual shares characteristics and behaviors with the ASD populations, can be important for parent and professional perceptions and attributions about behaviour, as well as for developing appropriate behavior management strategies and designing educational curricula (Howlin, 2000).

However, as noted above, the significant overlap between the phenomenology of ASD and the presentation of severe to profound intellectual disability gives rise to many difficulties. Both populations share, to some extent, delayed development in communication, presence of repetitive behaviours, and lack of imaginative play skills, in addition to impairments of social interaction. Stereotyped behaviors are reported in up to 67% of individuals with intellectual disability (Berkson & Davenport, 1962) and compulsive behavior has been reported to occur in up to 40% (Bodfish et al. 1995). As is the case for individuals with autism, a large proportion of individuals with intellectual disability fail to develop communication skills, and those who do are delayed in their development (Vig & Jedrysek, 1999). Development of nonverbal communication to accommodate this delay fails to be achieved in both populations (Lord & Pickles, 1996). It is because these areas of communication rely heavily on developmental level (Volkmar, Lord, Bailey, Schultz, & Klin, 2004) that these difficulties are not specific to individuals with autism. Thus, some individuals with intellectual disability may appear to fulfil criteria outlined in DSM-IV-TR (APA, 2000) and ICD-10 (WHO, 1992) for ASD, purely because they have not yet reached the developmental level required to acquire these behaviors. The current diagnostic criteria for autism do not take this developmental confound into account.

As is apparent from the discussion in the first section, it is important not to accept superficial similarities between the ASD triad of impairments and the problems in these domains that may be accounted for by other factors. Instead, it is imperative, for both theoretical and therapeutic reasons, to exam systematically where the similarities and differences lie.

Several subtle features may distinguish ASD symptomatology from deficits that arise purely because of severe intellectual disability. It has been suggested that some specific forms of nonverbal communication are relatively unaffected in individuals with intellectual disability. According to Lord and Paul (1997), individuals with intellectual disability show significantly more appropriate eye gaze and facial expression compared to individuals with ASD. Additionally, although both populations are characterized by delayed language development, Lord and Pickles (1996) report that children with ASD develop fewer words and are less likely to develop phrase speech than are individuals with intellectual disability without ASD. Jordan (2001) also suggests that impairments in communication in individuals with intellectual disability without ASD are likely to be caused primarily by difficulties in the acquisition of spoken language. Once effective, alternative means of communication are introduced, such as Makaton signing, objects of reference, or picture exchange, which individuals are often able to use for a number of functions. Thus, they have the motivation to communicate but not necessarily the means to do so. Conversely, individuals with ASD may not develop communication skills that can be generalized outside of specific teaching settings even when alternative modes of communication are introduced (Howlin, Gordon, Pasco, Wade, & Charman, 2007). Similarly, the marked discrepancy between expressive language level and communicative intent in verbal children with ASD suggests that communication impairments in individuals with ASD relate to underlying impairments in pragmatics and social-communication and a lack of motivation to communicate, rather than an inability to acquire communicative behaviors per se. This suggestion is supported by the fact that communication in individuals with autism is focused on the expression of demands and needs (protoimperatives) rather than the use of socially directed communication (protodeclaratives; Tager-Flusberg, 2000).

Assessment of ASD in Individuals with Intellectual Disability and Genetic Syndromes

Reliable and valid assessment of ASD is an ongoing challenge for clinicians and researchers. Alongside the diagnostic taxonomies, a variety of autism-specific assessment tools for screening and diagnosis of ASD have been developed. Each of these assessment tools is designed to be appropriate for individuals in different subgroups. The target age range, severity of ASD, and degree of disability is somewhat varied across these measures. Also, each assessment tool uses different methods of assessment including observation, interview, or informant ratings. Table 18.2 describes some of these assessment tools, their characteristics, psychometric properties, and whether they have been used to assess ASD in genetic syndromes. Note that this is not an exhaustive list of available assessments

but provides information about the most commonly employed measures. In this section, we will provide an overview of the methods and tools available for assessing ASD in individuals with intellectual disability, and we will critically explore the appropriateness of these assessments for identifying ASD in individuals with genetically determined syndromes associated with intellectual disability.

A number of the assessments described in Table 18.2 have been designed for individuals with intellectual disability of a particular level or for individuals of a particular age. For example, the Modified Checklist for Autism in Toddlers (M-CHAT; Robins, Fein, Barton, & Green, 2001); The Handicaps, Behaviour, and Skills Schedules (Wing, 1980); Social Responsiveness Scale (Constantino, 2002); and a range of other assessments are designed for use with individuals with mild intellectual disability or IQs within the normal range, and therefore are not suitable for assessing ASD in individuals with more severe intellectual disability. This presents a problem for the study of ASD in genetic syndromes. Heterogeneity of intellectual ability across and within genetic syndrome groups and the inclusion of broad age inclusion criteria in research studies means that it may be difficult to identify one single assessment of ASD that is suitable for assessing ASD across the whole range of ability and ages in a single population. Using ASD assessments that cover a broad range of ability and age would be most suitable for use in these groups.

Of the measures suitable for assessing ASD in both children *and* adults/adolescents with severe intellectual disability, the Scale for Pervasive Developmental Disorder in Mentally Retarded Persons (Kraijer, 1997) and the Autism Behavior Checklist (ABC; Krug, Arick, & Almond, 1980) may not have adequate psychometric properties. The PDD-MRS has been reported to have good discriminative validity; however, no reliability data have been reported on this measure (O'Brien, Pearson, Berney, & Barnard, 2001). The Gilliam Autism Rating Scale (GARS; Gilliam, 1995) was initially reported to have good psychometric properties (Gilliam, 1995); however, South et al. (2002) have suggested that the validity of this measure has been overestimated. South et al. (2002) found the GARS to misclassify 52% of their sample ($N = 119$) as not having ASD or having low likelihood of ASD. Similar findings regarding low sensitivity were reported by Lecavalier (2005) in addition to reporting lower levels of interrater reliability than had previously been reported in the manual. Overall, these findings suggest that

Table 18.2 Assessments of Autism Spectrum Disorder: Characteristics and psychometric properties*

Author	Measure	Format	Child	Adult/ Adolescent	SID	Time Taken	Reliability	Validity	Use in genetic syndromes**
Checklists/Questionnaires									
Krug et al., 1980	Autism Behavior Checklist (ABC)	Screening questionnaire	Yes	Yes	Yes	10–20 minutes	Interrater reliability variable for total score; internal consistency good for total score, poor on subscales	Diagnostic validity poor (Yirmiya et al., 1994); good concurrent validity with subscales on VABS, moderate concurrent validity with CARS	Yes
Matson et al., 2007	Autism Spectrum Disorders—Diagnosis Scale for Intellectually Disabled Adults (ASD—DA)	Informant questionnaire	No	Yes	Yes	31 items	Item test–retest and interrater reliability is low to moderate- average Kappa scores of 0.295 and 0.386 interrater and test–retest respectively	Moderate correlation with DSM-IV-TR and ICD-10 criteria	None identified
Ehlers and Gillberg (1993); Ehlers et al., (1999)	Autism Spectrum Screening Questionnaire	Informant questionnaire	Yes	No	No	Brief (27 items)	Test-retest reliability reported to be good (Posserud et al., 2006)	Cut-off score reported to have a specificity of .90 and sensitivity of .62 for parent report and .90 and .70 respectively for teacher reports	None identified
Nylander & Gillberg, 2001	Autistic spectrum disorder in adults screening questionnaire (ASDASQ)	Screening questionnaire	No	Yes	No	Brief (10 items)	Test–retest and interrater reliability are good (based on % agreement)	No published validity data	None identified
Robins et al., 2001	Modified Checklist for Autism in Toddlers (M-CHAT)	Simple screening questionnaire	Infants only	No	Mild ID only	Very brief	Internal reliability adequate for total and item level scores	Good discriminative validity for distinguishing autism from nonautistic individuals; Robins & Dumont-Mathieu (2006)	None identified

(Continued)

Table 18.2 Assessments of Autism Spectrum Disorder: Characteristics and psychometric properties[*] *(Continued)*

Author	Measure	Format	Child	Adult/ Adolescent	SID	Time Taken	Reliability	Validity	Use in genetic syndromes[**]
Checklists/Questionnaires ctd									
Allison et al., 2008	Quantitative-Checklist for Autism in Toddlers	Informant questionnaire	Yes (<2 yrs)	No	No (general population screener)	Brief (25 items)	Test–retest reliability is good.	ASD group scored significantly higher on the Q-CHAT compared to controls	None identified
Rimland, 1964	Rimland's Diagnostic Checklist for Behavior-Disturbed Children	Questionnaire	Unknown	Unknown	Unknown	Unknown	No published reliability	Discriminative validity has not been achieved despite several attempts	None identified
Rutter et al., 2003	Social Communication Questionnaire (SCQ; developed from the ASQ)	Screening questionnaire	Yes	Yes	Yes	Brief (40 items)	Good internal consistency	Good concurrent validity with the ADI-R and ADOS (Howlin & Karpf, 2004) Good discriminative validity (Rutter et al., 2003)	Yes
Constantino 2002	Social Responsiveness Scale	Informant Questionnaire	≤15 ys	No	No	Brief (65 items)	Test–retest good (.80)	Good concurrent validity with the ADI-R (Constantino et al., 2003)	None identified
Swinkels et al. 2006	The Early Screening of Autistic Traits Questionnaire	Informant questionnaire	Yes (<18 months)	No	No	Brief (14 items)	Test–retest reliability is good: r = .80	Good discriminant ability between typically developing children and children with ASD characteristics; may not discriminate well between ASD characteristics and developmental delay	None identified
Interviews									
Lord et al., 1994	Autism Diagnostic Interview–Revised (ADIR)	Interview	Yes	Yes	Yes (most valid for mild ID; O'Brien et al., 2001)	90–120 minutes	Reliability high at item level	Good discriminative validity for distinguishing autism from mild intellectual disability	Yes

Author/year	Instrument	Method				Time	Reliability	Validity	
Wing et al., 2002	Diagnostic Interview for Social and Communication Disorders (DISCO)	Semistructured interview	Yes	Yes	Yes	3 hours	Interrater and test–retest reliability good	Diagnostic cut-off scores significantly related to clinical diagnoses (Leekham et al., 2002)	Yes
Wing, 1980	Handicaps, Behaviour and Skills (HBS)	Semistructured interview	Yes	No	Mild-moderate ID only	45 minutes–2 hrs	Interrater reliability is high	Good convergent validity with the PEP (van Berckelaer-Onnes & van Dujin 1993)	Yes
Stone and Hogan, 1993	Parent Interview for Autism (PIA)	Interview	Yes	No	Yes	45 minutes	Test–retest reliability is satisfactory; internal consistency is adequate	Concurrent validity with the CARS	None identified
Kraijer, 1997	Scale for Pervasive Developmental Disorder in Mentally Retarded Persons (PDD-MRS)	Interview	From 2 yrs	Up to 55 yrs	Yes	30–60 minutes	No published reliability	Good sensitivity; only 9% misdiagnosis compared to clinical ratings using the PDD-MRS	None identified
Observations									
Lord et al., 2000	Autism Diagnostic Observation Schedule (ADOS)	Structured observations	Yes	Yes	Yes	30–45 minutes	Overall reliability good; reliability for individual items mixed	Good discriminative validity for distinguishing autism and PDD-NOS from nonspectrum disorders.	Yes
Bryson et al., 2007	Autism Observation Scale for Infants	Observational assessment	Yes (6–18 months)	No	No	18-item observation; 20 minutes	Interrater reliability good; test–retest reliability fair to good	Unknown	None identified
Freeman et al., 1978	Behavior Observation Scale (BOS)	Structured observations	Unknown	Unknown	Yes	Unknown	Interrater reliability adequate for 55 out of 67 coded behaviors	Good discriminative validity for distinguishing autism from intellectual disability	None identified

(*Continued*)

Table 18.2 Assessments of Autism Spectrum Disorder: Characteristics and psychometric properties *(Continued)*

Author	Measure	Format	Child	Adult/ Adolescent	SID	Time Taken	Reliability	Validity	Use in genetic syndromes**
Observations ctd.									
DiLavore et al., 1995	Pre-Linguistic Autism Diagnostic Observation Schedule (PLADOS)	Semistructured observations	<6 yrs	No	Mild ID only	30 minutes	Reliability good	Good discriminative validity for distinguishing autism from intellectual disability	None identified
Freeman et al., 1986	Ritvo Freeman Real Life Rating Scale	Observations	Unknown	Unknown	Unknown	Unknown	Satisfactory interrater reliability even with nonprofessional raters; internal consistency is variable	Unknown	None identified
Stone et al., 2000	Screening Tool for Autism in Two-year olds (STAT)	Observations	Yes	No	Unknown	20 minutes	No published reliability	Correctly classified 100% of children with autism and 97% of children with other intellectual disability	None identified
Combined Methods									
Ruttenberg et al., 1966	Behavior Rating Instrument for Autistic and Atypical Children (BRIAAC)	Unknown	Unknown	Unknown	Unknown	Unknown	Interrater reliability good; internal consistency good for all subscales	Comparison of total scores on the BRIAAC to clinical ratings indicated high correlations	None identified
Schopler et al., 1988	Childhood Autism Rating Scale (CARS)	Observation or questionnaire	Yes	Yes	Yes	30–60 minutes.	Internal consistency high; interrater reliability good; test–retest reliability good	Concurrent validity with clinical ratings is good	Yes

Combined Methods ctd.

Gilliam, 1995	Gilliam Autism Rating Scale (GARS)	Interview/Questionnaire	Yes	Up to 22 years only	Yes	5–10 minutes	Internal consistency strong	Good concurrent and discriminative validity found initially (Gilliam, 1995); recent studies indicate that sensitivity is very low (South et al., 2002)	Yes
Adrien et al., 1992	Infant Behavioral Summarized Evaluation (IBSE)	Questionnaire based on observations by professional	Infants only	No	Yes	Brief (29 items)	Global score reliability high; item reliability good for 31 out of 33 items	Good discriminative validity for distinguishing autism from intellectual disability and typically developing individuals	None identified

* Screening assessments of behavior that have subscales relevant to ASD are not included in this table since it was considered that such assessments, which are developed for their scope, contain too few items to provide the depth of information necessary to identify autistic phenomenology in detail. Measures of Asperger's syndrome have also not been included in the table since the focus of this chapter is on ASD in the intellectual disability population.

** Has this assessment been identified by the authors to have been used in studies of individuals with genetic syndromes to identify ASD?

caution should be exercised when using the GARS as a diagnostic tool. With regard to the ABC, initial reports of reliability and discriminative validity were high (Krug et al., 1980). The advantage of this measure is that it includes different score profiles for different chronological age ranges, therefore accounting for possible changes in the autistic profile with age. This may be particularly helpful for use in syndrome populations, given that there may be differences in the developmental trajectory of ASD characteristics in particular syndrome groups. Studies of FXS and CdLS have identified such differences, although this may not be considered for other syndrome groups. However, the original reliability figures were based on percentage agreement, which does not consider the influence of chance, and interraters were not blind to clinical diagnosis when discriminative validity was tested (Parks, 1983; Volkmar et al., 1988). Further studies using more stringent measures have indicated that internal consistency is good for total score but poor on subscales. This would make detailed investigation of specific behavioral profiles of ASD characteristics in individual syndrome groups difficult to interpret and would result in having to rely on the broad total score levels, which may mask syndrome specific behaviors, profiles, and phenomenology. The examples of FXS, RS, and CdLS demonstrate that broad scoring criteria may not be sufficient to fully understand the prevalence and phenomenology of ASD in genetic syndromes. Additionally, interrater reliability is poor (O'Brien et al., 2001; Sturmey, Matson, & Sevin, 1992; Volkmar et al., 1988) and discriminative validity is low. Although these measures are reported to be suitable for use with individuals with severe intellectual disability, their psychometric properties are weak and therefore the information derived from these assessments must be interpreted with caution.

Interview Measures Appropriate for Children and Adults with Intellectual Disability

The Diagnostic Interview for Social and Communication Disorders (DISCO; Wing, Leekham, Libby, Gould, & Larcombe, 2002) was designed to provide a systematic assessment of an individual's clinical history from birth and a description of current behavior. The measure is intended for use in obtaining information regarding ASD or other psychiatric disorders. Interrater reliability and discriminant validity according to ICD-10

diagnoses are reported to be good (Wing et al., 2002; Leekham, Libby, Wing, Gould, & Taylor, 2002). The DISCO was designed primarily to obtain a clinical history of information in a systematic way, rather than as a diagnostic instrument. The DISCO also includes items that cover a range of adaptive and developmental skills, including self-help skills and visuospatial skills, which may not be relevant to the diagnosis of ASD, in addition to information on other psychiatric disorders and forensic problems. Algorithms for identifying diagnostic categories have been devised to enable the DISCO to also be used for research purposes. Although these algorithms allow for use in research, the fact that the DISCO is largely intended for recording clinical history, and because of the length of time it takes to administer this interview, it may be more useful in the clinical setting.

The Autism Diagnostic Interview-Revised (ADI-R; Rutter et al., 2003) is an informant interview that can be used to diagnose ASD and autism in children and adults. Interrater and test–retest reliability is reported to be good. Reports of the concurrent validity between the ADI-R and a range of other autism-specific assessments including the SCQ, ADOS, CARS, and SRS have been good (Bishop & Norbury, 2002; Constantino et al., 2003; Perry, Condillac, Freeman, Dunn-Geier, & Belair, 2005), although de Bildt et al. (2004) reported the agreement between the ADI-R and the ADOS to be fair in individuals with intellectual disability. Studies have also reported lower levels of internal consistency than that originally reported by the authors (Saemundsen, Magnussen, Smari, & Sigurdardottir, 2003).

Diagnostic validity of the ADI-R is reported to be good. However, the ability of the ADI-R to discriminate between ASD and severe intellectual disability is thought to be somewhat limited (Charwaska, Klin, Paul, & Volkmar, 2007; Gray, Tongue, & Sweeney, 2008; Ventola et al., 2006), although other studies have reported validity and reliability of the ADI-R to be good across all ranges of intellectual ability (de Bildt et al., 2004). These findings suggest that the ADI-R may not be sensitive enough for use in individuals with severe and profound intellectual disability, and may be most valid for individuals with mild intellectual disability (O'Brien et al., 2001). The ADI-R should be used cautiously in syndrome groups such as RS, AS, and CdLS, in which degree of disability is typically severe to profound.

Questionnaire Measures Appropriate for Children and Adults with Severe Intellectual Disability

Of the measures described in Table 18.2, only one questionnaire is suitable for use in children and adults with severe intellectual disability. The Social Communication Questionnaire (SCQ; Rutter et al., 2003), originally designed as the Autism Screening Questionnaire (Berument et al., 1999), is a 40-item informant questionnaire that screens for the behaviors and features of communication and social interaction associated with autistic spectrum disorder. Items relate to three different domains: reciprocal social interaction, communication, and restricted, repetitive, and stereotyped patterns of behavior. Two forms of the SCQ have been developed. The Lifetime Version is completed with reference to the developmental history. The Current Version is completed with reference to behavior during the most recent 3-month period.

The discriminant ability of the SCQ is high in differentiating ASD from nonautism conditions and similarly good for differentiating between autism and intellectual disability. The authors identify a cut-off score of 15 as the standard optimal cut-off for distinguishing individuals with PDDs (including autism) from other diagnoses with good sensitivity and specificity for distinguishing individuals with autism from those with intellectual disability. A higher cut-off of 22 is reported by the authors to differentiate between individuals with autism and those with other PDDs. The discriminative ability of this higher cut-off score for distinguishing autism from intellectual disability is not reported in the manual. The measure has also been shown to have good concurrent validity with the ADI-R and with the ADOS (Berument et al., 1999; Howlin & Karpf, 2004). Internal consistency is also good (Berument et al., 1999). Validation of the SCQ with younger children has yielded inconsistent findings. Some studies have reported reduced sensitivity and specificity (Eaves, Wingert, Ho, & Mickelson, 2006; Eaves, Woods-Groves, Williams, & Fall, 2006; Snow & Lacavalier, 2008), whereas others have evidenced closer agreement with the original levels of sensitivity and specificity reported by the authors (Chandler et al., 2007). No interrater or test–retest reliability data for the SCQ have been reported by the authors.

Importantly, individuals who are nonverbal (and therefore likely to have a lower degree of intellectual disability) are not able to score on seven of the 39 items (18%) in the questionnaire. This scoring disadvantage is not taken into consideration at the level of total or subscale scores. This problem is particularly relevant to AS and CdLS and other syndrome groups in which the number of individuals with verbal skills is very limited, and it makes the use of this measure in cross-syndrome comparisons of ASD profiles and prevalence scoring above clinical cut-off scores very difficult. One further point of consideration is the fact that the SCQ was developed as a screening instrument and therefore the authors suggest that this assessment should not be used alone to identify and diagnose ASD.

Observational Measures Appropriate for Children and Adults with Intellectual Disability

Of the measures reported in Table 18.2, only one observational measure is appropriate for use with children and adults with severe intellectual disability. The ADOS (Lord et al., 2000) is a semistructured, standardized assessment of communication, social interaction, and play or imaginative use of materials. The assessment is suitable for individuals with a range of developmental levels, expressive language skills, and chronological ages. The ADOS consists of standardized activities that allow the examiner to observe behaviors that have been identified to be important for the diagnosis of ASD. The assessment incorporates the use of clear, planned social "presses," which provide the optimum opportunity for the participant to display certain behaviors or responses that are relevant to the diagnosis of ASD. The presence/absence and nature of these behaviors and responses are recorded. The assessment consists of four modules, each of which can be administered in 30–45 minutes. Each module has its own protocol. Selection of a particular module is based on the individual's expressive language skills and chronological age.

Good discriminative validity has been established (Lord et al., 2000). Although there have been some concerns regarding the discriminative ability of the ADOS in children with severe intellectual disability, diagnostic validity has been reported to be good across a range of ability levels (de Bildt et al., 2004; O'Brien et al., 2001). Concurrent validity with the ADI-R has largely been reported to be good, although de Bildt et al. (2004) reported only fair agreement with the

ADI-R in individuals with intellectual disability. The inconsistency of these findings regarding validity should be borne in mind when using this assessment for both clinical and research purposes. Checking reliability and validity of scoring methods within individual study samples has been conducted by Moss et al. (2008) in a study of individuals with CdLS and Cri du Chat syndrome that may be helpful particularly in groups associated with a more severe degree of disability, who are more likely to be affected by these validity and reliability issues.

The observational nature of the ADOS assessment is advantageous and allows for a detailed picture of autistic phenomenology. Importantly, the assessment provides the opportunity to identify some of the more subtle behavioral characteristics of ASD, enabling better differentiation of autistic phenomenology from global intellectual disability. The assessment also provides the opportunity to conduct real-time coding of behavioral characteristics or impairments within a standardized setting that can be used to help validate rating information (Moss et al., 2008) and provide a more detailed picture of subtle or atypical characteristics that may not be encompassed in the standardized ratings scales. This may be particularly useful for children and adults with genetic syndromes in which the profile is atypical. Although real-time coding could not be used to make clinical diagnoses, it may help to build a more detailed picture of the individual's strengths and difficulties. Given that the focus of the ADOS is on current behaviour, it is suggested by the authors that this should not be used without an accompanying diagnostic interview or screening tool to aid diagnosis and clinical judgement.

Combined Measures Appropriate for Children and Adults with Severe Intellectual Disability

The CARS (Schopler et al., 1988) assesses the severity of symptoms associated with ASD using a short parent/career interview and observation method that has been shown to be useful in individuals across the age range. Interrater and test–retest reliability are good, and internal consistency is reported to be high (Perry, Condillac, Freeman, Dunn-Geier, & Belair, 2005). Discriminative validity has been reported to be good across a number of studies (Schopler et al., 1988; Perry et al., 2005), and good concurrent validity with the ADI-R has also

been demonstrated. The main disadvantage of this instrument is that it does not take developmental level into account when scoring. Given the overlap between ASD and degree of disability, this oversight may have a significant impact on the utility of this measure for individuals with intellectual disability and particularly in those syndrome groups in which severe and profound intellectual disability is typical, such as AS. In particular, studies have shown that the CARS may be likely to misdiagnose young children with intellectual disability who do not have ASD. Other studies have identified that this measure may not be sensitive enough to diagnose autism correctly until children reach 3 years of age (Lord, 1995), and others report that scores on the CARS demonstrate a strong, negative correlation with level of IQ and adaptive level (Perry et al., 2005). Consequently, this assessment may not be suitable for assessing autism in young children or individuals with intellectual disability. The CARS has also been criticized for not being aligned with prevailing diagnostic criteria since it was published in 1988 and is therefore based on the DSM-III criteria. However, Perry et al. (2005) note that the CARS does include items that map onto the three core diagnostic areas outlined in the DSM-IV, although it does not include items referring to peer relationships, joint attention, or symbolic play, which may be important for early diagnosis. Rellini, Tortolani, Trillo, Carbone, and Montecchi (2004) also report a high level of agreement between DSM-IV clinician diagnosis and scores on the CARS, although the ability of the CARS to distinguish different subtypes of ASD is limited.

Summary

A number of different assessment tools are available that complement the use of expert clinical judgment for the diagnosis of ASD, and that can be used in the assessment of ASD in genetic syndromes associated with intellectual disability. These assessments include a range of formats (questionnaire, interview, or observation) and are designed for different purposes (screening vs. diagnosis) and for different age ranges and levels of intellectual ability. However, many were not designed for use with individuals with severe and profound degrees of intellectual disability, whereas others were developed for use with young children only and are therefore not appropriate for use with adolescents or adults. The fact that different measures are more or less suited to particular levels of intellectual disability and age ranges can be problematic for use in syndrome groups in which there may be a range of intellectual ability. Intellectual ability in TSC, for example, ranges from normal to severe. Finding a single measure of ASD that can be used across the board in a single syndrome group is difficult, potentially resulting in having to employ different measures of ASD within a single study population to cater for all levels of ability.

Of those that can be used in both children and adults with severe intellectual disability, findings regarding psychometric properties have been somewhat mixed, particularly with regard to their ability to distinguish ASD from severe intellectual disability in young children. Thus, when using ASD assessments in a research capacity, greater attention should be given to consider the validity of the assessment in relation to the specific study sample in which the assessment is being used. This is particularly important when using ASD assessments in syndrome groups, such as AS, in which the associated degree of disability (typically profound) makes this population more vulnerable to these issues of validity and reliability.

It is important to remember that standardized assessments are designed to *aid* the clinical diagnosis of ASD; they are not infallible. It is generally considered to be necessary in both clinical and research work to use a combination of assessments in addition to expert clinical judgment to accurately identify ASD in any individual, regardless of genetic status or degree of disability, although it is clear that even more caution is needed in such groups. Assessment tools like the ADI-R (Rutter et al., 2003) or ADOS (Lord et al., 2000) were developed to distinguish between children with ASD and typically developing children, or children with general intellectual disability. They were not designed to distinguish social-communication impairments in genetic syndromes that may be common but may also be complex, and present ASD profiles and characteristics that are somewhat different in nature, development, and etiology to those that are typical of idiopathic autism. At the broad level of diagnostic/clinical cut-off scores, autism-specific assessments may not be sensitive enough to identify the very subtle differences in ASD profiles, developmental trajectories that have been identified within the literature in some genetically determined syndromes, and any syndrome-specific characteristics that may be misidentified in an autism-specific assessment. This requires any assessment of ASD to demonstrate strong reliability and validity at both the subscale *and* item level, to enable researchers and clinicians to feel confident in their identification of ASD characteristics. For the purpose of considering subtle differences or unusual profiles in genetic syndromes, the use of the ADOS may be preferable as it allows for detailed observation of specific behaviors and characteristics within a standardized setting. In this way, detailed investigation of behaviors in genetic syndromes can go alongside the scoring and rating system that accompanies this assessment. The ADOS provides a standardized setting in which to observe and code real-time frequency and duration of core diagnostic characteristics and impairments in addition to the standardized and more clinically relevant scoring algorithm. This is not only useful for detailing phenomenology of ASD behaviors but also for providing further information about the validity of the assessment in the specific samples being investigated.

Conclusion

In this chapter, we have considered the prevalence and phenomenology of ASD in individuals with genetic syndromes associated with intellectual disability. It is clear that accurate identification and recognition of ASD phenomenology in individuals with genetic syndromes is extremely important in ensuring that they receive appropriate educational placement and behavior management strategies. However, research in this area has identified a number of methodological and conceptual issues that may impact on the way in which assessment and diagnosis of ASD in these individuals might be approached. The most prominent difficulty in accurately identifying ASD in these syndrome groups is the overlap between behaviors and impairments accounted for by associated intellectual disability and the behaviors and impairments associated with ASD. This is particularly difficult in the case of individuals with severe to profound intellectual disability. The diagnostic criteria outlined by the DSM-IV-TR (APA; 2000) and ICD-10 (Who, 1992) manuals may not be sensitive enough to distinguish between individuals who have not yet attained the appropriate level of development required to demonstrate a particular skill and those who show a genuine impairment in these skills. The difficulties in accurately recognizing and diagnosing ASD characteristics in this population are reflected in the inconsistent psychometric properties of a number of autism-specific assessments when used at these levels of ability.

We have highlighted the need to recognize that standardized ASD assessments were not designed for use in individuals with genetic syndromes who show a range of complex and often unusual behavioral and cognitive impairments. It is important to be aware of syndrome-specific behaviors and the risk of misidentification in autism-specific assessments. Caution is needed to avoid accepting superficial similarities or heightened scores on ASD assessments that may be accounted for by other syndrome-specific factors.

Finally, we have highlighted the importance of conducting detailed assessment of behavioral phenomenology. Studies in FXS, RS, and CdLS have identified unusual or atypical profiles of ASD phenomenology and differing developmental trajectories of behaviors and impairments. These in turn raise questions about the prevailing conceptualization of the triad of impairments and highlight the need to look beyond the level of diagnostic or clinical cut-off scores when identifying and assessing ASD characteristics. It is therefore important that assessments of ASD have good item-level reliability and validity, in addition to good psychometric properties at the domain or subscale level. Detailed and well-standardized observational assessments, such as the ADOS, may be particularly suited to the identification of more subtle social skills and impairments.

Notes

1. For the purposes of this review the term *autism spectrum disorder* (ASD) will be employed throughout the text to refer to all conditions classified by the *Diagnostic and Statistical Manual of Mental Disorders, 4th Edition, Text Revision* (DSM-IV-TR, 2000) within the category of Pervasive Developmental Disorder with the exception of RS and Child Disintegrative Disorder. When referring to particular studies, the terminology used by the authors of the study will be employed.
2. Throughout this chapter, we will use the terms *genetically determined syndromes* or *genetic syndromes* to refer to conditions that are associated with intellectual disability in which specific genetic etiology has been identified.
3. Some of the information in this chapter has been adapted from Moss & Howlin (2009).

References

Abrahams, B. S., & Geschwind, D. H. (2008). Advances in autism genetics: On the threshold of a new neurobiology. *Nature Reviews Genetics, 9*, 341–355.

Adrien, J. L., Barthelemy, C., Perrot, A., Roux, S., Lenoir, P., Hameury, L., et al. (1992). Validity and reliability of the Infant Behavioral Summarized Evaluation (IBSE): A rating scale for the assessment of young children with autism and developmental disorders. *Journal of Autism and Developmental Disorders, 22*, 375–394.

Allison, C., Baron-Cohen, S., Wheelwright, S., Charman, T., Richler, J., Pasco, G., & Brayne, C. (2008). The Q-CHAT (Quantitative Checklist for Autism in Toddlers): A normally distributed quantitative measure of autistic traits at 18–24 months of age: Preliminary report. *Journal of Autism and Developmental Disorders, 38*, 1414–1425.

American Psychiatric Association. (1987). *Diagnostic and statistical manual of mental disorders.* (3rd ed.). Washington, DC: Author.

American Psychiatric Association. (2000). *Diagnostic and statistical manual of mental disorders* (4th ed., text rev.). Washington, DC: Author.

Asano, E., Chugani, D. C., Muzik, O., Behen, M., Janisse, J., Rothermel, R., et al. (2001). Autism in tuberous sclerosis complex is related to both cortical and subcortical dysfunction. *Neurology, 57*, 1269–1277.

Baieli, S., Pavone, L., Meli, C., Fiumara, A., & Coleman, M. (2003). Autism and phenylketonuria. *Journal of Autism and Developmental Disorders, 33*, 201–204.

Bailey, D. B., Hatton, D. D., Skinner, M., & Mesibov, G. (2001). Autistic behavior, FMR1 protein, and developmental trajectories in young males with fragile X syndrome. *Journal of Autism and Developmental Disorders, 31*, 165–174.

Bailey, D. B., Mesibov, G. B., Hatton, D. D., Clark, R. D., Roberts, J. E., & Mayhew, L. (1998). Autistic behavior in young boys with fragile X syndrome. *Journal of Autism and Developmental Disorders, 28*, 499–508.

Baird, G., Simonoff, E., Pickles, A., Chandler, S., Loucas, T., Meldrum, D., et al. (2006). Prevalence of disorders of the autism spectrum in a population cohort of children in South Thames: The Special Needs and Autism Project (SNAP). *Lancet, 368*, 210–215.

Baker, P., Piven, J., & Sato, Y. (1998). Autism and tuberous sclerosis complex: Prevalence and clinical features. *Journal of Autism and Developmental Disorders, 28*, 279–285.

Barisnikov, K., Hippolyte, L., & van der Linden, M. (2008). Face processing and facial emotion recognition in adults with Down syndrome. *American Journal on Mental Retardation, 113*, 292–306.

Basile, E., Villa, L., Selicorni, A., & Molteni, M. (2007). The behavioural phenotype of Cornelia de Lange syndrome: A study of 56 individuals. *Journal of Intellectual Disability Research, 51*, 671–681.

Berkson, G., & Davenport, R. K. (1962). Stereotyped movements of mental defectives. I: Initial survey. *American Journal of Mental Deficiency, 66*, 849–852.

Berney, T. P., Ireland, M., & Burn, J. (1999). Behavioral phenotype of Cornelia de Lange syndrome. *Archives of Diseases in Childhood, 81*, 333–336.

Berument, S. K., Rutter, M., Lord, C., Pickles, A., & Bailey, A. (1999). Autism Screening Questionnaire: Diagnostic validity. *British Journal of Psychiatry, 175*, 444–451.

Bhuiyan, Z. A., Klein, M., Hammond, P., van Haeringen, A., Mannens, M. A. M., Van Berckelaer-Onnes, I., & Hennekam, R. C. M. (2006). Genotype-phenotype correlations of 39 patients with Cornelia de Lange syndrome: The Dutch experience. *Journal of Medical Genetics, 46*, 568–575.

Bishop, V. M., & Norbury, C. F. (2002). Exploring the borderlands of autistic disorder and specific language impairment: A study using standardized diagnostic instruments. *Journal of Child Psychology and Psychiatry, 43,* 917–929.

Bodfish, J. W., Crawford, T. W., Powell, S. B., Parker, D. E., Golden, R. N., & Lewis, M. H. (1995). Compulsions in adults with mental retardation: Prevalence, phenomenology, and comorbidity with stereotypy and self-injury. *American Journal of Mental Deficiency, 100,* 183–192.

Bolton, P., & Griffiths, P. D. (1997). Association of tuberous sclerosis of temporal lobes with autism and atypical autism. *The Lancet, 349,* 392–395.

Bolton, P. F., Park, R. J., Higgins, J. N. P., Griffiths, P. D., & Pickles, A. (2002). Neuro-epileptic determinants of autism spectrum disorders in tuberous sclerosis complex. *Brain, 125,* 1247–1255.

Bonati, M. T., Russo, S., Finelli, P., Valsecchi, M. R., Cogliati, F., Cavalleri F., et al. (2007). Evaluation of autism traits in Angelman syndrome: A resource to unfold autism genes. *Neurogenetics, 8,* 169–178.

Brown, W. T., Jenkins, E. C., Cohen, I. L., Fisch, G. S., Wolf-Schein, E. G., Gross, A., et al. (1986). Fragile X and autism: A multicenter survey. *American Journal of Medical Genetics, 23,* 341–352.

Bryson, S. E., Zwaigenbaum, L., Brian, J., Roberts, W., Szatmari, P., Rombough, V., & McDermott, C. (2007). A prospective case series of high-risk infants who developed autism. *Journal of Autism and Developmental Disorders, 37,* 12–24.

Capone, G. T., Grados, M. A., Kaufmann, W. E., Bernad-Ripoll, S., & Jewell, A. (2005). Down syndrome and comorbid autism-spectrum disorder: Characterization using the aberrant behavior checklist. *American Journal of Medical Genetics, 134A,* 373–380.

Chandler, S., Charman, T., Baird, G., Simonoff, E., Loucas, T., Meldrum, D., et al. (2007).Validation of the social communication questionnaire in a population cohort of children with autism spectrum disorders. *Journal of the American Academy of Child and Adolescent Psychiatry, 46,* 1324–1332.

Charman, T., Taylor, E., Drew, A., Cockerill, H., Brown, J., & Baird, G. (2005). Outcome at 7 years of children diagnosed with autism at age 2: Predictive validity of assessments conducted at 2 and 3 years of age and pattern of symptom change over time. *Journal of Child Psychology and Psychiatry, 46,* 500–513.

Charwarska, K., Klin, A., Paul, R., & Volkmar, F. (2007). Autism spectrum disorder in the second year: Stability and change in syndrome expression. *Journal of Child Psychology and Psychiatry, 48,* 128–138.

Cohen, I. L., Sudhalter, V., Pfadt, A., Jenkins, E. C., Brown, W. T., & Vietze, P. M. (1991). Why are autism and the fragile X syndrome associated? Conceptual and methodological issues. *American Journal of Human Genetics, 48,* 195–202.

Collis, L., Oliver, C., & Moss, J. (2006). Low mood and social anxiety in Cornelia de Lange syndrome. *Journal of Intellectual Disability Research, 50,* 791–800.

Constantino, J. N. (2002). *The Social Responsiveness Scale.* Los Angeles: Western Psychological Services.

Constantino, J. N., Davis, S. A., Todd, R. D., Schindler, M. K., Gross, M. M., Brophy, S. L., et al. (2003). Validation of a brief quantitative measure of autistic traits: Comparison of the Social Responsiveness Scale with the Autism Diagnostic Interview-Revised. *Journal of Autism and Developmental Disorders, 33,* 427–433.

Cornish, K., Turk, J., & Hagerman, R. (2008). The fragile X continuum: New advances and perspectives. *Journal of Intellectual Disability Research, 52,* 469–482.

Cornish, K., Turk, J., & Levitas, A. (2007). Fragile X syndrome and autism: Common developmental pathways? *Current Pediatric Reviews, 3,* 61–68.

de Bildt, A., Sytema, S., Ketelaars, C., Kraijer, D., Mulder, E., Volkmar, F., et al. (2004). Interrelationship between Autism Diagnostic Observation Schedule-Generic (ADOS-G), Autism Diagnostic Interview-Revised (ADI-R), and the Diagnostic and Statistical Manual of Mental Disorders (DSM-IV-TR) classification in children with mental retardation. *Journal of Autism and Developmental Disorders, 34,* 129–137.

de Vries, P. J., & Howe, C. J. (2007). The tuberous sclerosis complex proteins - A GRIPP on cognition and neurodevelopment. *Trends in Molecular Medicine, 13,* 319–326.

de Vries, P. J., Hunt, A., & Bolton, P. (2007). The psychopathologies of children and adolescents with tuberous sclerosis complex (TSC): A postal survey of UK families. *European Child and Adolescent Psychiatry, 16,* 16–24.

Deardorff, M. A., Kaur, M., Yaeger, D., Rampuria, A., Korolev, S., Pie, J., et al. (2007). Mutations in cohesion complex members SMC3 and SMC1A cause a mild variant of Cornelia de Lange syndrome with predominant mental retardation. *American Journal of Human Genetics, 80,* 485–494.

Deb, S., & Prasad, K. B. G. (1994). The prevalence of autistic disorder among children with a learning disability. *British Journal of Psychiatry, 165,* 395–399.

Demark, J. L., Feldman, M. A., & Holden, J. A. (2003). Behavioral relationship between autism and fragile X syndrome. *American Journal on Mental Retardation, 108,* 314–326.

Dennis, M., Lockyer, L., Lazenby, A. L., Donnelly, R. E., Wilkinson, M., & Schoonheyt, W. (1999). Intelligence patterns among children with high-functioning autism, phenylketonuria, and childhood head injury. *Journal of Autism and Developmental Disorders, 29,* 5–17.

DiLavore, P. C., Lord, C., & Rutter, M. (1995). The Pre-Linguistic Autism Diagnostic Observation Schedule. *Journal of Autism and Developmental Disorders, 25,* 355–379.

Dykens, E. M. (2007). Psychiatric and behavioral disorders in persons with Down syndrome. *Mental Retardation and Developmental Disabilities Research Reviews, 13,* 272–278.

Eaves, L. C., Wingert, H. D., Ho, H. H., & Mickelson, E. C. R. (2006). Screening for autism spectrum disorders with the social communication questionnaire. *Journal of Developmental and Behavioral Pediatrics, 27,* 95–103.

Eaves, R. C., Woods-Groves, S., Williams, T. O., & Fall, A. M. (2006). Reliability and validity of the Pervasive Developmental Disorders Rating Scale and the Gilliam Autism Rating Scale. *Education and Training In Developmental Disability, 41,* 300–309.

Ehlers, S., & Gillberg, C. (1993). The epidemiology of Aspergers syndrome: A total population study.

Ehlers, S., Gillberg, C., & Wing, L. (1999). A screening questionnaire for Asperger syndrome and other high-functioning autism spectrum disorders in school age children. *Journal of Autism and Developmental Disorders, 29,* 129–141.

Fombonne, E. (1999). The epidemiology of autism: A review. *Psychological Medicine, 29,* 769–786.

Fombonne, E. (2005). The changing epidemiology of autism. *Journal of Applied Research in Intellectual Disabilities, 18,* 281–294.

Freeman, B. J., Ritvo, E. R., Guthrie, D., Schroth, P., & Ball, J. (1978). The Behavior Observation Scale for Autism: Initial methodology, data analysis and preliminary findings on 89 children. *Journal of the American Academy of Child Psychiatry, 17,* 576–588.

Freeman, B. J., Ritvo, E. R., Yokota, A., & Ritvo, A. (1986). A scale for rating symptoms of patients with the syndrome of autism in real life settings. *Journal of the American Academy of Child and Adolescent Psychiatry, 25,* 130–136.

Ghaziuddin, M., Tsai, L. Y., & Ghaziuddin, N. (1992). Autism in Down's syndrome: Presentation and diagnosis. *Journal of Intellectual Disability Research, 36,* 449–456.

Gillberg, C., & Coleman, M. (2000). *The biology of the autistic syndromes.* (3rd ed.). London: McKeith Press.

Gillberg, C., Gillberg, I. C., & Ahlsen, G. (1994). Autistic behavior and attention deficits in tuberous sclerosis. *Developmental Medicine and Child Neurology, 36,* 50–56.

Gillberg, C., Pearson, E., Grufman, M., & Themner, U. (1986). Psychiatric disorders in mildly and severely mentally retarded urban children and adolescents: Epidemiological aspects. *British Journal of Psychiatry, 149,* 68–74.

Gilliam, J. E. (1995). *Gilliam autism rating scale.* Austin Texas: Pro-ed.

Gillis, L. A., McCallum, J., Kaur, M., DeScipio, C., Yaeger, D., Mariani, A., et al. (2004). NIPBL mutational analysis in 120 individuals with Cornelia de Lange syndrome and evaluation of genotype-phenotype correlations. *American Journal of Human Genetics, 75,* 610–623.

Goodban, M. T. (1993). Survey of speech and language skills with prognostic indicators in 116 patients with Cornelia de Lange syndrome. *American Journal of Medical Genetics, 47,* 1059–1063.

Grant, C. M., Apperly, I., & Oliver, C. (2007). Is theory of mind understanding impaired in fragile x syndrome? *Journal of Abnormal Child Psychology, 35,* 17–28.

Gray, K. M., Tongue, B., & Sweeney, D. J. (2008). Using the Autism Diagnostic Interview-Revised and the Autism Diagnostic Observation Schedule with young children with developmental delay: Evaluating diagnostic validity. *Journal of Autism and Developmental Disorders, 38,* 657–667.

Gutierrez, G., Smalley, S. L., & Tanguay, P. E. (1998). Autism in tuberous sclerosis complex. *Journal of Autism and Developmental Disorders, 28,* 97–103.

Hagerman, J., Jackson, A. W., Levitas, A., Rimland, B., & Braden, M. (1986). An analysis of autism in fifty males with the fragile X syndrome. *American Journal of Medical Genetics, 23,* 359–374.

Hagerman, R. J., Ono, M. Y., & Hagerman, P. J. (2005). Recent advances in fragile X: A model for autism and neurodegeneration. *Current Opinion in Psychiatry, 18,* 490–496.

Hall, S., deBernardis, M., & Reiss, A. (2006). Social escape behaviors in individuals with fragile X syndrome. *Journal of Autism and Developmental Disorders, 36,* 935–947.

Harrison, J. E., & Bolton, P. F. (1997). Annotation: Tuberous sclerosis. *Journal of Child Psychology and Psychiatry and Allied Disciplines, 38,* 603–614.

Hartshorne, T. S., Grialou, T. L., & Parker, K. R. (2005). Autistic-like behavior in CHARGE syndrome. *American Journal of Medical Genetics, 133A,* 248–256.

Hatton, D. D., Sideris, J., Skinner, M., Mankowski, J., Bailey, D. B., Roberts, J., et al. (2006). Autistic behavior in children with fragile X syndrome: Prevalence, stability, and the impact of FMRP. *American Journal of Medical Genetics, 140A,* 1804–1813.

Howlin, P. (2000). Autism and intellectual disability: Diagnostic and treatment issues. *Journal of the Royal Society of Medicine, 93,* 351–355.

Howlin, P. (2002). Autism related disorders. In G. O'Brien (Ed.), *Behavioural phenotypes in clinical practice* (2nd ed., pp. 31–43). Cambridge: Cambridge University Press.

Howlin, P., Gordon, R. K., Pasco, G., Wade, A., & Charman, T. (2007). The effectiveness of Picture Exchange Communication System (PECS) training for teachers of children with autism: A pragmatic, group randomised controlled trial. *Journal of Child Psychology and Psychiatry, 48,* 473–491.

Howlin, P., & Karpf, J. (2004). Using the Social Communication Questionnaire to identify "autistic spectrum" disorders associated with other genetic conditions: Findings from a study of individuals with Cohen syndrome. *Autism, 8,* 175–182.

Howlin, P., Wing, L., & Gould, J. (1995). The recognition of autism in children with Down syndrome: Implications for intervention and some speculations about pathology. *Developmental Medicine and Child Neurology, 37,* 398–414.

Humphrey, A., Neville, B. G. R., Clarke, A., & Bolton, P. F. (2006). Autistic regression associated with seizure onset in an infant with tuberous sclerosis. *Developmental Medicine and Child Neurology, 48,* 609–611.

Hunt, A., & Shepherd, C. (1993). A prevalence study of autism in tuberous sclerosis. *Journal of Autism and Developmental Disorders, 23,* 323–339.

Hyman, P., Oliver, C., & Hall, S. (2002). Self-injurious behavior, self-restraint, and compulsive behaviors in Cornelia de Lange syndrome. *American Journal of Mental Deficiency, 107,* 146–154.

Jackson, L., Kline, A. D., Barr, M., & Koch, S. (1993). de Lange syndrome: A clinical review of 310 individuals. *American Journal of Medical Genetics, 47,* 940–946.

Jambaque, I., Cusmai, R., Curatolo, P., Cortesi, F., Perrot, C., & Dulac, O. (1991). Neuropsychological aspects of tuberous sclerosis in relation to epilepsy and MRI findings. *Developmental Medicine and Child Neurology, 33,* 698–705.

Jeste, S. S., Sahin, M., Bolton, P., Ploubidis, G. B., & Humphrey, A. (2008). Characterization of autism in young children with tuberous sclerosis complex. *Journal of Child Neurology, 23,* 520–525.

Johansson, M., Rastam, M., Billstedt, E., Danielsson, S., Stromland, K., Miller, M., & Gillberg, C. (2006). Autism spectrum disorders and underlying brain pathology in CHARGE association. *Developmental Medicine and Child Neurology, 48,* 40–50.

Jordan, R. (2001). *Autism with severe learning difficulties: A guide for parents and professionals.* London: Souvenir Press (Educational and academic) Ltd.

Kau, A. S. M., Tierney, E., Bukelis, I., Stump, M. H., Kates, W. R., Trescher, W. H., et al. (2004). Social behavior profile in young males with fragile X syndrome: Characteristics and specificity. *American Journal of Medical Genetics, 126,* 9–17.

Kaufmann, W. E., Cortell, R., Kau, A. S. M., Bukelis, I., Tierney, E., Gray, R. M., et al. (2004). Autism spectrum disorder in fragile X syndrome: Communication, social interaction and specific behaviors. *American Journal of Medical Genetics, 129,* 225–234.

Kent, L., Evans, J., Paul, M., & Sharp, M. (1999). Comorbidity of autistic spectrum disorder in children with Down syndrome. *Developmental Medicine and Child Neurology, 41*, 158.

Kraijer, D. (1997). *Autism and autistic-like conditions in mental retardation.* Liss, The Netherlands: Swets & Zeitlinger.

Krantz, I. D., McCallum, J., DeScipio, C., Kaur, M., Gillis, L. A., Yaeger, D., et al. (2004). Cornelia de Lange syndrome is caused by mutations in NIPBL, the human homolog of Drosophila melanogaster Nipped–B. *Nature Genetics, 6*, 631–635.

Krug, D. A., Arick, J., & Almond, P. (1980). Behavior checklist for identifying severely handicapped individuals with high levels of autistic behavior. *Journal of Child Psychology and Psychiatry, 21*, 221–229.

La Malfa, G., Lassi, S., Bertelli, M., Salvini, R., & Placidi, G. F. (2004). Autism and intellectual disability: A study of prevalence on a sample of the Italian population. *Journal of Intellectual Disability Research, 48*, 262–267.

Laumonnier, F., Bonnet-Brilhault, F., Gomot, M., Blanc, R., David, A., Moizard, M. P. et al. (2004). X-linked mental retardation and autism are associated with a mutation in the NLGN4 gene, a member of the neuroligin family. *American Journal of Human Genetics, 74*, 554–557.

Lecavalier, L. (2005). An evaluation of the Gilliam Autism Rating Scale. *Journal of Autism and Developmental Disorders, 35*, 795–805.

Leekham, S. R., Libby, S. J., Wing, L., Gould, J., & Taylor, C. (2002). The diagnostic interview for social and communication disorders: Algorithms for ICD-10 childhood autism and Wing and Gould autistic spectrum disorder. *Journal of Child Psychology and Psychiatry and Allied Disciplines, 43*, 327–342.

Lesniak-Karpiak, K., Mazzocco, M. M. M., & Ross, J. L. (2003). Behavioral assessment of social anxiety in females with Turner or fragile X syndrome. *Journal of Autism and Developmental Disorders, 33*, 55–67.

Levitas, A., Hagerman, R. J., Braden, M., Rimland, B., Mcbogg, P., & Matus, I. (1983). Autism and the fragile-X syndrome. *Journal of Developmental and Behavioral Pediatrics, 4*, 151–158.

Loesch, D. Z., Bui, Q.M., Dissanayake, C., Clifford, S., Gould, E., et al,(2007). Molecular and cognitive predictors of the continuum of autistic behaviors in fragile X. *Neuroscience and Biobehavioral Reviews, 31*, 315–326.

Lord, C. (1995). Follow-up of two year olds referred for possible autism. *Journal of Child Psychology and Psychiatry, 36*, 1365–1382.

Lord, C., & Paul, R. (1997). Language and communication in autism. In D. J. Cohen, & F. R. Volkmar (Eds.), *Handbook of autism and pervasive developmental disorders* (2nd ed., pp. 195–225). New York: John Wiley & Sons Inc.

Lord, C., & Pickles, A. (1996). Language level and nonverbal social-communicative behaviors in autistic and language-delayed children. *Journal of the American Academy of Child and Adolescent Psychiatry, 35*, 1542–1550.

Lord, C., Risi, S., Lambrecht, L., Cook, E. H., Leventhal, B. L., DiLavore, P. C., et al. (2000). The Autism Diagnostic Observation Schedule-Generic: A standard measure of social and communication deficits associated with the spectrum of autism. *Journal of Autism and Developmental Disorders, 30*, 205–223.

Lord, C., Rutter, M., DiLavore, P. C., & Risi, S. (2000). *The Autism Diagnostic Observation Schedule (ADOS).* Los Angeles: Western Psychological Services.

Lord, C., Rutter, M., & Le Couteur, A. (1994). Autism Diagnostic Interview-Revised: A revised version of a diagnostic interview for caregivers of individuals with possible pervasive developmental disorders. *Journal of Autism and Developmental Disorders, 24*, 359–385.

Lowenthal, R., Paula, C. S., Schwartzman, J. S., Brunoni, D., & Mercadante, M. T. (2007). Prevalence of pervasive developmental disorders in Down's syndrome. *Journal of Autism and Developmental Disorders, 37*, 1394–1395.

Lund, J. (1988). Psychiatric aspects of Downs-syndrome. *Acta Psychiatrica Scandinavica, 78*, 369–374.

Matson, J. L., Boisjoli, J. A., Gonzalez, M. L., Smith, K. R., & Wilkins, J. (2007). Norms and cut off scores for the Autism Spectrum Disorders Diagnosis for Adults (ASD-DA) with intellectual disability. *Research in Autism Spectrum Disorders, 1*, 330–338.

Mazzocco, M. M., Kates, W. R., Baumgardener, T. L., Freund, L. S., & Reiss, A. L. (1997). Autistic behaviors among girls with fragile X syndrome. *Journal of Autism and Developmental Disorders, 27*, 415–433.

Miyake, N., Visser, R., Kinoshita, A., Yoshiura, K. I., Niikawa, N., Kondoh, T., et al. (2005). Four novel NIPBL mutations in Japanese patients with Cornelia de Lange syndrome. *American Journal of Medical Genetics, 135*, 103–105.

Moss, J., & Howlin, P. (2009). Invited annotation: Autism spectrum disorders in genetic syndromes: Implications for diagnosis, intervention and understanding the wider ASD population. *Journal of Intellectual Disability Research, 53*, 852–872.

Moss, J., Magiati, I., Charman, T., & Howlin, P. (2008). Stability of the Autism Diagnostic Interview-Revised from pre-school to elementary school in children with autism spectrum disorders. *Journal of Autism and Developmental Disorders, 38*, 1081–1091.

Moss, J., Oliver, C., Wilkie, L., Berg, K., Kaur, G., & Cornish, K. (2008). Prevalence of autism spectrum phenomenology in Cornelia de Lange and Cri du Chat syndromes. *American Journal of Mental Retardation, 113*, 278–291.

Moss, J., Oliver, C., Arron, K., Berg, K., Burbidge, C., Duffay, S., & Hooker, M. (2009). The prevalence and phenomenology of repetitive behavior in genetic syndromes. *Journal of Autism and Developmental Disorders, 39*, 572–588.

Mount, R. H., Charman, T., Hastings, R. P., Reilly, S., & Cass, H. (2003). Features of autism in Rett syndrome and severe mental retardation. *Journal of Autism and Developmental Disorders, 33*, 435–442.

Mount, R. H., Hastings, R. P., Reilly, S., Cass, H., & Charman, T. (2003). Towards a behavioral phenotype for Rett syndrome. *American Journal on Mental Retardation, 1*, 1–12.

Musio, A., Selicorni, A., Focarelli, M. L., Gervasini, C., Milani, D., Russo, S., et al. (2006). X-linked Cornelia de Lange syndrome owing to SMC1L1 mutations. *Nature Genetics, 38*, 528–530.

Naidu, S., Hyman, S., Piazza, K., Savedra, J., Perman, J., Wenk, G., et al. (1990). The Rett Syndrome: Progress report on studies at the Kennedy Institute. *Brain & Development, 12*, 5–7.

Nomura, Y., & Segawa, M. (2005). Natural history of Rett syndrome. *Journal of Child Neurology, 20*, 764–768.

Nordin, V., & Gillberg, C. (1996). Autism spectrum disorders in children with physical or mental disability or both. I: Clinical and epidemiological aspects. *Developmental Medicine and Child Neurology, 38*, 297–313.

Nylander, L., & Gillberg, C. (2001). Screening for autism spectrum disorders in adult psychiatric out-patients: A preliminary report. *Acta Psychiatrica Scandinavica, 103*, 428–434.

O'Brien, G., Pearson, J., Berney, T., & Barnard, L. (2001). Measuring behaviour in developmental disability: A review of existing schedules. *Developmental Medicine and Child Neurology, 43*, 1–70.

Oliver, C., Arron, K., Berg, K., Burbidge, C., Caley, A., Duffay, S., et al. (2005). A comparison of Cornelia de Lange, Cri du Chat, Prader-Willi, Smith-Magenis, Lowe, Angelman and fragile X syndromes. *Genetic Counseling, 13*, 363–381.

Oliver, C., Arron, K., Hall, S., Sloneem, J., Forman, D., & McClintock, K. (2006). Effects of social context on social interaction and self-injurious behavior in Cornelia de Lange syndrome. *American Journal on Mental Retardation, 111*, 184–192.

Oliver, C., Arron, K., Sloneem, J., & Hall, S. (2008). The behavioral phenotype of Cornelia de Lange syndrome: case control study. *British Journal of Psychiatry, 193*, 466–470.

Park, R. J., & Bolton, P. F. (2001). Pervasive developmental disorder and obstetric complications in children and adolescents with tuberous sclerosis. *Autism: International Journal of Research and Practice, 5*, 237–248.

Parks, S. L. (1983). The assessment of autistic children: A selective review of available instruments. *Journal of Autism and Developmental Disorders, 13*, 255–267.

Perry, A., Condillac, R. A., Freeman, N. L., Dunn-Geier, J., & Belair, J. (2005). Multi-site study of the Childhood Autism Rating Scale (CARS) in five clinical groups of young children. *Journal of Autism and Developmental Disorders, 35*, 625–634.

Persico, A. M., & Bourgeron, T. (2006). Searching for ways out of the autism maze: Genetic, epigenetic and environmental clues. *Trends in Neuroscience, 29*, 349–358.

Peters, S. U., Beaudit, A. L., Madduri, N., & Bacino, C. A. (2004). Autism in Angelman syndrome: Implications for autism research. *Clinical Genetics, 66*, 530–536.

Reiss, A. L., Feinstein, C., & Rosenbaum, K. N. (1986). Autism and genetic-disorders. *Schizophrenia Bulletin, 12*, 724–738.

Reiss, A. L., & Freund, L. S. (1990). Fragile X syndrome, DSM-III-R and autism. *Journal of the American Academy of Child and Adolescent Psychiatry, 29*, 885–891.

Reiss, S. S., Levitan, G. W., & Szyszko, J. (1982). Emotional disturbance and mental retardation: Diagnostic overshadowing. *American Journal on Mental Deficiency, 86*, 567–574.

Rellini, E., Tortolani, D., Trillo, S., Carbone, S., & Montecchi, F. (2004). Childhood Autism Rating Scale (CARS) and Autism Behavior Checklist (ABC) correspondence and conflicts with DSM-IV criteria in diagnosis of autism. *Journal of Autism and Developmental Disorders, 34*, 703–708.

Richards, C., Moss, J., O'Farrell, L., Kaur, G., & Oliver, C. (2009). Social anxiety in Cornelia de Lange syndrome. *Journal of Autism and Developmental Disorders, 39*, 1155–1162.

Rimland, B. (1964). *Infantile autism.* New York: Appleton-Century-Crofts.

Roberts, J. E., Weisenfeld, L. A. H., Hatton, D. D., Heath, M., & Kaufmann, W. E. (2007). Social approach and autistic behavior in children with Fragile X syndrome. *Journal of Autism and Developmental Disorders, 37*, 1748–1760.

Robins, D. L. & Dumont-Mathieu, T. M. (2006). Early screening for autism spectrum disorders: update on the modified checklist for autism in toddlers and other measures. *Journal of Developmental and Behavioral Pediatrics, 27*, S111–S119.

Robins, D. L., Fein, D., Barton, M. L., & Green, J. A. (2001). The modified checklist for autism in toddlers: An initial study investigating the early detection of autism and pervasive developmental disorders. *Journal of Autism and Developmental Disorders, 31*, 131–144.

Rumeau-Rouquette, C., Grandjean, H., Cans, C., Du Mazaubrun, C., & Verrier, A. (1997). Prevalence and time trends of disabilities in school-age children. *International Journal of Epidemiology, 26*, 137–145.

Ruttenberg, B. A., Dratman, R., Frakner, T. A., & Wenar, C. (1966). An instrument for evaluating autistic children. *Journal of the American Academy of Child and Adolescent Psychiatry, 5*, 453–478.

Rutter, M., Bailey, A., Lord, C., & Berument, S. K. (2003). *The Social Communication Questionnaire.* Los Angeles: Western Psychological Services.

Rutter, M., LeCouteur, A., & Lord, C. (2003). *Autism Diagnostic Interview-Revised (ADI-R).* Los Angeles: Western Psychological Services.

Sabaratnam, M., Murthy, N. V., Wijeratne, A., Buckingham, A., & Payne, S. (2003). Autistic-like behaviour profile and psychiatric morbidity in Fragile X Syndrome: a prospective ten-year follow-up study. *European Child & Adolescent Psychiatry, 12*, 172–177.

Sandberg, A. D., Ehlers, S., Hagberg, B., & Gillberg, C. (2000). The Rett syndrome complex: Communicative functions in relation to developmental level. *Autism: The International Journal of Research and Practice, 4*, 249–267.

Sarimski, K. (2007). Infant attentional behaviours as prognostic indicators in Cornelia de Lange syndrome. *Journal of Intellectual Disability Research, 51*, 697–701.

Schopler, E., Reichler, R. J. & Renner, B. R. (1988). The Childhood Autism Rating Scale (CARS). Los Angeles: Western Psychological Services.

Scriver, C. R., Eisensmith, R. C., Woo, S. L. C., & Kaufmann, S. (1994). The hyperphenylalaninemias of man and mouse. *Annual Review of Genetics, 28*, 141–165.

Skuse, D. H. (2007). Rethinking the nature of genetic vulnerability to autistic spectrum disorders. *Trends in Genetics, 23*, 387–395.

Saemundsen, E., Magnusson, P., Smari J., & Sigurdardottir, S. (2003). Autism Diagnostic Interview-Revised and the Childhood Autism Rating Scale: Convergence and discrepancy in diagnosing autism. *Journal of Autism and Developmental Disorders, 33*, 319–328.

Smalley, S. L. (1998). Autism and tuberous sclerosis. *Journal of Autism and Developmental Disorders, 28*, 407–414.

Smalley, S. L., Tanguay, P. E., Smith, M., & Gutierrez, G. (1992). Autism and tuberous sclerosis. *Journal of Autism and Developmental Disorders, 22*, 339–355.

Smith, I. M., Nichols, S. L., Issekutz, K., & Blake, K. (2005). Behavioral profiles and symptoms of autism in CHARGE syndrome: Preliminary Canadian epidemiological data. *American Journal of Medical Genetics, 133A*, 248–256.

Snow, A. V., & Lecavalier, L. (2008). Sensitivity and specificity of the Modified Checklist for Autism in Toddlers and the Social Communication Questionnaire in preschoolers suspected of having pervasive developmental disorders. *Autism, 12*, 627–644.

South, M., Williams, B. J., McMahon, M., Owley, T., Filipek, P. A., Shernoff, E., et al. (2002). Utility of the Gilliam Autism

Rating Scale in research and clinical populations. *Journal of Autism and Developmental Disorders, 32*, 593–599.

Swinkels, S. H., Dietz, C., van Daalen, E., Kerkhof, I. H., van Engeland, H., & Buitelaar, J. K. (2006). Screening for autistic spectrum in children aged 14–15 months. I: The development of the Early Screening of Autistic Traits Questionnaire (ESAT). *Journal of Autism and Developmental Disorders, 36*, 723–732.

Starr, E. M., Berument, S. K., Tomlins, M., Papanikolaou, K., & Rutter, M. (2005). Brief report: Autism in individuals with Down syndrome. *Journal of Autism and Developmental Disorders, 35*, 665–673.

Stone, W. L., & Hogan, K. L. (1993). A structured parent interview for identifying young children with autism. *Journal of Autism and Developmental Disorders, 23*, 639–652.

Stone, W. L., Coonrod, E. E., & Ousley, O. Y. (2000). Brief report: Screening tool for autism in two-year-olds (STAT): Development and preliminary data. *Journal of Autism and Developmental Disorders, 30*, 607–612.

Sturmey, P., Matson, J. L., & Sevin, J. A. (1992). Brief report: Analysis of the internal consistency of three autism scales. *Journal of Autism and Developmental Disorders, 22*, 321–327.

Sudhalter, V., Cohen, I. L., Silverman, W., & Wolfschein, E. G. (1990). Conversational analyses of males with fragile-X, Down syndrome, and autism: Comparison of the emergence of deviant language. *American Journal on Mental Retardation, 94*, 431–441.

Tager-Flusberg, H. (2000). Understanding the language and communicative impairments in autism. *International Review of Research in Mental Retardation, 23*, 185–205.

Tonkin, E. T., Wang, T., Lisgo, S., Bambshad, M. J., & Strachan, T. (2004). NIPBL, encoding a homolog of fungal Scc2-type sister chromatid cohesion proteins and fly Nipped-B, is mutated in Cornelia de Lange syndrome. *Nature Genetics, 6*, 636–641.

Trillingsaard, A., & Ostergaard, J. R. (2004). Autism in Angelman syndrome: An exploration of comorbidity. *Autism: International Journal of Research and Practice, 8*, 163–174.

Tsai, L. Y. (1992). Is Rett syndrome a subtype of pervasive developmental disorders. *Journal of Autism and Developmental Disorders, 22*, 551–561.

Turk, J., & Cornish, K. M. (1998). Face recognition and emotion perception in boys with fragile X syndrome. *Journal of Intellectual Disability Research, 42*, 490–499.

Turk, J., & Graham, P. (1997). Fragile X syndrome, autism and autistic features. *Autism, 1*, 175–197.

van Berckelaer, I. & van Duijn, G. (1993). A comparison between the handicaps behaviour and skills schedule and the psychoeducational profile. *Journal of Autism and Developmental Disorders, 23*, 263–272.

Ventola, P. E., Kleinman, J., Pandey, J., Barton, M., Allen, S., Green, J., et al. (2006). Agreement among four diagnostic instruments for autism spectrum disorders in toddlers. *Journal of Autism and Developmental Disorders, 36*, 839–847.

Vig, S., & Jedrysek, E. (1999). Autistic features in young children with significant cognitive impairment: Autism or mental retardation? *Journal of Autism and Developmental Disorders, 29*, 235–248.

Volkmar, F. R., Cicchetti, D. V., Dykens, E. M., Sparrow, S. S., Leckman, J. F., & Cohen, D. J. (1988). An evaluation of the Autism Behavior Checklist. *Journal of Autism and Developmental Disorders, 18*, 81–97.

Volkmar, F. R., Lord, C., Bailey, A., Schultz, R., & Klin, A. (2004). Autism and pervasive developmental disorders. *Journal of Child Psychology and Psychiatry, 45*, 135–170.

Walz, N. C., & Benson, B. A. (2002). Behavioral phenotypes in children with Down syndrome, Prader-Willi syndrome, or Angelman syndrome. *Journal of Developmental and Physical Disabilities, 14*, 307–321.

Walz, N. C. (2007). Parent report of stereotyped behaviors, social interaction, and developmental disturbances in individuals with Angelman syndrome. *Journal of Autism and Developmental Disorders, 37*, 940–947.

Webb, D. W., Clarke, A., Fryer, A., & Osborne, J. P. (1996). The cutaneous features of tuberous sclerosis: A population study. *British Journal of Dermatology, 135*, 1–5.

Williamson, D. A., & Bolton, P. (1995). Atypical autism and tuberous sclerosis in a sibling pair. *Journal of Autism and Developmental Disorders, 25*, 435–442.

Wing, L. (1980). *Schedule of handicaps, behavior and skills.* London: Medical Research Council.

Wing, L., Leekham, S. R., Libby, S. J., Gould, J., & Larcombe, M. (2002). The diagnostic interview for social and communication disorders: Background, inter-rater reliability and clinical use. *Journal of Child Psychology and Psychiatry, 43*, 307–325.

Wishart, J. G. (2007). Socio-cognitive understanding: A strength or a weakness in Down's syndrome? *Journal of Intellectual Disability Research, 51*, 996–1005.

Wishart, J. G., Cebula, K. R., Willis, D. S., & Pitcairn, T. K. (2007). Understanding of facial expressions of emotion by children with intellectual disabilities of differing aetiology *Journal of Intellectual Disability Research, 51*, 551–563.

Witt-Engerstrom, I., & Gillberg, C. (1987). Rett Syndrome in Sweden. *Journal of Autism and Developmental Disorders, 17*, 149–150.

Wong, V. (2006). Study of the relationship between tuberous sclerosis complex and autistic disorder. *Journal of Child Neurology, 21*, 199–204.

World Health Organization. (1992). *The ICD-10 classification of mental and behavioral disorders: Clinical descriptions and diagnostic guidelines.* Geneva: Author.

Yalaz, K., Vanli, L., Yilmaz, E., Tokatli, A., & Anlar, B. (2006). Phenylketonuria in pediatric neurology practice: A series of 146 cases. *Journal of Child Neurology, 21*, 987–990.

Yirmiya, N., Sigman, M., & Freeman, B. J. (1994). Comparison between diagnostic instruments for identifying high-functioning children with autism. *Journal of Autism and Developmental Disorders, 24*, 281–291.

Zappella, M., Gillberg, C., & Ehlers, S. (1998). The preserved speech variant: A subgroup of the Rett complex: A clinical report of 30 cases. *Journal of Autism and Developmental Disorders, 28*, 519–526.

Zappella, M., Meloni, I., Longo, I., Hayek, G., & Renieri, A. (2001). Preserved speech variants of the Rett syndrome: Molecular and clinical analysis. *American Journal of Medical Genetics, 104*, 14–22.

Zelazo, P. D., Burack, J. A., Benedetto, E., & Frye, D. (1996). Theory of mind and rule use in individuals with Down's syndrome: A test of the uniqueness and specificity claims. *Journal of Child Psychology and Psychiatry and Allied Disciplines, 37*, 479–484.

PART 6

Family and Context

Family Well-being and Children with Intellectual Disability

Laraine Masters Glidden

Abstract

This chapter examines the variability of parents' reactions to rearing children with intellectual and other developmental disabilities (IDD) in order to provide tentative conclusions regarding the factors that influence it. The intent is to update the review of published research, concentrating on the years since 1997 to avoid duplication with the 1998 reviews of Minnes and Shapiro et al. It highlights research with children with intellectual disability (ID), although evidence from studies of children with other developmental disabilities is included when it is conceptually and scientifically relevant. The chapter focuses on parental emotional responses and parent and family well-being, attending to positive emotions such as feelings of satisfaction, reward, pride, and happiness, as well as negative emotions such as depression, pessimism, anxiety, and anger.

Keywords: Intellectual disability, developmental disability, child-rearing, child care, parental emotional response, family well-being

People like him are there to show us something, they're not greedy, they don't want anything.
I wouldn't have missed having him for the world. (Quote from parent of son with profound impairments, Carr, 2005, p. 81)

Some days I feel like taking both babies in my arms and walking into the river. (Quote from parent of two children with profound intellectual disability, Garland, 1993, p. 68)

Parents have many stories; they are woven together in a tapestry of many hues from sorrow to joy. The fortunate ones grow to learn many things from the experience, learn to live life to the fullest and appreciate things that most people never even recognize. . . . (Quote from mother of a child with Rett syndrome, Hunter, 2002, p. 79)

The quotations that begin this chapter highlight the variability in reactions of parents to rearing children with intellectual and other developmental disabilities (IDD). This variability was highlighted in concluding remarks in two chapters in the first edition of this Handbook. Shapiro, Blacher, and Lopez (1998) wrote "family reaction to disability, and to mental retardation in particular, is highly variable, so that it is difficult and inaccurate to talk about 'families of children with retardation' in a general sense" (p. 625). Minnes (1998) similarly remarked, "Despite the wealth of information gathered during the past 30 years regarding the experiences of families with a developmentally disabled member, there is a surprising lack of consensus in the literature regarding the experiences of families of children with disabilities and the factors that contribute to successful coping and adaptation" (p. 704).

Although these conclusions emphasized variability of findings and lack of consensus in the empirical research, there were nonetheless also several noteworthy observations in these same chapters. They both acknowledged the importance of a developmental perspective and reviewed at least some research that was longitudinal in design (e.g., Blacher & Baker, 1994; Glidden, Kiphart, Willoughby, & Bush, 1993; Krauss & Seltzer, 1993). They also both recognized the family as a transactional system, with characteristics of the child with IDD influencing family members and family members influencing the characteristics of the child with IDD. Although both chapters considered adaptation and coping, Shapiro et al. quite explicitly summarized the move away from a pathology orientation to a much more complex conceptualization of adaptation, reflecting the growing realization that positive outcomes, rewards, and satisfactions had been too long ignored (Singer & Irvin, 1989; Trute & Hauch, 1988; Turnbull, Patterson, Behr, Murphy, Marquis, & Blue-Banning, 1993).

This emphasis on positive effects has continued, but not to the exclusion of a fully rounded view of both the satisfactions and difficulties of rearing a child with IDD. (Although see Cummins, 2001 for a different conclusion. He claims that the positive perspective has been overstated.) As I will document in this chapter, there is evidence of a continuum of effects, from the most adverse to the most beneficial, and some progress to understanding the basis of the variability in outcomes. One of the objectives of this chapter is to examine this variability and come to at least some tentative conclusions regarding the factors that influence it. The intent is to update the review of published research, concentrating on the years since 1997 to avoid duplication with the 1998 reviews of Minnes and Shapiro et al. I highlight research with children with intellectual disability (ID), although evidence from studies of children with other developmental disabilities is included when it is conceptually and scientifically relevant.

The focus is especially on parental emotional responses and parent and family well-being, attending to positive emotions, such as feelings of satisfaction, reward, pride, and happiness, as well as to negative emotions, such as depression, pessimism, anxiety, and anger. The emphasis is on parents and families with children rather than adults with disabilities, because another chapter in this volume focuses on later-life families. However, it is impossible to ignore the importance of a life-stage approach. Families are dynamic systems, and although some changes may seem haphazard and unpredictable, others are obviously systematic. The lives of parents and children are linked psychologically even after the children are adults (Greenfield & Marks, 2006). Thus, one of the goals of this chapter is to clarify the intensity and duration of emotional reactions and what precipitates them at different points in the family life cycle. Because mothers and fathers have frequently been studied separately, I plan to characterize the influences on each of them when appropriate, but also draw conclusions about the family as a whole.

Parents As Individuals
Positive Outcomes

Although there have been some reports of positive family outcomes for many years (e.g., Abbott & Meredith, 1986; Summers, Behr, & Turnbull, 1989; Trute & Hauch, 1988), the study of negative effects has dominated the field. Helff and Glidden (1998) reviewed research on family adjustment over a 20-year period, from the early 1970s to 1993 and concluded that, although the emphasis on negative outcomes had declined somewhat during this time period, there had been little increase in positive focus. In the ensuing years, models of stress and burden still dictated much of the research in parental adjustment to children with IDD, but more investigators began to include the measurement of positive outcomes in their assessments. This trend may have been accelerated by the positive psychology movement spearheaded by Martin Seligman when he was president of the American Psychological Association in 1998. Seligman guest-edited with Mihaly Csikszentmihalyi a special issue of the *American Psychologist* (Seligman & Csikszentmihalyi, 2000) devoted to articles on happiness, excellence, and optimal human functioning. Hastings and Taunt (2002) provided a review of research that directly measured positive perceptions and/or included at least some positive measures as one of their outcome variables. In studies using primarily qualitative designs, they were able to extract key themes such as growth in personal qualities (e.g., compassion, spirituality, confidence, purpose), experience of positive emotions (e.g., love, joy, satisfaction), and the development of new skills and social networks. Although the studies that Hastings and Taunt reviewed did not generally have comparison groups of families rearing children without disabilities, it is likely that these positive perceptions would characterize those families as well, suggesting that many of the positive aspects of parenting are present regardless of the child's abilities or disabilities.

It is useful to describe at some length a prototypical study cited in the Hastings and Taunt (2002) review. Scorgie and Sobsey (2000) used both a qualitative and quantitative design. They initially interviewed 15 parents about how their lives had changed because of the children with developmental disabilities (DD). The interview transcripts were qualitatively analyzed, resulting in nine themes, and three transformational outcomes—personal, relational, and perspectival—that they described. Subsequently, a survey was constructed with Likert-response items to explore these themes and outcomes with a different and larger sample of 80 parents. Although no comparison group was included in the survey, a comparison item did allow statistical testing. This item was: *to accept that my child's and family's outcome is entirely under the control of other people or external circumstance.* It represented a position that was opposite to the themes from the interview, and the prediction was that it would result in significantly less endorsement than the other items. This prediction was confirmed, and Scorgie and Sobsey concluded that parents perceive many positive life changes that result from rearing a child with a disability. Other investigators (Kearney & Griffin, 2001; Rehm & Bradley, 2005; Stainton & Besser, 1998) have come to similar conclusions.

I and my colleagues (Corrice & Glidden, 2009; Flaherty & Glidden, 2000; Glidden & Schoolcraft, 2003; Glidden, Bamberger, Turek, & Hill, 2010; Glidden, Billings, & Jobe, 2006; Glidden & Jobe, 2006, 2009; Jobe & Glidden, 2008) have studied positive and negative outcomes, using a research design that includes the unique comparison of families who have knowingly adopted children with IDDs and families with similar children born to them. Because the adoptive families were expecting positive outcomes, they were a frame that helped to illuminate those same outcomes in birth families. For example, in Flaherty and Glidden, we compared families who had knowingly adopted children with Down syndrome (DS) to families who were rearing their DS birth children. We reported that depression was low, and that family strengths, marital adjustment, and satisfaction with the child were high for both mothers and fathers, regardless of whether the child had been adopted by or born to the parents.

More recently, Trute and Hiebert-Murphy (2005) developed the Parenting Morale Index (PMI), designed to measure both positive and negative affect associated with daily parenting. Respondents, who were mothers and fathers who were receiving child disability services, were asked to endorse the extent to which they felt positive emotions such as optimism, contentment, and happiness, as well as negative emotions such as worry, frustration, and guilt. The PMI had adequate psychometric properties and predicted outcomes 1 year later for both mothers and fathers. Parents who more strongly endorsed experiencing positive emotions and less strongly endorsed experiencing negative ones, reported less stress and better family adjustment.

Well-being, frequently labeled *subjective well-being*, has been used as a summary measure in research studies, and it undoubtedly has both affective and cognitive components. Some scales have single items, e.g., "How do you feel about your life as a whole?," or "How do you feel about your life now?" Other scales have multiple items (Lucas, Diener, & Suh, 1996; Nachshen, Garcin, & Minnes, 2005). Diener (2000) reviewed recent work with this construct and concluded that personality and temperament, as well as actual life events and conditions, influence subjective well-being. If so, then parents with children with IDD should not systematically report lower well-being than would matched parents with children who do not have IDD as long as measurement is done long enough after diagnosis for the parents to have adapted to a changed life condition.

Although numerous studies report some type of well-being outcomes (e.g., Flaherty & Glidden, 2000; Hastings & Taunt, 2002; Nachshen & Minnes, 2005; Pakenham, Sofronoff, & Samios, 2004), definitive conclusions still elude us for varied reasons. Most important among them are that many studies do not include comparison samples of matched families rearing children without disabilities; when matched samples are included, sample sizes tend to be quite small and based on convenience; and the measurement of well-being is not standardized, with most investigators using different instruments (e.g., Duvdevany & Abboud, 2003; Glidden & Schoolcraft, 2007). Indeed, some investigators make the assumption that the absence of negative outcomes, such as low depression scores, is synonymous with well-being (Harris & McHale, 1989). However, it is far more likely that positive and negative reactions coexist and, although somewhat negatively correlated, are not polar opposites on the same continuum.

In an attempt to understand this coexistence, Grant and colleagues (Grant, Ramcharan, McGrath, Nolan, & Keady, 1998) administered two instruments—Carers' Assessment of Difficulties Index (CADI) and Carers' Assessment of Satisfactions Index (CASI). Although they found that satisfactions were more prevalent than stresses, they also reported a positive association between the two. One explanation that they offered for a seemingly contradictory finding is that the rewards were often based upon solving a problem satisfactorily—the development of mastery and control over an initially difficult situation. Perhaps we should not be too surprised at these results. After all, humanistic psychology has as one of its basic premises that human beings are motivated to become the best that they can be, or self-actualized (Maslow, 1968; Rogers, 1995). Despite being penetrated by the wounds and arrows of outrageous fortune, most not only survive, but also flourish. As humans, we endorse core values and principles and try to build a coherent life that adheres to these principles. Acting responsibly and confronting difficulties rather than ignoring or abandoning them is how we grow and self-actualize. Individuals who do this, then, would be aware of the negative aspects of rearing a child with IDD, but also would have achieved rewards and satisfactions from successfully adjusting to the situation. One mother, describing her husband's and her own reactions to the diagnosis of their child with DS, emphasized a sentiment consistent with this humanistic interpretation: "[T]his is a challenge that we have to meet, and we will do the best that we can to provide all that we can for him and to help him be all that he can be" (Poehlmann, Clements, Abbeduto, & Farsad, 2005, p. 262).

This Poehlmann et al. (2005) qualitative study reports results that are generally consistent with a humanistic view and with the results of Grant et al. (1998). Studying only 21 mothers of sons or daughters with either DS or fragile X syndrome, they documented both positive aspects of well-being as well as disruption and difficulties. Specifically, mothers focused on both positive and negative characteristics of their children. Positive themes included how well their children made connections with others, and their good humor and insightfulness. These positive attributes coexisted with a variety of challenging behaviors such as stubbornness, aggression, and anxiety.

In sum, there is little doubt that many families recognize that rearing a child with IDD will require adaptation and that, as a result of that adaptation, they may live a life that is atypical or unusual, but that has many positive aspects to it (Rehm & Bradley, 2005). Of course, they also recognize that the challenges are substantial and that negative outcomes may be more likely.

Negative Emotions

DEPRESSION

One of the most commonly measured emotional reactions to parenting children with IDD is depression.

It has been studied by many investigators in parents of young children soon after diagnosis (Eisenhower, Baker, & Blacher, 2005; Flaherty & Glidden, 2000) and throughout the family lifespan (Kim, Greenberg, Seltzer, & Krauss, 2003; Magaña, Schwartz, Rubert, & Szapocznik, 2006). Results from multiple research projects with diverse samples (Magaña & Smith, 2006; Blacher & McIntyre, 2006), and from different countries (Cho, Singer, & Brenner, 2000; Olsson & Hwang, 2001, 2003) come to the same conclusion: Depression is a common reaction of parents to the initial diagnosis of disability, but declines over time as families adjust and accommodate to an altered set of expectations and routines (Keogh, Garnier, Bernheimer, & Gallimore, 2000; Glidden & Schoolcraft, 2003; Glidden & Jobe, 2006). These findings from multiple studies converge with the conclusion from a meta-analysis of depression in mothers of children with and without IDD (Singer, 2006): Mothers of children with IDD experience significantly higher levels of depression than do mothers of children without IDD, but the effect moderates over time.

Glidden and Schoolcraft (2003) described this kind of trajectory over an 11-year period. Using the comparison design of adoptive and birth mothers described earlier, we found that, at initial diagnosis, birth mothers reported high depression scores in contrast to low depression of adoptive mothers when the child was first placed with the family. However, 5 and 11 years later, depression had declined substantially for the birth mothers, and their scores were no longer significantly different from those of adoptive mothers. Glidden and Jobe (2006) extended these results by an additional 6 years and found that depression remained low for both birth and adoptive mothers as their children approached adulthood. Results from the longitudinal research of Seltzer, Krauss, and colleagues (Krauss & Seltzer, 1998; Seltzer, Greenberg, Floyd, Pettee, & Hong, 2001) with parents of adult sons and daughters with ID corroborate this finding, with mean levels of maternal depression in the nonclinical range (e.g., Orsmond, Seltzer, Krauss, & Hong, 2003).

Because depression is, at least in part, a reaction to what is perceived as an adverse event, it may be amenable to change via interventions that change the perception of the event. Thus, intervention programs that focus on enhancing the development of children with IDD and improving family interactions could alleviate depression. Küçüker (2006) described such a program for children from

3–43 months of age in Ankara, Turkey. The Beck Depression Inventory was administered prior to the program and after its completion 8 months later. Data from 29 mothers and 27 fathers showed declines in BDI scores of approximately .5SD for both sets of parents over the 8-month interval. These results are promising with regard to the efficacy of early intervention for children, as well as an agent of change for parents. These changes may have altered the perceptions of parents, allowing them to view their children as more typical than atypical, or providing social or informational support in the form of other parents participating in the program. However, optimism must be tempered with the recognition that there was no control group. Given that the children were quite young at pretest, many of the parents might have been in the early stage of adjustment, when depression is a common reaction. Depression scores would have been expected to decline even without intervention during this 8-month interval.

OTHER NEGATIVE EMOTIONS

Although depression is by far the most frequently studied negative response of parents to a child with IDD, a variety of other negative emotions have been the subject of research. Anger, anxiety, and pessimism have all been investigated. Generally, the results conform to those found for depression. For example, Hodapp, Fidler, and Smith (1998) studied pessimism in parents of children with Smith-Magenis syndrome, a disorder caused by a deletion on the short arm of chromosome 17, and associated with ID and a variety of maladaptive behaviors. They found that pessimism, measured by a factor on the Friedrich Questionnaire on Resources and Stress, was higher in parents (mostly mothers) who were rearing children with lower levels of adaptive and higher levels of maladaptive behavior. Data from a similar study with parents of children with Prader-Willi syndrome (Hodapp, Dykens, & Masino, 1997) found that parental pessimism was significantly correlated with the child's internalizing behaviors, as well as with social and other problems.

In an intriguing program of research, Hall, Bobrow, and Marteau (2000) sampled parents who had prenatal testing but received reports that were falsely negative and later gave birth to babies with DS. Two to six years after the birth of their children, 179 mothers and 122 fathers were interviewed and assessments were conducted of their anxiety, depression, stress, attitudes toward the child, and the degree to which they blamed others. Parents were in one of three groups: they received a false negative prenatal serum test result; they were not offered a prenatal test; they were offered, but declined a test. Outcomes for all three groups were well within the normal ranges for levels of anxiety and depression, and there were no significant differences among groups on these two measures. However, parents who received false-negative results were more likely to report higher levels of parenting stress, hold more negative attitudes toward their child, and blame others for the child's condition than one or both of the other groups. Moreover, those parents who blamed others had generally poorer adjustment than those who did not. Hall and Marteau (2003) replicated the association between blame and poorer adjustment in a larger sample of mothers of children with DS.

In sum, individual positive and negative parental emotional response to developmental disability has been studied extensively since 1997. To a much greater degree than in earlier decades, this research has included measurement of positive emotions, although typically these positive emotions are conceptualized globally such as well-being or satisfaction, rather than individually such as joy, pride, and excitement. Nonetheless, most mothers and fathers do not live in isolation and therefore, in addition to studying parents individually, we must also consider them together. In the next section, I review research on the parental dyad and, in particular, the influence of rearing a child with IDD on marital adjustment and satisfaction.

The Parental Dyad: Marital Adjustment and Satisfaction

Original pathology-oriented views of the influence of a child with IDD on the family focused on marital strain, discord, and the likelihood of separation and divorce (Farber, 1959, 1960). Supposedly guilt-ridden parents blamed themselves and each other for the disability, and this psychological distress, compounded by the heavy burden of care, exacerbated strains and stresses that may have already been present in the marital relationship. The history of medical advice is replete with pediatricians warning parents that the child will "ruin their marriage," and recommending relinquishment. Although there has been some empirical literature to support this view of likely marital discord resulting from a child with IDD, it has been confirmed only in a much less extreme form. Particularly definitive is a meta-analysis by Risdal and Singer (2004). They included

13 empirical papers published between 1975 and 2003 that reported either divorce/separation rates or marital satisfaction/adjustment data from parents rearing children without and with disabilities such as ID, cerebral palsy, and autism. They combined the two types of measures to find a small effect size of $d = .21$, in favor of better adjustment by the parents of children without disabilities.

Some other studies, but not all, published in 1997 or later support this conclusion. For example, Joesch and Smith (1997) reported that children's chronic poor health or disability is associated with higher risk of divorce, but only for children with cerebral palsy, and not developmental delay. Reichman, Corman, and Noonan (2004) focused not on divorce only, but on whether the parents were living together and were more or less involved in their relationship. Children's poor health, measured as birthweight less than 4 pounds, a physical disability or ID, or not achieving developmental milestones, decreased the likelihood that parents would be married or cohabiting and increased the likelihood of lower involvement in the 12–18 months after the birth. They acknowledged, however, that although large, their sample was urban and not nationally representative, thus limiting the generalizability of the results. In contrast, moreover, Urbano and Hodapp (2007) found a slightly *lower* divorce rate for parents of children with DS, in comparison to those of children without disabilities.

A few studies have attempted to understand the relation between marital adjustment and children with disabilities. Willoughby and Glidden (1995) found that in 48 married couples rearing at least one child with DD, both mothers and fathers reported higher levels of marital adjustment when fathers participated more in child care. In fact, it was the only predictor of maternal marital satisfaction in a regression analysis that included family income, child level of functioning, amount of work outside the home, and maternal education. However, these data were somewhat limited because the measure of father participation was reported by mothers, and clearly could reflect maternal perceptions that might be biased by the mothers' views of the marital relationship.

Simmerman, Blacher, and Baker (2001) examined paternal level of involvement with the child, maternal satisfaction with paternal involvement, and the subsequent effects of paternal involvement on marital adjustment and caretaking burden. A total of 60 parents, all of whom were raising a child with severe ID, completed a variety of independent,

self-report measures during an in-home interview. The results revealed that two-thirds of all fathers were actively involved in playing with the child, nurturing the child, discipline, and child-related decision-making. On the other hand, only one-third of fathers were actively involved in feeding and dressing the child. Interestingly, fathers' actual level of involvement was not a significant predictor of mothers' burden. Rather, mothers' satisfaction with fathers' involvement, which was only moderately correlated with the actual paternal involvement, did significantly predict mothers' caretaking burden and mothers' marital adjustment. Thus, family functioning is most significantly influenced by a mother's satisfaction with the caretaking support she receives from the father.

Stoneman and Gavidia-Payne (2006) were also interested in explaining individual differences in marital adjustment, and focused on maternal and paternal coping strategies and daily stressors/hassles as predictors of marital adjustment scores. Their results supported the importance of using a family systems approach to understanding individual outcomes. They found that both mothers and fathers reported lower marital adjustment if they had more hassles. In addition, fathers who used more problem-focused coping reported higher marital adjustment, as did their wives. Maternal problem-focused coping did not significantly predict marital adjustment for either themselves or their husbands. These results are consistent with those of Simmerman et al. (2001), who found that mothers who perceived their husbands as more involved with child caretaking also had higher marital adjustment scores. Fathers who use problem-focused coping strategies are likely to be more involved with their children and families, in contrast to those who might use avoidance, denial, and distancing, all emotion-focused strategies that are generally associated with more negative outcomes.

In sum, based on the most recent research, as well as on studies reported earlier, the conclusion of previous reviewers (Glidden & Schoolcraft, 2007; Shapiro et al., 1998) appears to remain accurate: There is a small risk that marital adjustment will be lower for parents rearing a child with IDD rather than a child without IDD. However, many parents report positive effects on their relationships with their spouses, and these positive aspects of the changes in marital quality have not been studied extensively or systematically. Thus, this aspect of family well-being continues to be salient and in need of additional investigation, using a variety of methodologies that should include paper-and-pencil measures, direct observation, and large-*n* studies of divorce/separation rates.

The Family Unit

In the first edition of this handbook, Minnes was optimistic about the research moving toward a more systemic and transactional focus. The intervening 10 years have not justified this optimism. Glidden and Schoolcraft (2007) concluded that there was no widely accepted theory of family functioning, and therefore standards of healthy families were lacking. Without either one, it is difficult to diagnose dysfunction except in extreme cases. We also observed that the research on impact and functioning in families rearing children with IDD is mostly from the perspective of individual family members using self-report methodology. This research has serious limitations, and after reviewing it, we reached the conclusion that there was no reason to reject the null hypothesis with regard to systems characteristics of families with and without children with IDD. However, very few controlled studies have been completed and published.

Family Quality of Life

The quality-of-life concept, originally formulated with regard to individuals with disabilities, has been extended to families (Poston, Turnbull, Park, Mannan, Marquis, & Wang, 2003; Turnbull, Brown, & Turnbull, 2004). This work has a lot of promise, and it is important that it benefit from the mistakes of previous family-oriented measurement. Of necessity, if it is to be a true indication of family quality of life, it must first clearly define and determine who is a family member and then calibrate and in some way combine the data from individual family members, rather than rely on a single reporter, as is frequently done (e.g., Wheeler, Skinner, & Bailey, 2008).

Poston et al. (2003) grapple with these challenges in their qualitative study aimed at formulating domains of family quality of life, and suggesting indicators for each domain. In their conceptualization, the family defines its own membership. This strategy is problematic in a number of ways. It introduces substantial variance, and this variance is not likely to be random. Rather, the inclusion and exclusion of family members may be strongly related to family quality of life. Poston et al. does recognize the difference between individually and family-oriented family quality of life and recommends that the former be aggregated in some way to produce the latter.

A reliable and valid technique for combination is essential to move measurement forward, but thus far no published research has presented data on quality of life that is truly a family measure (Aznar & Castoñón, 2005; Jokinen & Brown, 2005; Summers et al., 2005).

Predicting Positive and Negative Outcomes

Even the earliest research studying parental emotional responses to a child with IDD attempted to explore individual differences. Farber (1959, 1960), for example, hypothesized that family integration was influenced by characteristics of the child such as age, sex, and degree of dependence; and by characteristics of the parents such as religious affiliation, social status, and degree of community participation. Shapiro et al. (1998), in the first edition of this handbook, reviewed multiple predictors and correlates of maternal adaptation to child disability. Based on the extant evidence, they were unable to draw conclusions about the role of child age, sex, or degree or type of child disability. Similarly, socioeconomic status (SES), maternal age, maternal employment, and marital SES were not consistently related to either more positive or more negative well-being. On the other hand, a number of investigators had linked various kinds of positive family functioning, such as adaptability and cohesion, with better individual well-being. Also, Shapiro et al. concluded that there was ample evidence for the positive effects of social support. In the ensuing decade, considerable additional research has been devoted to predicting individual differences, and some progress has been made.

Time Since, and Until, Diagnosis

The first few decades of research on family reaction to disability used mostly cross-sectional or retrospective methods to study parental reaction. Exceptions, such as the work of Ann Gath (1977, 1993) and Janet Carr (2005), both with families of children with DS, were notable. Cross-sectional and retrospective data are likely to be weaker than prospective and longitudinal data, and their methodological limitations may result in misleading conclusions. Most importantly, retrospective methods rely on memory, notoriously fragmented and selective, especially after long periods of time. Cross-sectional data, of course, represent only a small slice of experience in what is an ongoing and dynamic process. Because of the need for large and continuing resources, long-term longitudinal research projects, especially those with substantial samples, are dependent on stable funding sources. Some of these longitudinal studies have been funded in recent years, and their results are important in understanding the time course of parental emotional reactions.

There is little doubt that initial reactions to the recognition and/or diagnosis of disability are more likely to be negative and that most families are likely to demonstrate improved adjustment over time (Glidden & Schoolcraft, 2003; Glidden & Jobe, 2006, 2009; Poehlmann et al., 2005). Time until diagnosis is also a factor in determining the family experience. Some conditions, like DS, are diagnosed early, whereas others may take years before a definitive diagnosis is made. In the Poehlmann et al. study the mothers of children with fragile X syndrome talked about the difficulties they had in dealing with the uncertainty of the child's condition, and several mothers actually found that the diagnosis was a relief. This same diagnostic certainty also benefited mothers of children with DS in comparison to mothers of children with ID for unknown reasons (Lenhard, Breitenback, Ebert, Schindelhauer-Deutscher, & Henn, 2005). The mothers who received a certain diagnosis of DS reported lower levels of anxiety, worry, regret, and general emotional strain.

Demographic Characteristics

Shapiro et al. (1998) were unable to reject the null hypothesis with regard to the influences of SES, parental age, or culture/ethnicity on parental reactions to rearing children with DD. The situation has not changed more than a decade later. Generally, the research methods that have been used by family researchers have not been amenable to studying these variables. Although samples have frequently been diverse with regard to SES and racial/ethnic composition, they have been mostly small samples and convenient, whereas large population-based data sets are more appropriate to study demographic characteristics. Population-based research has been done to estimate the prevalence of IDD in different SES and racial/ethnic groups (Avchen, Bhasin, Braun, & Yeargin-Allsopp, 2007), but not to ascertain the parental or family reaction to it. However, the increasing interest in developmental epidemiology (Hodapp & Urbano, 2007) should translate to more use of these techniques in the next decade.

Child Behavior Problems

There seems to be little doubt at this point that child behavior problems result in a variety of negative outcomes for parents (Baker, Blacher, Crnic, & Edelbrock, 2002; Baker, McIntyre, Blacher, Crnic, Edelbrock, & Low, 2003; Hastings, 2003; Hastings & Brown, 2002; Ricci & Hodapp, 2003). There also seems little doubt that children with IDD are at greater risk for behavior problems than are children without IDD (Baker et al., 2002; Douma, Dekker, & Koot, 2006). Several published studies from an ongoing longitudinal project comparing delayed and nondelayed children have consistently reported this finding. Baker et al. found significantly higher total Child Behavior Checklist (CBCL) scores for delayed than for nondelayed 3-year-olds. Moreover, behavior problems accounted for more than triple the variance in maternal negative impact scores and more than quadruple the variance in paternal negative impact than did intellectual functioning. A year later, Baker et al. (2003) reported follow-up information for these children. Findings were similar. Mother and father reports were stable over time, and parents reported more behavior problems among the children with delays than among those without. Most importantly for this conclusion, they found that increases in behavior problems over the 1-year period were associated with increases in negative impact scores (although, interestingly, not decreases in positive impact). As with Baker et al. (2002), it was behavior problems, not delay per se, that was associated much more strongly with negative outcomes.

Floyd and Gallagher (1997) reported similar results with different samples of children with and without behavior problems, ID, or chronic illness. For a wide range of negative reactions, including depression, they found that behavior problems alone or in conjunction with ID or chronic illness resulted in significantly more negative impact than did either condition without behavior problems. Moreover, families with children with behavior problems were heavier users of a variety of community support services, indicating that these diagnosed conditions have implications that go far beyond the family.

My colleagues and I have corroborated these findings in a sample of families with 1,865 children adopted from the child welfare system in Florida. We found that both internalizing and externalizing behavior problems mediated the relation between learning disorders and parental satisfaction with the adoption. When the variable of child behavior problems was used to predict parental satisfaction, the previously significant effect of learning disorders was reduced and no longer significant

(Nalavany, Glidden, & Ryan, 2009). This replication in an adoptive sample expands the strength and scope of the effect, as adoptive families who made a voluntary decision to rear a child with special needs are likely to be better prepared for a difficult child than are birth families.

Beck, Hastings, Daley and Stevenson (2004) also reported that behavior problems in children with IDD resulted in more negative outcomes for mothers. However, their measure of negative outcome was the total score of the Parenting Stress Index-Short Form (Abidin, 1990). Because this scale contains items that are child behavior problems, their results may be little more than one measure of behavior problems correlating with a different measure of behavior problems.

Given the preponderance of evidence, it is time for the field to advance beyond merely demonstrating that child behavior problems are linked to more negative parental outcomes. Certainly, much remains to be done in terms of understanding this cause–effect relation and designing interventions to attack it. Interventions might target the behavior problems, the parental reaction to them, or the link between the two. Thus, successful interventions could reduce the problems, shift the parental reaction, and/or disentangle the reaction from the problem behavior.

However, the design of successful interventions is dependent on far more detailed information about all three aspects of this relation. First, we need to know a lot more about the behavior problems themselves. What triggers them? How are their intensities and durations maintained or reduced? Are some behaviors more probable for some types of disability? Relevant to this last question is the promising study of the topographies of maladaptive behaviors (Dykens, 1999), which has accelerated in recent years. For example, the Rebruary 2011 issue of the *Journal of Intellectual Disability Research* focused on mental health and intellectual disability and included several articles on maladaptive behavioral phenotypes (e.g., Arron, Oliver, Moss, Berg, & Burbridge, 2011; Teixeira, Emerich, Orsati, Rimério, Gatto, Chappaz, & Kim, 2011; and others). The results of these studies and others like them have clear implications for our understanding of the etiology of behavior problems and also for their treatment. In addition to understanding the behavior problems, we must also learn more about the parental responses to them. Elements of these responses include how parents think about the causes of the behavior problems. Investigation based on attribution theory has found that when the source of the condition is uncontrollable (i.e., a child with IDD), the person usually will have an attitude of pity, lack of anger, and help-giving. When the source of the condition is thought to be controllable (i.e., a child behaving poorly), anger is the typical response (Weiner, Perry, & Magnusson, 1988). When the child who is behaving poorly has IDD, his or her poor behavior might actually be "excused" as uncontrollable because of the disability. Chavira, López, Blacher, and Shapiro (2000) reported results consistent with this prediction in a sample of Latina mothers. Mothers of children and adolescents with severe to profound ID were interviewed about the problematic behaviors of their sons and daughters, and completed a measure about whether the children were responsible for these behaviors. The mothers also reported their emotional reactions when the problem behaviors occurred. Mothers reported significantly more negative emotions such as anger, desperation, frustration, sadness and embarrassment, when they indicated that the child was responsible for the problem behavior than when the child was not responsible for the behavior.

Despite the conclusive main effect of behavior problems and parental response, there are individual differences among parents. One source of difference is parental disposition, which can moderate the relation between behavior problems and well-being. Baker, Blacher, and Olsson (2005) found that mothers (but not fathers) with high levels of optimism in comparison to those with low levels of optimism, reported lower depression and negative impact, and more positive marital adjustment even when children had high levels of behavior problems. These results are consistent with other findings on dispositional optimism and adjustment (Chang, 1998).

Parental Personality

Shapiro et al. (1998) concluded that internal locus of control, hardiness, and positive appraisal of the situation were all associated with increased well-being. Additional research relating personality to adjustment has extended these earlier findings. With regard to emotions, it is well documented that individuals differ in the intensity and quality of their emotional reactivity. For example, a woman may be warm and affectionate, love large gatherings and be gregarious in them, enjoy being busy and active, and feel mostly positive emotions such as joy and enthusiasm. Such a person would tend to experience positive emotions more than negative ones, and would experience these emotions somewhat intensively. She would score high on a personality variable of Extraversion (Costa & McCrae, 1992). In contrast, another woman may be vulnerable to anxiety and depression, easily stressed, quick to anger, and frequently react with hostility to others. She would score high on a personality variability of Neuroticism. Personality influences the ways in which individuals respond to events in their lives, including the adaptation to a child with IDD.

I and my colleagues have demonstrated this relation with regard to both depression and subjective well-being. In Glidden and Schoolcraft (2003), mothers who had either knowingly adopted or given birth to children with DD and were participating in a longitudinal study provided data on personality, depression, and subjective well-being related to the child. For both adoptive and birth mothers, the personality variable of neuroticism significantly predicted depression scores, even after controlling for earlier levels of depression. Thus, mothers who scored higher on neuroticism also reported higher levels of depression. This was not, however, the case for subjective well-being related to the child. For birth mothers only, higher levels of agreeableness—i.e., individuals who were more trusting, altruistic, and compliant—predicted significantly more positive regard for the child. This pattern of results suggests the importance of measuring different constructs related to family adaptation, recognizing that adaptation is a multidimensional and complex process, linked to many variables that may influence it in different ways. One of these variables that has received some attention from family researchers in the last decade is parental coping strategies.

Parental Coping Strategies and Styles

Research on coping has generally demonstrated that individuals who use coping strategies that have focused on problem solving and social support have reported more positive adjustment outcomes, in contrast to those with relatively high use of strategies that have focused on denial, escape, and avoidance of difficulties (Altshuler & Ruble, 1989; Levy-Shiff, Dimitrovsky, Shulman, & Har-Even, 1998; Reichman, Miller, Gordon, & Hendricks-Munoz, 2000). Although there has not been complete consistency across studies with samples of parents rearing children with IDD, the findings generally show a similar pattern (Abbeduto, Seltzer, Shattuck, Krauss, Orsmond & Murphy, 2004; Essex, Seltzer & Krauss, 1999; Glidden et al.,

2006; Judge, 1998; Stoneman & Gavidia-Payne, 2006).

Although individual differences in the use of coping strategies have not been studied extensively, a few investigators have compared mothers and fathers. Both mothers and fathers report using problem-focused coping to a much greater extent than emotion-focused coping (Glidden et al., 2006), and differences between mothers and fathers in their use of these two types of strategies seem to be small and often not significant (Abbeduto et al., 2004; Stoneman & Gavidia-Payne, 2006). However, Essex et al. (1999) reported that mothers used more problem-focused strategies than did fathers, and Glidden et al. (2006) also reported small but statistically significant differences as a function of parental role. Mothers described seeking social support more than did fathers for two different coping events. Mothers also reported using more problem solving strategies than did fathers, but only for one of two coping situations.

The comparison of mothers and fathers is one small dimension of the overall debate with regard to degree to which coping is determined by context (i.e., state-related) versus determined by individual preference or style (i.e., trait-related; Lazarus, Lazarus, Campos, Tennen, & Tennen, 2006). In adults more generally, it has been demonstrated that personality is strongly related to the use of coping strategies. In a summary of much of the research linking personality and coping, Costa, Somerfield, and McCrae (1996) concluded that each of the five personality factors—Neuroticism, Extraversion, Openness, Agreeableness, and Conscientiousness—is related to some facets of coping. Neuroticism, for example, was strongly related to emotion-focused coping mechanisms that were generally ineffective, whereas Extraversion was associated with rational action, positive thinking, and seeking support. In parents of children with IDD, Glidden et al. (2006) reported that, even after controlling for the effect of personality traits, coping strategies still predicted depression and subjective well-being for both mothers and fathers. For example, for mothers, escape-avoidance coping predicted higher levels of depression, and positive reappraisal predicted higher levels of subjective well-being. Subjective well-being was higher for fathers when they used more planful problem solving and less distancing.

Although the two global dimensions of problem- versus emotion-focused coping may be a simple way to summarize coping strategies, their use also poses some problems. For example, in the widely used

Ways of Coping (Folkman & Lazarus, 1988), the factor of Seeking Social Support has both problem- and emotion-focused facets. Moreover, at least one emotion-focused strategy in the Ways of Coping inventory, Positive Reappraisal, has been associated with good adjustment (Glidden et al., 2006), in contrast to the generally adverse outcomes associated with other emotion-focused strategies. Hastings, Allen, McDermott, and Still (2002), using the F-COPES, also reported that the strategy of Reframing, similar to Positive Reappraisal, was associated with a variety of positive perceptions in mothers of children with IDD.

The study of coping suffers from problems similar to those present in the measurement of other facets of family well-being. It is difficult to compare results across research studies because different investigators often use different instruments to operationalize the construct of coping. Indeed, confusion exists because many investigators have used the term *coping* generically, as a response to stress, and have not standardized its measurement. For example, Scorgie, Wilgosh, and McDonald (1998) reviewed 25 studies that they classified as stress and coping, but very few of the studies actually directly measured coping as a process. Rather, it was assumed that coping was more effective when respondents reported lower levels of stress.

Discussion
Advances
Progress has been made in the years since the first edition of this handbook. The three most important developments in these years have been the continuing shift away from a pathology-only orientation to a more nuanced understanding of both the positive and negative emotional reactions in parents, the confirmation of the role of child maladaptive behavior in influencing those parental responses, and the increased emphasis on a lifespan approach in understanding the dynamic and transactional nature of the impact of child disability on parents.

Limitations
Despite the decade of progress, much remains to be done. Advances are often haphazard rather than systematic, and they will continue to be so until agreement is reached on fundamental research issues. Foremost is that learning more about parental responses requires standardizing construct measurement. Whereas the Achenbach Child Behavior Checklist (1991) seems to have emerged as a gold standard for the measurement of behavior problems,

no instruments have similar status in the measurement of parental emotional responses. Indeed, the constructs to be measured span a wide range and, frequently, inventories are used that clearly mix constructs (Glidden, 1993). Notably, Glidden and Schoolcraft (2007), reviewing research on family demands, burden, and stress, identified 25 articles that had been published from 1997 to 2002 in three leading journals that publish research related to ID: *American Journal on Mental Retardation* (now *American Journal on Intellectual and Developmental Disabilities*), *Journal on Intellectual Disability Research,* and *Mental Retardation* (now *Intellectual and Developmental Disabilities*). The most frequently used instrument was used in only 16% of the articles, and 19 different instruments were used to operationalize one or more of these constructs. Glidden and Schoolcraft concluded that it was impossible, therefore, to determine the reason for inconsistent results. Measurement differences could almost never be eliminated as a possible explanation.

Another difficulty related to definition and measurement is the problem of the level of analysis. Cook and Kenny (2006) argue cogently that individual self-report assessments that purport to measure dyadic or family factors must account for variance, in addition to that which explains individual-level characteristics. If the assessments at the dyadic or family levels do not contribute significant variance, then even though an individual is supposedly rating a marriage or a family, the assessment can only be interpreted as being at the level of the individual.

Although we must standardize measurement, we must also recognize that the complexity of families and lives means that we should be far-ranging in deciding what to measure. A Swedish study demonstrated that a small percentage of parents with DS children had very high job absentee rates, mostly the result of the sickness of their children, and that these same parents had a lower sense of coherence than did parents with lower missed days of work (Hedow, Wikblad, & Annerén, 2006). Although this study did not establish cause and effect, it did establish the far-ranging implications of caring for a child with a disability.

Conclusion
Hurley and Levitas (2004) reinvoke the Olshansky (1962) concept of chronic sorrow as they describe elements that should be included in therapy for parents of individuals with IDD. However, they do so

with a 21st-century sensibility. They recommend that, when professionals engage parents, they should do so in a balanced way, being certain to focus on strengths and not just problems, on praise for parent efforts, not just prescriptions—whether pharmaceutical or psychological. Their argument for balance, however, is countered by the cautionary conclusions of Cummins (2001) in a review of the subjective well-being of caretakers. He points out that much of the research emphasizing the positive aspects of caretaking is fueled by economic rationalism because family caretaking is less expensive than institutional care. The research, he argues, tends to exaggerate positive influences on the caretaking family. Many investigators assume that because caretakers do report some rewards, that therefore family quality of life is not compromised in comparison to persons who are not caretakers. Cummins' caution is well-advised, but it should not be rationalism that leads us to definitive answers. Effects on quality of life and other outcomes are researchable issues. Answers will come only from well-controlled research with large samples of multiple family members that examine a full range of outcomes, both positive and negative, over the lifespan. We have made progress, but are still inching our way to understanding an impact that is complex and dynamic.

Acknowledgments

The preparation of this manuscript was supported, in part, by Grant No. HD 21993 from NICHD to Laraine Glidden, and by St. Mary's College of Maryland.

References

Abbeduto, L., Seltzer, M. M., Shattuck, P., Krauss, M. W., Orsmond, G., & Murphy, M. M. (2004). Psychological well-being and coping in mothers of youths with autism, Down syndrome, or fragile X syndrome. *American Journal on Mental Retardation, 109*, 237–254.

Abidin, R. R. (1990). *Parenting stress index—manual* (3rd ed.). Charlottesville, VA: Pediatric Psychology Press.

Abbott, D. A., & Meredith, W. H. (1986). Strengths of parents with retarded children. *Family Relations, 35*, 371–375.

Achenbach T. (1991). *Manual for the child behavior checklist 4–18*. Burlington, VT: University of Vermont, Department of Psychiatry.

Arron, K., Oliver, C., Moss, J., Berg, K., & Burbridge, C. (2011). The prevalence and phenomenology of self-injurious and aggressive behavior in genetic syndromes. *Journal of Intellectual Disability Research, 55*, 109–120.

Altshuler, J. L., & Ruble, D. N. (1989). Developmental changes in children's awareness of strategies for coping with uncontrollable stress. *Child Development, 60*, 1337–1349.

Avchen, R. N., Bhasin, T. K., Braun, K. V. N., & Yeargin-Allsopp, M. (2007). Public health impact: Metropolitan Atlanta developmental disabilities surveillance program. In R. C. Urbano, & R. M. Hodapp (Eds.), *International review of research in mental retardation* Vol. 33 (pp. 149–190). San Diego: Elsevier.

Aznar, A. S., & Castañón, D. G. (2005). Quality of life from the point of view of Latin American families: A participative research study. *Journal of Intellectual Disability Research, 49*, 784–788.

Baker, B. L., Blacher, J., Crnic, K. A., & Edelbrock, C. (2002). Behavior problems and parenting stress in families of three-year-old children with and without developmental delays. *American Journal on Mental Retardation, 107*, 433–444.

Baker, B. L., Blacher, J., & Olsson, M. B. (2005). Preschool children with and without developmental delay: Behaviour problems, parents' optimism and well-being. *Journal of Intellectual Disability Research, 49*, 575–590.

Baker, B. L., McIntyre, L. L., Blacher, J., Crnic, K., Edelbrock, C., & Low, C. (2003). Pre-school children with and without developmental delay: Behaviour problems and parenting stress over time. *Journal of Intellectual Disability Research, 47*, 217–230.

Beck, A., Hastings, R. P., Daley, D., & Stevenson, J. (2004). Pro-social behaviour and behaviour problems independently predict maternal stress. *Journal of Intellectual & Developmental Disability, 29*, 339–349.

Blacher, J, & Baker, B. L. (1994). Out-of-home placement for children with retardation: Family decision-making and satisfaction. *Family Relations, 43*, 10–15.

Blacher, J., & McIntyre, L. L. (2006). Syndrome specificity and behavioral disorders in young adults with intellectual disability: Cultural differences in family impact. *Journal of Intellectual Disability Research, 50*, 184–198.

Carr, J. (2005). Families of 30–35-year olds with Down's syndrome. *Journal of Applied Research in Intellectual Disabilities, 18*, 75–84.

Chang, E. C. (1998). Dispositional optimism and primary and secondary appraisal of a stressor: Controlling for confounding influences and relations to coping and psychological and physical adjustment. *Journal of Personality and Social Psychology, 74*, 1109–1120.

Chavira, V., López, S. R., Blacher, J., & Shapiro, J. (2000). Latina mothers' attributions, emotions, and reactions to the problem behaviors of their children with developmental disabilities. *Journal of Child Psychology & Psychiatry & Allied Disciplines, 41*, 245–252.

Cho, S., Singer, G. H. S., & Brenner, M. (2000). Adaptation and accommodation to young children with disabilities: A comparison of Korean and Korean American parents. *Topics in Early Childhood Special Education, 20*, 236–249.

Cook, W. L., & Kenny, D. A. (2006). Examining the validity of self-report assessments of family functioning: A question of the level of analysis. *Journal of Family Psychology, 20*, 209–216.

Corrice, A. M., & Glidden, L. M. (2009). The Down syndrome advantage: Fact or fiction? *American Journal on Intellectual and Developmental Disabilities, 114*, 254–268.

Costa, P. T., & McCrae, R. (1992). *Revised NEO Personality Inventory (NEO- PI-R) and NEO Five Factor Inventory (NEO-FFI) professional manual*. Odessa, FL: Psychological Assessment Resources.

Costa, P., Somerfield, M., & McCrae, R. (1996). Personality and coping: A reconceptualization. In M. Zeidner, & N. S. Endler (Eds.), *Handbook of coping* (pp. 44–61). New York: John Wiley.

Cummins, R. A. (2001). The subjective well-being of people caring for a family member with a severe disability at home: A review. *Journal of Intellectual & Developmental Disability, 26*, 83–100.

Diener, E. (2000). Subjective well-being: The science of happiness and a proposal for a national index. *American Psychologist, 55*, 34–43.

Douma, J. C. H., Dekker, M. C., & Koot, H. M. (2006). Supporting parents of youths with intellectual disabilities and psychopathology. *Journal of Intellectual Disability Research, 50*, 570–581.

Duvdvany, I., & Abboud, S. (2003). Stress, social support and well-being of Arab mothers of children with intellectual disability who are served by welfare services in northern Israel. *Journal of Intellectual Disability Research, 47*, 264–272.

Dykens, E. M. (1999). Direct effects of genetic mental retardation syndromes: Maladaptive behavior and psychopathology. In L. M. Glidden (Ed.), *International review of research in mental retardation* Vol. 22 (pp. 1–26). San Diego: Academic Press.

Eisenhower, A. S., Baker, B. L., & Blacher, J. (2005). Preschool children with intellectual disability: Syndrome specificity, behaviour problems, and maternal well-being. *Journal of Intellectual Disability Research, 49*, 657–671.

Essex, E. L., Seltzer, M. M., & Krauss, M. W. (1999). Differences in coping effectiveness and well-being among aging mothers and fathers of adults with mental retardation. *American Journal on Mental Retardation, 104*, 545–563.

Farber, B. (1959). Effects of a severely mentally retarded child on family integration. *Monographs of the Society for Research in Child Development, 24*(2, Serial No. 71).

Farber, B. (1960). Family organization and crisis: Maintenance of integration in families with a severely mentally retarded child. *Monographs of the Society for Research in Child Development, 25* (1, Serial No. 75).

Flaherty, E. M., & Glidden, L. M. (2000). Positive adjustment in parents rearing children with Down syndrome. *Early Education & Development, 11*, 407–422.

Floyd, F. J., & Gallagher, E. M. (1997). Parental stress, care demands, and use of support services for school-age children with disabilities and behavior problems. *Family Relations, 46*, 359–371.

Folkman, S., & Lazarus, R. (1988). *Ways of coping questionnaire sampler set.* Palo Alto, CA: Mind Garden.

Garland, C. W. (1993). Beyond chronic sorrow: A new understanding of family adaptation. In A. Turnbull, D. Murphy, J. Patterson, J. Marquis, S. Behr, & M. Blue Banning (Eds.), *Cognitive coping, families, & disability* (pp.67–80). Baltimore: Paul H. Brookes.

Gath, A. (1977). The impact of an abnormal child upon the parents. *The British Journal of Psychiatry, 130*, 405–410.

Gath, A. (1993). Changes that occur in families as children with intellectual disability grow up. *International Journal of Disability, Development and Education, 40*, 167–174.

Glidden, L. M. (1993). What we do *not* know about families with children who have developmental disabilities: Questionnaire on Resources and Stress as a case study. *American Journal on Mental Retardation, 97*, 481–495.

Glidden, L. M., Bamberger, K. T., Turek, K. C., & Hill, K. L. (2010). Predicting mother/father-child interactions: Parental personality and well-being, socioeconomic variables and child disability status. *Journal of Applied Research in Intellectual Disabilities, 23*, 3–13.

Glidden, L. M., Billings, F. J., & Jobe, B. M. (2006). Personality, coping style and well-being of parents rearing children with developmental disabilities. *Journal of Intellectual Disability Research, 50*, 949–962.

Glidden, L. M. & Jobe, B. M. (2006). The longitudinal course of depression in adoptive and birth mothers of children with intellectual disabilities. *Journal of Policy and Practice in Intellectual Disabilities, 3*, 139–142.

Glidden, L. M., & Jobe, B. M. (2009). By choice or by chance: Longitudinal perspectives on resilience and vulnerability in adoptive and birth parents of children with developmental disabilities. In L. M. Glidden & M. M. Seltzer (Eds.), *International review of research in mental retardation* (pp. 61–93). San Diego: Academic Press/Elsevier.

Glidden, L. M., Kiphart, M., Willoughby, J., & Bush, B. (1993). Family functioning when rearing children with developmental disabilities. In A. Turnbull, D. Murphy, J. Patterson, J. Marquis, S. Behr, & M. Blue Banning (Eds.), *Cognitive coping, families, & disability* (pp.183–194). Baltimore: Paul H. Brookes.

Glidden, L. M., & Schoolcraft, S. A. (2003). Depression: its trajectory and correlates in mothers rearing children with intellectual disability. *Journal of Intellectual Disability Research, 47*, 250–263.

Glidden, L. M., & Schoolcraft, S. A. (2007). Family assessment and social support. In J.W. Jacobson, J. A. Mulick, & J. Rojahn (Eds.) *Handbook of intellectual and developmental disabilities* (pp. 391–422). New York: Springer.

Grant, G., Ramcharan, P., McGrath, M., Nolan, M., & Keady, J. (1998). Rewards and gratifications among family caregivers: Towards a refined model of caring and coping. *Journal of Intellectual Disability Research, 42*, 58–71.

Greenfield, E. A., & Marks, N. F. (2006). Linked lives: Adult children's problems and their parents' psychological and relational well-being. *Journal of Marriage and Family, 68*, 442–454.

Hall, S., Bobrow, M., & Marteau, T. M. (2000). Psychological consequences for parents of false negative results on prenatal screening for Down's syndrome: Retrospective interview study. *British Medical Journal, 320*, 407–412.

Hall, S., & Marteau, T. M. (2003). Causal attributions and blame: Associations with mothers' adjustment to the birth of a child with Down syndrome. *Psychology, Health & Medicine, 8*, 415–423.

Harris, V. S., & McHale, S. M. (1989). Family life problems, daily caregiving activities, and the psychological well-being of mothers of mentally retarded children. *American Journal on Mental Retardation, 94*, 231–239.

Hastings, R. P. (2003). Child behaviour problems and partner mental health as correlates of stress in mothers and fathers of children with autism. *Journal of Intellectual Disability Research, 47*, 231–237.

Hastings, R. P., Allen, R., McDermott, K., & Still, D. (2002). Factors related to positive perceptions in mothers of children with intellectual disabilities. *Journal of Applied Research in Intellectual Disabilities, 15*, 269–275.

Hastings, R. P., & Brown, T. (2002). Behavior problems of children with autism, parental self-efficacy, and mental health. *American Journal on Mental Retardation, 107*, 222–232.

Hastings, R. P., & Taunt, H. (2002). Positive perceptions in families of children with developmental disabilities. *American Journal on Mental Retardation, 107*, 116–127.

Hedov, G., Wikblad, K., & Annerén, G. (2006). Sickness absence in Swedish parents of children with Down's syndrome: Relation to self-perceived health, stress and sense of coherence. *Journal of Intellectual Disability Research, 50*, 546–552.

Helff, C., & Glidden, L. M. (1998). More positive or less negative? Trends in research on adjustment of families rearing children. *Mental Retardation, 36*, 457–465.

Hodapp, R. M., Dykens, E. M., & Masino, L. L. (1997). Families of children with Prader-Willi syndrome: Stress-support and relations to child characteristics. *Journal of Autism and Developmental Disorders, 27*, 11–24.

Hodapp, R. M., Fidler, D. J., & Smith, A. C. M. (1998). Stress and coping in families of children with Smith-Magenis syndrome. *Journal of Intellectual Disability Research, 42*, 331–340.

Hodapp, R.M., & Urbano, R. C. (2007). Developmental epidemiology of mental retardation/developmental disabilities: An emerging discipline. In R. C. Urbano, & R. M. Hodapp (Eds.), *International review of research in mental retardation* Vol. 33 (pp. 3–24). San Diego, CA: Academic Press/Elsevier.

Hunter, K. (2002). Looking from inside out: A parent's perspective. *Mental Retardation and Developmental Disabilities Research Review, 8*, 77–81.

Hurley, A., & Levitas, A. S. (2004). Therapeutic engagement of the family for treatment of individuals with intellectual disability: Chronic sorrow. *Mental Health Aspects of Developmental Disabilities, 7*, 77–80.

Jobe, B. M., & Glidden, L. M. (2008). Predicting maternal rewards and worries for the transition to adulthood of children with developmental disabilities. *Journal on Developmental Disabilities, 4*, 423–432.

Joesch, J. M., & Smith, K. R. (1997). Children's health and their mothers' risk of divorce or separation. *Social Biology, 44*, 159–169.

Jokinen, N. S., & Brown, R. I. (2005). Family quality of life from the perspective of older parents. *Journal of Intellectual Disability Research, 49*, 789–793.

Judge, S. L. (1998). Parental coping strategies and strengths in families of young children with disabilities. *Family Relations, 47*, 263–268.

Kearney, P. M., & Griffin, T. (2001). Between joy and sorrow: Being a parent of a child with developmental disability. *Issues and Innovations in Nursing Practice, 34*, 582–592.

Kim, H. W., Greenberg, J. S., Seltzer, M. M., & Krauss, M. W. (2003). The role of coping in maintaining the psychological well-being of mothers of adults with intellectual disability and mental illness. *Journal of Intellectual Disability Research, 47*, 313–327.

Keogh, B. K., Garnier, H. E., Bernheimer, L. P., & Gallimore, R. (2000). Models of child-family interactions for children with developmental delays: Child-driven or transactional? *American Journal on Mental Retardation, 105*, 32–46.

Krauss, M., & Seltzer, M. (1993). Coping strategies among older mothers of adults with retardation: A life-span developmental perspective. In A. P. Turnbull, J. M. Patterson, S. K. Behr, D. L. Murphy, J. G. Marquis, M. J. Blue-Banning, (Eds.), *Cognitive coping, families, and disability* (pp. 173–182). Baltimore, MD: Paul H. Brookes.

Krauss, M. W., & Seltzer, M. M.(1998). Life course perspectives in mental retardation research: The case of family caregiving. In J. A. Burack, R. M. Hodapp, & E. Zigler (Eds.), *Handbook of mental retardation and development*. New York: Cambridge University.

Küçüker, S. (2006). The family-focused early intervention programme: Evaluation of parental stress and depression. *Early Child Development and Care, 176*, 329–341.

Lazarus R., Lazarus B., Campos, J., Tennen, R., & Tennen, H. (2006). Emotions and interpersonal relationships: Toward a person-centered conceptualization of emotions and coping. *Journal of Personality, 74*, 9–46.

Lenhard, W., Breitenbach, E., Ebert, H., Schindelhauer-Deutscher, H. J., & Henn, W. (2005). Psychological benefit of diagnostic certainty for mothers of children with disabilities: Lessons from Down syndrome. *American Journal of Medical Genetics, 133*, 170–175.

Levy-Shiff, R., Dimitrovsky, L., Shulman, S., & Har-Even, D. (1998). Cognitive appraisals, coping strategies, and support resources as correlates of parenting and infant development. *Developmental Psychology, 34*, 1417–1427.

Lucas, R. E., Diener, E., & Suh, E. (1996). Discriminant validity of well-being measures. *Journal of Personality and Social Psychology, 71*, 616–628.

Magaña, S., Schwartz, S. J., Rupert, M. P., & Szapocznik, J. (2006). Hispanic caregivers of adults with mental retardation: Importance of family functioning. *American Journal of mental Retardation, 111*, 250–262.

Magaña, S., & Smith, M. J. (2006). Health outcomes of midlife and older Latina and Black American mothers of children with developmental disabilities. *Mental Retardation, 44*, 224–234.

Maslow, A. H. (1968). *Toward a psychology of being* (2nd ed.). New York: Nostrand.

Minnes, P. (1998). Mental retardation: The impact upon the family. In J.W. Jacobson, & J. A. Mulick (Eds.), *Handbook of mental retardation and developmental disabilities*. New York: Kluwer/Plenum.

Nachshen, J. S., & Minnes, P. (2005). Empowerment in parents of school-aged children with and without developmental disabilities. *Journal of Intellectual Disability Research, 49*, 889–904.

Nachshen, J. S., Garcin, N., & Minnes, P. (2005). Problem behavior in children with intellectual disabilities: Parenting stress, empowerment and school services. *Mental Health Aspects of Developmental Disabilities, 8*(4), 105–114.

Nalavany, B. A., Glidden, L. M., & Ryan, S. (2009). Parental satisfaction in the adoption of children with learning disorders: The role of behavior problems. *Family Relations, 58*, 621–633.

Olshansky, S. (1962). Chronic sorrow: A response to having a mentally defective child. *Social Casework, 43*, 191–194.

Olsson, M. B., & Hwang, C. P. (2001). Depression in mothers and fathers of children with intellectual disability. *Journal of Intellectual Disability Research, 45*, 535–543.

Olsson, M. B., & Hwang, C. P. (2003). Influence of macrostructure of society on the life situation of families with a child with intellectual disability: Sweden as an example. *Journal of Intellectual Disability Research, 47*, 328–341.

Orsmond, G. I., Seltzer, M. M., Krauss, M. W., & Hong, J. (2003). Behavior problems in adults with mental retardation and maternal well-being: Examination of the direction of effects. *American Journal on Mental Retardation, 108*, 257–271.

Pakenham, K. I., Sofronoff, K., & Samios, C. (2004). Finding meaning in parenting a child with Asperger syndrome: Correlates of sense making and benefit finding. *Research in Developmental Disabilities, 25*, 245–264.

Poehlmann, J., Clements, M., Abbeduto, L., & Farsad, V. (2005). Family experiences associated with a child's diagnosis of fragile X or Down syndrome: Evidence for disruption and resilience. *Mental Retardation, 43*, 255–267.

Poston, D., Turnbull, A., Park, J., Mannan, H., Marquis, J., & Wang, M. (2003). Family quality of life: A qualitative inquiry. *Mental Retardation, 41*, 313–328.

Rehm, R. S., & Bradley, J. F. (2005). Normalization in families raising a child who is medically fragile/technology dependent and developmentally delayed. *Qualitative Health Research, 15*, 807–820.

Reichman, N. E., Corman, H., & Noonan, K. (2004). Effects of child health on parents' relationship status. *Demography, 41*, 569–584.

Reichman, S., Miller, A. C., Gordon, R., & Hendricks-Munoz, K. (2000). Stress appraisal and coping in mothers of NICU infants. *Children's Health Care, 29*, 279–293.

Ricci, L. A., & Hodapp, R. M. (2003). Fathers of children with Down's syndrome versus other types of intellectual disability: Perceptions, stress and involvement. *Journal of Intellectual Disability Research, 47*, 273–284.

Risdal, D., & Singer, G. H. S. (2004). Marital adjustment in parents of children with disabilities: A historical review and meta-analysis. *Research & Practice for Persons with Severe Disabilities, 29*, 95–103.

Rogers, C. R. (1995). *A way of being.* Boston: Houghton Mifflin.

Scorgie, K., & Sobsey, D. (2000). Transformational outcomes associated with parenting children who have disabilities. *Mental Retardation, 38*, 195–206.

Scorgie, K., Wilgosh, L., & McDonald, L. (1998). Stress and coping in families of children with disabilities: An examination of recent literature. *Developmental Disabilities Bulletin, 26*, 22–42.

Seligman, M. E. P., & Csikszentmihalyi, M. (Eds.) (2000). Positive psychology [Special issue]. *American Psychologist, 55*.

Seltzer, M. M., Greenberg, J. S., Floyd, F. J., Pettee, Y., & Hong, J. (2001). Life course impacts of parenting a child with a disability. *American Journal on Mental Retardation, 106*, 265–286.

Shapiro, J., Blacher, J., & Lopez, S. R. (1998). Maternal reactions to children with mental retardation. In J. W. Jacobson, & J. A. Mulick (Eds.), *Handbook of mental retardation and developmental disabilities.* New York: Kluwer/Plenum.

Simmerman, S., Blacher, J., & Baker, B. L. (2001). Fathers' and mothers' perceptions of father involvement in families with young children with a disability. *Journal of Intellectual & Developmental Disability, 26*, 325–338.

Singer, G. H. (2006). Meta-analysis of comparative studies of depression in mothers of children with and without developmental disabilities. *American Journal on Mental Retardation, 111*, 155–169.

Singer, G. H., & Irvin, L. K. (Eds.) (1989). *Support for caregiving families: Enabling positive adaptation to disability.* Baltimore: Paul Brookes.

Stainton, T., & Besser, H. (1998). The positive impact of children with an intellectual disability on the family. *Journal of Intellectual & Developmental Disability, 23*, 57–70.

Stoneman, Z., & Gavidia-Payne, S. (2006). Marital adjustment in families of young children with disabilities: Associations with daily hassles and problem-focused coping. *American Journal on Mental Retardation, 111*, 1–14.

Summers, J. A., Behr, S. K., & Turnbull, A. P. (1989). Positive adaptation and coping strength in families who have children with disabilities In G. H. S. Singer, & L. K. Irvin (Eds.), *Support for caregiving families: Enabling positive adaptation to disability* (pp. 27–40). Baltimore: Brookes.

Teixeira, M. C. T. V., Emerich, D. R., Orsati, R. C., Rimério, K. R., Gatto, Chappaz, I. O., & Kim, C. A. (2011). A description of adaptive and maladaptive behavior in children and adolescents with Cri-du-chat syndrome. *Journal of Intellectual Disability Research, 55*, 132–137.

Trute, B., & Hauch, C. (1988). Building on family strength: A study of families with positive adjustment to the birth of a developmentally disabled child. *Journal of Marital and Family Therapy, 14*, 185–193.

Trute, B., & Hiebert-Murphy, D. (2005). Predicting family adjustment and parenting stress in childhood disability services using brief assessment tools. *Journal of Intellectual & Developmental Disability, 30*, 217–225.

Turnbull, A., Brown, I., & Turnbull, H. R. (Eds.) (2004). *Families and people with mental retardation and quality of life: International perspectives.* Washington DC: American Association on Mental Retardation.

Turnbull, A. P., Patterson, J. M., Behr, S. K., Murphy, D. L., Marquis, J. G., & Blue-Banning, M. J. (1993). *Cognitive coping, families, & disability.* Baltimore: Brookes.

Urbano, R. C., & Hodapp, R. M. (2007). Divorce in families of children with Down syndrome: A population-based study. *American Journal on Mental Retardation, 112*, 261–274.

Weiner, B., Perry, R. P., & Magnusson, J. (1988). An attributional analysis of reactions to stigmas. *Journal of Personality and Social Psychology, 55*, 738–748.

Wheeler, A. C., Skinner, D. G., & Bailey, D. B. (2008). Perceived quality of life in mothers of children with fragile X syndrome. *American Journal on Mental Retardation, 113*, 159–177.

Willoughby, J. C., & Glidden, L. M. (1995). Fathers helping out: Shared child care and marital satisfaction in parents of children with disabilities. *American Journal on Mental Retardation, 99*, 399–406.

Dyadic Interaction Between Mothers and Children with Down Syndrome or Williams Syndrome: Empirical Evidence and Emerging Agendas

Penny Hauser-Cram, Angela N. Howell-Moneta, *and* Jessica Mercer Young

Abstract

This chapter highlights the theoretical foundations that have guided research on mother–child interaction. It discusses the physical and behavioral characteristics of children with Down syndrome (DS) that influence their social interactions, then reviews research findings on mother–child interaction in these dyads. It discusses research conducted during the past decade since the review in the last *Handbook of Mental Retardation* (Marfo, Dedrick, & Barbour, 1998) and proposes an agenda for future research. The chapter also describes the behaviors and processes related to Williams syndrome that are likely to be relevant to mother–child interaction. It proposes a research agenda that both builds on and is distinct from that related to children with DS.

Keywords: Mother–child interaction, developmental disability, Down syndrome, Williams syndrome, social interaction

From a developmental systems perspective, the relational processes that occur between a mother and her young child are central to the child's cognitive and socioemotional development (Shonkoff & Phillips, 2000). A large body of research exists on mother–child interaction in dyads in which a child is developing typically. Such research emanates from several theoretical perspectives. In this chapter, we highlight the theoretical foundations that have guided research on mother–child interaction, and review research relevant to mother–child interaction in dyads in which a child has a specific genetically based disability, either Down syndrome (DS) or Williams syndrome (WS). We have selected to focus on these two syndromes because each has distinct behavioral phenotypes that contribute to patterns of strength and vulnerability in aspects of social interaction.

An understanding of how such patterns relate to mother–child interaction holds promise for service providers, as well as for scholars seeking to portray the full range of developmental patterns. As Hodapp and Burack (1990) contended, learning about typical

development is advanced by the study of those with intellectual disabilities because developmental processes can be scrutinized to determine both necessary and sufficient behaviors for adaptive functioning. In this chapter, we discuss the physical and behavioral characteristics of children with DS that influence their social interactions, followed by a review of the research findings on mother–child interaction in these dyads. Research conducted during the past decade since the review in the last *Handbook of Mental Retardation* (Marfo, Dedrick, & Barbour, 1998) is discussed, and an agenda for future research is proposed. We also focus on WS, a rare genetically based disability, which has a growing research base that provides descriptive information about children's genotypic and phenotypic profiles. In that section, we describe the behaviors and processes related to WS that are likely to be relevant to mother–child interaction. We propose a research agenda that both builds on and is distinct from that related to children with DS. The similarities and contrasts between the profiles of children with each syndrome are informative for those who seek possible avenues of intervention for promoting optimal mother–child interactions when a child has a disability of genetic etiology.

Theoretical Perspectives on Mother–Child Interaction

The history of theoretical perspectives on mother–child interaction has followed its own developmental course, with mother–child interaction seen as a key developmental context critical for the healthy development of all children. Although the attachment between the mother and the infant serves as the core of most perspectives on mother–child interaction, an understanding of the transactional dimensions of the mother–child relationship and the cultural context that guides parenting behaviors broadens and deepens the theoretical and empirical base. Each of these perspectives is briefly reviewed in the following sections.

Attachment Theory

Bowlby (1969/1982) originally theorized that an attachment system was formed through infants' interactions with their mothers. Attachment behaviors are demonstrated when a young child who is frightened, sick, or stressed is then comforted when an attachment figure provides protection, help, and soothing (Bretherton, 1985). Knowing that the attachment figure is available and would be responsive to the child in situations of stress provides the child with a sense of security (Bowlby, 1969/1982). The attachment system also provides a crucial biological function; it protects the attached person from both physical and psychological harm (Bretherton, 1985). Bowlby (1969/1982) suggested that, through the attachment system, an internal working model is formed that guides the child's action in all future relationships and allows the child to understand both the self and others.

To investigate dimensions of attachment, developmental psychologists often have employed the Strange Situation paradigm (Ainsworth, Blehar, Waters, & Wall, 1978; Main & Solomon, 1990), which classifies children into either securely attached or insecurely attached categories. More recent studies, however, have focused less attention on children's behaviors during episodes of separation and reunion, and more attention on the sensitive and responsive behaviors of mothers. In particular, maternal responsiveness, conceptualized as the contingent, prompt, and appropriate reactions of mothers to their infants' cues, has been studied extensively in relation to children's developing competencies

(Bornstein, 2006). The affective quality of maternal responsiveness includes maternal warmth and sensitivity and has been postulated to reflect the extent to which the mother expresses positive affect when she responds to her infant's needs and abilities (Bornstein & Tamis-LeMonda, 2001). Empirical evidence regarding mothers' sensitive and responsive behaviors indicates that these qualities are related to typically developing children's later cognitive and language competencies (Bornstein, Tamis-LeMonda, & Baumwell, 2001; Frankel & Bates, 1990; Landry, Smith, Swank, & Miller-Loncar, 2000; Pianta & Harbers, 1996) as well as social competencies (Elicker, Englund, & Sroufe, 1992; Morrison, Rimm-Kaufman, & Pianta, 2003).

Transactional Theory

Researchers working from the basis of attachment theory tend to emphasize the importance of a mother's responses to her child, yet three decades ago Bell (1968) posited that the child's role in this dyadic interaction was an active and equally critical factor. Infants bring dispositional tendencies to the interaction and demonstrate these both in responses to mothers as well as when initiating interactive episodes. Much research, therefore, builds on the recognition of the bidirectional and transactional nature of mother–child interaction (Sameroff & MacKenzie, 2003). Derived from the developmental systems theory, those operating from the view of the transactional model posit that members of the dyad react to each other in a manner that mutually creates developmental pathways. Interactions within dyads have also been described in terms of their synchrony, where interaction within synchronistic dyads has been likened to an interactive dance (Barnard, Hammond, Booth, Bee, Mitchell, & Spieker, 1989). Such synchrony is "an observable pattern of dyadic interaction that is mutually regulated, reciprocal, and harmonious" (Harrist & Waugh, 2002, p. 557). From the perspective of the transactional model, if one partner is off beat or off tempo, the whole interaction may suffer. Thus, an asynchronistic pattern of interaction may have serious implications for children's development, resulting in an insecure attachment relationship (Isabella & Belsky, 1991) and deleterious child functioning (Sameroff & Fiese, 2000).

Consistent with the recognition of the transactional nature of the mother–child dyadic relationship, and stimulated by the co-constructivist model (Bruner, 1982; Vygotsky, 1978), many researchers have focused on how both members of the dyad engage the other toward shared or joint activity. According to Tomasello (1995), the dyadic interaction typical of mother–child interaction during the early months changes during the end of the first year to triadic interaction, in which the child and mother coordinate their attention to objects or other individuals. Aspects of shared activities involve the mother's actions in supporting the child's efforts, the child's actions in viewing the mother's responses, and the dual accommodations made by the mother and child during episodes of joint attention.

Derived from the work of Vygotsky (1978), the co-constructivist perspective emphasizes both the cognitive and emotional benefits that accrue in the young child through maternal efforts to understand and build on the child's intentions. Emphasizing the cognitive benefits of mother–child co-construction, Heckhausen (1993) described how a toddler develops mastery of behavior–event contingencies through maternal scaffolding of the child's attempts to attain a goal, such as nesting a series of cups. According to Heckhausen, children develop more positive cognitive trajectories if mothers understand the capabilities of the child and stretch those capabilities by providing "one step ahead" scaffolding.

The dyad also co-constructs knowledge through social referencing. Children use social referencing by taking cues from mothers' emotional reactions in ambiguous or potentially fearful situations; children then use these cues to determine their own responses (Repacholi, 1998). In this way, children to some extent appropriate maternal emotional reactions, using the mother's emotional state to judge the safety of a situation. By referencing back to his or her mother, the child develops an emotional foundation for dealing with novel situations, objects, and people.

Some researchers focus extensively on the role of joint attention during mother–child exchanges. The behaviors of both the mother and child that lead to moments of coordinated attention are considered. Legerstee and Weintraub (1997) proposed that joint attention occurs in a developmental sequence. During the first 6 months, infants tend to focus on either a person or an object when presented with both. A mother, however, advances this behavior toward shared activity by following the infant's line of vision and commenting on what the infant sees. The infant in turn develops sufficient awareness to track the mother's gaze (Corkum & Moore, 1998). Around 9–12 months of age, the child can intentionally attempt to coordinate his or her regard with that of another individual (e.g., the mother)

on an object or another person (Bakeman & Adamson, 1984), resulting in triadic, rather than exclusively dyadic, interaction. Such joint attention between a child and mother to an object, individual, or action facilitates the child's language acquisition, through, for example, learning appropriate language labels (Carpenter, Nagel, & Tomasello, 1998). Through joint attention, the mother maintains the child's focus on the shared activity and, in doing so, limits the cognitive demands on the child, thus enabling the word and object (or activity) to be more easily associated with each other (Bruner, 1983). Despite similarities in the developmental sequence of joint attention across mother–child dyads, individual differences in child–caregiver episodes of joint attention are evident and have been found to predict children's expressive language development (Markus, Mundy, Morales, Delgado, & Yale, 2000).

Cultural Theory

The mother–child transactional dyadic relationship occurs within a larger context that includes cultural values and ideologies about optimal mother–child interaction. Sameroff and Fiese (2000) delineated how transactions involving the mother–child dyad are related to genotype, phenotype, and environment (which they term "environtype"), with the latter including cultural codes of child rearing and family codes related to group belonging. Cultural psychologists (e.g., Harkness & Super, 1996; Rogoff, 2003) indicate that behaviors and actions on the part of mothers have roots in culturally sanctioned beliefs and values. Moreover, beliefs about the nature of a developmental disability are often culturally based and lay the foundations for maternal actions, expectations, and interpretations of a child's behavior (Fadiman, 1997; Garcia, Coll, & Magnuson, 2000). Although analyses of cultural codes are beyond the scope of this chapter, the larger framework that includes such codes is valuable to consider when interpreting the current research on mother–child interaction in dyads in which a child has a developmental disability.

Down Syndrome
Down Syndrome: Mother–Child Attachment Research

In a review of the socioemotional development of typically developing children, Thompson, Easterbrooks, and Padilla-Walker (2003) posit that individual differences in mother–child secure attachment relate to the child's psychobiology, as well as to mothers' sensitive responsiveness to the child. Children with DS, a genetic disorder that affects cognitive development, also display phenotypic characteristics or behaviors that may directly influence the mother–child relationship. For example, health impairments common among children with DS include thyroid dysfunction, congenital heart defects, and ear infections, which can limit children's energy to engage in sustained interactions. In addition, sleep problems, such as obstructive sleep apnea, are prevalent among infants with DS and contribute to frequent awakening and daytime sleepiness (American Academy of Pediatrics: Committee on Genetics, 2001). The lethargic quality of infant behavior may create a challenge for mothers to engage their children in interactions and sustain their children's attention during learning tasks. Phenotypic behaviors may also indirectly influence the attachment relationship by requiring mothers to expend time and energy to obtain information and resources and by evoking expectations from mothers regarding their children's vulnerability (Guralnick, 1998). Such associations suggest that secure mother–child attachment may be difficult to achieve.

Amid speculations that arise about the relation of phenotypic characteristics of children with DS to mother–child attachment, a few such studies have been conducted during the last decade. The studies have revealed similar results, but also have led to important questions about the validity of measures typically used, especially the Strange Situation (Ainsworth et al., 1978), when applied to children with DS and their mothers.

In a meta-analysis of the relative effects of maternal and child problems on the quality of attachment as evidenced by the Strange Situation, van IJzendoorn, Goldberg, Kroonenberg, and Frenkel (1992) analyzed studies of children from clinical samples and typically developing samples. The 34 studies of clinical samples included those drawn from populations identifying a child problem, specifically utilizing the child's diagnosis as the identifying criteria (e.g., DS); populations identified by maternal problems (e.g., mental illness, maltreatment); and populations that were difficult to classify and were considered "other." The data from typically developing children came from 21 samples with children aged 12–24 months; children in the clinical samples tended to be older, ranging in age from 12–50 months. Overall, the researchers found that the mother appeared to play a more important role than the child in shaping the quality of the infant–mother attachment relationship, as maternal

problems increased the likelihood of an insecure attachment classification. Of the "child problem" group, only children with DS were found to be significantly overrepresented in one insecure attachment classification, the disorganized attachment category. Van IJzendoorn et al. (1992) suggested that the coding scheme utilized by the Strange Situation may not be valid for children with DS since the original classification scheme was constructed for a typically developing, middle-class population; therefore, the interpretation of the reaction of children with similar genetically based disabilities who show delayed or muted responses to social situations like the Strange Situation is not readily understood.

In an effort to test the validity of the Strange Situation as an assessment of attachment for children with DS, Vaughn, Goldberg, Atkinson, Marcovitch, MacGregor, and Seifer (1994) investigated the attachment ratings of 138 children with DS taken from three independent studies. All of the children recruited to the three studies were in some form of early intervention services. Children ranged in chronological age (CA) from 24–54 months (developmental age of 10–36 months), from 12–36 months (developmental age from 8.5 months to 23.6 months), and from 21–37 months (average developmental age of 16.2 months) in the three studies, respectively. A comparative sample of 146 typically developing children was available from an independent study of infants and toddlers between 12 and 14 months of age (Vaughn, Lefer, Seifer, & Barglow, 1989). For this study, Vaughn et al. (1994) chose to categorize cases that might have been otherwise classified as insecure-disorganized as insecure-unclassifiable.

Although Vaughn et al. (1994) found that, overall, more children with DS were classified as insecurely attached in comparison to the typically developing group, they attributed this finding to the larger number of children with DS who were categorized as "unclassifiable" and insecure. The developmentally and chronologically younger children with DS were the most likely to be considered insecure-unclassifiable. When these insecure-unclassifiable cases were dropped from the analysis, Vaughn et al. (1994) found that the proportions of secure versus insecurely attached cases were no longer significantly different, and in fact a larger proportion of cases from the DS group were assigned to the secure classification than the typically developing group. They speculated that the Strange Situation itself may produce a lower level of stress reactions in children with DS as compared to typically developing children, as they noted that the children with DS rarely showed distress during the episodes of separation and reunion. Children with DS also did not seek to maintain contact in the reunion episodes, and even if they did seek proximity to the mother, they required little or no comforting. Vaughn et al. (1994) proposed that the Strange Situation may not provide sufficient attunement to the unique behavioral profile of children with DS and thus is not a valid measure of attachment quality for children with DS.

The results of a more recent study (Moore, Oates, Goodwin, & Hobson, 2008) add more evidence to the prior speculation that children with DS exhibit less intense emotional responsiveness than other children under situations of stress. Moore and colleagues investigated the responses of infants with DS when their mothers employed the Still-Face procedure of Tronick, Als, Adamson, Wise, and Brazelton (1978). During this procedure, mothers stop expressing positive emotions and maintain a neutral expression even when their infants attempt to elicit positive affect. Although typically developing infants usually display some form of dysregulation during the Still Face procedure, infants with DS were found to show significantly less fussing than their typical peers in both the still phase and the re-engagement phase.

In an effort to determine whether the lack of distress reactions in children with DS is related to attachment quality, Ganiban, Barnett, and Cicchetti (2000) investigated the relation of low versus high negative reactivity and attachment classification in 30 children with DS at 19 and 27 months of age (average Bayley Mental Developmental Index was 62 [SD = 13] at 19 months and 62 [SD = 12] at 24 months). As in prior studies, the researchers found a high frequency of insecure-disorganized type or insecure-unclassifiable attachments, specifically 30% of the children displayed this attachment pattern. Additionally, contrary to Vaughn et al.'s (1994) hypothesis, Ganiban et al. (2000) reported that low negative reactivity was not consistently related to insecure attachment classifications. Both high and low negative reactivity groups displayed increases in proximity seeking, contact maintenance, resistance, and avoidance during the course of the Strange Situation. The researchers posited that, in contrast to the speculations of Vaughn et al. (1994), the attachment system of children with DS is in fact being activated by the separations and reunions of the Strange Situation.

Ganiban et al. (2000) also found increasing rates of attachment insecurity in the children with DS over the 8-month period from the time children were 19–27 months old. The researchers speculated that reciprocal synchronous interactions may be difficult to establish in these mother–child dyads. This may create a cumulative effect on the overall quality of the interaction over time, leading to higher rates of attachment insecurity as the children grow older. The researchers continued to question why an elevated rate of attachment insecurity occurs in children with DS and suggested that the attachment patterns described by Ainsworth et al. (1978) may actually be different for children with DS.

Atkinson et al. (1999) investigated the influence of child intellectual/adaptive functioning and maternal sensitivity, and their interaction, on attachment security. They examined 53 infants and toddlers with DS between the CAs of 14 and 30 months, with developmental ages of 12–23 months at first observation. Mothers and children were assessed four times at home and two times in the lab over a 2-year period. The researchers found a similar pattern to that reported in other investigations, with fewer children with DS displaying secure attachments (40%) and a higher proportion displaying unclassifiable (47%) attachment patterns in the Strange Situation at 26 months. The researchers maintained, however, that the unclassifiable group's security status was unclear. They investigated whether characteristics of the child and mother were related to attachment security status and found that children with lower cognitive functioning were less likely to be classified as securely attached. They also found that maternal sensitivity, defined as the mother's prompt and appropriate response to the child's cues, was positively related to children's security status. Thus, both maternal sensitivity and child cognitive performance predicted attachment security, where relatively high levels of both factors increased the probability of the child being classified as securely attached whereas low levels of either decreased that likelihood.

Researchers are still trying to explain the finding that children with DS are more likely than typically developing children to be classified as insecure-disorganized or as insecure-unclassifiable in relation to the attachment categories based on the Strange Situation. Some investigators have questioned the validity of this paradigm and classification system for studying mother–child relations in dyads in which a child has DS (e.g., Ganiban et al., 2000; van IJzendoorn et al., 1992). Even if further research determines that the paradigm is not suitable for studying attachment in this constellation, the overall findings from studies on attachment suggest that both the child and the mother contribute to their relationship.

Investigating the overall dyadic synchrony of the mother–child dyad may be crucial to understanding children with DS's attachment classifications as research with typically developing populations suggests that a relation exists between synchronistic dyads and secure attachment (Isabella & Belsky, 1991). Since dyadic synchrony differs by the contribution of the child to the interaction, the phenotypic characteristics of children with DS, especially health-related issues, low motor tone, and less readable preverbal cues (Hyche, Bakeman, & Adamson, 1992), may lead to asynchrony affecting attachment. Nevertheless, the mother–child attachment relationship is likely to vary as a function of maternal sensitivity as well as the child's behaviors and their bidirectional influences on each other.

Down Syndrome: The Learning Context of Mother–Child Interactions

Early interactions between mothers and their infants provide a vital context for learning (Kelly & Barnard, 2000). Researchers have shown a strong correlation between the interactive behaviors of mothers and children with DS during exchanges, suggesting that children with DS attend and respond to their mother's interactive behaviors, and mothers are able to respond to the cues of their children with DS (Cielinski, Vaughn, Siefer, & Contreras, 1995; Roach, Barratt, Miller, & Leavitt, 1998).

The importance of mother–child interaction to the learning context is underscored by the finding that a relation between maternal interactive behaviors and child functioning has been found for children with DS. Observations of sensitive and responsive maternal behaviors during early mother–child interactions predicted growth in the adaptive functioning of children with DS over the first 5 years of life (Hauser-Cram, Warfield, Shonkoff, Krauss, Upshur, & Sayer, 1999) as well as over the first 10 years of life in the areas of social and communication skills (Hauser-Cram, Warfield, Shonkoff, Krauss, Sayer, & Upshur, 2001). Thus, mother–child exchanges during the first few years of life appear to set trajectories of adaptive functioning for children with DS.

A predominant challenge faced by mothers of children with DS, however, is engaging and sustaining their children's attention toward environmental stimuli that can promote learning. Optimal learning contexts during infancy require that a mother be able to engage her infant when the infant is calm but attention is high (Barnard & Sumner, 2002). Phenotypic characteristics associated with DS, such as hypothyroidism and hypotonia, generally lower metabolic rate, and slow digestion, cause lethargy and inattentiveness, potentially reducing the time that the infant is in an alert state. Slonims and McConachie (2006) observed the interactions of 23 mothers and their infants with DS and 23 mothers and their typically developing infants matched on CA. At 8 weeks, infants with DS were significantly less alert and communicative than typically developing infants, but by 20 weeks, although they continued to be rated as less "lively," infants with DS did not show differences from other infants in their interactive behaviors. Mothers of children with DS were rated as displaying lower quality of interactions with their child at the 20-week assessment but also showed improving interactions associated with the improving communicative skills of the child.

The limits regarding appropriate behavior set by mothers play a critical role in the initial development of self-regulation among infants (Crockenberg & Litman, 1990). Heightened maternal control over the child's actions may reduce an infant's opportunities to exert autonomy, contributing over time to lower motivation for exploration. In a study of young children with DS, Hauser-Cram (1993) found that high levels of direct parent engagement in structuring children's play led to children's less active independent motivation on problem-posing tasks. In a recursive manner, lower levels of motivation to explore may contribute to less frequent spontaneous play, which has been observed among children with DS (Brooks-Gunn & Lewis, 1984). Over time, diminished playfulness and less persistence in problem solving activities may prevent children with DS from developing a sense of mastery of their environment. This may eventually weaken the child's sense of internal control over challenging problems (Bundy, 1997).

Toddlers with DS have been found to have specific deficits related to nonverbal instrumental requests (e.g., eye gaze or pointing with the intention of regulating another's behavior) during problem solving tasks. In contrast, they display adequate nonverbal gestures in the context of social routines (e.g., tickling) in comparison to mental age (MA)-matched peers (Fidler, Philofsky, Hepburn, & Rogers, 2005). Thus, differences in communication patterns emerge between children with DS and those developing typically mainly in the context of cognitive problem solving situations. As early as preschool, children with DS tend to show a dependence on adults when presented with challenging tasks. Kasari and Freeman (2001) presented children with DS aged 5–12 years with both solvable and unsolvable puzzles. They found that children with DS frequently used adults for help by looking at the experimenter's face and puzzle during unsolvable tasks, but they did not make many verbal requests for help. Children with DS also took longer to start and complete all tasks compared to children with intellectual impairment of unknown etiology (MA 30–77 months) and typically developing children (MA 43–67 months). Similarly, Pitcairn and Wishart (1994) found that children aged 3–5 years with DS exhibited a high rate of nonverbal help-seeking during challenging tasks and attempted to engage the experimenter in social activities, possibly as a means to evade completing the task. These findings suggest that young children with DS may require finely tuned support from their caregivers to develop the persistence and mastery skills necessary to complete problem-posing tasks.

In a detailed review of mother–child interaction, Marfo, Dedrick, and Barbour (1998) analyzed a series of studies that suggested that mothers tend to be highly directive with their children with intellectual disabilities. They emphasized that although maternal directives have been considered to be intrusive (e.g., Cielinski, Vaughn, Seifer, & Contreras, 1995), many such directives may instead be purposeful and adaptive, especially in dyads in which children display inappropriate use of objects or noncompliant behavior. Roach, Barratt, Miller, and Leavitt (1998) examined mother–child interactions among 28 toddlers with DS aged 11–30 months with a developmental age of 10–17 months. Comparison groups of typically developing children were matched on chronological or developmental age. Roach et al. found that mothers of all three groups were contingently responsive to their children's behavioral signals, but that mothers of children with DS engaged in more directive behaviors than did mothers of children in the other two groups. Roach et al. further reported that mothers of children with DS also used more supportive behaviors (e.g., vocal praise or scaffolding by holding an object) and that directives (e.g., "Find the red one") were often embedded within a series of supportive behaviors. Therefore, the behavioral context of directives deserves consideration, as does their role in structured as opposed to unstructured situations (Marfo

et al., 1998). Marfo (1990) posited that directives are multidimensional and require examination within a broader view of maternal adaptation. Such a perspective is necessary as we develop a deeper understanding of the challenges posed by children with DS during shared activities with their mothers.

Down Syndrome: The Influence of Behavioral Phenotypes on Shared Activity

Children with DS demonstrate behavioral profiles that create significant challenges for mothers as they help their toddlers explore the environment and learn to communicate effectively. Although eye contact between the child and caregiver occurs at a later age for children with DS, the general sequence of gaze development appears to be similar (Carvajal & Iglesias, 2002). Nevertheless, in confirmation of earlier research (e.g., Kasari, Mundy, Yirmiya, & Sigman, 1990), Carvajal and Inglesias (2000) have documented that infants with DS (aged 3.2–13.6 months) in comparison to typically developing children of the same age generally display longer gazes to their social partners, although patterns of the two groups are similar in considering the relation between looking and smiling. Researchers studying the movement from face-to-face interaction to triadic interaction point to areas of specific difficulty for the toddler with DS. In a comparison of children with DS to children developing typically matched on MA (from 6 to 20 months MA), Legerstee and Fisher (2008) found that children with DS displayed less coordinated attention (e.g., gaze from an object attended to by both the child and the mother, toward the mother's face, back to the object) until the MA of 20 months. Children with DS, similar to typically developing children, also began to use declarative pointing (i.e., communicating to share an interesting aspect of an object) after the onset of coordinated attention, although they showed lower levels of such pointing. Children with DS, however, did not vary from their MA-matched peers in their use of imperative pointing (i.e., communicating to obtain an object) which, Legerstee and Fisher contend, is not as closely linked with children's understanding of the mental states of others as is declarative pointing.

In a study of children's attention to novel objects, Brown, Johnson, Paterson, Gilmore, Longhi, and Karmiloff-Smith (2003) reported that infants with DS aged 24–37 months (12–21 months developmental age) exhibited fewer and shorter periods of sustained attention toward such objects compared to children matched for either CA or developmental age. Toddlers with DS also showed less interest in playing with objects and more interest in engaging in play with people (Carvajal & Iglesias, 2000; Kasari, Mundy, Yirmiya, & Sigman, 1990; Landry & Chapieski, 1990). Legerstee, Varghese, and van Beek (2002) found that toddlers with DS had particular difficulty shifting attention from person to object, thereby delaying the development of coordinated joint attention. Researchers have not yet determined whether this difficulty relates to an innate preference for social activities, as suggested by Kasari and Freeman (2001) or whether such shifts challenge the information processing capabilities of children with DS, as postulated by Tomasello and Farrar (1986).

Observations of mothers and their children with DS have revealed that mothers alter their behavior in different ways to accommodate their child's attentional difficulties (Harris, Kasari, & Sigman, 1996). For example, during an unstructured play observation of mothers with their toddlers with DS (aged 12–41 months), Harris et al. (1996) found that some mothers responded to their child's lack of sustained attention by redirecting the child to maternally selected objects in an effort to engage the child's interest. Other mothers followed their child's gaze to an object that appeared to catch their infant's attention and then successfully sustained their child's attention by animating the object and talking about it. Toddlers whose mothers engaged in shared attention with their child on an object selected by the child were found to have higher receptive language skills 13 months later compared to those whose mothers attempted to redirect the child's attention to an object that the caregiver selected (Harris et al., 1996). These findings raise important questions about the timing of maternal redirection of children's gaze in efforts to facilitate joint attention. Legerstee and Weintraub (1997) reported that, in their study of two groups of infants and toddlers with DS (mean MAs of 8.6 months and 16.5 months), compared to typically developing children of the same MAs, those with DS displayed less play with objects and less coordinated attention. When mothers of children with DS supported their children's efforts to interact with an object by integrating it into social play and by repeating patterns of play, they facilitated the infant's ability to attend alternatively to object and to mother. Nevertheless, even with such support, infants with DS showed lower amounts of coordinated joint attention.

The degree of support that mothers provide to their infants is related to the developmental skills of the infant. Legerstee et al. (2002) found similarities in the type of strategies used by mothers of children (both typically developing and DS) based on the child's developmental age (mean MAs of 8.6 months or 16.5 months). During interactions with children of toddler MA, mothers were more likely to use strategies to maintain their children's attention to an object, attempting to engage their children in coordinated attention. In contrast, mothers of children with MAs below 1 year attempted to redirect the attention of their children but often followed that redirection by using behaviors to maintain the children's attention. Although redirection alone appeared to suppress the referential behaviors necessary for joint attention, the subsequent maintaining behaviors supported joint attention. This finding suggests that mothers of children with DS, like mothers of typically developing children, adjust their supportive strategies to match their child's developmental competence and provide scaffolding to foster their child's attention skills.

Children are often in situations that involve more than one potential interactive partner, and some research has indicated that such situations pose challenges for preschoolers with DS. In a study in which preschoolers with and without DS reacted to a novel object, O'Neill and Happe (2000) found that children with DS (mean age 45 month) in comparison to peers (mean age 22 months) and to children with autism (mean age 55 months) directed behavior to their mothers less often than typically developing children (and similar to children with autism) in the presence of both a toy and an experimenter. O'Neill and Happe (2000) interpreted these findings as indicative of the challenges encountered by children with DS during triadic interactions when two possible partners are present. This interpretation again points to the difficulty that children with DS have making attentional shifts.

Social referencing, another aspect of shared activity, contrasts with coordinated joint attention because it occurs in situations that are ambiguous for the child (e.g., is this novelty a threat or amusing?) and occurs for the purpose of information seeking rather than information sharing (Kasari, Freeman, Mundy, & Sigman, 1995). Some differences in social referencing patterns of children with DS have been noted. When presented with a mechanical robot, toddlers with DS (aged 13–42 months) shifted their attention less from a person (either the parent or experimenter) to an object than did children in the comparison group (composed of typically developing children of similar MA, 9–27 months) (Kasari et al., 1995). Kasari et al. speculated that children with DS have more difficulty cognitively appraising the ambiguous situation than do typically developing children. Knieps, Walden, and Baxter (1994), however, found that toddlers with DS engaged in referential looking when ambiguous novel objects were presented to them (e.g., remote-controlled mechanical toys), but the toddlers' affective responses to the toys frequently did not match the affective responses displayed by mothers. This finding further supports the hypothesis that toddlers with DS have difficulty regulating their attention from person to object and may not attend or encode social information provided by mothers as efficiently as do typically developing children. In turn, mothers of children with DS may have greater difficulty interpreting and responding to their children's affective expressions when they do not match the ongoing situation. Consequently, mothers may experience challenges in teaching their children with DS about novel objects.

Down Syndrome: Future Research on Mother–Child Interaction

Several parallel streams of research have occurred during the last decade in relation to interactions between mothers and their children with DS. We have described research on mother–child attachment within dyads in which a child has DS. The results of those studies, however, leave many questions unanswered about the value of using the Strange Situation for measuring attachment in children with DS. In our view, this work should continue only if it is demonstrated to have predictive power for later relationships, both mother–child and child–peer, and if the results are directed toward areas of intervention designed to benefit mother–child relationships.

Another stream of research, aligned with co-constructivist and transactional theories, has been focused on mother and child behaviors during sequences of interaction. Shared activity serves as the proximal social context in which cognitive, social, emotional, and communicative domains of development are broadened and enhanced (Iarocci, Virji-Babul, & Reebye, 2006). Scholarly work on such sequences has moved away from concern about mothers being overly directive to a more nuanced understanding of those directives and their adaptability within the bidirectional mother–child relationship (Marfo et al., 1998). The research reviewed

here indicates that the last decade's work has produced a deeper understanding of the cognitive load placed on children with DS during mother–child exchanges, especially when such exchanges require the child to make attentional shifts. As suggested by Iarocci, Virji-Babul, and Reebye (2006), the shifts from dyadic to triadic interactions are foundational steps in the development of social competence of all children, including those with DS. Obtaining a greater understanding of the delays or difficulties that children with DS demonstrate when shifting their attention, especially in situations involving triadic interactions, deserves increased focus by researchers. The field would benefit from future research that addresses strategies that mothers of children with DS can use to assist children in making attentional shifts within the context of interactions characterized by the sensitivity and warmth known to be advantageous to the mother–child relationship.

Williams Syndrome
Williams Syndrome: Research Relevant to Dyadic Interaction

Williams syndrome is a rare genetic disorder that affects children's cognitive and social development. The cognitive phenotype is characterized by an uneven profile of skills, such as lower problem solving, planning, spatial, and numerical processing skills (Bellugi, Lichtenberger, Jones, Lai, & St. George, 2000) with perceptual functioning more impaired than memory function (Einfeld, 2005) and higher verbal ability relative to perceptual functioning (Tager-Flusberg & Sullivan, 2000). Children with WS present with a unique personality style, often considered to be hypersocial (Doyle, Bellugi, Korenberg, & Graham, 2004; Jones et al., 2000), as well as shy, tense, sensitive, empathic, gregarious and people-oriented compared to children with intellectual disabilities from mixed etiologies (Järvinen-Pasley Bellugi, Reilly, Mills, Galaburda, Reiss, & Korenberg, 2008; Klein-Tasman & Mervis, 2003).

Based on this profile, one might expect that dyadic interactions between mothers and children with WS would benefit from such social tendencies. A complex understanding of WS has been achieved in regard to the strengths that children with WS have in facial recognition and expressive language acquisition relative to their other cognitive skills. Patterns of behaviors in both of these domains have implications for mother–child interaction.

First, in relation to the interest in faces and the facial recognition skills displayed by children with WS, research has primarily been conducted in laboratory settings. The results of several studies (e.g., Bellugi, Wang, & Jernigan, 1994; Fidler, Hepburn, Most, Philofsky, & Rogers, 2007; Wang, Doherty, Rourke, & Bellugi, 1995) have indicated that, despite impairments in visual–spatial skills and in general cognitive performance, individuals with WS show typical performance on facial recognition tasks. That skill does not seem to extend to all aspects of facial recognition, such as emotional labeling of facial expressions. Young children with WS also show difficulty interpreting emotional expressions and in using this information to make social decisions (Fidler et al., 2007). In a study focused on labeling facial emotions, Plesa-Skwerer, Faja, Schofield, Verbalis, and Tager-Flusberg (2006) compared children and adults with WS (ages 12–32 years) to those with intellectual disabilities, as well as to those with typical development. They found that individuals with WS and adults with intellectual disabilities (matched for age, IQ, and language performance) had poorer performance than age-matched individuals in the typical comparison group in identifying negative emotions. Children and adults in all three groups, however, were able to accurately label positive emotions. Thus, the skills that children with WS have in the recognition of faces and positive emotions would seem to benefit the family system as a whole and possibly the mother–child dyad in particular. The child's accurate recognition of positive emotions may create a synergy of positive bidirectional effects.

In addition to intact facial recognition skills, children with WS, in comparison to other children, tend to gaze more at faces, which might establish a positive context for interactions between children and mothers but also could interfere with that relationship in situations in which other individuals are also present. Jones et al. (2000) studied children with WS (mean age of 18.5 months) in comparison to their typically developing same-aged peers and reported that children with WS "looked excessively at the experimenter's face, often at the expense of performing the task at hand" (p. 39) during both warm-up tasks and cognitive testing. Mervis et al. (2003) reported two studies in which infants and toddlers with WS, in comparison to those of the same age developing typically, were found to spend significantly more time looking at their mothers or a stranger. These findings may suggest an innate predisposition toward social interaction. Such a predisposition can enhance dyadic interaction but also is likely to interfere with the development of the joint attention that occurs in triadic interactions

between mother, infant, and objects (Doyle et al., 2004; Laing et al., 2002). In an extensive review, Järvinen-Pasley and colleagues (2008) summarized research that indicates that children with WS spend more time looking at a novel adult than at their parent when involved in triadic situations. As a result, they often turn triadic interactions into dyadic ones by attempting to "hook" the engagement of the novel adult. Therefore, joint attention with a parent and object can readily become interrupted by the child's predilection to focus on novel persons, with a concomitant lack of attention to the parent or the selected object. Although the effects of such actions have not been fully investigated, it is probable that such behaviors reduce the child's ability to learn language skills through dyadic interaction with a parent as well as to learn about the properties of objects.

The long gazes toward people displayed by children with William syndrome may also indicate a slower rate of processing information about faces. Mobbs, Garrett, Menon, Rose, Bellugi, and Reiss (2004) studied the performance of 11 adults with WS in comparison to other similar-aged adults on gaze following during facial processing. They found that those with WS were less accurate in determining the direction of gaze and had longer response latencies, as well as a different pattern of cortical activation. Thus, longer gazes during the infant and toddler years may relate to the need for increased time to process facial features.

Another interpretation of the long gazes displayed by infants and toddlers with WS is that they are due to difficulties in disengaging attentional focus. Brown et al. (2003) found that infants and toddlers (ages 23–37 months) with WS in comparison to those with DS, as well as with those with similar CAs or similar developmental ages (12–21 months), had difficulty with disengagement from the stimulus. It is possible that mothers (and other caregivers) attribute such fixation on faces as indicative of interest in social interaction. Alternatively, the attentional focus on faces may challenge maternal efforts to engage her child in joint attention toward objects outside the mother–child dyad.

The highly social tendencies of children with WS might be expected to assist such children in the development of friendships, but it appears that they have difficulty developing and maintaining friendships (Gosh & Pankau, 1994; Udwin & Yule, 1991). A potential reason for such difficulties derives from the proposal by Tager-Flusberg and Sullivan (2000) that the acquisition of theory of mind (i.e., social knowledge) is comprised of two components, and children with WS show a weakness in one of these components. Such children are relatively successful with the social-perceptual component, which involves the perception of people and evaluation of their affective (especially positive) states. This claim is supported by studies indicating that children with WS express high levels of empathy (Tager-Flusberg & Sullivan, 2000) and abnormally positive ratings of the approachability of human faces (Bellugi, Adolphs, Cassady, & Chiles, 1999). Thus, success in the social-perceptual component underlies children's tendencies to readily attempt to engage others. In contrast, children with WS appear to be much less successful with the social-cognitive components of social knowledge, which involves understanding the representational aspects of mind (Fidler et al., 2007; Järvinen-Pasley et al., 2008; Tager-Flusberg & Sullivan, 2000). Representational understanding is crucial for recognizing the intentions of others, a necessary skill for friendship maintenance.

Researchers have also focused on another domain of development—expressive language—which, similarly to facial recognition, has been associated with an area of relative strength for children with WS. Although children with WS show delays of 24 months in vocabulary acquisition during early childhood (at levels similar to those of children with DS), they improve rapidly and display a relative strength in language skills (in relation to spatial skills) by school age. Bellugi, Lichtenberger, Jones, Lai, and St. George (2000) described children with WS as "talkative to the point of being loquacious" (p. 11) and indicated that they have a proclivity for understanding and using vocabulary that is unusual (e.g., "canine, abrasive, solemn," p. 14) given their general cognitive functioning. Various studies have found that adolescents with WS use unusual vocabulary and social evaluative devices to enrich narrative content (e.g., "He was *so* sad") as well as vocal prosody (e.g., pitch changes) when telling a story. They also found that even during middle childhood, individuals with WS tend to use social engagement devices to attract the listener ("Lo and behold . . .") (Järvinen-Pasley et al., 2008; Jones et al., 2000). Although children with WS appear to have strengths in the use of social evaluative language, they show deficits in pragmatic language skills, such as appropriate initiation of topics (La Croix, Bernicot, & Reilly, 2007). Moreover, the quality of their conversations suggests a lack of understanding of the perspective of their conversational partners (LaCroix, Bernicot, & Reilly, 2007).

Children with WS display an unusual sequence in the use of gestures and language, and this sequence raises questions about the essential role of mother–child joint attention in language development (Laing et al., 2002). In typically developing children, as in children with DS, speech production follows the use of specific gestures, such as pointing, yet the opposite sequence has been found to occur for children with WS (Mervis, Morris, Bertrand, & Robinson, 1999). Unlike other children, it appears that, in children with WS, aspects of joint attention, such as referential gestures, occur only after vocabulary is well developed (Laing et al., 2002). Mervis and Bertrand (1997) posited that this developmental sequence may partially reflect the visual–spatial deficits of children with WS, since pointing requires rudimentary spatial skills. Nevertheless, the unusual sequencing of the acquisition of verbal expression before referential gestures in children with WS is puzzling and deserves extensive research. It raises questions about the role of joint attention and perspective taking in the overall development of children with WS.

Williams Syndrome: Studies on Mother–Child Interaction

The studies reviewed in this section illustrate points of entry into investigations of dyadic interactions of mothers of children with WS. Researchers in the first study consider children's reactions during separation from the parent, and those in the second study focus on maternal directives. The results of each study are suggestive of areas of future investigation.

Jones et al. (2000) used a parent separation task to examine attachment styles among children with WS aged 15–58 months, matched on CA and gender to one comparison group and on developmental age and gender to a second group of comparison children (mean MA of 18.5 months). They found that the children with WS exhibited negative facial expressions less frequently, and showed less intense vocal and facial distress as their parents left the room in comparison to both groups. Upon being reunited with their parents, the children reengaged in play and needed less consoling than did their typically developing peers. Similar to speculations about the behavior of children with DS during separations, these findings suggest either that signals of distress might be muted and less readable in such children, or that situations of separation are not as stressful for children with WS as they are for typically developing children. Future studies may help to determine the interpretation of these findings.

Ly and Hodapp (2005) examined the role of directives in parent interactions with children with WS. In a comparison of children with WS to children with Prader-Willi syndrome, parents (primarily mothers) and children were observed during a puzzle completion task. Contrasts were expected as children with WS tend to exhibit relative weaknesses in visual–spatial tasks such as puzzles, whereas children with Prader-Willi syndrome have relative strengths in this domain. Parents of children with WS engaged in a more directive style of interaction, and provided more help and reinforcement, although within both groups, parents provided more directives to children with lower puzzle skills. Ly and Hodapp (2005) reasoned that parents of children with WS may have provided more helping behaviors and reinforcement as strategies to engage the child in an area of perceived weakness. They speculated that these findings illustrate not only the direct effects of a syndrome on a child's behavior and parents' perceptions of their child's competence, but also the indirect effect of etiology on children's behaviors through parental attributions.

Williams Syndrome: An Agenda for Research on Mother–Child Interaction

Despite having intellectual disabilities, children with WS tend to have patterns of relative strengths in areas that have implications for mother–child interaction. Such strengths might be enhanced or diminished through interactions with caregivers, and research is needed to determine the extent to which this occurs, as well as to delineate the process by which this occurs. For example, the role of maternal directives and the situations in which such directives appear to be beneficial to the development of children with WS deserves careful attention. Additionally, investigations on the avenues to joint attention between children with WS and their caregivers are likely to yield information about the role of shared activities in children's developmental trajectories. How does such activity serve to enhance the development of children with WS? What types of scaffolding or instructional strategies are used by parents, and in what contexts is this most beneficial for learning? Do children with WS display attentional disengagement difficulties in a variety of situations, or only within certain contexts? What interventions can occur to assist children with WS with such disengagement?

In relation to attachment research, the same questions about the validity of the Strange Situation paradigm are likely to emerge for children with WS

as they have for children with DS. Other approaches to measuring attachment have been developed. In particular, the Q-sort relies on ratings of mothers' interactions with children when asked to attend to a task not involving the child (Pederson & Moran, 1996). This may provide a more ecologically valid approach than the Strange Situation in measuring the attachment of mothers and children with WS. Because of their relevance to application, the qualities that mothers bring to the interaction, especially warmth and sensitive responsiveness, deserve to be further studied in relation to predicting the development of children with WS. Research that also captures the child's contributions to the interaction and the transactional waves of interaction would advance understanding of mutually adaptive dyads (Sameroff & MacKenzie, 2003). Finally, examination of how mothers advance a child's development through scaffolding and other forms of cognitive and socioemotional growth promotion would contribute to an understanding of potential sources of intervention support for mothers and their children with WS.

Research on Mother–Child Interaction: Neglected Avenues and Future Paths

Consideration of the research literature reviewed in this chapter reveals several prominent themes that deserve more attention. Mothers are not the only caregivers of young children, and the extent to which knowledge about mother–child interactions is relevant to other caregiver–child interactions needs careful investigation. Although in this chapter we have focused on research involving mothers and their children, a few studies have also been conducted with fathers. For example, in a comparison of both mothers and fathers of toddlers with DS, cleft lip and/or palate and typically developing children, Pelchat, Bisson, Bois, and Saucier (2003) found that the child's type of disability predicted variance in sensitivity only for fathers of children with DS. Even less studied than father–child interaction is the three-way interactions that frequently take place involving mother, father, and child. A promising model for studying such complexity has been suggested by Frascarolo et al. (Frascarolo, Favez, Carneiro, & Fivaz-Dépeursinge, 2004). This model includes an analysis of the functions necessary to co-construct three-way play episodes, including participation of all parties, organization of roles, focalization of attention, and affective contact.

A second prominent concern regarding the research base on mother–child interaction in families in which a child has a disability is the chasm created between the knowledge we have and that which we need to acquire about a range of families with diverse backgrounds, cultural codes, and beliefs about parenting a child with a disability. Most research has focused on white middle-income families, making generalizations to other families questionable. Indeed, data from the National Early Intervention Longitudinal Study (Hebbeler, Spiker, Mallik, Scarborough, & Simeonsson, 2004) indicates that, in the United States, only 53% of children entering early intervention services are Caucasian. The ethnic and cultural codes related to parenting practices vary considerably based on parents' perceptions of developmental disabilities (García Coll & Magnusson, 2000), parenting ethno-theories (Harkness & Super, 1996), and the role of spirituality or religiosity in the family (Raghavan, Weisner, & Patel, 1999; Rogers-Dulan & Blacher, 1995). Much research is needed that focuses on the wide range of families, including single-parent families, extended families, and blended families who have children with developmental disabilities.

Finally, during the last two decades research has certainly moved from the laboratory to the settings in which children actually learn and grow. Although studies on children with disabilities have followed this trend, a gap still exists in our knowledge base about the interactional styles of children and their caregivers in a range of normative environments. From an ecological perspective (Bronfenbrenner, 1986), policies, programs, and practices at federal, state, and community levels affect families and ultimately influence the opportunities and settings available to parents. Such broad maps are rarely captured in research studies, yet those operating from the perspective of developmental systems models highlight the multifaceted context within which caregiver–child interactions occur (Guralnick, 2005).

Future research on mother–child interaction will develop based on the theoretical perspectives of the researchers and on trends in the general field of developmental psychology. A central developmental principle that guides the field is that the proximal relationship between children and their caregivers is central to children's development. If that principle is valid, it should hold for children with biologically based syndromes. Indeed, the research on children with DS suggests that although some dyads may experience difficulties, most children are well attached to their mothers and derive developmental benefits from warm and sensitive interactions.

Fundamental research needs to occur to understand the extent to which interactions among dyads in which a child has WS operate according to the same principles as those of other dyads.

Research on children with either DS or WS would benefit from more knowledge of the role that shared activity between a child and caregiver plays in the development of language, cognitive, and social skills. Further studies may help illuminate the importance of joint attention for the later language and cognitive development of children with DS and WS, and whether such children develop a means of self-regulation through social referencing or through other processes. This research is important not only for its potential to advance the development of children with DS or WS, but also for its contribution to the understanding of the full range of human development. By studying children with biologically based disabilities like DS and WS, we gain an understanding of the role of essential processes, such as attachment, but we also learn about the potential of alternative pathways to development, such as the role of gestures to speech production. Investigations of mother–child interaction provide an important avenue to such understanding.

Acknowledgments

The preparation of this chapter was supported in part by grant R40 MC08956 from the Maternal and Child Health Bureau (Title V, Social Security Act), Health Resources and Services Administration, U.S. Department of Health and Human Services.

References

Ainsworth, M. D. S., Blehar, M. C., Waters, E., & Wall, S. (1978). *Patterns of attachment.* Hillsdale, NJ: Lawrence Erlbaum.

American Academy of Pediatrics: Committee on Genetics (2001). Health supervision for children with Down syndrome. *Pediatrics, 107,* 442–449.

Atkinson, L., Chisholm, V. V., Scott, B., Goldberg, S., Vaughn, B. F., Blackwell, J., et al. (1999). Maternal sensitivity, child functional level, and attachment in Down syndrome. In J. I. Vondra, & D. Barnett (Eds.), Atypical attachment in infancy and early childhood among children at developmental risk. *Monographs of the Society for Research in Child Development, 64* (3) (Serial No. 258).

Bakeman, R., & Adamson, L. B. (1984). Coordinating attention to people and objects in mother-infant and peer-infant interaction. *Child Development, 54,* 1278–1289.

Barnard, K. E., Hammond, M. A., Booth, C. L., Bee, H. L., Mitchell, S. K., & Spieker, S. J. (1989). Measurement and meaning of parent-child interaction. In F. J. Morrison, C. Lord, & D. P. Keating (Eds.), *Applied developmental psychology* Vol. 3 (pp. 39–79). New York: Academic Press.

Barnard, K. E., & Sumner, G. A. (2002). Promoting awareness of the infant's behavioral patterns: Elements of anticipatory guidance for parents. In J. Gomes-Pedro, K. J. Nugent,

G. J. Young, & B. T. Brazelton (Eds.), *The infant and the family in the twenty-first century* (pp. 139–157). New York: Brunner-Routledge.

Bell, R. Q. (1968). A reinterpretation of the direction of effects in studies of socialization. *Psychological Review, 75*, 81–95.

Bellugi, U., Adolphs, R., Cassady, C., & Chiles, M. (1999). Towards the neural basis for hypersociability genetic syndrome. *NeuroReport, 10*(8), 1–5.

Bellugi, U., Lichtenberger, L., Jones, W., Lai, Z., & St. George, M. (2000). The neurocognitive profile of Williams syndrome: A complex pattern of strengths and weaknesses. *Journal of Cognitive Neuroscience, 12*(Supplement), 7–29.

Bellugi, U., Wang, P. P., & Jernigan, T. L. (1994). Williams syndrome: An unusual neuropsychological profile. In S. H. Broman, & J. Grafman (Eds.), *Atypical cognitive deficits in developmental disorders* (pp. 22–83). Hillsdale, NJ: Erlbaum.

Bornstein, M. H. (2006). Parenting science and practice. In K. A. Renninger, & I. E. Sigel (Eds.), *Child psychology in practice:* Vol. 4 *Handbook of child psychology* (6th ed., pp. 893–949). Editors-in-chief: W. Damon, & R. M. Lerner. Hoboken, NJ: Wiley.

Bornstein, M. H., & Tamis-LeMonda, C. S. (2001). Mother-infant interaction. In G. Bremner, & A. Fogel (Ed.), *Blackwell handbook of infant development* (pp. 269–295). Malden, MA: Blackwell Publishing.

Bornstein, M. H., Tamis-LeMonda, C. S., & Baumwell, L. (2001). Maternal responsiveness and children's achievement of language milestones. *Child Development, 72*, 748–767.

Bowlby, J. (1969/1982). *Attachment and loss:* Vol. 1. *Attachment.* New York: Basic Books.

Bretherton, I. (1985). Attachment theory: Retrospect and prospect. *Monographs of the Society for Research in Child Development, 50*, 3–35.

Bronfenbrenner, U. (1986). Ecology of the family as a context for human development: Research perspectives. *Developmental Psychology, 22*, 723–742.

Brooks-Gunn, J., & Lewis, M. (1984). Maternal responsivity in interactions with handicapped infants. *Child Development, 55*, 782–793.

Brown, J. H., Johnson, M. H., Paterson, S. J., Gilmore, R., Longhi, E., & Karmiloff-Smith, A. (2003). Spatial representation and attention in toddlers with Williams syndrome and Down syndrome. *Neuropsychologia, 41*, 1037–1046.

Bruner, J. S. (1982). The organization of action and the nature of adult-infant transaction. In M. von Cranach, & R. Harre (Eds.), *The analysis of action* (pp.313–328). Cambridge, UK: Cambridge University Press.

Bruner, J. S. (1983). *Child's talk: Learning to use language.* New York: Norton.

Bundy, A. C. (1997). Play and playfulness: What to look for. In L. D. Parham, & L. S. Fazio (Eds.), *Play in occupational therapy for children* (pp. 52–66). St. Louis: Mosby.

Carpenter, M., Nagel, K., & Tomasello, M. (1998). Social cognition, joint attention, and communicative competence. *Monographs of the Society for Research in Child Development, 63* (4, Serial No. 255).

Carvajal, F., & Iglesias, J. (2000). Looking behavior and smiling in Down syndrome infants. *Journal of Nonverbal Behavior, 24*, 225–236.

Carvajal, F., & Iglesias, J. (2002). Face-to-face emotion interaction studies in Down syndrome infants. *International Journal of Behavioral Development, 26*, 104–112.

Cielinski, K. L., Vaughn, B. E., Seifer, R., & Contreras, J. (1995). Relations among sustained engagement during play, quality of play, and mother-child interaction in samples of children with Down syndrome and normally developing toddlers. *Infant Behavior and Development, 18*, 163–176.

Corkum, V. L., & Moore, C. (1998). The origins of joint attention. *Developmental Psychology, 34*, 28–38.

Crockenberg, S., & Litman, C. (1990). Autonomy as competence in 2-year-olds: Maternal correlates of child defiance, compliance, and self-assertion. *Developmental Psychology, 26*, 972–977.

Doyle, T. F., Bellugi, U., Korenberg, J. R., & Graham, J. (2004). "Everybody in the world is my friend": Hypersociability in young children with Williams syndrome. *American Journal of Medical Genetics, 124*, 263–273.

Einfeld, S. (2005). Behaviour problems in children with genetic disorders causing intellectual disability. *Educational Psychology, 25*, 341–346.

Elicker, J., Englund, M., & Sroufe, L. A. (1992). Predicting peer competence and peer relationships in childhood from early parent-child relationships. In R. D. Parke, & G. W. Ladd (Eds.), *Family-peer relationships: Modes of linkage* (pp. 77–106). Hillsdale, NJ: Lawrence Erlbaum.

Fadiman, A. (1997). *The spirit catches you and you fall down: An Hmong child, her American doctors, and the collision of two cultures.* New York: Farrar, Strauss and Giroux.

Fidler, D. J., Hepburn, S. L., Most, D. E., Philofsky, A., & Rogers, S. J. (2007). Emotional responsivity in young children with Williams syndrome. *American Journal on Mental Retardation, 112*, 194–206.

Fidler, D. J., Philofsky, A., Hepburn, S. L., & Rogers, S. J. (2005). Nonverbal requesting and problem-solving by toddlers with Down syndrome. *American Journal on Mental Retardation, 110*, 312–322.

Frankel, K. A., & Bates, J. E. (1990). Mother-toddler problem solving: Antecedants in attachment, home behavior, and temperament. *Child Development, 61*, 810–819.

Frascarolo, F., Favez, N., Carneiro, C., & Fivaz-Dépeursinge, E. (2004). Hierarchy of interactive functions in father-mother-baby three-way games. *Infant and Child Development, 13*, 301–322.

Ganiban, J., Barnett, D., & Cicchetti, D. (2000). Negative reactivity and attachment: Own syndrome's contribution to the attachment-temperament debate. *Development and Psychopathology, 12*, 1–21.

García Coll, C., & Magnuson, K. (2000). Cultural differences as sources of developmental vulnerabilities and resources. In J. P. Shonkoff, & S. J. Meisels (Eds.). *Handbook of early childhood intervention* (2nd ed., pp. 94–114). New York: Cambridge University Press.

Guralnick, M. J. (1998). The effectiveness of early intervention for vulnerable children: A developmental perspective. *American Journal on Mental Retardation, 102*, 319–345.

Guralnick, M. J. (2005). An overview of the developmental systems model for early intervention. In M. J. Guralnick (Ed.), *The developmental systems approach to early intervention* (pp. 3–28). Baltimore: Paul H. Brookes.

Harkness, S., & Super, C. M. (1996). *Parents' cultural belief systems: Their origins, expressions, and consequences.* New York: The Guilford Press.

Harris, S., Kasari, C., & Sigman, M. (1996). Joint attention and language gains in children with Down syndrome. *American Journal on Mental Retardation, 100*, 608–619.

Harrist, A. W., & Waugh, R. M. (2002). Dyadic synchrony: Its structure and function in children's development. *Developmental Review, 22,* 555–592.

Hauser-Cram, P. (1993). Mastery motivation in 3-year-old children with Down syndrome. In D. Messer (Ed.), *Mastery motivation in early childhood* (pp. 230–250). London: Routledge.

Hauser-Cram, P., Warfield, M. E., Shonkoff, J. P., Krauss, M. W., Upshur, C. C., & Sayer, A. (1999). Family influences on adaptive development in young children with Down syndrome. *Child Development, 70,* 979–989.

Hauser-Cram, P., Warfield, M. E., Shonkoff, J. P., Krauss, M. W., Sayer, A., & Upshur, C. C. (2001). Children with disabilities: A longitudinal study of child development and parent well-being. *Monographs of the Society for Research in Child Development, 66* (Serial no. 266).

Hebbeler, K., Spiker, D., Mallik, S., Scarborough, A., & Simeonsson, R. (2004). National Early Intervention Longitudinal Study: Birth history and health status of children entering early intervention. Retrieved from www.sri.com/neils/pdfs/EFI_1_Exec_Summary_10_15_dpww.pdf

Heckhausen, J. (1993). The development of mastery and its perception within caretaker- child dyads. In D. Messer (Ed.), *Mastery motivation in early childhood* (pp. 55–79). London: Routledge.

Hodapp, R. M., & Burack, J. A. (1990). What mental retardation tells us about typical evelopment: The examples of sequences, rates, and cross-domain relations. *Developmental Psychopathology, 2,* 213–225.

Hyche, J. K., Bakeman, R., & Adamson, L. B. (1992). Understanding communicative cues of infants with Down syndrome: Effects of mothers' experience and infants' age. *Journal of Applied Developmental Psychology, 13,* 1–16.

Iarocci, G., Virji-Babul, N., & Reebye, P. (2006). The learn at play program (LAAP): Merging family, developmental research, early intervention, and play goals for children with Down syndrome. *Journal of Policy and Practice in Intellectual Disabilities, 3,* 11–21.

Isabella, R. A., & Belsky, J. (1991). Interactional synchrony and the origins of infant- mother attachment: A replication study. *Child Development, 62,* 373–384.

Järvinen-Pasley, A., Bellugi, U., Reilly, J., Mills, D. L., Galaburda, A., Reiss, A. L., & Korenberg, J. R. (2008). Defining the social phenotype in Williams syndrome: A model for linking gene, the brain, and behavior. *Development and Psychopathology, 20,* 1–35.

Jones, W., Bellugi, U., Lai, Z., Chiles, M., Reilly, J., Lincoln, A., & Adolphs, R. (2000). Hypersociability in Williams syndrome. *Journal of Cognitive Neuroscience, 12*(Supplement), 30–46.

Kasari, C., & Freeman, S. F. N. (2001). Task-related social behavior in children with own syndrome. *American Journal on Mental Retardation, 106,* 253–264.

Kasari, C., Freeman, S., Mundy, P., & Sigman, M. (1995). Attention regulation by hildren with Down syndrome: Coordinated joint attention and social referencing looks. *American Journal on Mental Retardation, 100,* 128–136.

Kasari, C., Mundy, P., Yirmiya, N., & Sigman, M. (1990). Affect and attention in hildren with Down syndrome. *American Journal on Mental Retardation, 95,* 5–67.

Kelly, J. F., & Barnard, K. E. (2000). Assessment of parent-child interaction: Implications for early intervention. In J. P. Shonkoff, & S. J. Meisels (Eds.), *Handbook of early childhood intervention*

(2nd ed., pp. 258–289). New York: Cambridge University Press.

Klein-Tasman, B. P., & Mervis, C. B. (2003). Distinctive personality characteristics of 8-, 9-, and 10-year-olds with Williams syndrome. *Developmental Neuropsychology, 23,* 269–290.

Knieps, L. J., Walden, T. A., & Baxter, A. (1994). Affective expressions of toddlers with and without Down syndrome in a social referencing context. *American Journal on Mental Retardation, 99,* 301–312.

LaCroix, A., Bernicot, J., & Reilly, J. (2007). Narration and collaborative conversation in French-speaking children with Williams syndrome. *Journal of Neurolinguistics, 20,* 445–461.

Laing, E., Butterworth, G., Ansari, D., Gsödl, M., Longhi, E., Panagiotaki, G., et al. (2002). Atypical development of language and social communication in toddlers with Williams syndrome. *Developmental Science, 5*(2), 233–246.

Landry, S. H., & Chapieski, M. L. (1990). Joint attention of six-month-old Down syndrome and preterm infants: I. Attention to toys and mother. *American Journal n Mental Retardation, 94,* 488–498.

Landry, S. H., Smith, K. E., Swank, P. R., & Miller-Loncar, C. L. (2000). Early maternal and child influences on children's later cognitive and social functioning. *Child Development, 71,* 358–375.

Legerstee, M., & Fisher, T. (2008). Coordinated attention, declarative and imperative pointing in infants with and without Down syndrome: Sharing experiences with adults and peers. *First Language, 28,* 281–331.

Legerstee, M., Varghese, Y., & van Beek, J. (2002). Effects of maintaining and redirecting infant attention on the production of referential communication in infants with and without Down syndrome. *Journal of Child Language, 29,* 23–48.

Legerstee, M., & Weintraub, J. (1997). The integration of person and object attention in infants with and without Down syndrome. *Infant Behavior and Development, 20,* 1–82.

Ly, T. M., & Hodapp, R. M. (2005). Parents' attributions of their child's jigsaw-puzzle performance: Comparing two genetic syndromes. *Mental Retardation, 43,* 135–144.

Main, M., & Solomon, J. (1990). Procedures for identifying infants as disorganized/disoriented during the Ainsworth strange situation. In M. T. Greenberg, D. Cicchetti, & E. M. Cummings (Eds.), *Attachment in the preschool ears: Theory, research, and intervention.* (pp. 121–160). Chicago: University of Chicago Press.

Marfo, K. (1990). Maternal directiveness in interactions with mentally handicapped children: An analytical commentary. *Journal of Child Psychology and Psychiatry, 31*(4), 531–549.

Marfo, K., Dedrick, C. F., & Barbour, N. (1998). Mother-child interactions and the evelopment of children with mental retardation. In J. A. Burack, R. M. Hodapp, & E. Zigler (Eds.), *Handbook of mental retardation and development* (pp. 637–668). Cambridge, UK: Cambridge University Press.

Markus, J., Mundy, P., Morales, M., Delgado, C. E. F., & Yale, M. (2000). Individual differences in infant skills as predictors of child-caregiver joint attention and language. *Social Development, 9,* 302–315.

Mervis, C. B., & Bertrand, J. (1997). Developmental relations between cognition and language: Evidence from Williams syndrome. In L. B. Adamson, & M. A. Romski (Eds.), *Communication and language acquisition: Discoveries from atypical development* (pp. 75–106). Baltimore: Paul. H. Brookes.

Mervis, C. B., Morris, C. A., Bertrand, J., & Robinson, B. F. (1999). Williams syndrome: Findings from an integrated program of research. In H. Tager-Flusberg (Ed.), *Neurodevelopmental disorders* (pp. 65–110). Cambridge, MA: MIT Press.

Mervis, C. B., Morris, C. A., Klein-Tasman, B. P., Bertrand, J., Kwitny, S., Appelbaum, L. G., & Rice, C. E. (2003). Attentional characteristics of infants and toddlers with Williams syndrome during triadic interactions. *Developmental Neuropsychology, 23*, 243–268.

Mobbs, D., Garrett, A. S., Menon, V., Rose, F. E., Bellugi, U., & Reiss, A. L. (2004). Anomalous brain activation during face and gaze processing in Williams syndrome. *Neurology, 62*, 2070–2076.

Moore, D. G., Oates, J. M., Goodwin, J., & Hobson, R. P. (2008). Behavior of mothers and infants with and without down syndrome during the still-face procedure. *Infancy, 13*, 75–89.

Morrison, E. F., Rimm-Kaufman, S., & Pianta, R. C. (2003). A longitudinal study of other-child interactions at school entry and academic outcomes in middle school. *Journal of School Psychology, 41*, 185–200.

O'Neill, D. K., & Happe, F. G. E. (2000). Noticing and commenting on what's new: Differences and similarities among 22-month-old typically developing children, children with Down syndrome and children with autism. *Developmental Science, 3*, 457–478.

Pederson, D., & Moran, G. (1996). Expressions of the attachment relationship outside of he strange situation. *Child Development, 67*, 915–927.

Pelchat, D., Bisson, J., Bois, C., & Saucier, J, F. (2003). The effects of early relational antecedents and other factors on the parental sensitivity of mothers and fathers. *Infant and Child Development, 12*, 27–51.

Pianta, R. C., & Harbers, K. L. (1996). Observing mother and child behavior in a problem-solving situation at school entry: Relations with academic achievement. *Journal of School Psychology, 34*, 307–322.

Pitcairn, T. K., & Wishart, J. G. (1994). Reactions of young children with Down syndrome to an impossible task. *British Journal of Developmental Psychology, 2*, 485–490.

Plesa-Skwerer, D., Faja, S., Schofield, C., Verbalis, A., & Tager-Flusberg, H. (2006). Perceiving facial and vocal expressions of emotion in individuals with Williams syndrome. *American Journal on Mental Retardation, 111*, 15–26.

Raghavan, C., Weisner, T. S., & Patel, D. (1999). The adaptive project of parenting: South Asian families with children with developmental delays. *Education and Training in Mental Retardation and Developmental Disabilities, 34*(3), 281–292.

Repacholi, B. M. (1998). Infants' use of attentional cues to identify the referent of another person's emotional expression. *Developmental Psychology, 34*, 1017–1025.

Roach, M. A., Barratt, M, S., Miller, J. F., & Leavitt, L. A. (1998). The structure of mother-child play: Young children with Down syndrome and typically developing children. *Developmental Psychology, 34*, 77–87.

Rogers-Dulan, J., & Blacher, J. (1995). African American families, religion, and disability: A conceptual framework. *Mental Retardation, 33*(4), 226–238.

Rogoff, B. (2003). *The cultural nature of human development.* Oxford, UK: Oxford University Press.

Sameroff, A. J., & Fiese, B. H. (2000). Transactional regulation: The developmental ecology of early intervention. In J. P. Shonkoff, & S. J. Meisels (Eds.), *Handbook of early childhood intervention* (2nd ed., pp. 135–159). New York: Cambridge University Press.

Sameroff, A. J., & MacKenzie, M. J. (2003). Research strategies for capturing transactional models of development: The limits of the possible. *Development and Psychopathology, 15*, 613–640.

Shonkoff, J. P., & Phillips, D. A. (2000). *From neurons to neighborhood: The science of early childhood development.* Washington, D.C.: National Research Council and Institute of Medicine.

Slonims, V., & McConachie, H. (2006). Analysis of mother-infant interaction in infants with Down syndrome and typically developing infants. *American Journal on Mental Retardation, 111*, 273–289.

Tager-Flusberg, H., & Sullivan, K. (2000). A componential view of theory of mind: Evidence from Williams syndrome. *Cognition, 76*, 59–89.

Thompson, R. A., Easterbrooks, M. A., & Padilla-Walker, L. (2003). Social and motional development in infancy. In R. M. Lerner, M. A. Easterbrooks, & J. Mistry (Eds.), *Handbook of psychology* Vol. 6. *Developmental psychology* (pp. 91–112). New York: Wiley.

Tomasello, M. (1995). Joint attention as social cognition. In C. Moore, & P. J. Dunham Eds.), *Joint attention: Its origins and role in development* (pp. 103–130). Hillsdale, NJ: Lawrence Erlbaum.

Tomasello, M., & Farrar, J. (1986). Joint attention and early language. *Child Development, 57*, 1454–1463.

Tronick, E., Als, H., Adamson, L., Wise, S., & Brazelton, T. B. (1978). The infant's response to entrapment between contradictory messages in face-to-face interaction. *Journal of the American Academy of Child Psychiatry, 17*, 1–13.

Udwin, O., & Yule, W. (1991). A cognitive and behavioral phenotype in Williams syndrome. *Journal of Clinical and Experimental Neuropsychology, 13*, 232–144.

van IJzendoorn, M. H., Goldberg, S., Kroonenberg, P. M., & Frenkel, O. J. (1992). The relative effects of maternal and child problems on the quality of attachment: A meta-analysis of attachment in clinical samples. *Child Development, 63*, 840–858.

Vaughn, B. E., Goldberg, S., Atkinson, L., Marcovitch, S., MacGregor, D., & Seifer, R. (1994). Quality of toddler-mother attachment in children with Down syndrome: Limits to interpretation of Strange Situation behavior. *Child Development, 65*, 95–108.

Vaughn, B. E., Lefever, G. B., Seifer, R., & Barglow, P. (1989). Attachment behavior, attachment security, and temperament during infancy. *Child Development, 60*, 728–737.

Vygotsky, L. S. (1978). *Mind in society.* Cambridge, MA: Harvard University Press.

Wang, P. P., Doherty, S., Rourke, S. B., & Bellugi, U. (1995). Unique profile of visuo-perceptual skills in a genetic syndrome. *Brain and Cognition, 29*, 54–65.

Parenting and Intellectual Disability: An Attachment Perspective

Rinat Feniger-Schaal, David Oppenheim, Nina Koren-Karie, *and* Nurit Yirmiya

Abstract

This chapter begins with a brief review of attachment theory. It describes how attachment is assessed using the Strange Situation Procedure (SSP), and reviews the studies of attachment in children with Intellectual Disability (ID). It introduces two issues pertinent to attachment and ID: the first involves the cognitive prerequisites for the development of attachment; the second involves the factors contributing to the development of secure (or insecure) attachments in typically developing children, as well as in the development of children with ID. In addition to factors relating to the children, the chapter considers factors relating to the parents, including both parents' behavior with their children as reflected in their sensitivity, and parents' representations of their children, as reflected in their insightfulness into the experience of the child and their reactions to the diagnosis of the child.

Keywords: Attachment theory, children with Intellectual Disability, parental behavior, parenting, cognitive delay

Attachment theory is a powerful theoretical and empirical framework for the investigation of the socioemotional development of children (Cassidy & Shaver, 1999). In this chapter, we employ this framework for the conceptualization and understanding of the social and emotional development of children with Intellectual Disability (ID) and the parenting processes that contribute to this development. An attachment perspective can enrich our understanding of the development of children with ID, leading to a greater appreciation of both the child's and the parent's experience. Furthermore, beyond providing a fuller theoretical and empirical account, this knowledge may also have significant importance for interventions designed to enhance the emotional well-being of children with ID and their families. Our application of attachment theory is informed by Zigler (1967), one of the first to introduce a developmental approach to ID. He proposed that persons with ID proceed through the same sequence of developmental phases as do typically developing children, but more slowly. If so, theories that have made major contributions to our understanding of typical development—in our case, attachment theory—may be equally relevant for our understanding of the development of children with ID (Hodapp, Burack & Zigler, 1998). Zigler also argued that research on persons with ID should give greater attention to their social and emotional experiences, and that these might play an important role in their adjustment to the everyday world (Zigler, 2001, 2002). In the examination of the development of children with ID through the lens of attachment theory, we heed Zigler's call.

We will first provide a brief review of attachment theory, describe how attachment is assessed using the Strange Situation Procedure (SSP), and review the studies of attachment in children with ID. In this context two issues pertinent to attachment and ID will be introduced: The first involves the cognitive prerequisites for the development of attachment, and the second involves the factors contributing to the development of secure (or insecure) attachments in typically developing children, as well as in the development of children with ID. In addition to factors relating to the children, we will focus on factors relating to the parents, including both parents' behavior with their children as reflected in their sensitivity, and parents' representations of their children, as reflected in their insightfulness into the experience of the child and their reactions to the diagnosis of the child. *Insightfulness* refers to the parent's ability to "see things from the child's point of view," and *resolution* refers to coming to terms with the child's diagnosis and working through the emotional reactions that accompany receiving a diagnosis for the child. Both are hypothesized to impact the caregiving behavior and the attachment that children form to their parents, and research on insightfulness and resolution will be reviewed, together with excerpts from interviews designed to assess these processes.

Attachment Theory: A Brief Overview

One of the central tenets of Bowlby's theory of attachment (1982) is that forming attachments is a species-wide characteristic that has evolved through evolution and has survival value, and therefore all children form attachments to their caregivers. The only exception is extreme cases of institutionalized or severely deprived children. Attachments are not present at birth but develop during the first year of life, and their appearance is contingent on cognitive attainments that all typically developing children make by the age of 1 year. This point is particularly pertinent in the case of attachment among children with ID, whose cognitive development is delayed, and will be discussed further below.

Bowlby's additional premise was that the nature of the child's attachment to the caregiver, and more specifically the degree to which the child feels secure about the caregiver's availability to relieve the child's distress and provide a secure base for exploration, depends on that child's specific experiences with that caregiver. Thus, although the propensity to form attachments does not depend on the child's specific experiences and is "experience expectant," the security of the attachment that the child forms depends on the child's specific experiences with each of the child's caregivers and is "experience dependent" (Greenough & Black, 1992).

With respect to the study of attachment in children with ID, Zigler (2001, 2002) recently underscored the need to investigate social experiences that

give rise to emotional and motivational features that constitute their personality structure. Specifically, Zigler claimed that emotional and motivational factors, and not only IQ and cognitive processes, play a significant role in the adjustment of persons with ID. This approach is consistent with Bowlby's emphasis on the role of socioemotional development in general and the early mother–child relationship more specifically in children's development.

An additional tenet of attachment theory (Bowlby, 1982) is that early attachments provide the basis for the child's subsequent socioemotional development (Main, Kaplan, & Cassidy, 1985; Thompson, 1999). This idea has received support in numerous studies of children with typical development. For example, in a 30-year longitudinal study, Sroufe and colleagues (Sroufe, Egeland, Carlson, & Collins, 2005) found that securely attached children, by comparison with insecurely attached ones, develop into more competent toddlers and preschoolers, demonstrate better relationships with their peers; and express emotions more adaptively. Moreover, the authors found that the link between secure attachment and general measures of social competence continues, throughout development, from early childhood to adulthood (Sroufe, Egeland, Carlson, & Collins. 2005). By contrast, insecure attachments, and particularly disorganized attachment is a strong predictor of later psychopathology (Lyons-Ruth, 1996; Sroufe, Carlson, Levy, & Egeland, 1999).

The Strange Situation Procedure

Based on Bowlby's theorizing about attachment, Ainsworth devised the "Strange Situation Procedure" (SSP), a laboratory procedure that assesses individual differences in the quality of infant–caregiver attachment (Ainsworth, Blehar, Waters, & Wall, 1978). The SSP entails a structured observation of infants and their mothers, as well as an unfamiliar female in a laboratory playroom. The central events include two brief, 3-minute-long mother–infant separations. During the first separation, the infant is left with the stranger; during the second separation the infant is first alone, then with the stranger, and only subsequently is reunited with the mother. The procedure has proven to be extraordinarily informative and has been used to assess attachment patterns in a large number of studies in a wide range of cultures (van IJzendoorn & Kroonenberg, 1988; van IJzendoorn & Sagi, 2008), and within a wide range of clinical populations (e.g., Ganiban, Barnett, & Cicchetti, 2000).

Based on children's behavior during the SSP, and particularly based on their responses during the two reunion episodes, children are classified into one of four attachment patterns that reflect individual differences in the security of the child's attachment to the caregiver (Ainsworth et al., 1978): secure (B), insecure-avoidant (A), insecure-ambivalent (C), and insecure-disorganized (D). Infants who are securely attached (B) use their mothers as a secure base from which to explore; in her absence, they reduce their exploration and might be distressed, but greet her positively upon her return and soon resume exploring. This pattern is shown by 65%–70% of infants in normative samples. Infants whose attachment pattern is insecure-avoidant (A) explore with minimal reference to the mother, are minimally distressed by her departure, and ignore or avoid her on return. In normative samples, this pattern characterizes between 20%–25% of infants. Infants whose attachment pattern is insecure-ambivalent/resistant (C) explore minimally, showing high distress during separations and difficulty settling upon reunion. In normative samples, approximately 10% of infants show this pattern (Colin, 1996; van-IJzendoorn, Goldberg, Kroonenberg, & Frenkel, 1992). Finally, infants whose attachment pattern is insecure-disorganized (D) show disorganized or disoriented behaviors, indicating momentary lapses in their capacity to manage the stress of separation and reunion. In contrast to the previous three patterns, which are characterized by a coherent strategy for managing arousal in the strange situation (albeit an insecure strategy in the case of avoidant and resistant/ambivalent attachment), the salient feature of this group involves the breakdown of the child's strategy for dealing with the separations from the mother during the SSP In a non-clinical sample, 10-15% of infants fit the group D criteria (van IJzendoorn, Schuengel, & Bakermans-Kranenburg, 1999).

The SSP was developed and validated with typically developing children. Reviewing the corpus of studies supporting the validity of the SSP is beyond the scope of this chapter, but generally this research has shown that SSP classifications are associated with the history of the interactions between the infant and his or her caregivers. Mothers of infants classified as secure were observed throughout the first year of life as responding sensitively and appropriately to their infant's emotional signals when compared with infants who were not classified secure. In addition, SSP classifications were found to predict children's socioemotional development during childhood and adolescence, as mentioned above (Thompson, 1999, Sroufe, Egeland, Carlson, & Collins, 2005).

Strange Situation Behavior of Children with Intellectual Disability

The success of research using the SSP with typically developing children prompted studies using this procedure for children with atypical development, including ID. The subgroup that attracted the most research attention among children with ID involved children with Down Syndrome (DS), possibly because it is the most common genetically-based ID syndrome, and therefore most of the studies reviewed below concern this group.

Atkinson and colleagues (Atkinson, Chisholm, Scott, Goldberg, Vaughn, Blackwell, Dickerns, & Tam, 1999) observed 53 children with DS using the SSP and found that 40% were classified as secure at 26 months and 48% at 42 months. They also reported that a similar proportion was unclassifiable (it was unclear to the researchers whether they were insecure or lacked secure base behavior). Vaughn and colleagues (Vaughn, Goldberg, Atkinson, Marcovitch, MacGregor, & Seifer, 1994) compared the SSP classifications of 138 children with DS aged 14-54 months (from three different samples) and those of a sample of typically developing children aged 12-14 months. More children were classified secure in the typically developing group than in the DS group, and more children were unclassifiable in the DS group than in the group of typically developing children. Nevertheless, 48% of children with DS were classified as secure, although the authors pointed out that these children's reunion behavior was often difficult to interpret or categorize according to Ainsworth's traditional classification. Vaughn et al. (1994) were among the first to find an over-representation of disorganized attachment among children with DS. Similar rates of secure attachment were found by Ganiban, Barnett and Cicchetti (2000), who observed 30 infants with DS using the SSP at 19 and 27 months and found that many of the children were securely attached to their mothers (43% at 19 months and 53% at 27 months). Consistent with Vaughn and colleagues, Ganiban and colleagues (Ganiban, Barnett, & Cicchetti, 2000) also found elevated rates of disorganized attachment behaviour among children with DS.

An important limitation of this body of research is that the conclusions of these studies cannot be assumed to apply to children with ID who do not have DS. Although some studies suggest that the development of children with DS is the same as that of other groups of children with ID (Pino, 2000), others suggest that children with DS have higher levels of adaptive behavior including receptive, leisure and play skills (Canepa, Barbagna, Millepiedi, & Marcheschi, 2000), and that the mother-child interactions are better in the case of children with DS than in other groups of children with ID (Marcheschi, Millepiedi, & Barbagna, 1996), possibly because children with DS generally display a more cheerful and sociable personality (Hodapp, 2002) which may impact their behavior in the SSP. Unfortunately, there is a paucity of research on the attachment of children with ID who do not have DS.

Goldberg (1988) conducted one of the few attachment studies in children with developmental delay with unknown etiology. Goldberg used the SSP to study three groups of preschoolers with developmental delays: 40 children with DS, 29 children with neurological disorder, and 40 children with delay of unknown etiology. The author reported that the distribution of attachment classifications among all children in the study that could be classified using the conventional classification system did not differ from normative data, but one third of the SSPs could not be classified using the conventional classification system, and were classified as Avoidant (A) and Resistant (C) because of a mixture of proximity seeking, anger, and avoidance toward the mother. Furthermore, there were no significant differences in the distribution of attachment classifications between the diagnostic subgroups.

Recently, we conducted a study of 40 children with ID with unknown etiology whose ages ranged between 2.5 and 5.5 years. We used the SSP to assess children' attachment and found that 40% of the children were classified as secure, 35% were classified as insecure-organized and 25% were classified as insecure-disorganized (Feniger-Schaal, 2010). Taken together with the studies reviewed above, this study indicated that a considerable proportion of children with ID develop secure attachment relationships to their mothers. However, when compared with typically developing children, the rates of attachment insecurity in this group appear elevated, and we discuss next possible factors that might account for this elevation.

Applicability of the SSP for Children with ID

Trying to explain the relatively high rate of insecure attachment among children with ID it is important to note that some of the studies reviewed above called attention to the challenges involved in applying the conventional attachment classification system to children with ID. Therefore one issue is whether children with ID react to the stress in the SSP similarly to typically developing children and whether the "attachment system" – that is, the behavioral system governing the child's attachment behaviors in times of distress – is evoked by the separations in the SSP. This issue has been controversial. Some researchers found that children with DS appear to be less distressed by the SSP (Thompson, Cicchetti, Lamb, & Malkin, 1985; van IJzendoorn, 1994), whereas a study by Berry, Gunn and Andrews (1980) showed that children with DS became distressed during the SSP. Although children with DS are less likely to signal attachment needs, approach their mothers, or make physical contact on reunion, they evinced awareness of the changes during the SSP (Berry, Gunn, & Andrews, 1980; Cicchetti & Serafica, 1981). Vaughn et al. (1994) added that children with DS show clear evidence of awareness of the separation, conveyed by changes in the quality of their play and expressive behaviour, but indicated that the behaviour at the time of the reunion is more difficult to interpret.

The most programmatic effort to extend the use of the SSP and its classification to children with DS has been the series of studies by Cicchetti and associates (e.g. Ganiban, Barnett, & Cicchetti, 2000; Cicchetti & Ganiban, 1990; Cicchetti & Serafica, 1981; Cicchetti & Sroufe, 1978; Ganiban & Barnett, 1991), who adopted a broad organizational perspective of development in their interpretation of the behavior of children with DS during the SSP. Based on these studies, Cicchetti and colleagues concluded that between the ages of 12 and 24 months of developmental age (DA) attachment becomes consolidated among children with DS (Cicchetti & Beeghly, 1990), with an organization of SSP responses similar to that of typically developing children and with secure attachment as the normative pattern (Cicchetti & Ganiban, 1990; Ganiban & Barnett, 1991).

One way of resolving the discrepant views about the applicability of the SSP to children with ID is to examine the associations between SSP classifications and observations of mother-child interactions in a variety of contexts and over time. The validity of the SSP for use with typically developing children is based chiefly on the numerous studies that reported associations between mother–infant interactions during the first year of life, particularly in terms of maternal sensitivity to the infant's signals, and that child's attachment (De Wolff & van IJzendoorn, 1997). Sensitive maternal behavior, that is, behavior that is based on accurate reading of the child's emotional signals and on prompt and appropriate responses to these signals, has been consistently linked with the secure SSP classification. Data such as these—that is, sensitivity-attachment associations—with regard to children with ID would help support the validity of the SSP in ID. Unfortunately, there are only few studies on this issue, yet the findings are encouraging. Atkinson et al. (1999) examined attachment among children with DS and reported that children's attachment classifications were related to measures of maternal sensitivity obtained over a 2-year period under varying conditions, with mothers of secure children rated as more sensitive than mothers of insecure children. Similarly, Moran, Pederson, Petit, and Krupka (1992) found positive associations between maternal sensitivity and attachment security within a group of toddlers with DS, although in their study security was assessed by Waters and Deane's (1985) Attachment Behavior Q-Sort (AQS) and not by SSP. In the AQS observers conduct extended observations of the child and mother and following these observations sort a set of cards describing a wide range of child behaviors into a forced distribution ranging from most- to least-characteristic of the child. The correlation between the resultant profile and an "ideal" sort of a securely attached child provided by the Q-sort developers is the child's security score. The AQS is considered to be a valid assessment of attachment in infancy and is associated with the SSP (Waters et al., 1985). Therefore, the above findings linking maternal sensitivity with secure attachment support the application of attachment constructs and measures to children with ID.

In a more recent study, van IJzendoorn and colleagues (van IJzendoorn, Rutgers, Bakermans-Kranenburg, van Daalen, Dietz, Buitelaar, Swinkels, Naber, & England, 2007) examined maternal sensitivity and attachment among children with autism. Using a group of children with ID as one of the comparison groups, the authors found positive associations between security of attachment and parental sensitivity among children with ID and their mothers. The generalizability of the results is limited, however, because of the small number of participants in the ID group (n = 10). The association between maternal sensitivity and security of attachment was also reported in studies of children with autism, many of whom are also intellectually disabled (Capps, Sigman, & Mundy, 1994; Koren-Karie, Oppenheim, Dolev, & Yirmiya, 2009).

In a recent study, we examined the association between maternal sensitivity and security of attachment among 40 children with ID with unknown etiology (Feniger-Schaal, 2010). We found that securely attached children had mothers who were rated as more sensitive than those of children with insecure attachment. These finding reinforce the notion that maternal sensitivity fosters the development of secure attachment not only in typically developing children but also in children with ID. By linking child security to its hypothesized antecedent, maternal sensitivity, these findings also contribute to the validity of the SSP with children with ID.

To summarize, the association between maternal sensitivity and security of attachment in children with ID has been examined only in very few studies, and clearly, more research is needed on this matter. Taken together, the body of research on attachment in children with ID, particularly those with DS, show that a significant proportion—in some studies the majority—develops secure attachment. This finding is remarkable when considering the cognitive limitations of children with ID and the stress involved in raising a child with special needs—factors that may contribute to the difficulties in developing secure attachment. However, it is also noteworthy that the rate of security for the ID samples is lower than in nonclinical samples, whereas the rate of disorganized attachment is similar to that of clinical (e.g., maltreatment) samples (Ganiban et al., 2000).

Determinants of Attachment in Intellectual Disability

Next, we discuss the various determinants of attachment among children with ID. Our discussion first addresses the child's side of the attachment relationship, and more specifically the impact of cognitive delays and other characteristic of children with ID on the development of attachment. We then discuss studies that focus on the interactions between children with ID and their parents, and the implications of these for the development of attachment. Finally, we discuss the parental side of the relationship, particularly in terms of the significance of insightfulness into the experience of the child and of parents' coming to terms with the child's diagnosis and resolving its emotional impact.

Cognitive Delays and Attachment

The development of attachment depends on cognitive attainments such as object permanence, discrimination learning, and selective attention and memory that typically developing children achieve by the end of the first year of life (Bowlby, 1982; Cassidy, 1999; Main et al., 1985; Waters, Kondo-Ikemura, Posada, & Richters, 1991). Children with ID develop these skills later, and some have specific delays or deficits in these domains (Janssen, Schuengel, & Stolk, 2002). For example, Cicchetti's early work on attachment in children with DS (e.g., Cicchetti & Serafica, 1981) showed that these children developed attachments to their mothers in ways that resemble typically developing children but at a later chronological age, when their cognitive development was sufficiently advanced. Cicchetti's findings support the *sequence hypothesis*, which states that the development of children with ID progresses along the same developmental sequence as typically developing children but at a slower pace (Zigler, 1967).

Atkinson et al. (1999) investigated the quality of the attachment of higher versus lower functioning children with DS and found that low-functioning children with DS were less frequently classified as secure in the SSP than were high-functioning children. These findings suggest that the cognitive delay characteristic of children with ID may not only postpone the CA in which they develop attachments, but may also contribute to the increased rates of insecurity once attachment is formed. This is a slightly different conclusion than the one based on Cicchetti's studies, as it suggests that cognitive delays increase the likelihood that an insecure attachment will develop.

One possible way in which cognitive delay may impact the security of attachment is revealed in studies showing that cognitive impairments in children with ID lead to greater vulnerability to stress and the use of less effective coping strategies (Janssen et al., 2002). Jahromi, Gulsrud, and Kasari (2008) found that children with DS use a limited repertoire of strategies for coping with frustration, and the authors suggest that this may contribute to the behavior problems exhibit by children with DS. Janssen and his colleagues suggested that the vulnerability to stress and the limitations in coping strategies may mediate the link between children's cognitive impairments and insecure attachment (Janssen et al., 2002). Thus, the child may be using less effective strategies to deal with attachment-related stress, and this may be reflected in insecure attachment.

The cognitive delays, as well as other difficulties characterizing children with ID, are also manifested in the interactions between these children and their parents. In general, children with ID are described as less reactive and cooperative and less clear in their signaling behavior, which makes it more difficult for parents to be sensitive, and to find interactions with their child to be appealing or rewarding (Janssen et al., 2002). For example, Bridges and Cicchetti (1982) proposed that muted affect or ambiguous affective cues due to poor muscle tone may make it difficult to accurately interpret the cues of children with DS. In addition, Berger (1990) noted that key social cues are delayed in their onset within DS population. Walden and Knieps (1996) reported that toddlers with DS have difficulties in decoding their mother facial expression, and Kasari, Freeman, and Hughes (2001) found that children with DS have difficulties in understanding and labeling of emotions. In their summary of studies on the social and emotional development of children with ID, Kasari and Bauminger (1998) conclude that children with ID have difficulties in emotion responsivity, emotion recognition, and prosocial behavior.

Studies that investigated the interaction between children with ID and their mothers from mothers' point of view found that mothers have difficulties in correctly understanding their children's behavior and in accurately evaluating their own parenting skills, due to lack of clear feedback from their child (Blacher, 1984; Bruchin, 1990; Marom, 1990; Weissman, 1991). Thus, the cognitive delays, as well as the social and emotional difficulties of children with ID, may impede the establishment of synchronous, reciprocal interaction between these children and their parents, possibly accounting for the lower rates of secure attachment found in this population.

Parenting Children with Intellectual Disability

Beyond the child's contribution to the quality of attachment, the parenting that the child receives is considered in attachment theory as the other major determinant of the security of the child's attachment to the parent (Weinfield, Sroufe, Egeland, & Carlson, 1999). Among the parental characteristics that may contribute to child attachment, our review will focus on parental stress, parental insightfulness, and parental resolution of the child's diagnosis.

Parenting a child with ID presents unique difficulties. Bruchin (1990) and others (e.g., Beckman, 2002; Donenberg & Baker, 1993; Hauser-Cram, Warfield, Shonkoff, & Krauss, 2001) found that having a child with developmental delays is associated with increased stress for parents. Baker and his colleagues (Baker, Blacher, Crnic, & Edelbrock, 2002) reported a negative impact on mothers' and fathers' stress levels as early as the child's age of 3 years. Weissman (1991) reported that parents of children with mental disabilities showed more depression, helplessness, and burnout than did two groups of parents of typically developing children, one matched on CA and the other on mental age (MA). The divorce rate among couples who have a child with ID was shown to be higher than in couples who have only typically developing children (Gath, 1977; Schell, 1981). In addition, financial worries (Meyer, Vadasy, Fewell, & Schell, 1982) and negative effects on the siblings (Hannah & Midlarsky, 1999; Levy-Shiff, 1986; Zaider, 1987) add to the distress of a family raising a child with ID. Thus, having a child with ID can introduce substantial stress to parents and the entire family. Because parental stress may reduce parental emotional availability to the child (Belsky, 1984), the stress experienced by parents of children with ID may be one of the contributors to the lower rate of secure attachment among these children.

Other studies have shown that having a child with ID may have positive effects on families. For example, Cuskelly and Gunn (2003) have shown that siblings of children with DS show less unkindness and more empathy toward their siblings with DS, and they participate in more caregiving activities than do siblings of typically developed children. In addition, longitudinal studies have shown that while families may experience elevated stress initially, over time the negative impact of the child's condition decreases and parent's well-being increases (Barnett et al. 2006; Keogh, Garnier, Bernheimer, & Gallimore, 2000). Thus, raising a child with ID may have both positive and negative effects on families. Additionally, not all families experience the same amount of stress, and families may respond differently to similar stressors, thus yielding important individual differences among parents and children, including the individual differences in attachment security reviewed earlier.

From an attachment point of view, the main mechanism thought to account for individual differences in children's attachment is the caregiver's sensitivity to the child's emotional signals (Ainsworth et al., 1978). As mentioned earlier, this mechanism received support from numerous studies with typically developing children (Weinfield et al., 1999) and from a few studies involving children with ID (Feniger-Schaal, 2010). The link between maternal sensitivity and attachment also emerged from studies of children with autism, many of whom are also mentally retarded (Capps, Sigman, & Mundy, 1994; Koren-Karie, Oppenheim, Dolev, & Yirmiya, 2009). Additional, although less direct evidence for the impact of parenting on children's attachment comes from a meta-analysis conducted by van IJzendoorn et al. (1992). For 34 clinical samples in which attachment data were available, these researchers compared studies with "maternal problems" (e.g., mental illness, drug abuse) versus "child problems" (e.g., deafness, premature birth, ID). Results showed that groups with "maternal problems" revealed more insecure child attachments compared to the nonclinical population, whereas the "child problems" groups revealed rates of insecurity that resembled the distributions of nonclinical samples.

Taken together, both theory and research support the notion that caregiving plays an important role in shaping children's attachment security, with sensitive caregiving associated with secure child–parent attachment. What accounts for individual differences in parental sensitivity? Attachment theory postulates a caregiving behavioral system (George & Solomon, 1999) that organizes parent's caregiving and is based on mental representations of the child. These representations play an important role in shaping caregiving behavior and are central to the parents' ability to detect and respond sensitively to the child's emotional needs. For example, Zeanah and his colleagues found that coherent and balanced representations of the child were related to parental behavior that promoted the development of secure attachment in studies with normally developing samples (e.g., Benoit, Parker, & Zeanah, 1997; Zeanah, Benoit, Hirshberg, Barton, & Regan, 1995). We turn next to two important aspects of parents' representations of their children that are at the focus of our research on parenting children with ID: parental insightfulness and parents' resolution regarding the child's diagnosis.

Parental Insightfulness

According to Ainsworth (1978), the prompt, accurate, and appropriate responses characterizing sensitive parenting are based on the capacity to "see things from the child's point of view," referred to recently by Oppenheim and Koren-Karie (2002) as *insightfulness* into the child's inner world. We discuss the assessment of insightfulness next, followed by excerpts from insightfulness assessment interviews with mothers of children with ID.

The assessment of insightfulness involves two steps. The parent and the child are first observed in several contexts to yield video vignettes that will serve as the basis for interviewing the parents. Second, after viewing each vignette, parents are interviewed regarding their perceptions of their children's thoughts and feelings during the segments, as well as their own thoughts and feelings. They are asked what they think the child was thinking and feeling in the video segment, whether this is typical for the child and says something more general about the child's personality, and what they were feeling when watching the segment. Interviews are transcribed, rated on ten scales, and subsequently classified into one of four groups. The first group, labeled *positively insightful*, indicates the capacity for insightfulness, whereas the remaining three (labeled *one-sided, disengaged,* and *mixed*) indicate a lack of insightfulness.

Parental insightfulness involves three central components: considering the motives underlying the child's behavior, holding on to an emotionally complex view of the child, and showing openness regarding new and unexpected information regarding the child. All three aspects provide the basis for reading children's emotional signals accurately and responding to them appropriately, in a way that enhances the child's emotion regulation and sense of security (Oppenheim & Koren-Karie, 2002).

Considering motives underlying the child's behavior is based on accepting the child as a separate person with plans, needs, and wishes of his or her own. The parent sees it as his or her role to explain observed behavior by referring to the thoughts, emotions, and motivations that underlie the child's behavior in a way that matches the behavior they are intended to explain.

Second, an emotionally complex view of the child involves a believable, convincing portrayal of the child as a whole person, with both positive and negative features. Positive features are described openly and are supported by convincing examples from everyday life, and typically outweigh negative descriptions. Negative descriptions are provided in a nonblaming, frank way, so that frustrating, unflattering, and upsetting aspects of the child are discussed within an accepting framework and in the context of attempts to find explanations for the child's behavior.

Third, openness is also central to insightfulness. Rather than imposing a preconceived notion of who their child is, insightful parents are not only open to see the familiar and comfortable aspects of their children but also to see unexpected behaviors without distortion. Openness also involves the parent's attitude toward herself: Parents can utilize observations of themselves and of the child to take a new, fresh look at themselves without excessive criticism or, on the other hand, defensiveness.

In our research with typically developing children, we found associations between maternal insightfulness and infants' security of attachment (Koren-Karie, Oppenheim, Dolev, Sher, & Etzion-Carasso, 2002; Oppenheim & Koren-Karie, 2002). Children whose mothers' were classified as positively insightful were most likely to be securely attached compared to children whose mothers were classified in one of the other, noninsightful groups. Results also showed that mothers classified as positively insightful were more sensitive to their children's signals during interactions when compared with mothers not so classified (Koren-Karie et al., 2002.) In an additional study (Oppenheim, Goldsmith, & Koren-Karie, 2004), we examined insightfulness in a clinical sample of preschool children who had been referred to treatment for various emotional and behavioral problems. Results revealed that children showed improvements in their behavior problems only when their mothers showed improvements in their insightfulness toward their children during treatment. Taken together, these findings support the hypothesis that insightfulness provides a basis for the development of secure child–parent attachments and optimal emotion regulation among typically developing children.

Insightfulness is likely to be as important for child–parent attachment when children with ID are concerned and the results of a recent study we conducted indicate that this might be the case. In the study we found a positive association between maternal insightfulness and security of attachment among children with ID (Feniger-Schaal, Oppenheim & Koren-Karie, 2011). These results suggest that maternal insightfulness promotes the development of secure attachment among children with ID as it does in typically developing children.

Children with ID may at times be more challenging, less rewarding, and more difficult to read compared to typically developing children, but an attachment-based approach suggests that their needs for security are no different. Furthermore, the insightfulness framework is particularly relevant for children with ID because it emphasizes understanding of the uniqueness of the individual child that goes beyond general perceptions and diagnostic labels such as ID. In addition, insightfulness is held to be a mental process residing "inside" the parent, one that depends less on the child's objective features such as temperament, gender, or in this case, ID (Oppenheim & Koren-Karie, 2009).

We turn next to excerpts from insightfulness interviews (regarding previously video taped mother–child structured interactions) from a study of mothers of children aged 2.5–5 years who have ID (Feniger-Schaal, Oppenheim, & Koren-Karie, 2011). Various features of insightfulness emerged in these mothers, similar to those found among parents of normally developing children. Some parents were able to see things from their child's unique point of view. For example, after being asked "what was going on in her child's head," one mother attempted to explain her child's thoughts and feelings when playing a game that involves inserting balls into holes:

> He wasn't frustrated that he failed the game, because he was concentrating on something else, he was not concentrating on the rules of the game as we see it. . . . As far as he's concerned, the "fun" part is when the ball falls and "clicks" into the hole. If it falls, he sees it as a success. The colors and all that—he doesn't care about that. . . .

This insightful mother is able to understand what her child experiences as pleasurable even though the pleasure is not derived from the conventional use of the toy (i.e., inserting the balls into the holes). She is not frustrated when the child does not play with the toy as expected but rather shows acceptance of his perspective as she focuses on his experience:

> He is looking for ways for using this toy to make him happy. That is his motivation—to have fun. He loves sounds, so when the ball is falling and makes a sound, it makes him happy—you can actually see how happy he is. . . . The cognitive part he finds less interesting. . . .

As can be seen in this example, insightful parents realistically describe the challenging aspects of their child's behavior, yet can nonetheless see positive aspects as well:

> Obviously, there is a lot of frustration, many things that he cannot do. . . . But together with that, there is the way he finds the positive in everything. . . . One of his unique characteristics is that he takes things lightly, not heavily. An optimistic kid in his soul. Many grownups could learn from him [laughs].

In contrast, parents who are classified as not insightful find it difficult to think about the child in terms of his or her internal experience, as illustrated in the following example:

> I have no idea what goes on in her head; it's a mystery for me. She does not say much. . . . I don't know if she has something in her head like "leave me alone," or if she doesn't even have that in her head.

Such parents experience difficulties understanding the child's motives and seeing things from the child's point of view. In the following excerpt, a mother rigidly adheres to her own point of view and seems to not understand her daughter's perspective:

> She plays games, but not according to the rules that I explain. For example, when I read her a story, she likes looking at the pictures at her own pace. She turns the pages, singing to herself and looking at the pictures. But when I read her a story, she should listen, there needs to be some order and not just looking at the pictures.

Note the contrast between this mother and the one presented earlier. The earlier excerpt highlighted the mother's capacity to both understand and accept the child's joy in play even though the game was used in an unconventional and "inappropriate" way. The same child behavior—i.e., playing not according to the rules—elicits in this mother an opposite reaction: lack of acceptance and irritation. As our findings regarding the associations between maternal insightfulness and child attachment suggest, differences in parents' construction of their children's behavior and experience, such as those illustrated above, appear to be not only reflections of internal processes in the mind of the parent, but also to have an effect on the child's feelings of being understood and secure.

When children carry a diagnosis such as ID, part of insightfulness involves seeing the unique characteristics of the child beyond the diagnostic label. This requires that the parent come to terms, or "resolve," the child's diagnosis, and we discuss this issue next.

Resolution of the Child's Diagnosis

Seeing things from the child's point of view requires acceptance of the child's diagnosis, so that the parent incorporates that diagnosis and its current and future implications into his or her representations of the child (Marvin & Pianta, 1996). The process of parental adaptation to the child's diagnosis was examined in the early writings of Blacher (1984) and more recently in the work of Pianta and Marvin within the context of attachment research. These researchers describe receiving a diagnosis such as ID for one's child as equivalent to a loss—the loss of the hoped for, typically developing child.

Blacher (1984) reviewed research that investigated parental reactions to receiving diagnoses of various medical conditions for their children, including ID, DS, and heart defects. She found that parents reported similar emotional reaction patterns, which she described as progressive stages. The first stage involved shock, denial, and a search for a reason. The second stage, *emotional disorganization*, was primarily characterized by feelings of guilt, and the third, *emotional adjustment*, included adaptation and acceptance. Blacher emphasized that parents do not necessarily progress in a linear fashion from stage to stage, and can move back and forth among them. Transitions and crises related to the child, such as changing schools or other stressful life events, can trigger a return to prior stages. Although the emotional reactions Blacher described are commonly observed, there is less agreement regarding the validity of the stage-like sequence she described. For example, more recent literature suggests that the three stages can be seen as main categories of response rather than as clearly defined stages (e.g., Dichfield, 1992).

Important understanding concerning parents' resolution of the difficult feelings associated with receiving a diagnosis for their child has emerged from the work of Marvin and Pianta (1996). They interviewed parents of children with diagnoses such as cerebral palsy or epilepsy using the Reaction to Diagnosis Interview (RDI), and asked these parents to reflect on their experiences and on the processes they have undergone since receiving the diagnosis. Specifically, parents were asked to describe when they began to notice their child's difficulty and their response at the time; their feelings, thoughts, and actions surrounding the time that they received the child's diagnosis; the changes in their feelings from the day of getting the diagnosis until the present; and any thoughts they may have about why their child has difficulties. Similar to Blacher (1984), Marvin and Pianta viewed the experience of receiving a serious diagnosis for one's child as a metaphorical loss that triggers an emotionally painful process with many similarities to grief and mourning.

Bowlby (1980, 1982) in his writing about loss and mourning, conceptualized the ultimate goal of the grief process as "reorganization", which includes accepting the irreversible nature of the loss, working through and discarding old patterns of thinking, feeling, and acting, and a gradual acceptance that the loss is permanent and that life must be shaped. Following Bowlby, Marvin and Pianta (1996) defined "resolution" as an integration of the experience of the diagnosis into the parent's representations, which allows for a reorientation and refocus of attention and problem solving on present reality. Resolved parents, as defined by Marvin and Pianta, reveal recognition of the changes they experienced since the diagnosis, an assertion of moving on in life, an accurate representation of the child's ability, suspension of the search for a reason, and balanced statements regarding the experience's benefits to the self. Unresolved parents are characterized by a focus away from the reality of the child's needs, feelings, and signals; and the lack of a coherent, organized mental strategy, which impedes accurate interpretation of the child's cues or selection of appropriate caregiving behaviors. The following excerpts were taken from an ongoing study of parents with children with ID that employed the RDI. When interviewed, all parents have known about the diagnosis of their children for at least 6 months.

As demonstrated in the following excerpt, resolved parents express the difficulty related to receiving the diagnosis but simultaneously reveal that they have not remained "stuck" in the past. The following mother, classified as "resolved," described how her emotional reaction to her child's diagnosis has changed over time. This mother not only showed the sense of "moving on" but also acceptance of her daughter's condition while maintaining hope for the future:

> I used to think: "Why me? Why *my* daughter, when I have only one daughter?" I don't think that way anymore, I look at things differently. This is my child, I am proud of her, we love her dearly and that's it. I hope she can develop in a way that will enable her to be a bit more independent.

Not all resolved parents are alike, and Marvin and Pianta (1996) described three orientations toward the adaptation process: thinking, feeling, and action orientations. We provide first an example of a resolved mother who is thinking-oriented:

> I decided to keep thinking positively, so that I can keep on living. Anything new she does, every new word, is a celebration. You try to think with reason instead of being depressed.

Another mother exemplifies an "action-oriented" strategy:

> In the beginning, it was mainly running to the Internet to find out information . . . that's our way

of coping . . . to look for information, to look for experts.

In her action-oriented way, this mother expressed her acceptance of the child's difficulties and needs:

My husband and I discussed it, and we decided that it would be best for him to go to a special nursery school, where he can get all the treatments he needs.

Unresolved parents show difficulties in revising their mental representations of their child in light of the diagnosis. Marvin and Pianta (1996) described four types of unresolved parents: neutralizing, emotionally overwhelmed, angrily preoccupied, and depressed and cognitively distorted or confused. We turn to an example of an angrily preoccupied parent.

When asked to describe her emotional reaction to receiving the diagnosis, this mother expressed her rage toward the doctor who gave her child the diagnosis. Importantly, the rage seems to be as strong in the present as it was when the diagnosis was given, several years prior to the interview.

I was confused, shocked, hysterical. . . . First of all, the assessment he performed was a failure, as far as I am concerned. His personality and his lack of ability to communicate with children. . . . How dare you, after 20 minutes of looking at the child across the desk, when she did not cooperate with you, say that she is mentally retarded? I almost wanted him to die; even today I wish that will happen. I met him one day at the mall, and I wanted to push him into the elevator pit, I just despise this man, and I also know that he was wrong.

According to Marvin and Pianta (1996), it is not so much the anger per se that indicates lack of resolution but its overwhelming, persistent nature. Marvin and Pianta suggest that such preoccupation may limit the parent's capacity to focus attention to the child's present needs.

Other parents are overwhelmed by grief rather than anger. One mother cried in response to each of the RDI questions, appearing overwhelmed by the feelings involving her daughter's diagnosis, as if she were in the midst of mourning the loss of the child she hoped for:

I keep asking: "Why does it have to be this way?" I say maybe I was punished, I don't know. . . . I find it difficult to accept this. . . . I have a child who looks normal and she is really not. . . . I can't accept it. I feel a lot of frustration, as if . . . I don't know . . . I am angry. I try to understand and to ask, I don't

know who, why? How can this be? Such a sweet girl, why? What's wrong with her?

The patterns of thought and feeling revealed in the RDI are thought to be important not only because of what they reveal about the parent's inner experience but also because of their associations with parental behavior. Resolved parents, whose representations of the child are aligned with the child's functioning, are likely to be sensitive to the child's signals and to match their behavior to the child's strengths, as well as the child's vulnerabilities (Marvin & Pianta, 1996; Pianta, Marvin, Britner, & Borowitz, 1996). Consequently, children of resolved parents are expected to develop secure attachments to them. Conversely, unresolved parents' difficulties in revising their representations of the child in light of the child's diagnosis may limit their capacity to adjust their caregiving to the child and to respond in a way that is appropriate and matched to the child, leading to an insecure attachment between the child and the parent. Support for this hypothesis comes from Marvin and Pianta's report of the association between mothers' reaction to their children's diagnoses (of cerebral palsy) on the RDI and the children's security of attachment (Marvin & Pianta, 1996, Pianta, Marvin, & Morog, 1999). The researchers found that 82% of the mothers who were classified as resolved with regard to their child's diagnosis had securely attached children, and 81% of mothers classified as unresolved had insecurely attached children. In a recent study, Barnett et al. (2006) provided additional support to Marvin and Pianta's results: Maternal resolution of the child's diagnosis of congenital anomalies (including ID) was associated with the child's secure attachment. Importantly, resolution was not associated with the severity of the child's diagnosis, suggesting that resolution is not simply a reflection of milder impairment in the child. The resolution–attachment links are presumably due to the enhanced sensitivity of mothers classified resolved. Dolev (2006) found support for this hypothesis in her study of preschoolers diagnosed with autism spectrum disorder (ASD), many of whom also had ID. Dolev found that mothers classified as resolved on the RDI showed greater sensitivity to their children during interactions with the child and structured the interaction more optimally, compared to mothers classified as unresolved. Similar to Dolev (2006), Feniger-Schaal (2010) used the RDI with mothers of preschool children diagnosed with ID and found a positive association between maternal resolution and maternal sensitivity: Mothers who were resolved were more sensitive than those classified as unresolved. Like Barnett et al. (2006), Feniger-Schaal (2010) reported that resolution was not associated with children's severity of the diagnosis, thus supporting the notion that the RDI captures how parents manage the emotions and thoughts related to the child's diagnosis and is not simply a reflection of the severity of the child's condition.

Conclusion

The literature on attachment and ID (and particularly DS) reviewed in this chapter indicates that many children exhibit secure, organized attachment relationships to their parents. This finding is particularly significant when the challenges presented by ID are considered. The substantial rate of security notwithstanding, an elevated rate of attachment insecurity and disorganization was found in the ID population when compared with typically developing children, and this chapter reviewed some of the mechanisms responsible for these findings. These include (but are not limited to) the child's cognitive impairments, parent's difficulties reading the interactional cues of children with ID, and mothers' difficulties in attaining insightfulness into the child's inner experience and "resolving" their emotional responses to the child's diagnosis. Further studies on these issues are clearly needed, particularly regarding parental sensitivity, insightfulness, and the reaction to the diagnosis—topics about which there is very little empirical research. In addition, the vast majority of studies on attachment and ID involved children with DS. Expanding the research to other groups with ID will broaden our understanding of the relations between cognitive and behavioral impairment and emotional development. These research directions are also important because they highlight individual differences within groups rather than between-group differences. Much of the research in this field involves comparing children with ID with comparison groups, but the research reviewed in this chapter suggests that within-group differences exist and are important. A better understanding of the roots of such individual differences can increase our ability to support the development of children with ID.

Finally, perhaps the most striking lacuna in this field involves the absence of studies on child–father attachment in ID and its contributions to children's development. Children's attachments to their fathers are important because through such attachments children may benefit from an additional, potentially secure relationship beyond their attachments to their mothers. Such an attachment may supplement a secure attachment with mother or compensate for an insecure attachment with her. Additionally, several authors (e.g., Grossmann, Grossmann, Fremmer-Bombik, Kindler, & Zimmermann, 2002; Oppenheim, Sagi, & Lamb, 1988) have suggested that children's attachments to their fathers may promote different aspects of development compared to those promoted by their attachments to their mothers, and thus neglecting to study the child–father attachment leaves the developmental picture incomplete. In both cases, and particularly due to the challenges faced by children with ID, there is great need to study their attachments to their fathers.

Attachment theory and research may also have implications for intervention with children with ID and their families. For example, based on the findings regarding the importance of parental resolution, Barnett and his colleagues (Barnett, Clements, Kaplan-Estrin, & Fialka, 2003) designed a group intervention program to promote parental adaptation to the child's disability. They view resolution broadly as psychosocial adaptation, which involves updating or rebuilding a new representation of the child in line with the child's diagnosis. This adaptation fosters both acceptance of the child and, importantly, an accurate perception of both the child's abilities and difficulties, thus providing the basis for interactions that are matched to the child's developmental needs and are likely to direct the child onto a positive developmental pathway. Other clinical implications of an attachment approach involve the importance of enhancing parents' capacity for insightfulness by helping them understand the roots of their children's behaviors—including those that are challenging—in the child's inner experience. Additionally, supporting a complex view of the child and his or her difficulties that goes beyond the child's ID diagnosis and appreciates the individuality of each child's experience is likely to enhance the parent's capacity to respond sensitively and appropriately to the child's signals and support the child's feelings of security and sense of being understood. Such emotional experiences are likely to promote the development of children with ID and help them maximize their developmental potential.

References

Ainsworth, M. D. S., Blehar, M. C., Waters, E., & Wall, S. (1978). *Patterns of attachment: A psychological study of the strange situation.* Hillsdale, NJ: Lawrence Erlbaum.

Atkinson, L., Chisholm, V. C., Scott, B., Goldberg, S., Vaughn, B. E., Blackwell, J., Dickerns, S., & Tam, F. (1999). Maternal sensitivity, child functional level, and attachment in Down syndrome. *Monographs of the Society for Research in Child Development, 64,* 45–66.

Baker, B. L., Blacher, J., Crnic, K. A., & Edelbrock, C. (2002). Behavior problems and parenting stress in families of three year old children with and without developmental delays. *American Journal on Mental Retardation, 107,* 433–444.

Barnett, D., Clements, M., Kaplan-Estrin, M., & Fialka, J. (2003). Building new dreams; supporting parents' adaptation to their child with special needs. *Infants and Young Children, 16,* 184–200.

Barnett, D., Clements, M., Kaplan-Estrin, M., McCaskill, W. J., Hill Hunt, K., Butler, M. C., Schram, L. J., & Jenisse, C. H. (2006). Maternal resolution of the child diagnosis: Stability and relationship with child attachment across the toddler to preschooler transition. *Journal of Family Psychology, 20,* 100–107.

Beckman, P. J. (2002). Influence of selected child characteristic on stress in families of handicapped infants. In J. Blacher, & B. B. Baker (Eds.), *The best of AAMR. Families and mental retardation: A collection of notable AAMR journal articles across the 20th century* (pp. 71–79). Washington: American Association for Mental Retardation. (Original work published 1983).

Berger, J. (1990). Interactions between parents and their children with Down syndrome. In D. Cicchetti, & M. Beeghly (Eds.). *Children with Down syndrome: A developmental perspective* (pp. 101–146). New York: Cambridge University Press.

Benoit, D., Parker, K. C. H., & Zeanah, C. H. (1997). Mother's representation of their infants assessed prenatally: Stability and association with infants' attachment classification. *Journal of Child Psychology and Psychiatry, 38,* 307–313.

Belsky, J. (1984). The determinants of parenting: A process model. *Child Development, 55,* 83–96.

Berger, J. (1990). Interactions between parents and their infants with Down syndrome. In D. Cicchetti, & M. Beeghly (Eds.), *Children with Down syndrome: A developmental perspective* (pp. 101–146). New York: Cambridge University Press.

Berry, P., Gunn, P., & Andrews, R. (1980). Behavior of Down's syndrome infants in a strange situation. *American Journal of Mental Deficiency, 85,* 213–218.

Blacher, J. (1984). The sequential stages of parental adjustment to the birth of a child with handicaps: Fact or artifact. *Mental Retardation, 22,* 55–68.

Bowlby, J. (1980). *Attachment and loss: Vol. III. Loss.* New York: Basic Books.

Bowlby, J. (1982). *Attachment and loss: Vol. 1. Attachment* (2nd ed.). London: Penguin Books.

Bridges, F. A., & Cicchetti, D. (1982). Mother's rating of the temperament characteristics of Down syndrome infants. *Developmental Psychology, 18*(2), 238–244.

Bruchin, A. (1990). *Behaviour of parents to children with mental retardation: Stress level and perception of parental role.* Unpublished doctoral dissertation, Bar-Ilan University, Israel.

Canepa, G., Barbagna, S., Millepiedi, S., & Marcheschi, M. (2000). Il funzionamento sociale nella syndrome di down. studio preliminare. / adaptive behavior in children with down's syndrome. preliminary study. *Minerva Psichiatrica, 41,* 2, 103–110

Capps, L., Sigman, M., & Mundy, P. (1994). Attachment security in children with autism. *Development and Psychopathology, 6,* 249–261.

Cassidy, J. (1999). The nature of the child's ties. In J. Cassidy, & P. R. Shaver (Eds.), *Handbook of attachment theory, research and clinical application* (pp. 3–21). New York: Guilford Press.

Cicchetti, D., & Beeghly, M. (1990). An organizational approach to the study of Down syndrome: Contribution to an integrative theory of development. In D. Cicchetti, & M. Beeghly (Eds.), *Children with Down syndrome: A developmental perspective* (pp. 29–62). New York: Cambridge University Press.

Cicchetti, D., & Ganiban, J. (1990). The organization and coherence of developmental processes in infants and children with Down syndrome. In R. M. Hodapp, J. A. Burack, & E. Zigler (Eds.), *Issues in the developmental approach to mental retardation* (pp. 1–28). New York: Cambridge University Press.

Cicchetti, D., & Serafica, F. C. (1981). Interplay among behavioral systems: Illustrations from the study of attachment, affiliation, and wariness in young children with Down's syndrome. *Developmental Psychology, 17,* 36–49.

Cicchetti, D., & Sroufe, L. A. (1978). An organizational view of affect: Illustration from the study of Down syndrome infants. In M. Lewis, & L. A. Rosenblum (Eds.), *The development of affect* (pp. 309–350). New York: Plenum.

Colin, V. L. (1996). *Human attachment.* Philadelphia: Temple University Press.

Cuskelly, M., & Gunn, P. (2003). Siblings relationship of children with Down syndrome: Perspectives of mothers, fathers, and siblings. *American Journal on Mental Retardation, 108,* 234–244.

De Wolff, M. S., & van IJzendoorn, M. H. (1997). Sensitivity and attachment: A meta-analysis on parental antecedents of infant attachment. *Child Development, 68,* 571–591.

Dichfield, H. (1992). The birth of a child with a mental handicap: Coping with loss? In A. Waitman, & S. Conboy-Hill (Eds.), *Psychotherapy and mental handicap* (pp. 9–24). London: Sage.

Dolev, S. (2006). *Insightfulness and the reaction to diagnosis in mothers of children with Autism: Associations with maternal sensitivity.* Unpublished doctoral dissertation, Haifa University, Israel.

Donenberg, G., & Baker, B. L. (1993). The impact of young children with externalizing behaviors on their families. *Journal of Abnormal Child Psychology, 21,* 179–198.

Feniger-Schaal, R. (2010). *Mothers' Resolution of the Diagnosis of Intellectual Disability given to their children: Association with Maternal Sensitivity and Children's Security of Attachment.* Unpublished doctoral dissertation, Haifa University, Israel.

Feniger-Schaal, R., & Oppenheim, D. (2009). *Mothers' Reactions to their Children's Diagnosis of Intellectual Disability: Relations to Maternal Sensitivity.* Poster presented at the annual meeting of the Society for Research in Child Development, Denver, Colorado.

Feniger-Schaal, R., Oppenheim D., & Koren-Karie N. (2011). *Maternal Insightfulness and Security of Attachment among Children with Intellectual Disability.* Poster presented at the annual meeting of the Society for Research in Child Development, Montreal, Canada.

Freeman, S. F. N., & Kasari, C. (2002). Characteristics and quality of the play dates of children with Down syndrome: Emerging or true friends? *American Journal of Mental Retardation, 107,* 16–31.

Ganiban, J., & Barnett, D. (1991). *Emotion regulatory strategies of securely and insecurely attached infants with Down syndrome in the strange situation.* Poster presented at the meeting for Research in Child Development, Seattle.

Ganiban, J., Barnett, D., & Cicchetti, D. (2000). Negative reactivity and attachment: Down syndrome's contribution to the attachment-temperament debate. *Development and Psychopathology, 12,* 1–21.

George, C., & Solomon, J. (1999). Attachment and caregiving: The caregiving behavioral system. handbook of attachment: Theory, research, and clinical applications. In J. Cassidy & P. R. Shaver, (Eds.), *Handbook of attachment: Theory, research, and clinical applications.* (pp. 649–670). New York, NY, US: Guilford Pres.

Goldberg, S. (1988). Risk factors in attachment. *Canadian Journal of Psychology, 42,* 173–188.

Gath, A. (1977). The impact of an abnormal child upon the parents. *British Journal of Psychiatry, 130,* 405–410.

Greenough, W. T., & Black, J. E. (1992). Induction of brain structure by experience: Substrates for cognitive development. In M. R. Gunnar, & C. A. Nelson (Eds.), *Developmental behavior neuroscience* (pp. 155–200). Hillsdale, NJ: Lawrence Erlbaum.

Grossmann, K., Grossmann, K. E., Fremmer-Bombik, E., Kindler, H., & Zimmermann, P. (2002). The uniqueness of the child-father attachment relationship: Fathers' sensitive and challenging play as a pivotal variable in a 16-year longitudinal study. *Social Development, 11,* 307–331.

Hannah, M. E., & Midlarsky, E. (1999). Competence and adjustment of siblings of children with mental retardation. *American Journal on Mental Retardation, 104*(1), 22–37.

Hauser-Cram, P., Warfield, M. E., Shonkoff, J. P., & Krauss, M. W. (2001). Children with disabilities: A longitudinal study of child development and parent well-being. *Monographs of the Society for Research in Child Development, 66,* 1–131.

Hodapp, R. M., Burack, J. A., & Zigler, E. (1998). Developmental approaches to mental retardation: A short introduction. In J. A. Burack, R. M. Hodapp, & E. Zigler (Eds.), *Handbook of mental retardation and development* (pp. 3–19). Cambridge, UK: Cambridge University Press.

Hodapp, R. (2002). Parenting children with mental retardation. In M. H. M. Bornstein (Ed.), *Handbook of parenting: Children and parenting* (pp. 355–381). Mahwah, NJ, US: Lawrence Erlbaum Associates Publishers.

Jahromi, L. B., Gulsrud, A., & Kasari, C. (2008). Emotional competence in children with Down syndrome: Negativity and regulation. *American Journal on Mental Retardation, 113*(1), 32–43.

Janssen, C. G. C., Schuengel, C., & Stolk, J. (2002). Understanding challenging behavior in people with severe and profound intellectual disability: A stress-attachment model. *Journal of Intellectual Disability Research, 46,* 445–453.

Kasari, C., & Bauminger. N. (1998). Social and emotional development in children with mental retardation. In J. A. Burack, R. M. Hodapp, & E. Zigler (Eds.), *Handbook of mental retardation and development* (pp. 411–434). Cambridge, UK: Cambridge University Press.

Kasari, C., Freeman, S. F., & Hughes, M. A. (2001). Emotion recognition by children with Down syndrome. *American Journal on Mental Retardation, 106,* 59–72.

Keogh, B. K., Garnier, H. E., Bernheimer, L. P., & Gallimore, R. (2000). Models of child-family interactions for children with developmental delays: Child-driven or transactional? *American Journal on Mental Retardation, 105,* 32–46.

Koren-Karie, N., Oppenheim, D., Dolev, S., Sher, E., & Etzion-Carasso, A. (2002). Mothers' insightfulness regarding their infants' internal experience: Relations with maternal sensitivity and infant attachment. *Developmental Psychology, 38,* 534–542.

Koren-Karie, N., Oppenheim, D., Dolev, S., & Yirmiya, N. (2009). Mothers of securely attached children with Autism Spectrum Disorder are more sensitive than mothers of insecurely attached children. *Journal of Child Psychology and Psychiatry. 50,* 643–650.

Levy-Shiff, R. (1986). Mother father child interactions in families of a mentally retarded young child. *American Journal of Mental Deficiency, 91,* 141–149.

Lyon-Ruth, K. (1996). Attachment relationships among children with aggressive behavior problems: The role of disorganized early attachment patterns. *Journal of Consulting and Clinical Psychology, 64,* 32–40.

Main, M. (1983). Exploration, play, and cognitive functioning related to infant-mother attachment. *Infant Behavior and Development, 6,* 167–174.

Main, M., Kaplan, N., & Cassidy, J. (1985). Security in infancy, childhood and adulthood: A move to the level of representation. In I. Bretherton, & E. Waters (Eds.), *Growing points of attachment theory and research* (pp. 66–104). Chicago: University of Chicago Press.

Marom, A. (1990). *Behaviour of parents to children with developmental delay and its relation to marital life and family atmosphere.* Unpublished doctoral dissertation, Bar-Illan University, Israel.

Marvin, R. S., & Pianta, R. C. (1996). Mothers' reactions to their child's diagnosis: Relations with security of attachment. *Journal of Clinical Child Psychology, 25,* 436–445.

Meyer, D. J., Vadasy, P. F., Fewell, R. R., & Schell, G. (1982). Involving fathers of handicapped infants: Translating research into program goals. *Journal of the Division of Early Childhood, 5,* 64–72.

Moran, G., Pederson, D. R., Pettit, P., & Krupka, A. (1992). Maternal sensitivity and infant attachment in a high-risk sample. *Infant Behavior and Development, 15,* 427–442.

Oppenheim, D., Goldsmith, D., & Koren-Karie, N. (2004). Maternal insightfulness and preschoolers' emotion and behavior problems: Reciprocal influences in a day-treatment program. *Infant Mental Health Journal, 25,* 352–367.

Oppenheim, D., & Koren-Karie, N. (2002). Mother's insightfulness regarding their children's internal world: The capacity underlying secure child-mother relationships. *Infant Mental Health Journal, 23,* 593–605.

Oppenheim, D., & Koren-Karie, N. (2009). Infant-parent relationship assessment: Parent insightfulness regarding their young children's internal worlds. In C. Zeanah, (Ed.), *Handbook of infant mental health* (pp. 266–280). New York: Guilford.

Oppenheim, D., Sagi, A., & Lamb, M. E. (1988). Infant-adult attachments in the Kibbutz and their relation to socioemotional development four years later. *Developmental Psychology, 24,* 427–433.

Pianta, R. C., Marvin, R. S., Britner, P. A., & Borowitz, K. C. (1996). Mothers' resolution of their children's diagnosis: Organized patterns of caregiving representations. *Journal of Infant Mental Health, 17,* 239–256.

Pianta, R. C., Marvin, R. S., & Morog, M. C. (1999). Resolving the past and present: Relations with attachment disorganization.

In J. Solomon, & C. George (Eds.), *Attachment disorganization* (pp. 379–398). New York: Guilford.

Schell, G. C. (1981). The young handicapped child: A family perspective. *Topics in Early Childhood Special Education, 1,* 21–27.

Sroufe, L. A. (1979). The coherence of individual development early care, attachment, and subsequent developmental issues. *American Psychologist, 34,* 834–841.

Sroufe, L. A, Carlson, E. A., Levy, K., & Egeland, B. (1999). Implications of attachment theory for developmental psychopathology. *Development and Psychopathology, 11,* 1–13.

Sroufe, L. A., Egeland, B., Carlson, E., & Collins, W. A. (2005). Placing early attachment experiences in developmental context: The Minnesota longitudinal study. In K. E. Grossmann, K. Grossmann & E. Waters (Eds.), *Attachment from infancy to adulthood: The major longitudinal studies.* (pp. 48–70). New York, NY, US: Guilford Publications.

Thompson, R. A., Cicchetti, D., Lamb, M. E., & Malkin, C. (1985). Emotional responses of Down syndrome and normal infants in the strange situation: The organization of affective behavior in infants. *Developmental Psychology, 21,* 828–841.

Thompson, R. A. (1999). Early attachment and later development. In J. Cassidy, & P. R. Shaver (Eds.), *Handbook of attachment: Theory, research, and clinical applications* (pp. 265–286). New York: Guilford Press.

van IJzendoorn, M. H., Goldberg, S., Kroonenberg, P. M., & Frenkel, O. J. (1992). The relative effects of maternal and child problems on the quality of attachment: A meta-analysis of attachment in clinical samples. *Child Development, 63,* 840–858.

van IJzendoorn, M. H., & Kroonenberg, P. M. (1988). Cross-cultural patterns of attachment: A meta-analysis of the strange situation. *Child Development, 59,* 147–156.

van IJzendoorn, M. H., Rutgers, A. H., Bakermans-Kranenburg, M. J., van Daalen, E., Dietz, C., Buitelaar, J. K., et al. (2007). Parental sensitivity and attachment in children with autism spectrum disorder: Comparison with children with mental retardation, with language delays, and with typical development. *Child Development, 78,* 2, 597–608.

van IJzendoorn, M. H., & Sagi, A. (2008). Cross-cultural patterns of attachment: Universal and contextual dimensions. In J. Cassidy & P. R. Shaver (Eds.), *Handbook of attachment: Theory, research, and clinical applications* (pp. 713–734). New York, NY, US: Guilford Press.

van IJzendoorn, M. H., Schuengel, C., & Bakermans-Kranenburg, M. K. (1999). Disorganized attachment in early childhood: Meta-analysis of precursors, concomitants

and sequelae. *Development and Psychopathology, 11,* 225–249.

Vaughn, B., Goldberg, S., Atkinson, L., Marcovitch, S., MacGregor, D., & Seifer, R. (1994). Quality of toddler-mother attachment in children with Down's syndrome: Limits to interpretation of strange situation behavior. *Child Development, 65,* 95–108.

Waters, E., & Deane, K. E. (1985). Defining and assessing individual differences in attachment relationships: Q-methodology and the organization of behavior in infancy and early childhood. In I. Bretherton, & E. Waters (Eds.), *Growing points of attachment theory and research* (pp. 41–65). *Monographs of the Society for Research in Child Development, 50* (1–2, Serial No. 209).

Walden, T., & Knieps, L. (1996). Reading and responding to social signals. In S. M. W. Sullivan, & M. Lewis (Eds.), *Emotional development in atypical children* (pp. 29–42). Hillsdale, NJ: Lawrence Erlbaum Associates.

Waters, E., Kondo-Ikemura, K., Posada, G., & Richters, J. (1991). Learning to love: Mechanisms and milestones. In M. Gunner, & A. Sroufe (Eds.), *Minnesota symposium on child psychology: Vol. 23. Self processes and development* (pp. 217–255). Minneapolis: University of Minnesota Press.

Weinfield, N. S., Sroufe, L. A., Egeland, B., & Carlson, E. (1999). The nature of individual differences in infant-caregiver attachment. In J. Cassidy, & P. Shaver (Eds.), *Handbook of attachment: Theory, research, and clinical application* (pp. 73–95). New York: Guilford Press.

Weissman, D. (1991). *Parents of children with a mental disability: Their behavior, perception of parenting role and burnout.* Ramat-Gan, Israel: Bar-Ilan University.

Zaider, J. (1987). *The normal siblings of the exceptional child.* Jerusalem, Israel.

Zigler, E. (1967). Familial mental retardation: A continuing dilemma. *Science, 155,* 292–298.

Zigler, E. (2001). Looking back 40 years and still seeing the person with mental retardation as a whole person. In H. N. Switzky (Ed.), *Personality and Motivational Differences in Persons with Mental Retardation* (3–55).

Zigler, E. (2002). A veteran worker urges renewed research on personality factors in mental retardation. *Japanese Journal of Special Education, 39,* 1–13.

Zeanah, C. H., Benoit, D., Hirshberg, L., Barton, M., & Regan, C. (1995). Mothers' representations of their infants are concordant with infant attachment classifications. *Developmental Issues in Psychiatry, 1,* 1–14.

Children with Down Syndrome: Parents' Perspectives

Michal Al-Yagon *and* Malka Margalit

Abstract

This chapter reviews research focusing on two major themes regarding parents and children with Down syndrome: the shift from a pathology perspective to a stress and coping approach, and the study of parent–child interactions, attachment, and relationships. It calls for the additional future exploration of the inconsistent findings regarding parents' stress, family-focused programs, parental personal resources, fathers' perspectives, and coping resources.

Keywords: Down syndrome, pathology perspective, stress and coping, parent–child interactions

When interviewed at the end of the first year of an early intervention program at Shalva Center in Jerusalem, Ruth (an assumed name), mother to a 13-month-old boy with Down syndrome, concluded: "My son has developed during this year far beyond my expectations. Indeed, the therapists were wonderful, very helpful and knowledgeable. I don't have enough words to express how grateful I am. I almost feel like I've found an extended family." Then, she continued very quietly, almost to herself: "But the Down did not go away." This quote exemplifies some important questions and dilemmas regarding the impact of children with Down syndrome on their parents and families, as well as the bidirectional effects and child–family transactions.

The general consensus from a comprehensive survey of international studies (Hodapp, 2002) suggests that parenting a child with mental retardation (MR) is a challenge to any parent. Yet, the experience of raising a child with Down syndrome (DS) adds uniquely to understanding this challenge, pinpointing attention to distinctive trends and dilemmas and to interventional implications (e.g., Hodapp, 2002; Hodapp, Ricci, Ly, & Fidler, 2003). Thus, the goals of this chapter are to provide a survey of research focusing on the impact of children with DS on their families, in an attempt to characterize families' sources of stressors and coping, and to highlight future research directions and interventional implications.

Down syndrome is the most common disorder resulting from chromosomal abnormalities.

Many individuals with DS function at a moderate level of retardation (Mash & Wolfe, 2005). As suggested by the *Diagnostic and Statistical Manual of Mental Disorders, 4th Edition, Text Revision* (DS DSM-IV-TR; American Psychiatric Association, 2000), children with moderate MR (an IQ level of 40–54) show delays in reaching early developmental milestones and are unlikely to progress beyond the second-grade level in academic subjects. By adulthood, individuals with DS may adapt well to living in the community, and may perform unskilled or semiskilled work in general workplaces or sheltered workshops (Mash & Wolfe, 2005).

The number of children with DS has gradually decreased from 1 in 700 births to 1 in 1,000 births over the last two decades, due to increased prenatal screening and terminated pregnancies diagnosed with DS (Roizen & Patterson, 2003). Studies have indicated that although DS affects relatively few families directly, it is discussed with millions of women and couples when they are offered prenatal screening (Wapner et al., 2003). Therefore, researchers have also examined parents' experience with delivering and receiving a diagnosis of DS (Alderson, 2001).

The difficulties of children with DS in early childhood have been documented, showing standard cognitive performance scores at least 2 standard deviations below the normative means (e.g., Carr, 1995; Hauser-Cram et al., 1999), as well as communication difficulties, especially in expressive language abilities (e.g., Dykens, Hodapp, & Evans, 1994). Conversely, impairments are relatively less pronounced in social development, as well as in the mastery of adaptive skills associated with the tasks of daily living (e.g., Tingey, Mortensen, Matheson, & Doret, 1991). Children and adults with DS show lower rates of emotional and behavior problems when compared to individuals with other intellectual disabilities (Rosner, Hodapp, Fidler, Sagun, & Dykens, 2004). For example, young children with DS show relative strengths in gestural-symbolic activities such as "talking" into a toy telephone and manifest higher levels of social competence when compared to individuals with either Prader-Willi or Williams syndromes (Beeghly, 1998; Harris, Bellugi, Bates, Jones, & Rossen, 1997). These children were often described as friendly, yet their attention difficulties, stubbornness, and noncompliance problems were noted (Dykens, Shah, Sagun, Beck, & King, 2002; Rosner et al., 2004). In our survey, we focused the discussion on two major themes: the shift from a pathology perspective to a stress and coping approach, and the study of parent–child interactions, attachment, and relationships.

From a Pathology Perspective to a Stress and Coping Approach

Over the last 40 years, studies examining parents and families of children with MR have shifted from a focus on the expressions of crisis and pathology (Blacher, Neece, & Paczkowski, 2005) to the dynamic approach within the stress and coping paradigm (Abery, 2006; Margalit, Al-Yagon, & Kleitman, 2006; Van Riper, 2003). This change may reflect the shift from a reductionistic, problem-oriented approach to a perspective accentuating nurturing and strengths (Richardson, 2002). An overview of

the family studies (Hodapp, 2002; Hodapp, Ly, Fidler, & Ricci, 2001) revealed the negative impact of a child with MR on parents' functioning and well-being, as well as on various aspects of family climate and functioning. These early studies indicated that such mothers showed more depression and greater difficulties handling anger toward their children, in comparison to mothers of typically developing children (e.g., Cummings, Bayley, & Rie, 1966; Friedrich & Friedrich, 1981). Similarly, fathers of children with MR showed more depression and neuroticism, as well as lower levels of dominance, self-esteem, and enjoyment of their children with MR in comparison to fathers of typically developing children (e.g., Erickson, 1969; Friedrich & Friedrich, 1981). Families of children with MR reported lower levels of marital satisfaction, as well as increased levels of marital conflict and divorce (Friedrich & Friedrich, 1981; Gath, 1977). In these families, mothers tended to become overinvolved with their children with MR, whereas fathers manifested high levels of withdrawal behaviors, either emotional or physical (Levy, 1970). In general, the focus of their scientific involvement was on exploring crisis and distress.

Since the 1980s, researchers shifted from considering the child with disabilities as a cause of psychopathology, to a conceptualization of stressors within the family system (Hodapp, 2002). According to this change in perspective, stressors within the family system may lead to negative parental and familial effects such as psychiatric difficulties, but can also strengthen parents and the family system, as reflected in positive outcomes such as a high level of family cohesion, appreciation of personal strengths, and initiation of family advocacy groups (Crnic, Friedrich, & Greenberg, 1983; Hodapp et al., 2001).

This change in empirical perspectives vis à vis parents of children with DS also led to the adaptation of theoretical models from other areas of MR (Hoddap, 2002). Studies that examined parents of children with MR adopted the double ABCX model (McCubbin & Patterson, 1983). This model consists of stressor elements that interact with family resources and with the meaning assigned by the family members to their situation to meet the increased demands and needs caused by that stressor, with outcome factors in the form of family crisis and post-crisis adaptation. The effects of the "crisis" of having a child with MR (i.e., X in the model) are influenced by the child's specific characteristics (i.e., the "stressor event" or A in the model) and are mediated by the family's internal and external resources (i.e., B in the model) and by the family's perception of the child and the disability (i.e., C in the model). This model explained both negative and positive consequences of parenting a child with MR and also emphasized the role of children's level of emotional problems, difficult temperament, and physical caring needs in families' adaptation, as well as the contribution of families' internal/external resources in mediating the impact of the crisis (e.g., Minnes, 1988).

STRESS AND COPING AMONG PARENTS OF CHILDREN WITH DOWN SYNDROME

Parental stress may affect not only the well-being of the parents, but also the adjustment of their children. Family research showed increased stress as an outcome of having a child with disabilities (Margalit, 1994). As defined by Boss (1988), parent and family stress refers to the pressure or tension in the family system that creates a disturbance in the family. More recent definitions refer to the difficulties that emerge from the demands of being a parent, which affect parents' behaviors and well-being, as well as children's adjustment (Anthony et al., 2005). Parental stress remains relatively stable across children's preschool period in families of children with typical development, suggesting that stressed parents tend to remain stressed, and that cumulative stress may build up across developmental stages to create increased risk for parents' and children's functioning (Crnic, Gaze, & Hoffman, 2005).

Stress experiences are often considered a major concern among families of children with disabilities, manifested sometimes as social isolation, emotional depression, or relationship conflict (Keller & Honig, 2004; Margalit, Leyser, Ankonina, & Avraham, 1991). This stress appears to stem from a combination of the increased caring needs of the child with atypical development, along with the family's emotional reactions to the disability (McCubbin & Patterson, 1983). For example, Saloviita, Italinna, and Leinonen (2003) reported that the most important predictor of parental stress among parents of children with intellectual disabilities was parents' negative definition of the situation; yet, this definition differentiated mothers and fathers. For mothers, the negative definition was associated with the child's behavioral problems, whereas for the fathers, it was connected with the experienced social acceptance of the child.

Comparisons of parental stress between parents of children with DS and parents of children with various other disabilities yielded inconsistent results.

Several studies indicated the "DS advantage," reporting lower stress levels among parents of children with DS as compared to parents of children with autism or psychiatric disorders (Hodapp et al., 2001; Holroyd & MacArthur, 1976; Kasari & Sigman, 1997; Sanders & Morgan, 1997). A similar "advantage" for the DS group emerged in comparison to parents of children with other types of MR. For example, Fidler, Hodapp, and Dykens (2000) revealed that parents of children with DS between the ages of 3 to 10 years compared to parents of children with either Williams syndrome or Smith-Magenis syndrome experienced lower stress level. Moreover, fathers of children with DS experienced less child-related stress than did fathers of children with other types of intellectual disability, particularly in the areas of acceptability, adaptability, and demand requests (Ricci & Hodapp, 2003). Ricci and Hodapp emphasized the role of fathers' positive personality traits and children's fewer maladaptive behaviors in explaining these fathers' lower levels of stress.

The focus on mothers' experiences provided a different perspective. For example, Lenhard et al. (2005) examined three groups of mothers: mothers of children with DS, mothers of typically developing children, and mothers of children with a diagnostically unassigned intellectual disability, with regard to maternal levels of anxiety, feelings of guilt, and the experience of emotional burden (Lenhard, Breitenbach, Ebert, Schindelhauer-Deutscher, & Henn, 2005). The mothers of children with DS scored comparably to the mothers of typically developing children, whereas the findings showed broad psychoemotional disadvantages for mothers of children with intellectual disabilities of unknown etiology.

The distress due to increased amounts of everyday demands for time and work required from the parents of children with DS, because of the special medical and psychosocial needs of their handicapped child, was the only identified difference between them and the mothers of typical developing children. Inasmuch as the two groups of mothers of children with disabilities were otherwise similar, diagnostic uncertainty appears to constitute a strong independent determinant of long-lasting emotional burden for parents. Conversely, the definite diagnosis of a common, sporadic genetic anomaly such as DS, with its usually good prognosis and functional network of self-support groups, enabled parents to do nearly as well emotionally as parents of nondisabled children. Similar findings emerged for parents of adults with DS. For example, Seltzer,

Krauss, and Tsunematsu (1993) reported that mothers of 35-year-old adults with DS experienced lower levels of parenting stress as compared to mothers of adults with other types of MR.

In contrast to the aforementioned research outcomes, several studies did not find an "advantage" for DS, instead highlighting that parents of children with DS and parents of children with other forms of intellectual disability reported comparable levels of stress (e.g., Cahill & Glidden, 1996; Gosch, 2001). In these studies, mothers in the latter group (regardless of the disability's etiology) expressed more stress than did mothers of nondisabled children. Yet, specific behavior problems and challenging behaviors associated with the behavioral phenotype of a syndrome also influence the level of mothers' and fathers' stress (Gosch, 2001; Ricci & Hodapp, 2003). Children's characteristics in terms of their appearance, difficulties in developing expressive language, articulation, and linguistic grammar (Fowler, 1990; Miller, Leddy, Miolo, & Sedey, 1995), as well as additional developmental and health difficulties, may contribute to increased parental stress (Roizen & Patterson, 2003).

Reports of parental stress levels among parents of children with DS versus parents of typically developing children were inconsistent. Several studies did not find differences between these two parent groups (Lenhard et al., 2005; Sanders & Morgan, 1997; Wolf, Noh, Fisman, & Speechley, 1989), whereas others demonstrated a higher level of parental stress among parents of children with DS as compared to parents of typically developing children (Roach, Orsmond, & Barratt, 1999; Scott, Atkinson, Minton, & Bowman, 1997). Research on the impact of parenting a child with DS on parents' life satisfaction and nonwork activities reveal no significant differences between these parents and parents of typically developing children (Branholm & Degerman, 1992).

It can be concluded that studies of the stress expressed by parents of children with DS yielded inconsistent findings when compared to parents of children with typical development or with other disabilities (Hodapp et al., 2001). These inconsistent findings call for more refined and in-depth explorations and raise some questions regarding the roots of the commonly acknowledged "DS advantage."

Parenting Children with Down Syndrome: Is It a Different Experience?
In examining possible explanations for the aforementioned "DS advantage" regarding parental

stress, several aspects of the syndrome suggest that these parents' experiences differ from that of parents with children who have other disabilities. First, as the most common genetic cause of intellectual disabilities, DS is well known to professionals and parents alike, and boasts many active parent support and advocacy groups (Hodapp et al., 2001). Perhaps these features of the syndrome may lead parents to a greater sense of familiarity, control, and support than is available for parents of children with less known, more infrequent, and vaguer diagnoses. Second, even with the increased availability of screening procedures, the positive correlation between the mother's increasing age and higher rates of DS in her fetus continues (Olsen, Cross, Gensburg, & Hughes, 1996). The stronger likelihood that DS babies will be born to older and more mature mothers may explain this group's predominant maternal characteristics, such as greater experience as a parent and higher level of socioeconomic status (SES; Cahill & Glidden, 1996).

Third, the "DS advantage" might stem from these children's characteristic behavioral functioning. For example, the trajectory of symptoms among children with DS is quite distinct and quite stable over the life course (Greenberg, Seltzer, Krauss, Chou, & Hong, 2004; Zigman, Seltzer, & Silverman, 1994), which may possibly promote parents' sense of predictability, control, and manageability. Thus, during childhood and adolescence, parents of a child with DS generally sense a warm exchange of emotion with their child and can realistically expect this type of relationship to continue into the future (Greenberg et al., 2004). Similarly, mothers of adults with DS reported better relationships with their son or daughter than did mothers of adults with autism or mothers of adults with schizophrenia (Greenberg et al., 2004).

Children with DS tend to have fewer and less severe behavior problems (Dykens & Kasari, 1997; Meyers & Pueschel, 1991), which may constitute an "advantage" considering that children's level of maladaptive behaviors was found to best predict parental stress in families of children with MR (Hodapp, Dykens, & Masino, 1997; Hodapp, Wijma, & Masino, 1997). For example, parents of children with DS reported more child-related rewards than did parents of children with other disabilities, with rates similar to parents of same-age typically developing children (Hodapp et al., 2001). *Rewardingness* refers to the feelings of gratification and reinforcement brought about by parenting a child, and involves feeling love and appreciated by the child as well as feeling that the child returns the parents' love and attention

The children's relatively high capacity for socially oriented behaviors may also contribute to the "DS advantage" (Hodapp et al., 2001). Although debates are raised about the "DS personality" (e.g., Wishart & Johnston, 1990), these children have a relatively less pronounced impairment in social development aspects (Hauser-Cram et al., 1999). Compared to typically developing children of the same mental ages, toddlers with DS, as a group, spent more time looking at an interesting adult than at surrounding toys (Kasari, Mundy, Yirmiya, & Sigman, 1990). During the school years, these children continue to look more at adults during problem-solving tasks than do their peers with other types of MR (Kasari & Freeman, 2001). Thus, it is not surprising that parents tend to describe their children with DS as manifesting a high level of sociable and cheerful behavior, using terminology such as "affectionate," "lovable," "nice," and "gets on well with problems" (Carr, 1995). Similar descriptions were given by fathers of 7 - to 14-year-old children with DS, such as "sociable," "friendly," "lovable," and "cheerful" (Hornby, 1995). Moreover, parents' view of their children with DS as highly sociable appears to contradict with studies indicating that such children tend to have difficulties in high-level social skills, as manifested on hypothetical empathy tasks and on assignments requiring emotion labeling or understanding (Kasari, Freeman, & Bass, 2001; Kasari, Freeman, & Hughes, 2001).

Moreover, as emphasized by Fidler and Hodapp (1999), the baby-face characteristics of children with DS may also be related to parental judgments. Children with DS were viewed as more honest, naïve, warm, compliant, and sociable than were children with another genetic MR disorder, as well as same-aged typically developing children. Fidler and Hodapp (1999) argued that these children's faces may ultimately be related to adults' perceptions.

Stress Specific to Receiving the Diagnosis
As mentioned above, researchers examined parents' experience with the stressful event of receiving their child's diagnosis of DS (Alderson, 2001; Wapner et al., 2003). For example, Hall, Bobrow, and Marteau's (2000) study of three subgroups of parents of children with DS provided additional insight into the stressful psychological consequences associated with prenatal screening tests. These three groups of parents were those who received a false-negative result from prenatal screening, those who

were not offered the screening, and those who declined the test. Overall, all three groups of parents adjusted well to having a child with DS. Their levels of anxiety, depression, and parental stress, as well as their attitudes toward their disabled child were similar to those of parents of typically developing children. However, a false-negative prenatal screening result, one that did not detect the affected pregnancy, undermined parents' adjustment. For mothers and fathers alike, a false-negative result was associated with higher parenting stress, a stronger tendency to blame others for the birth of the child, and more negative attitudes toward the child, in comparison with those who declined a test. A false-negative result was also associated with higher anxiety among the mothers.

Mothers who received a prenatal diagnosis of DS for their fetus but decided to continue the pregnancy expressed lower levels of distress, probably because they gradually came to terms with their decision (Skotko, 2005). Women who chose to continue their pregnancy after a prenatal diagnosis of DS did so primarily because of personal beliefs and values. The majority of these mothers approached the screening feeling confident that they would continue the pregnancy no matter what the results indicated. Others who felt undecided about continuing the pregnancy wanted to gather more information if the results indicated the fetus had DS. Moreover, the majority of these mothers expressed frustration from their interactions with physicians and emphasized the need for more up-to-date printed materials on DS and for referral to local support groups (Skotko, 2005).

Parents experience strong feelings of depression at the time of the baby's birth and diagnosis with DS (Emde & Brown, 1978; Zahn-Waxler, Duggal, & Gruber, 2002). After the initial period of depression, parents often do better until the baby reaches approximately 4 months of age. At this point, a second wave of depression occurs when mothers realize the developmental implications of DS, as their infant shows more dampened affect and less consistent social smiles than typically developing children. Several waves of depression may also occur in the preschool period, when mothers are concerned about children's developmental milestones, such as walking, talking, and toilet training, and also through puberty and the onset of adulthood. Maternal emotions may be most intense directly after the birth of the child, but later milestones may also elicit strong reactions (Zahn-Waxler et al., 2002).

Stress Related to Other Variables

Researchers have examined parental stress in socio-economically matched samples (Roach et al., 1999). In this comparison, parents of children with DS perceived more caregiving difficulties, child-related stress (distractibility, demandingness, unacceptability), and parent-related stress (incompetence, depression, health problems, role restriction) than did parents of typically developing children. For both groups of parents, mothers' stress was associated with children's caregiving difficulties, whereas fathers' stress was related to the presence of a child with DS. Mothers who reported more responsibilities for childcare experienced more health difficulties, less spousal support, and role restrictions. Fathers who reported more responsibilities for childcare experienced fewer difficulties with parental competence. These parents also reported distress in relation to their limited available time for leisure, which changed their choices of recreational activity and increased the need to plan leisure pursuits. In examinations of parents' satisfaction with the manner in which they allocated their time, these parents of children with DS frequently noted the potential benefits of incorporating more leisure into their daily lives (Wayne & Krishnagiri, 2005).

Sources of Stress

Stress represented not only a single mechanism but may represent several interrelated ones. This differentiation is valuable not only for the in-depth comprehension of parental experience, but is especially needed to plan differential and individually adapted empowering approaches (Cacioppo, Hawkley, & Berntson, 2003):

- The *added-stress hypothesis* assumes that the number of stressors render a cumulative impact. Thus, having children with DS may add further unique stressors to preexisting normative hassles and stressors in the lives of individuals and families.
- The *differential-exposure hypothesis* assumes that parents of children with DS may be exposed to stressful events more frequently than other parents, and thus they may experience stressors more often. Over time, they may experience greater "wear and tear" on their personal regulatory mechanisms.
- The *differential-reactivity hypothesis* posits that the stressors to which the parents are exposed may not actually be more frequent than the stressors met by other parents, but having a

child with DS may increase these parents' vulnerability to those objectively equivalent stressors. Thus, stressors may be subjectively viewed as more intense and may elicit stronger reactions from these parents.

- The *differential-stress buffering hypothesis* posits that these parents are less likely than their counterparts with typically developing children to believe they have other people to whom they can turn for assistance. Without the adequate relief emerging from supportive relations, the stressors to which these parents are exposed may be perceived as more severe.

Abidin (1995) made a distinction between two sources of parenting stress. The first, *child-related stress,* refers to child behaviors and characteristics that cause difficulties for parents and contribute to parenting stress. Such characteristics include the child's diagnosis, maladaptive behavior, specific developmental difficulties, additional health problems, and difficult temperament. The second source of parental stress, *parent-related stress,* refers to characteristics, attitudes, and experiences of the parent that do not directly involve the child. These variables may also refer to parental self-efficacy, trust in professional help, feelings of competence, and parents' beliefs, values, and expectations (Bukowski, Adams, & Santo, 2006).

COPING AMONG PARENTS OF CHILDREN WITH DOWN SYNDROME

There is wide agreement that parents' coping style contributes to their cognitive, emotional, and behavioral reactions (Turnbull et al., 1993). However, only a few studies examined in-depth unique coping patterns among families of individuals with DS, calling for future explorations. Coping was defined as the thoughts and behaviors used to manage the internal and external demands of stressful situations (Folkman & Moskowitz, 2004). Two types of coping strategies were identified. First, *problem-oriented coping* refers to efforts to deal with the sources of stress by changing the individual's behaviors, by changing the environmental conditions, or both. Second, *emotional regulation coping* refers to coping efforts aimed at reducing emotional distress and maintaining a satisfactory internal state (Folkman & Lazarus, 1988). These types of coping responses are interrelated as well as complementary, and are closely associated with emotional reactions. Overall, parents had better well-being (i.e., lower levels of depressive and physical symptoms, higher levels of environmental mastery and self-acceptance) if they used accommodative coping (flexibly adjusting one's goals in response to a persistent problem) (Seltzer, Frank, Floyd, Greenberg, & Hong, 2004).

Mothers who use problem-oriented coping strategies tend to essentially address their child's MR as a practical, concrete problem to be managed (e.g., Turnbull et al., 1993). Thus, they make plans to handle everyday problems and feel that they have learned from their experiences. Conversely, mothers who use emotion-focused coping tend to either totally deny their feelings about their child and his or her disabilities or, instead, become overly concerned or even almost obsessed with their own feelings of depression and grief. A greater proportion of active problem-oriented mothers seem to be considerably better adjusted than emotion-focused mothers (Abbeduto et al., 2004; Glidden, Billings, & Jobe, 2006).

Parents of children with disabilities have often reported a greater use of avoidance as a coping style (e.g., Al-Yagon, 2007; Margalit, Raviv, & Ankonina, 1992). An increased use of avoidant coping, in families of children with and without disabilities alike, predicted higher levels of negative and distressed parental affect, pinpointing attention at the crucial maladaptive role played by parents' attempts to deny a stressful reality (Al-Yagon, 2007; Margalit & Ankonina, 1991). Parental active coping is often expressed through requesting and allocating help and support within and outside the family. For example, participation in valued life activities, when used as a coping method, can help one to manage feelings of depression and loneliness, structure time, avoid rumination, and restore a sense of purpose and mastery (Lent, 2004). Realistic goal setting (e.g., shifting to more reachable goals or more accessible routes to goal pursuit) may also be a viable coping method in the face of difficult circumstances.

The few studies that focused on parental coping strategies among parents of children with DS reported similar findings to those revealed by previous studies on children with other disabilities (Lam & Mackenie, 2002; Sullivan, 2002; Van Riper, 1999). For example, Lam and Mackenie (2002) examined Chinese mothers' experiences of parenting a child with DS. According to their results, this group of mothers frequently used coping strategies characterized by high levels of avoidance, self-reliance, and seeking of social support. The comparisons between fathers and mothers of children with DS revealed several gender differences in parental coping strategies (Sullivan, 2002). Women scored significantly higher than men in seeking instrumental and emotional support, in focusing on and venting emotions, and in suppression of competing activities.

In examination of the association between mothers' cognitive coping style (approach-avoidance), affective state, and sensitivity, 56 mothers and their children with DS were followed for 2 years (Atkinson et al., 1995). Cognitive coping and affective distress inventories were administered, and sensitivity was rated on the basis of mother–child observations. Results indicated that approach and avoidance were stable across the 2 years. These coping variables mediated the distress of parenting children with DS in complex ways. Mothers with a strong tendency to monitor stressors reported greater affective distress than did mothers who adopt a less vigilant coping style. At the same time, cognitive avoidance of stressors and affective distress reduced the behavioral sensitivity of mothers toward their children.

The Role of Social Support

Constant coping challenges enhance the importance of available social support options (Friedrich, Wilturner, & Cohen, 1985). Social support refers to the information leading individuals to believe that they are cared for, esteemed, and members of a network with mutual obligations (Dunst, Trivette, & Deal, 1988). Social support conveys many benefits, not the least of which is the transmission of significant others' beliefs about one's efficacy, which may play a key role in rebuilding morale in the face of parental efficacy-deflating conditions (Lent, 2004).

Social support can exist in the forms of companionship, material support, and informational support. Companionship refers to spending time together with others, feeling mutually close, expressing appreciation, and regarding the person as valued. Material support is related to the provision of resources and actual assistance, whereas informational support involves the availability of advice and counseling. Support and assistance may be provided in different styles, such as formal help (e.g., from psychologists or teachers) and informal support (e.g., from a friend or another parent). However, virtual Internet connections challenge the classical conceptualization of social supports in terms of style and proximity.

The characteristics of the parent who is requesting and receiving help may contribute to the type and style of the different supports he or she needs. To take advantage of available possibilities within the community, parents must be able to accept help and to maintain interpersonal relations. Gender differences were also noted in parental expectations for support, with mothers scoring significantly higher than fathers in attempts to seek emotional support and to focus on and vent emotions, and with fathers emphasizing the need for instrumental support and problem solving (Sullivan, 2002). The study of satisfaction from support provides an important index regarding not only the quality of the support provided, but also the ability of the parent to cope effectively with his or her own loneliness and to benefit from that support (Dunst et al., 1988). Moreover, children's characteristics also contributed to parental satisfaction, as documented by the similarities in needs, yet the differences in satisfaction, with social support in comparisons between parents of children with autism and children with DS (Siklos & Kerns, 2006).

In an intervention study of infants with developmental disabilities (Margalit et al., 2006), mothers' expectations for support and for direct help with their infants revealed interactions between maternal perceptions of personal strength and of family cohesion. Strong mothers who felt confident in themselves but felt their families to be noncohesive and unsupportive viewed the early intervention staff as a family substitute, saying, as it were: "I found a new family." Mothers who did not feel confident in themselves but felt they had highly cohesive families were not looking for a "new family;" yet, they expressed satisfaction from the program's personal empowerment, saying, as it were: "They help me believe that I can help my child." Parental support was also related to parents' experience of isolation; only a few studies have investigated parental isolation, but their results were consistent. For example, Florian and Krulik (1991) reported that negative correlations were found between the availability of social support and mothers' feelings of loneliness.

In line with ecological models that focused attention on the interactions between individuals and their environment (Bronfenbrenner, 1979; Bronfenbrenner & Ceci, 1994), the experience of stress has been examined in different cultures to identify the unique cultural dynamics related to community attitudes and parents' interrelations within those communities.

Cultural Context of Stress and Coping
Mothers of different ethnicities seem to react differently to rearing a child with MR, reflecting contextual conditions and cultural emphases. For example,

Heller and his colleagues (1994) reported on varied contextual and cultural emphases and demonstrated that Hispanic mothers considered raising a child with MR as a religious duty. Mothers from the African American community reported the high benefit they received from the support of church members (Rogers-Dulan, 1998). In Greece, mothers of children with DS reported greater stress and more frequent and lengthy time demands that affected their recreational and educational activities, due to children's increased dependency, in comparison to mothers of nondisabled children (Padeliadu, 1998). Furthermore, these Greek mothers of children with DS perceived the time they spent with their children as a source of stress.

Regardless of cultural differences, Chinese mothers in Hong Kong also reported that the presence of a child with DS in the family represented a significant ongoing source of stress for mothers (Lam & Mackenzie, 2002). Major themes related to maternal stress were the unexpected birth of an abnormal child, struggles related to the acceptance of the child, special needs of the child, worries about the future, effects on the marital relationship, and social restrictions. The types of stressors changed over time according to the child's age and to the availability of help and support systems. Coping strategies varied accordingly, with avoidance, self-reliance, and seeking social support as the most frequent strategies. The particular problems faced by mothers of children with DS in Hong Kong were discussed against the sociocultural background of the region and the highly competitive nature of its society. In another study that examined Taiwanese mothers' descriptions of interactions with their babies with DS, two themes emerged (McCollum & Chen, 2003). The first theme highlighted how mothers talked about their babies' abilities and limitations, and the second described mothers' expectations (pessimistic and optimistic) with respect to raising a baby with DS, thus providing a potential way to understand mothers' beliefs about their own roles in supporting their babies' development.

Studies have also examined the association between parents' stress, support, and well-being among parents of children with DS (e.g., Hauser-Cram et al., 1999). The results indicated that social-emotional support predicted enhanced well-being. Mothers who reported high levels of stress felt less able to meet day-to-day demands (McDowell, Saylor, Taylor, Boyce, & Stokes, 1995; Webster-Stratton, 1990). Maternal stress was negatively associated with mental health, but was not associated with physical health or social functioning, even when controlling for demographic status, disability type, and functional independence (Wallander, Pitt, & Mellins, 1990). The results' comparisons revealed that, in different cultures, parents of children with DS reported an experience of increased stress as well as a need for updated information on their children's syndrome and for meaningful support. These parents expressed pessimistic as well as optimistic future expectations, and community support played a critical role in the quality of parental experiences.

The Role of the Community: Social Capital

Social capital is the aggregate construct of resources (information, opportunities, and instrumental support) that arise from reciprocal social networks and relationships and that emerge from participation in formal and informal settings (Mancini, Bowen, & Martin, 2005). Considering the increased need of the family for social support, the community context should have a more prominent place in research about families of children with disabilities. Community context factors, including transactions with other families and institutions and social capital, can be expected to constitute significant elements in understanding and strengthening families. The actions of civic and social advocacy groups, local faith communities, various community-based membership groups, and online support and self-help groups are sources for effective support.

Elements of community capacity include organizational resources (Chaskin, Brown, Venkatesh, & Vidal, 2001) that provide the understanding of norms, networks, and associated processes within the community life (Mancini et al., 2005). Social organization accounts for a wide range of influences on family life, including both specific groups of people whom we know well and others with whom we share norms rather than relationships. Culturally based attitudes and perceptions of disabilities include norms related to acceptance/rejection of behavior patterns, which may further affect children's adjustment and growth. The development of virtual communities provides an extension of the classic social organization conceptualization that enables new options of support, and parental coping patterns have to be explored in these new types of relations.

Virtual Social Support

There is a growing appreciation to social support provided through the Internet (Baum, 2004; Colvin, Chenoweth, Bold, & Harding, 2004; Eastin & LaRose, 2005). Individuals of various ages, from diverse cultures, with different needs and sources of distress, present themselves online, sharing their past experiences and future expectations (Kanayama, 2003). Individuals send messages to e-communities that share a common interest, in order to get advice, communicate concerns and dilemmas, and develop meaningful relations. Two main support functions were identified in online groups (Zaidman-Zait & Jamieson, 2007). First, informational support is based on the knowledge and experience of the participants, who may also refer fellow users to other resources and websites containing information about the issue of interest (Sarkadi & Bremberg, 2005). Second, emotional support may also be a significant aspect of online groups (Scharer, 2005).

Paradoxically, these connections provide users with feelings of close proximity and intimacy, regardless of their anonymity and objective distances (Chan & Cheng, 2004). For example, Jones and Lewis (2000) used content analysis to explore the function of an Internet discussion group used by the parents of people with DS. The parents required information that they needed for problem solving and decision making. At the same time, parents communicated a sense of achievement celebration and advocated a focus on the child rather than on the handicap. They shared hopes for becoming the agents of change. The analysis of messages sent by parents of children with autism also indicated that the e-group functioned as a support group in making sense of autism (Huws, Jones, & Ingledew, 2001). This study identified major categories in these messages, such as their searching for a meaning, adjusting to changes, and providing support and encouragement to other members of the group.

It seems that, for parents who already struggle with increased time demands related to the increased needs of their children, the time flexibility provided by Internet communities is extremely valuable. In an interview, a mother of a 1-year-old girl with DS reported connecting to the Internet almost every night, but during a late hour. She related: "That is the only available time to be in contact with the other mothers who have similar difficulties and become my friends . . . I never met with them, but I feel very close to them. I know everything about their struggle. It helps."

In conclusion, parents of children with disabilities such as DS find social support online, not only seeking information about effective parenting and problem solving but also developing close supportive interactions with other parents who share similar conflicts, challenging conditions, and dilemmas (Baum, 2004; Jones, & Lewis, 2000; Leonard, 2004; Sarkadi & Bremberg, 2005; Scharer, 2005). The conceptual move from pathogenic approaches to DS to the stress and coping paradigm clarified sources of stress, indicating possibilities for support and the importance of interpersonal relations for empowering parents (Van Riper, 2003). A different approach for examining interpersonal relations within these families is rooted in the attachment conceptualization.

Parent–Child Interactions and Attachment Relationships

The early parent–infant relationship has been conceptualized primarily within the framework of attachment theory (Ainsworth, Blehar, Waters, & Wall, 1978; Bowlby, 1973, 1982/1969, 1988). Briefly, attachment theory emphasizes that, over the course of the first year of life, infants develop a specific and enduring relationship with their primary caretakers (Ainsworth & Wittig, 1969). Infants' strong tendency to seek proximity to caregivers is the overt manifestation of the attachment behavioral system, an inborn system designed to restore or maintain proximity to supportive others in times of need. Proximity to an available, supportive, and responsive caregiver "attachment figure" provides the infant with a sense of "secure base," which refers to a set of expectations about others' availability and responsiveness in times of stress.

Attachment figures play a central role in the infant's cognitive, social, and emotional development, as well as in the development of a sense of self (Bowlby, 1988; Waters & Cummings, 2000). Children's experiences with attachment figures are internalized into "working models of attachment"—a mental representation of the significant other and the self. These result in unique attachment styles— stable patterns of cognitions and behaviors that are manifested in other close relationships and social interactions. Many studies have examined the relations between attachment patterns and children's socioemotional and behavioral adjustment (for a review, see Thompson, 1999). Securely attached children clearly revealed better mental health and functioning, higher levels of psychological well-being, and more optimal signs of social and emotional adjustment than did children with an insecure style (e.g., Erickson, Sroufe, & Egeland, 1985; Greenberg, Speltz, & DeKlyen, 1993; Lyons-Ruth, 1996; Sroufe, 1983).

During the Strange Situation Laboratory Observation (Ainsworth et al., 1978), children with DS display separation distress that is less intense and of shorter duration, compared to control groups of typically developing children matched for mental age (MA) and for chronological age (CA) (Cicchetti & Serafica 1981; Thompson, Ciccheti, Lamb, & Malkin, 1985; Vaughn et al., 1994). Ainsworth's laboratory-based observation focuses on the infant's response to two brief separations from the caretaker and to reunion. Infant responses to this situation are customarily classified into one of three patterns of behavior, one considered secure and the other two (avoidant and anxious-ambivalent) considered insecure. Each of these represents a primary strategy for maintaining the attention of the attachment figure. A fourth pattern—disorganized—(also considered insecure) was added later by Main and Solomon (1986). Infant responses to a particular parent in this situation are considered to reflect the history of the interactions the infant has experienced with that parent in the home and to predict important differences in later functioning (see Bretherton, 1985 for a review). In normative samples, 65% of infants showed secure attached pattern (van IJzendoorn & Kroonenberg, 1988).

Focusing on the attachment behaviors of children with DS, Vaughn et al. (1994) conducted an extensive study that examined 133 toddlers with DS aged 14–54 months. Their results demonstrated that these children manifested lower levels of proximity seeking, contact maintenance, and resistance than found among comparison groups. Vaughn et al. also reported low percentages of securely attached children as compared to typically developing children. Their study showed that only 46% of these children were classified as securely attached to their mothers. A large proportion of the insecurely attached children (42%) were classified as Type D, the insecure/ disorganized attachment type. These Type D percentages were higher than those observed among nonclinical samples, but similar to other clinical groups (e.g., van Ijzendoorn, Goldberg, Kroonenberg, & Frenkel, 1992). Similar attachment classification distributions emerged in two other studies of DS (Atkinson et al., 1999; Ganiban, Barnett, & Cicchetti, 2000).

Some researchers (e.g., Atkinson et al., 1999; Ganiban et al., 2000; Vaughn et al., 1994) have suggested that these findings may possibly stem from low validity levels for both the Strange Situation Procedure and the attachment patterns described by Ainsworth and her colleagues (1978) vis à vis these children with DS. Low validity could perhaps be related to these children's ambiguous affective reactions due to poor muscle tone, which may impede accurate measurement and interpretation of their attachment cues. Importantly, studies have emphasized the possible negative impact of these children's motor and neurological dysfunction on the development of their attachment relationships (Bridges & Cicchetti, 1982; Ganiban et al., 2000).

In line with this perspective, studies reported that many caregivers of children with DS are highly directive and intrusive with their children (e.g., Crawley & Spiker, 1983; Marfo, Dedrick, & Barbour, 1998). Some researchers suggested a link between the characteristics of infants with DS and the development of maternal interaction strategies that reveal more sensitivity and greater directedness compared to control groups (Crawley & Spiker, 1983; Mahoney, Fors, & Wood, 1990). Inasmuch as these infants have been depicted as more lethargic and hypotonic and as providing fewer and less clear interactive cues to their caregivers than in typical development (Hyche, Bakeman, & Adamson, 1992), these children may be less "readable" for their parents and thus may elicit more direct and intrusive parental behaviors to fill the interaction gap (Sorce & Emde, 1982).

The context of language development provides an additional perspective on mother–child interactions for children with DS. There is wide agreement that mothers of children with DS provide their children with similar language modeling, the same amount of information per sentence, and similar grammatical complexity as provided by mothers of nonretarded children of the same language age or MA (see Hodapp, 2002 for a review). However, as described above, studies have also indicated that these mothers manifest very different styles in their interactions than do mothers of typically developing children. Mothers of children with DS were reported to be more didactic, to take longer and more frequent instructive turns during interactions with their children, and to more frequently speak at the same time as their children (Marfo et al., 1998; Tannock, 1988). Perhaps these mothers considered verbal interactions to be an opportunity for "teaching sessions" in their effort to intervene and cope effectively with their children's deficits (Cardoso-Martins & Mervis, 1984; Hodapp, 2002), although such roles may be less fulfilling for parents. As suggested by Marfo et al. (1998), a directive/intrusive style of interaction may serve as an effective coping style to foster short-term cognitive development

among toddlers with DS, but this strategy may not be a sensitive response to these children's emotional needs.

Taken together, these findings show that, as a group, mothers of children with DS manifested some similar but many different strategies while interacting with their children, in comparison to mothers of typically developing children. The two groups of mothers showed similar aspects of communication and language complexity. However, as a group, mothers of children with DS demonstrated more intrusive, didactic, directive, and sensitive interaction strategies than did their counterparts with typically developing children. In line with attachment theory assumptions (Bowlby, 1988; Waters & Cummings, 2000), a consistent history of such asynchronous-intrusive or insensitive interactions may offer fewer opportunities to develop organized and coherent attachment strategies and may dispose these toddlers with DS to display insecure patterns of attachment behaviors. These findings call for additional exploration regarding parental interaction style's contribution to these children's cognitive and socioemotional development.

Discussion and Future Directions

This chapter provided a survey of research focusing on two major themes with regard to this group of parents and children with DS: the shift from a pathology perspective to a stress and coping approach, and the study of parent–child interactions, attachment, and relationships. The outcomes of this survey call for additional future exploration of several aspects.

THE INCONSISTENT FINDINGS REGARDING PARENTS' STRESS

The current survey of research on the stress expressed by parents of children with DS yielded inconsistent findings when compared to parents of children with typical development or with other disabling conditions (Lewis et al., 2006; Seltzer, Abbeduto, Krauss, Greenberg, & Swe, 2004), thus pointing to the need for more refined and in-depth explorations, as well as an intragroup approach. Life cycle perspectives further support the outcomes of the research on families of adults with DS to younger studies. These studies examined maternal stress among mothers of adults with DS (Carr, 2005; Heller & Caldwell, 2005) and reported the importance of family control on support and respite programs as predictors of well-being and health. These studies also demonstrated that these parents did not experience greater stress or health problems than did comparison groups of same age parents.

FAMILY-FOCUSED PROGRAMS

General consensus emerged from large numbers of programs, as well as research studies, asserting the significant contribution of family functioning to childhood development and adjustment (e.g., Patterson, 2002; Campbell, 1998). Research findings emphasizing the contribution of family diversity to children's later maladjustment (Campbell, 1994, 1998; Denham et al., 2000; Greenberg et al., 1993) clearly suggest the need to establish more systematic services for the families, and to provide them with increased structuring control of the programs to meet their changing needs at various age stages (Heller & Caldwell, 2005). For example, with regard to studies' recommendations that focused on secure early attachment as a protective factor for at-risk children (Al-Yagon, 2003; Svanberg, 1998; Werner, 1993), as well as the low percentages of securely attached children with DS as compared to typically developing children (e.g., Atkinson et al., 1999; Ganiban et al., 2000), family-focused interventions may offer parents training to improve the quality of parent–child relationships and the formation of a secure attachment style with their children.

PARENTAL PERSONAL RESOURCES

A variety of research supported the prediction that parents' psychological resources, as well as their developmental histories, directly influence child rearing quality and, through parenting, child development (Belsky, 1984; Belsky & Barends, 2002; Parke, 2004). Moreover, Belsky (1984) argued that parental psychological resources comprise the most important determinant, being more influential than the child's individual characteristics or the contextual sources. Research has been conducted on parental personal resources that are assumed to play a substantial role in child development, including parental well-being and psychopathology (e.g., Campbell, 2003; Goodman & Gotlib, 2002; Greenberg et al., 1993; Luthar & Cicchetti, 2000; Werner, 1993), parental personality (Belsky & Barends, 2002), and parental ego-resiliency (van Bakel & Riksen-Walraven, 2002), among others. However, despite the growing awareness regarding the contribution of parents' psychological resources, as well as their developmental histories to child rearing quality and, through parenting, child development among typically developing children

(Belsky, 1984; Belsky & Barends, 2002; Parke, 2004), studies examining these factors among parents of children with DS are rare.

FATHERS' PERSPECTIVES

There is a growing awareness regarding the contribution of fathers to children's development and adjustment (e.g., Marsiglio, Amato, Day, & Lamb, 2000; Parke, 2004), yet the vast majority of the studies have examined maternal factors and perspectives, thus calling for further examination of fathers' roles and influences. Gender differences in parental characteristics, levels of involvement, perceptions of children with DS, and their coping resources may contribute to an in-depth conceptualization of the family construct.

TECHNOLOGY INTEGRATION AND INTERNET CHALLENGES

The technology revolution has crucial ramifications for almost all facets of modern society. Computers and the Internet have become integrated into our everyday lives within work, home, and leisure environments, and they transcend the boundaries of time and place during social interactions and information sharing.

However, there is a strong need to investigate in-depth the emotional meaning of support provided by virtual communities—other parents who share similar difficulties—and of empowerment via online resources, as well as the ability for information processing among parents with lower educational levels and among highly distressed parents. Sitting a parent in front of a computer may not suffice. Planned instruction and supported experimentation can enhance parents' effective utilization of such sites, so that parents can begin to realize the potential of such technologies within intervention programs, and to promote their accessibility to parents with different levels of education and emotional distress. There is a need for future studies to identify ways of integrating these extended options into the current intervention procedures and parental support and monitoring.

COPING RESOURCES

Only a few studies were devoted uniquely to exploring parental coping resources and strategies among parents of children with DS (Atkinson et al., 1995; Lam & Mackenie, 2002; Sullivan, 2002; Van Riper, 1999). This an important theoretical and interventional issue that requires extended attention. Family studies of different disabilities provided insight into processing and outcomes (Al-Yagon, 2007; Turnbull et al, 1993). The examination of parental sense of coherence, and their expectations for hope within the hope theory (Snyder, 2002), enhanced the conceptualization of a dynamic developmental paradigm. Future studies will have to explore the specific characteristics of DS to the notion of parental coping.

Finally, the growing recognition of the importance of family-centered support programs and community capital within different cultures, as well as the beginning explorations of the promises of new technology, call for future international research to promote the well-being and life quality of fathers and mothers of individuals with DS and to empower their coping abilities.

Acknowledgments

The author would like to express her appreciation to Dee B. Ankonina for her editorial contribution.

References

Abbeduto, L., Seltzer, M. M., Shattuck, P., Krauss, Wyngaarden, M., Orsmond, G., & Murphy, M. M. (2004). Psychological well-being and coping in mothers of youths with autism, Down syndrome, or fragile X syndrome. *American Journal on Mental Retardation, 109,* 237–254.

Abery, B. H. (2006). Family adjustment and adaptation with children with Down syndrome. *Focus on Exceptional Children, 38,* 1–19.

Abidin, R. (1995). *Parenting stress index: Manual* (3rd ed.). Odessa, FL: Psychological Assessment Resources.

Ainsworth, M. D., Blehar, M. C., Waters, E., & Wall, S. (1978). *Patterns of attachment: A psychological study of the strange situation.* Hillside, NJ: Erlbaum.

Ainsworth, M. D., & Wittig, B. A. (1969). Attachment and exploratory behavior of one-year-olds in a strange situation. In B. M. Foss (Ed.), *Determinants of infant behavior* Vol. 4 (pp. 113–136). London: Methuen.

Al-Yagon, M. (2003). Children at-risk for developing learning disorders: Multiple perspectives. *Journal of Learning Disabilities, 36,* 318–335.

Al-Yagon, M. (2007). Socioemotional and behavioral adjustment among school-age children with learning disabilities: The moderating role of maternal personal resources. *Journal of Special Education., 40,* 205–217.

Alderson, P. (2001). Down's syndrome: Cost, quality and value of life. *Social Science & Medicine, 5,* 627–638.

American Psychiatric Association. (2000). *Diagnostic and statistical manual of mental disorders* (text revision). Washington, DC: Author.

Anthony, L. G., Anthony, B. J., Glanville, D. N., Naiman, D. Q., Waanders, C., & Shaffer, S. (2005). The relationships between parenting stress, parenting behavior and preschoolers social competence and behavior problems in the classroom. *Infant and Child Development, 14,* 133–154.

Atkinson, L., Chisholm, V. C., Scott, B., Goldberg, S., Vaughn, B. E., Blackwell, J., et al. (1999). Maternal sensitivity, child function level, and attachment in Down syndrome. *Monographs of the Society for Research in Child Development, 64,* 45–66.

Atkinson, L., Scott, B., Chisholm, V., Blackwell, J., Dickens, S., Tam, F., et al. (1995). Cognitive coping, affective distress, and maternal sensitivity: Mothers of children with Down syndrome. *Developmental Psychology, 31,* 668–676.

Baum, L. S. (2004). Internet parent support groups for primary caregivers of a child with special health care needs. *Pediatric Nursing, 30,* 381–390.

Beeghly, M. (1998). Emergence of symbolic play: Perspectives from typical and atypical development. In J. A. Burack, R. M. Hodapp, & E. Zigler (Eds.), *Handbook of mental retardation and development* (pp. 240–289). Cambridge, UK: Cambridge University Press.

Belsky, J. (1984). The determinants of parenting: A process model. *Child Development, 55,* 83–96.

Belsky, J., & Barends, N. (2002). Personality and parenting. In M. H. Bornstein (Ed.), *Handbook of parenting* Vol. 3 (2nd ed., pp. 415–438). Mahwah, NJ: Lawrence Erlbaum.

Blacher, J., Neece, C. L., & Paczkowski., E. (2005). Families and intellectual disability. *Current Opinion in Psychiatry, 18,* 507–515.

Boss, P. (1988). *Family stress management.* Newbury Park, CA: Sage.

Bowlby, J. (1982/1969). *Attachment and loss: Attachment.* New York: Basic Books.

Bowlby, J. (1973). *Attachment and loss: Anxiety, anger, and separation.* New York: Basic Books.

Bowlby, J. (1988). *A secure base: Clinical applications of attachment theory.* London: Routledge.

Branholm, I., & Degerman, E. (1992). Life satisfaction and activity preferences in parents of Down's syndrome children. *Scandinavian Journal of Social Medicine, 20,* 37–44.

Bretherton, I. (1985). Attachment theory: Retrospect and prospect. In I. Bretherton, & E. Waters (Eds.), Growing points in attachment theory and research. *Monographs of the Society for Research in Child Development, 50* (1–2, Serial no. 209), 3–35.

Bridges, F., & Cicchetti, D. (1982). Mothers' ratings of temperament characteristics of Down's syndrome infants. *Developmental Psychology, 18,* 238–244.

Bronfenbrenner, U. (1979). *The ecology of human development.* Cambridge, MA: Harvard University Press.

Bronfenbrenner, U., & Ceci, S. J. (1994). Nature-nurture reconceptualized in developmental perspective: A bioecological model. *Psychological Review, 101,* 568–586.

Bukowski, W.M., Adams, R.E., & Santo, J.B. (2006). Recent advances in the study of development, social and personal experience, and psychopathology. *International Journal of Behavioral Development, 30,* 26–30.

Cacioppo, J. T., Hawkley, L. C., & Berntson, G. G. (2003). The anatomy of loneliness. *Current Direction in Psychological Science, 12,* 71–74.

Cahill, B. M., & Glidden, L. M. (1996). Influence of child diagnosis on family and parent functioning: Down syndrome versus other disabilities. *American Journal on Mental Retardation, 101,* 149–160.

Campbell, S. B. (1994). Hard-to-manage preschool boys: Externalizing behavior, social competence, and family context at two-year follow-up. *Journal of Atypical Child Psychology, 22,* 147–166.

Campbell, S. B. (1998). Developmental perspectives. In T. H. Ollendick, & M. Hersen (Eds.), *Handbook of child psychopathology* (pp. 3–35). New York: Plenum Press.

Campbell, S. B. (2003). *Behavior problems in preschool children: Clinical and developmental issues*. New York: Guilford Press.

Cardoso-Martins, C., & Mervis, C. (1984). Maternal speech to prelinguistic children with Down syndrome. *American Journal of Mental Deficiency, 89*, 451–458.

Carr, J. (1995). *Down's syndrome: Children growing up*. Cambridge, UK: Cambridge University Press.

Carr, J. (2005). Families of 30–35-year olds with Down's syndrome. *Journal of Applied Research in Intellectual Disabilities, 18*(1), 75–84.

Chan, D. K. -S., & Cheng, G. H. -L. (2004). A comparison of offline and online friendship qualities at different stages of relationship development. *Journal of Social and Personal Relationships, 21*, 305–320.

Chaskin, R. J., Brown, P., Venkatesh, S., & Vidal, A. (2001). *Building community capacity*. New York: Aldine De Gruyter.

Cicchetti, D., & Serafica, F. (1981). The interplay among behavioral systems: Illustrations of the study of attachment, affiliation, and wariness in young children with Down's syndrome. *Developmental Psychology, 17*, 36–49.

Colvin, J., Chenoweth, L., Bold, M., & Harding, C. (2004). Caregivers of older adults: Advantages and disadvantages of Internet-based social support. *Family Relations, 53*, 49–57.

Crawley, S., & Spiker, D. (1983). Mother-child interactions involving two-year-olds with Down syndrome: A look at individual differences. *Child Development, 54*, 1312–1323.

Crnic, K., Friedrich, W., & Greenberg, M. (1983). Adaptation of families with mentally handicapped children: A model of stress, coping, and family ecology. *American Journal of Mental Deficiency, 88*, 125–138.

Crnic, K. A., Gaze, C., & Hoffman, C. (2005). Cumulative parenting stress across the preschool period: Relations to maternal parenting and child behavior at age 5. *Infant and Child Development, 14*, 117–132.

Cummings, S., Bayley, H., & Rie, H. (1966). Effects of the child's deficiency on the mother: A study of mentally retarded, chronically ill, and neurotic children. *American Journal of Orthopsychiatry, 36*, 595–608.

Denham, S. A., Workman, E., Cole, P. M, Weissbrod, C, Kendziora, T., & Zahn-Waxler, C. (2000). Prediction of externalizing behavior problems from early to middle childhood: The role of parental socialization and emotional expression. *Development and Psychopathology, 12*, 23–45.

Dunst, C. J., Trivette, C. M., & Deal, A. G. (1988). *Enabling and empowering families*. Cambridge, MA: Brookline.

Dykens, E. M., Hodapp, R. M., & Evans, D. W. (1994). Profiles and development of adaptive behavior in children with Down syndrome. *American Journal on Mental Retardation, 98*, 580–587.

Dykens, E. M., & Kasari, C. (1997). Maladaptive behavior in children with Prader-Willi syndrome, Down syndrome, and nonspecific mental retardation. *American Journal on Mental Retardation, 102*, 228–237.

Dykens, E. M., Shah, B., Sagun, J., Beck, T., & King, B. Y. (2002). Maladaptive behavior and psychiatric disorders in persons with Down's syndrome. *Journal of Intellectual Disabilities Research, 46*, 484–492.

Eastin, M. S., & LaRose, R. (2005). Alternative support: Modeling social support online. *Computers in Human Behavior, 21*, 977–992.

Emde, R., & Brown, C. (1978). Adaptation to the birth of a Down's syndrome infant: Grieving and maternal attachment. *Journal of the American Academy of Child Psychiatry, 17*, 299–323.

Erickson, M. (1969). MMPI profiles of parents of young retarded children. *American Journal of Mental Deficiency, 73*, 727–732.

Erickson, M. F., Sroufe, L. A., & Egeland, B. (1985). The relationship between quality of attachment and behavior problems in a preschool high-risk sample. In I. Bretherton, & E. Waters (Eds.), Growing points in attachment theory and research. *Monographs of the Society for Research in Child Development, 50*(1–2, Serial No. 209), 147–166.

Fidler, D. J., & Hodapp, R. M. (1999). Craniofacial maturity and perceived personality in children with Down syndrome. *American Journal on Mental Retardation, 104*, 410–421.

Fidler, D. J., Hodapp, R. M., & Dykens, E. M. (2000). Stress in families of young children with Down syndrome, Williams syndrome, and Smith-Magenis syndrome. *Early Education and Development, 11*, 395–406.

Florian, V., & Krulik, T. (1991). Loneliness and social support of mothers of chronically ill children. *Social Science and Medicine, 32*, 1291–1296.

Folkman, S., & Lazarus, R. S. (1988). Coping as a mediator of emotions. *Journal of Personality and Social Psychology, 54*, 466–475.

Folkman, S., & Moskowitz, J. T. (2004). Coping: Pitfalls and promise. *Annual Review in Psychology, 55*, 745–774.

Fowler, A. (1990). Language abilities in children with Down's syndrome: Evidence for a specific syntactic delay. In D. Cicchetti, & M. Beeghly (Eds.), *Children with Down's syndrome: A developmental approach* (pp. 302–328). New York: Cambridge University Press.

Friedrich, W. L., & Freidrich, W. N. (1981). Psychosocial assets of parents of handicapped and nonhandicapped children. *American Journal of Mental Deficiency, 85*, 551–553.

Friedrich, W. N., Wilturner, L. T., & Cohen, D. S. (1985). Coping, resources and parenting mentally retarded children. *American Journal of Mental Deficiency, 90*, 130–139.

Ganiban, J., Barnett, D., & Ciccetti, D. (2000). Negative reactivity and attachment: Down syndrome's contribution to the attachment-temperament debate. *Development and Psychopathology, 12*, 1–21.

Gath, A. (1977). The impact of an abnormal child upon the parents. *British Journal of Psychiatry, 130*, 405–410.

Glidden, L. M., Billings, F. J., & Jobe, B. M. (2006). Personality, coping style and well-being of parents rearing children with developmental disabilities. *Journal of Intellectual Disability Research, 50*(12), 949–962.

Goodman, S. H., & Gotlib, I. H. (2002). *Children of depressed parents*. Washington, DC: American Psychology Association.

Gosch, A. (2001). Maternal stress among mothers of children with Williams-Beuren syndrome, Down's syndrome and mental retardation of non-syndromal etiology in comparison to mothers of non-disabled children. *Zeitschrift für Kinder- und Jugendpsychiatrie und Psychotherapie, 29*, 285–295.

Greenberg, J. S., Seltzer, M. M., Krauss, M. W., Chou, R., & Hong, J. H. (2004). The effect of quality of the relationships between mothers and adult children with schizophrenia, autism, or Down syndrome on maternal well-being: The mediating role of optimism. *American Journal of Orthopsychiatry, 74*, 14–25.

Greenberg, M. T., Speltz, L., & DeKlyen, M. (1993). The role of attachment in the early development of disruptive behavior problems. *Development and Psychopathology, 5*, 191–213.

Hall, S., Bobrow, M., & Marteau, T. M. (2000). Psychological consequences for parents of false negative results on prenatal screening for Down's syndrome: Retrospective interview study. *British Medical Journal, 320,* 407–412.

Harris, N. G. S., Bellugi, U., Bates, E., Jones, W., & Rossen, M. (1997). Contrasting profiles of language development in children with Williams and Down's syndromes. *Developmental Neuropsychology, 13,* 345–370.

Hauser-Cram, P., Warfield, M. E., Shonkoff, J. P., Krauss, M. W., Upshur, C. C., & Sayer, A. (1999). Family influences on adaptive development in young children with Down syndrome. *Child Development, 70,* 979–989.

Heller, T., & Caldwell, J. (2005). Impact of a consumer-directed family support program on reduced out-of-home institutional placement. *Journal of Policy and Practice in Intellectual Disabilities, 2,* 63–65.

Heller, T., Markwardt, R., Rowitz, L., & Farber, B. (1994). Adaptation of Hispanic families to a member with mental-retardation. *American Journal on Mental Retardation, 99,* 289–300.

Huws, J., Jones, R. S., & Ingledew, D. K. (2001). Parents of children with Autism using an Email group: A grounded theory study. *Journal of Health Psychology, 6,* 569–584

Hodapp, R. M. (2002). Parenting children with mental retardation. In M. H. Bornstein (Ed.), *Handbook of parenting* Vol. 1 (2nd ed., pp. 355–382). Mahwah, NJ: Lawrence Erlbaum.

Hodapp, R. M., Dykens, E. M., & Masino, L. L. (1997). Families of children with Prader-Willi syndrome: Stress-support and relations to child characteristics. *Journal of Autism and Developmental Disorders, 27,* 11–24.

Hodapp, R. M., Ly, T. M., Fidler, D. E., & Ricci, L. A. (2001). Less stress, more rewarding: Parenting children with Down syndrome. *Parenting: Science and Practice, 1,* 317–337.

Hodapp, R. M., Ricci, L. A., Ly, T. M., & Fidler, D. J. (2003). The effects of the child with Down syndrome on maternal stress. *British Journal of Developmental Psychology, 21,* 137–151.

Hodapp, R. M., Wijma, C. A., & Masino, L. L. (1997). Families of children with 5p-(cri du chat) syndrome: Familial stress and sibling reactions. *Developmental Medicine and Child Neurology, 39,* 757–761.

Holroyd, J., & MacArthur, D. (1976). Mental retardation and stress on parents: A contrast between Down's syndrome and childhood autism. *American Journal of Mental Deficiency, 80,* 431–436.

Hornby, G. (1995). Fathers' views of the effects on their families of children with Down syndrome. *Journal of Child and Family Studies, 4,* 103–117.

Hyche, J., Bakeman, R., & Adamson, L. (1992). Understanding communicative cues of infants with Down syndrome: Effects of mothers' experience and infants' age. *Journal of Applied Developmental Psychology, 13,* 1–16.

Jones, R. S. P., & Lewis, H. (2000). Debunking the pathological model: The functions of an Internet discussion group. *Down Syndrome Research and Practice, 6,* 126–131.

Kanayama, T. (2003). Ethnographic research on the experience of Japanese elderly people online. *New Media Society, 5,* 267–288.

Kasari, C., & Freeman, S. F. N. (2001). Task-related social behavior in children with Down syndrome. *American Journal on Mental Retardation, 106,* 253–264.

Kasari, C., Freeman, S. F. N, & Bass, W. (2001). Empathy and response to distress in children with Down syndrome. *Journal of Child Psychology and Psychiatry, 44,* 424–431.

Kasari, C., Freeman, S. F. N., & Hughes, M. (2001). Emotion recognition of children with Down syndrome. *American Journal on Mental Retardation, 106,* 59–72.

Kasari, C., Mundy, P., Yirmiya, N., & Sigman, M. (1990). Affect and attention in children with Down syndrome. *American Journal on Mental Retardation, 95,* 55–67.

Kasari, C., & Sigman, M. (1997). Linking parental perceptions to interactions in young children with autism. *Journal of Autism and Developmental Disorders, 27,* 39–57.

Keller, D., & Honig, A. S. (2004). Maternal and paternal stress in families with school-aged children with disabilities. *American Journal of Orthopsychiatry, 74,* 337–348.

Lam, L. W., & Mackenzie, A. E. (2002). Coping with a child with Down syndrome: The experiences of mothers in Hong Kong. *Qualitative Health Research, 12*(2), 223–238.

Lenhard, W., Breitenbach, E., Ebert, H., Schindelhauer-Deutscher, H. J., & Henn, W. (2005). Psychological benefit of diagnostic certainty for mothers of children with disabilities: Lessons from Down syndrome. *American Journal of Medical Genetics Part A, 133,* 170–175.

Lent, R. W. (2004). Toward a unifying theoretical and practical perspective on well-being and psychosocial adjustment. *Journal of Counseling Psychology, 51,* 482–509.

Leonard, H. (2004). How can the Internet help parents of children with rare neurologic disorders? *Journal of Child Neurology, 19,* 902–908.

Levy, D. (1970). The concept of maternal overprotection. In E. J. Anthony, & T. Benedek (Eds.), *Parenthood* (pp.387–409). Boston: Little, Brown.

Lewis, P., Abbeduto, L., Murphy, M., Richmond, E., Giles, N., Bruno, L., et al. (2006). Psychological well-being of mothers of youth with fragile X syndrome: Syndrome specificity and within-syndrome variability. *Journal of Intellectual Disability Research, 50*(12), 894–904.

Luthar, S. S., & Cicchetti, D. (2000). The construct of resilience: Implications for interventions and social policies. *Development and Psychopathology, 12,* 857–885.

Lyons-Ruth, K. (1996). Attachment relationships among children with aggressive behavior problems: The role of disorganized early attachment patterns. *Journal of Consulting and Clinical Psychology, 64,* 64–73.

Mahoney, G., Fors, S., & Wood, S. (1990). Maternal directive behavior revisited. *American Journal on Mental Retardation, 94,* 398–406.

Main, M., & Solomon, J. (1986). Discovery of an insecure-disorganized/disoriented attachment pattern. In T. B. Brazelton, & M. W. Yogman (Eds.), *Affective development in infancy* (pp. 95–124). Norwood, NJ: Ablex.

Mancini, J. A., Bowen, G. L., & Martin, J. A. (2005). Community social organization: A conceptual linchpin in examining families in the context of communities. *Family Relations, 54,* 570–582.

Marfo, K., Dedrick, C., & Barbour, N. (1998). Mother-child interactions and the development of children with mental retardation. In J. Burack, R. Hodapp, & E. Zigler (Eds.), *Handbook of mental retardation and development* (pp.637–668). New York: Cambridge University Press.

Margalit, M. (1994). *Loneliness among children with special needs: Theory, research, coping and intervention.* New York: Springer-Verlag.

Margalit, M., Al-Yagon, M., & Kleitman, T. (2006). Family subtyping and early intervention. *Journal of Policy and Practice in Intellectual Disabilities, 3,* 33–41.

Margalit, M., & Ankonina, D. B. (1991). Positive and negative affect in parenting disabled children. *Counseling Psychology Quarterly, 4*, 289–299.

Margalit, M., Leyser, Y., Ankonina, D. B., & Avraham, Y. (1991). Community support in Israeli kibbutz and city families of disabled children: Family climate and parental coherence. *Journal of Special Education, 24*, 427–440.

Margalit, M., Raviv, A., & Ankonina, D. B (1992). Coping and coherence among parents with disabled children. *Journal of Clinical Child Psychology, 2*, 202–209.

Marsiglio, W., Amato, P., Day, R. D., & Lamb, M. E. (2000). Scholarship on fatherhood in the 1990s and beyond. *Journal of Marriage and the Family, 62*, 1172–1191.

Mash, E. J., & Wolfe, D. A. (2005). Mental retardation. In E. J. Mash, & D. A. Wolfe (Eds.), *Abnormal child psychology* (pp. 254–282). Belmont, CA: Wadsworth.

McCollum, J. A., & Chen, Y. J. (2003). Parent-child interaction when babies have Down syndrome: The perceptions of Taiwanese mothers. *Infants & Young Children, 16*, 22–32.

McCubbin, H., & Patterson, J. (1983). Family transitions: Adaptations to stress. In H. McCubbin, & C. Figley (Eds.), *Stress and the family* Vol.1 (pp.5–25). New York: Brunner Mazel.

McDowell, A. D., Saylor, C. F., Taylor, M. J., Boyce, G. C., & Stokes, S. J. (1995). Ethnicity and parenting stress change during early intervention. *Early Child Development and Care, 111*, 131–140.

Meyers, B. A., & Pueschel, S. M. (1991). Psychiatric disorders in persons with Down syndrome. *Journal of Nervous and Mental Disease, 179*, 609–613.

Miller, J., Leddy, M., Miolo, G., & Sedey, A. (1995). The development of early language skills in children with Down's syndrome. In L. Nadel, & D. Rosenthal (Eds.), *Down's syndrome: Living and learning in the community* (pp. 115–120). New York: Wiley-Liss.

Minnes, P. (1988). Family stress associated with a developmentally handicapped child. *International Review of Research on Mental Retardation, 15*, 195–226.

Olsen, C. L., Cross, P. K., Gensburg, L. J., & Hughes, J. P. (1996). The effects of prenatal diagnosis, population aging, and changing fertility rates on the live birth prevalence of Down syndrome in New York State, 1983–1992. *Prenatal Diagnosis, 16*, 991–1002.

Padeliadu, S. (1998). Time demands and experienced stress in Greek mothers of children with Down's syndrome. *Journal of Intellectual Disability Research, 42*, 144–153.

Parke, D. R. (2004). Development in the family. *Annual Review of Psychology, 55*, 365–399.

Patterson, J. M. (2002). Understanding family resilience. *Journal of Clinical Psychology, 58*, 233–246.

Ricci, L. A., & Hodapp, R. M. (2003). Fathers of children with Down's syndrome versus other types of intellectual disability: Perceptions, stress and involvement. *Journal of Intellectual Disability Research, 47*, 273–284.

Richardson, G. E. (2002). The metatheory of resilience and resiliency. *Journal of Clinical Psychology, 58*, 307–321.

Roach, M. A., Orsmond, G. I., & Barratt, M. S. (1999). Mothers and fathers of children with Down syndrome: Parental stress and involvement in childcare. *American Journal on Mental Retardation, 104*, 422–436.

Rogers-Dulan, J. (1998). Religious connectedness among urban African American families who have a child with disabilities. *Mental Retardation, 36*, 91–103.

Roizen, N. J., & Patterson, D. (2003). Down's syndrome. *Lancet, 361*, 1281–1289.

Rosner, B. A., Hodapp, R. M., Fidler, D. J., Sagun, J. N., & Dykens, E. M. (2004). Social competence in persons with Prader-Willi, Williams and Down's syndromes. *Journal of Applied Research in Intellectual Disabilities, 17*, 209–217.

Saloviita, T., Italinna, M., & Leinonen, E. (2003). Explaining the parental stress of fathers and mothers caring for a child with intellectual disability: A double ABCX model. *Journal of Intellectual Disability Research, 47*, 300–312.

Sanders, J. L., & Morgan, S. B (1997). Family stress and adjustment as perceived by parents of children with autism or Down syndrome: Implications for intervention. *Child and Family Behavior Therapy, 19*, 15–32.

Sarkadi, A., & Bremberg, S. (2005). Socially unbiased parenting support on the Internet: A cross-sectional study of users of a large Swedish parenting website. *Child: Care, Health and Development, 31*, 43–52.

Scharer, K. (2005). Internet social support for parents: The state of science. *Journal of Child and Adolescent Psychiatric Nursing, 18*, 26–35.

Scott, B. S., Atkinson, L., Minton, H. L., & Bowman, T. (1997). Psychological distress of parents of infant with Down syndrome. *American Journal of Mental Retardation, 102*, 161–171.

Seltzer, M., Krauss, M. W., & Tsunematsu, N. (1993). Adults with Down syndrome and their aging mothers: Diagnostic group differences. *American Journal on Mental Retardation, 97*, 496–508.

Seltzer, M. M., Abbeduto, L., Krauss, M. W., Greenberg, J., & Swe, A. (2004). Comparison groups in autism family research: Down syndrome, Fragile X syndrome, and schizophrenia *Journal of Autism and Developmental Disorders, 34*, 41–48.

Seltzer, M. M., Frank J. Floyd, P., Greenberg, J. S., & Hong, J. (2004). Accommodative coping and well-being of midlife parents of children with mental health problems for developmental disabilities. *American Journal of Orthopsychiatry, 74*, 187–195.

Siklos, S., & Kerns, K. A. (2006). Assessing need for social support in parents of children with autism and Down syndrome. *Journal of Autism and Developmental Disorders, 36*, 921–933.

Skotko, B. G. (2005). Prenatally diagnosed Down syndrome: Mothers who continued their pregnancies evaluate their health care providers. *American Journal of Obstetrics and Gynecology, 192*, 670–677.

Snyder, C. R. (2002). Hope theory: Rainbow in the mind. *Psychological Inquiry, 13*(4), 249–275.

Sorce, J., & Emde, R. (1982). The meaning of infant emotion and expressions: Regularities in caregiving responses of normal and Down's syndrome infants. *Journal of Child Psychology and Psychiatry, 23*, 145–158.

Sroufe, L. A. (1983). Infant-caregiver attachment and patterns of adaptation in preschool: The roots of maladaption and competence. In M. Perlmutter (Ed.), *Minnesota symposium in child psychology* Vol. 16 (pp. 41–81). Hillsdale, NJ: Erlbaum.

Sullivan, A. (2002). Gender differences in coping strategies of parents of children with Down syndrome. *Down Syndrome Research and Practice, 8*, 67–73.

Svanberg, P. O. G. (1998). Attachment, resilience, and prevention. *Journal of Mental Health, 7*, 543–578.

Tannock, R. (1988). Mothers' directiveness in their interactions with children with and without Down syndrome. *American Journal on Mental Retardation, 93*, 154–165.

Thompson, R. A. (1999). Early attachment and later development. In J. Cassidy, & P. R. Shaver (Eds.), *Handbook of attachment: Theory, research, and clinical applications* (pp. 265–286). New York: Guilford Press.

Thompson, R., Cicchetti, D., Lamb, M., & Malkin, C. (1985). The emotional responses of Down syndrome and normal infants in the strange situation: The organization of affective behavior in infants. *Developmental Psychology, 21*, 828–841.

Tingey, C., Mortensen, L., Matheson, P., & Doret, W. (1991). Developmental attainment of infants and young children with Down syndrome. *International Journal of Disability, Development and Education, 38*, 15–26.

Turnbull, A. P., Patterson, J. M., Behr, S. K., Murphy, D. L., Marquis, J. G., & Blue-Banning, M. J. (Eds.) (1993). *Cognitive coping, families, and disability.* Baltimore: Brookes.

van Bakel, H. J., & Riksen-Walraven, J. M. (2002). Parenting and development of one-year-olds: Links with parental, contextual, and child characteristics. *Child Development, 73*, 256–273.

van IJzendoorn, M., Goldberg, S., Kroonenberg, P. M., & Frenkel, O. J. (1992). The relative effects of maternal and child problems on quality of attachment: A meta-analysis of attachment in clinical samples. *Child Development, 63*, 840–858.

van IJzendoorn, M., & Kroonenberg, P. M. (1988). Cross-cultural patterns of attachment: A meta-analysis of the strange situation. *Child Development, 59*, 147–156.

Van Riper, M. (1999). Maternal perceptions of family-provider relationships and well-being in families of children with Down syndrome. *Research in Nursing & Health, 22*, 357–368.

Van Riper, M. (2003). A change of plans: The birth of a child with Down syndrome doesn't have to be a negative experience. *American Journal of Nursing, 103*, 71–74.

Vaughn, B., Goldberg, S., Atkinson, L., Marcovitch, S., MacGregor, D., & Seifer, R. (1994). Quality of toddler-mother attachment in children with Down syndrome: Limits to interpretation of strange situation behavior. *Child Development, 65*, 95–108.

Wallander, J., Pitt, L. C., & Mellins, C. A. (1990). Child functional independence and maternal psychosocial stress as risk factors threatening adaptation in mothers of physically or sensorially handicapped children. *Journal of Consulting and Clinical Psychology, 58*, 818–824.

Wapner, R., Thorn, E., Simpson, J. L., Pergament, E., Silver, R., Filkins, K., et al. (2003). First- trimester screening for trisomies 21 and 18. *New England Journal of Medicine, 349*, 1405–1413.

Waters, E., & Cummings, E. M. (2000). A secure base from which to explore close relationships. *Child Development, 71*, 164–172.

Wayne, D. O., & Krishnagiri, S. (2005). Parents' leisure: The impact of raising a child with Down syndrome. *Occupational Therapy International, 12*, 180–194.

Webster-Stratton, C. (1990). Stress: A potential disrupter of parent perceptions and family interactions. *Journal of Clinical Child Psychology, 4*, 302–312.

Werner, E. E. (1993). Risk, resilience, and recovery: Perspectives from the Kauai longitudinal study. *Development and Psychopathology, 5*, 503–515.

Wishart, J. G., & Johnston, F. H. (1990). The effects of experience on attribution of a stereotyped personality of children with Down's syndrome. *Journal of Mental Deficiency Research, 34*, 409–420.

Wolf, L. C., Noh, S. Fisman, S. N. & Speechley, M. (1989). Psychological effects of parenting stress on parents of autistic children. *Journal of Autism and Developmental Disorders, 19*, 157–166.

Zahn-Waxler, C., Duggal, S., & Gruber, R. (2002). Parental psychopathology. In M. H. Bornstein (Ed.), *Handbook of parenting* Vol. 4 (2nd ed., pp. 295–327). Mahwah, NJ: Lawrence Erlbaum.

Zaidman-Zait, A., & Jamieson, J. R. (2007). Providing web-based support for families of infants and young children with established disabilities. *Infants & Young Children, 20*, 11–25.

Zigman, W. B., Seltzer, G. B., & Silverman, W. P. (1994). Behavioral and mental health changes associated with aging in adults with mental retardation. In M. M. Seltzer, M. W. Krauss, & M. P. Janicki (Eds.), *Life course perspectives on adulthood and old age* (pp. 67–92). Washington, DC: American Association on Mental Retardation.

Child Eliciting Effects in Families of Children with Intellectual Disability: Proximal and Distal Perspectives

Deborah J. Fidler

Abstract

This chapter describes two potential frameworks for examining child effects in families of children with intellectual disability. The first framework is an etiology-specific framework, which is rooted in Hodapp's (1997) notion of direct and indirect effects in families of children with intellectual disability (ID) of different etiologies. This approach offers a proximal account of how a specific child factor—child diagnosis—can be linked to patterns of parent and family functioning. The second framework places the child effects phenomenon within a bio-anthropological paradigm. This paradigm offers a more distal account of child eliciting factors in children with disabilities, and takes into account evolutionary influences on parent–child relationships.

Keywords: Child eliciting effects, intellectual disability, families, etiology, parent–child relationship

A great deal of evidence suggests that raising a child with intellectual disability (ID) has an impact on family functioning that is not observed in families of children without disabilities.

These effects can be adverse, in the form of social isolation (Birenbaum, 1970), sibling role tensions (Farber & Kirk, 1959), parent depression (Cummings, Bayley, & Rie, 1966), and neurotic-like constriction (Cummings, 1976). Parents have been described as grieving over the loss of the "ideal child" for which they had been prepared (Drotar, Baskiewicz, Irvin, Kennel, & Klaus, 1975; Solnit & Stark, 1961), and have been thought to move through stages of denial, emotional disorganization (depression, blame, anger), and emotional reorganization (realistic acceptance of situation; see Blacher, 1984).

Other effects on families of children with disabilities have been shown to take more positive forms. Recent studies have acknowledged the stresses and strains associated with this experience, but they also explore the ways in which parents enjoy and are rewarded by raising their child with disabilities (Hastings & Taunt, 2002; Van Riper,

Ryff & Pridham, 1992; Yau & Li-Tsang, 1999). Grant et al. (1998) note that "[t]he co-existence of stresses and rewards can be viewed as 'push–pull' factors which create tensions for caregivers in everyday life: the very circumstances which generate problems may also create moments or enduring periods of gratification" (p. 59). Wikler, Wasow, and Hatfield (1983) found that, although the majority of families in their study also reported that they experienced chronic sorrow related to raising a child with disabilities, 75% of parents also reported that the experience made them stronger. One parent noted that her family "hit many peaks and valleys. I would say that there is some sorrow, but our happy moments over-shadow the sad time, our daughter has been a joy and a sorrow" (p. 314).

Thus, at present, there is a great deal of evidence that raising children with disabilities elicits specific positive and negative responses in families that are not observed in families of children without disabilities. Yet, there are also studies that report findings of "no differences" between families of children with and without disabilities. "No differences" outcomes have been observed in parents of children with developmental disabilities and comparison groups for self-esteem (Harris & McHale, 1989), depression (Gowen, Johnson-Martin, Goldman, & Appelbaum, 1989; Harris & McHale, 1989), overall family functioning (Dyson, 1993; Trute, 1990), and self-perceived parenting competence (Gowen et al., 1989). These studies suggest that, under some conditions, children with disabilities do not seem to have as pronounced an impact on family outcomes. Given the somewhat mixed evidence for the effects of children with disabilities on families, it is unclear whether and under which circumstances children with disabilities elicit specific reactions from parents, and the nature of those responses.

This chapter includes a description of two potential frameworks for examining child effects in families of children with ID. The first framework is an etiology specific framework, which is rooted in Hodapp's (1997) notion of direct and indirect effects in families of children ID of different etiologies. This approach will offer a proximal account of how a specific child factor—child diagnosis—can be linked to patterns of parent and family functioning. The second framework places the child effects phenomenon within a bio-anthropological paradigm. This paradigm will offer a more distal account of child eliciting factors in children with disabilities, and will take into account evolutionary influences on parent–child relationships.

Child Eliciting Effects: A Brief History

The study of child eliciting characteristics is rooted in Richard Q. Bell's (1968) work on "reinterpreting the direction of effects" in parent–child relationships, which challenged the assumption that the parent–child relationship only had one direction of influence. Around the same time that Bell examined this topic, Lawrence Harper similarly began to criticize the unidirectional view of parent–child relationships that pervaded most child development research. Harper (1975) observed that, at that time, the main focus of research on parent–child relationships concerned the way that "every aspect of the child's functioning is affected by the behavior of the caregiver" (p.784). Both Bell and Harper were critiquing the same phenomenon, in which approaches in research on normative child development seemed to focus only on one direction of influence—the influence of the environment on the child.

According to Bell (1968) and Harper (1975), children are not simply recipients of the influence of family and environment. Instead, children actively interact with their environments and often exert strong influences on others, eliciting specific parenting responses that are associated with their behaviors and personalities. Subsequent decades of child development research adopted more "transactional" approaches to the interaction between child and environment (Sameroff & Chandler, 1975), and the effects of children on their parents have been incorporated into larger models of parenting behavior (Belsky, 1984).

The approaches of Bell and Harper helped shape research on families of children with ID over the past several decades. Children with ID show greater complexity in their profiles beyond simple delays in development. In addition to a delayed timetable for reaching developmental milestones, many children with ID show maladaptive behaviors, uneven learning profiles, and atypical socioemotional functioning. The presence of these non-normative outcomes brings into focus the role that the child plays in eliciting parental responses. In a way, the special case of children with ID may make it possible to explore dynamics that may be more invisible in typical parent–child dyads. Indeed, Glidden (2002) notes that this child effects model took hold more quickly in research on families of children with disabilities than in research on families of typically developing children.

Yet, within this child effects framework, the identification of outcomes linked consistently to specific child characteristics has been elusive. In some cases, such as maladaptive behavior, clear evidence of a link between child behavior and parental response can be identified (Baker, Blacher, Crnic, & Edelbrock, 2002; Floyd & Gallagher, 1997; Hayden & Goldman, 1996; Stores, Stores, Fellows, & Buckley, 1998). In other cases, such as child gender (Frey, Greenberg, & Fewell, 1989; Trute, 1990) and severity of impairment (Hanson & Hanline, 1990; McKinney & Peterson, 1987; Haldy & Hanzlik, 1990; Bristol, Gallagher, & Schopler, 1988; Kazak & Clark, 1986), this link is less observable, suggesting a need for a more systematic framework from which to generate better hypotheses regarding child effects in families of children with ID.

Proximal Framework: Etiology-specific Effects on Families

Among the most important factors that impact a child's developmental trajectory is the cause, or the etiology, of a child's ID. There is now substantial evidence that different genetic disorders predispose children to specific profiles of strength and weakness throughout their development (Dykens, 1995; Dykens, Hodapp, & Finucane, 2000; Hodapp, 1997). These profiles, or behavioral phenotypes, can involve a wide range of areas of behavior, including cognition, language, social-emotional functioning, motor development, and psychopathology (see Dykens et al., 2000). The discovery of these profiles has led some to question whether phenotypic outcomes have implications for family outcomes as well. Hodapp (1997) argued that syndrome-specific profiles indirectly affect families in specific ways. Within this framework, genetic disorders not only predispose children to particular behavioral outcomes or behavioral phenotypes, but they also indirectly predispose children to elicit certain perceptions, reactions, and responses from others.

Etiology-related Findings: Phenotypic Characteristics

The overall nature of a child's disability, for example the presence of cognitive impairment versus the presence of motor impairment, has specific implications for families. In one study, when parenting stress (as measured by the Questionnaire on Resources and Stress [QRS]) was compared in families of children with fragile X syndrome (FXS), families of children with spinal muscular atrophy, and a control group of families of children without disabilities, significantly higher rates of Child Characteristic-related stress and Total stress were observed in the FXS group than in the other groups (von Gontard et al., 2002). This suggests that the factors associated with a developmental disability such as FXS elicit greater family stress than do the factors associated with a motor impairment such as spinal muscular atrophy. Additional comparisons of family coping (using the F-COPES) in this study demonstrated that families of children with FXS reported significantly greater difficulty mobilizing their families to acquire and accept help.

In addition to broad distinctions between families of children with different areas of impairment, differences in family outcome are also observed between groups of children who share the status of having a disability that impairs behavioral development, but who fall into different diagnostic categories. Holroyd and McArthur (1976) found that parents of children with autism, a pervasive developmental disorder, reported significantly higher levels of stress (measured by the QRS) than did families of children with Down syndrome (DS), a genetic disorder, and families of children with of a nonspecific psychiatric clinic control group.

Specifically, mothers of children with autism were more upset and disappointed by their child, more aware of their child's inadequacies, worried about family integration, and more concerned about vocational issues. Several other studies have also found worse outcomes for families of children with autism than for other disability groups (Donovan, 1988; Dumas, Wolf, Fisman, & Culligan, 1991; Olsson & Hwang, 2001; Sander & Morgan, 1997).

But, beyond the general distinctions between cognitive and motor impairments, or between pervasive developmental disorders and genetic disorders, Hodapp's (1997) model suggests that children with different types of genetic disorders may elicit different parental responses and family stress profiles. In one study, when stress in families of children with DS, Williams syndrome, and Smith-Magenis syndrome were compared using the QRS-F, between-etiology differences were observed for parent and family problems and parental pessimism, with lower levels reported in the DS group (Fidler, Hodapp, & Dykens, 2000). Between-group differences were observed in another study comparing families of children with DS and FXS (both with and without autism; Lewis et al., 2007). Specifically, higher rates of pessimism as measured by the QRS Pessimism scale were observed in both FXS groups when compared with the mothers of children with DS. In another cross-syndrome study that compared Parenting Stress Inventory scores, Sarimski (1997) found that overall rates of stress were elevated in all three syndrome groups studied. However, higher rates of depression were reported in the Prader-Willi syndrome (PWS) group and the Williams syndrome group than in the FXS group (Sarimski, 1997).

Down Syndrome "Advantage"

Although additional work is needed to characterize these cross-syndrome comparisons, one set of findings has been reported consistently since the earliest studies of stress in families of children with disabilities. Numerous studies have shown that parents of children with DS show more optimal outcomes than do families of children with other types of disabilities (Fidler et al., 2000; Kasari & Sigman, 1997; Mink, Myers, & Nihira, 1984; Noh, Dumas, Wolf, & Fisman, 1989; Seltzer, Krauss, & Tsunematsu, 1993; Stoneman, 2007). This finding has been demonstrated when families of children with DS are compared to other groups using a variety of measures, including various versions of the QRS (Fidler et al., 2000; Holroyd & McArthur, 1976;

Sanders & Morgan, 1997; Seltzer et al., 1993), the Parenting Stress Inventory (Most, Fidler, Booth-LaForce, & Kelley, 2006; Hanson & Hanline, 1990; Kasari & Sigman, 1997), and the Beck Depression Inventory (Scott, Atkinson, Minton, & Bowman, 1997). The phenomenon is also observed when families of children with DS are compared to families of children with many different types of disabilities, including idiopathic IDs (Kasari & Sigman, 1997; Hodapp, Ricci, Ly, & Fidler, 2003; Olsson & Hwang, 2003), children with other genetic disorders (Fidler et al., 2000), and autism (Holroyd & McArthur, 1976; Kasari & Sigman, 1997). Over time, this phenomenon has been referred to as the "DS advantage" (Stoneman, 2007) and has been the topic of much discussion and debate.

The "DS advantage" is not just measured in terms of the lower levels of negative affect or family stress, but it has also been observed in terms of the presence of positive experiences reported as well (Hodapp, Ly, Fidler, & Ricci, 2001). For example, several studies have demonstrated that parents of children with DS report equal or higher levels of *rewardingness* (in the form of lower levels of "rewardingness stress" on the PSI) when compared with families of typically developing children (Noh et al., 1989; Roach, Orsmond, & Barratt (1999). Another study has demonstrated that mothers of children with DS report higher scores on the Maternal Gratification Scale when compared to mothers of children with autism (Hoppes & Harris, 1990).

The source of this "DS advantage" is the subject of debate. Some hypothesize that children with DS may elicit less stress and more rewardingness from their parents because of specific phenotypic features associated with the disorder. Candidate features that have been proposed include personality characteristics (Hodapp et al., 2001), lower levels of maladaptive behavior (Dykens & Kasari, 1997), perceived immaturity (Fidler & Hodapp, 1999; Fidler 2003), and temperament (Stoneman, 2007). However, others argue that demographic characteristics, rather than child characteristics, are likely to account for much of the well-being reported in parents of children with DS (Cahill & Glidden, 1996; Stoneman, 2007). Because parents of children with DS tend to be older, it may be that demographic dimensions, such as income and other resources, may serve as a protective factor for these families. This suggestion is in line with reports of associations in the literature between parenting, mental health dimensions, and income in families of children with disabilities (Emerson, 2003). In two studies in

which demographic differences, such as income, were controlled for, the "DS advantage" was no longer observable (Cahill & Glidden, 1996; Stoneman, 2007).

Child Psychopathology

A closer examination of the pattern of associations in family stress studies suggests that certain child behaviors that are associated with these disorders may account for large percentages of the stress observed. In two studies of genetic syndromes with clinically high levels of maladaptive behavior, PWS (Hodapp, Dykens, & Masino, 1997), and 5p syndrome (Hodapp, Wijma. & Masino, 1997), the strongest predictor of family stress was the child's score on the Achenbach's Child Behavior Checklist, a measure of child maladaptive behavior. Specifically, Hodapp et al. (1997) found that families of children with PWS report higher levels of parent and family problems as measured by the QRS-F when compared to published reports of stress levels in families of children with ID of mixed etiology. Child psychopathology (as measured by the Total CBCL score) was the only statistically significant predictor of total stress on the QRS-F, even when child body mass index, IQ, and age were entered into the equation. In addition, the "other problems" domain of the CBCL, which contains items particularly relevant to PWS, such as skin-picking and hoarding, was strongly associated with all dimensions of stress.

In another study of mothers of children with FXS, child psychopathology (as measured by total CBCL score and/or the SCL-90-R) predicted Isolation stress, Competence stress, Acceptability stress, and Parenting stress domains. Similarly, using structural equation modeling, Hall, Burns, and Reiss (2007) demonstrated that child behavior problems were associated with increases in maternal distress in families of children with FXS. Child IQ effects in this study were mediated by the relationship between IQ and behavior problems.

Other Comparisons

As our understanding of the genetic underpinnings of specific disorders advances, new questions are beginning to emerge regarding family outcomes in different disorders. In a study that examined dimensions such as depression, loss of control, uncertainty about the future, and coping in parents of children with PWS and Angelman syndrome (AS), important syndrome-related differences were observed (van den Borne et al., 1999). Both PWS and AS are linked to a deletion on the long arm of chromosome 15, but because they are imprinting disorders (involving either the maternally or the paternally derived chromosome 15), they lead to very different phenotypic profiles. Children with AS are known to be quite impaired cognitive, linguistic, and motorically, whereas individuals with PWS show mild or borderline cognitive impairments amid a profile of obsessive-compulsive behaviors and hyperphagia.

In this study, parents of children with AS experienced a higher level of loss of control and were more likely to report that they were not able to handle their responsibilities as they were before their child with disabilities was born. In addition, parents of children with AS showed a pattern of increased concern regarding negative consequences for themselves, whereas parents of children with PWS showed a pattern of concern regarding the psychosocial issues facing their child.

Etiology-related Findings: Nonphenotypic Factors

In addition to the behavioral profiles associated with specific disorders, it may be important to consider an additional set of factors that surround a child's diagnosis of a particular genetic disorder in eliciting responses from families (see Seltzer, Abbeduto, Krauss, Greenberg, & Swe, 2004, for a discussion). Issues such as time-to-diagnosis, practitioner familiarity with the diagnosis, maternal risk associated with age, heritability of the diagnosis, and other family demographic factors are known to vary by syndrome group (Seltzer et al., 2004). These factors, beyond the direct impact of the syndrome on a child's developmental trajectory, may also play a role in the responses parents show in relation to their child's disability.

Time-to-diagnosis is a factor that may play a large role in the family experience during the early years of a child's life. Some disorders, such as DS, spina bifida, phenylketonuria (PKU), and thyroid-related IDs are routinely screened for prenatally or immediately after birth (American Academy of Pediatrics et al., 2000; Koch, 1999). As a result, families receiving routine prenatal care are most likely to receive the diagnosis of DS as early as the first trimester of pregnancy, through the use of the latest technology such as nuchal translucency screening and/or chorionic villi sampling (Malone et al., 2005; Wapner et al., 2003). Van Riper (1999) described that, for some families of children with DS in their sample, the prenatal diagnosis process allowed them a period of adjustment in which they could experience a "chance to grieve" (p. 3) and prepare themselves for the arrival of their child with DS in a positive way.

In contrast, many other genetic disorders are not a part of routine screening procedures, and thus families often undergo a process of uncertainty during the early years of their child's life (Huang, Sadler, O'Riordan, & Robin, 2002). In particular, families may begin to suspect an atypical pattern of development in their child as early as the second half of the first year of life (Bailey, Skinner, Hatton, & Roberts, 2000; Carmichael, Pembrey, Turner, & Barnicoat, 1999). For families of children with FXS, for example, Bailey et al. (2000) reported that concerns regarding development began on average at age 9 months, whereas the mean age of diagnosis in their sample was 35 months. This leaves a substantial period of uncertainty for parents, who may receive a range of different diagnoses for their child before finally arriving at the correct genetic diagnosis. Poehlmann et al. (2005) found that over half of the children with FXS in their sample had received one or more previous diagnoses, including seizure disorder, anxiety disorder, autism, speech/language disorder, and learning disability.

Such a period of uncertainty may have far-ranging impact on family stress, as well as a parent's ability to plan effectively for current and future educational and related child needs. There is evidence that time to diagnosis rates are becoming shorter (Carmichael et al., 1999), especially with the advent of techniques such as DNA microarray analysis (Ward, 2005). Yet, these factors may continue to be important as there will likely remain a distinction between families of children who receive prenatal diagnoses and those families who identify a delayed pattern of development and search for a diagnosis in the first year or two of life.

Etiology group also seems to influence the types of attributions of blame that parents make about the causes of their child's disability. Parents of children with DS are likely to attribute their child's outcome to a genetic fluke, and parents of children with nonspecific etiologies for their developmental disabilities identify possible causes such as pregnancy stress and other related issues, whereas parents of children with autism attribute their child's outcome to an interaction between genes and environment (Mickelson, Wroble, & Helgeson, 1999). In cases such as X-linked disorders, in which a syndrome is known to be heritable and one parent is known to be a carrier of the disorder, higher rates of guilt have been reported in parents when considering their child's condition (Kay & Kingston, 2002). Syndrome heritability can also impact decisions regarding future pregnancies within a nuclear family, as well as members of the extended family, who may or may not be willing to engage in the testing process (Bailey, Skinner, & Sparkman, 2003).

Summary

The literature on outcomes in specific syndrome groups presented in this section provides evidence that factors such as child maladaptive behavior and time-to-diagnosis may play a role in shaping the experiences reported by families. Although taking an etiology-specific approach has furthered the field of study in families of children with disabilities and its clinical implications, some limitations remain with taking a proximal approach to interpreting family responses to children with disabilities. The etiology-specific approach does not provide a comprehensive, unifying account of why parenting a child with disabilities might elicit the psychological and emotional responses that have been reported. In the following section, we turn our attention to a more distal account of parenting children with ID by examining recent theory in field of bio-anthropology. Within this framework, it might be possible to generate a new set of hypotheses regarding the specific child characteristics that are likely to play a role in eliciting different parenting responses in families of children with ID.

Distal Framework
Bio-Anthropological Approaches and Parenting Children with Disabilities

The study of evolutionary influences on parenting and child development has been of interest since the strongly influential works of John Bowlby (1969), Robert Hinde (1987), and Nicholas Blurton Jones (1972). Over the past decade, there has been a renewed movement toward understanding evolutionary influences on child development in general, and parenting in particular, in the growing fields of evolutionary psychology, biological anthropology, and human behavioral ecology. David Bjorklund and his colleagues have begun to develop a new line of research on *evolutionary developmental psychology* (Bjorklund & Pellegrini, 2002), an exploration of "evolutionary and biological influences on human development . . . and the social and ecological conditions that will necessarily affect the development and expression of social and cognitive competencies" (Geary & Bjorklund, 2000, p. 63).

Although not limited to mammals, parenting behavior is a hallmark feature of mammals, and across many mammalian species, a variety of parenting strategies can be observed (Stern, 1997). It has long been hypothesized that natural selection favors parenting behaviors that covary with offspring survival and reproduction, but only recently has this work been applied to humans (Geary & Flinn, 2001; Price, 1970). Recent theoretical accounts have offered new insights into the role that evolution may have played in shaping parenting behavior in humans (Bjorklund & Pellegrini, 2002).

Of particular note for research on parenting children with ID is the notion of parental investment behavior, and more importantly, differential parental investment (Trivers, 1972). Parental investment theory, a seminal theory first delineated by Trivers (1972), involves hypotheses regarding how parents in a wide range of species devote time, resources, and energy to their dependent offspring (Bjorklund, Yunger, & Pellegrini, 2002). Within this understanding, parents in different species may show different levels of investment in offspring depending on various situational characteristics, such as the availability of resources to the parents to support their parenting behavior (food, shelter, a dependable mate), as well as characteristics in the offspring, such as signs of health and potential reproductive fitness. Bjorklund et al. (2002) explain that, "parents often choose to invest differentially in their offspring, investing the most in those who have the greatest chance of reaching reproductive age and thus carrying forth the parents' genes" (p. 15, Bjorklund et al., 2002). Thus, *differential* parental investment refers to the varying degrees with which parents within a given species invest in their offspring, and the circumstances in which parents may be more or less likely to invest.

Although this approach has the potential to shed light on the issue of parental responses to children with disabilities, it is important to address a common question regarding humans versus other animal species. It seems imaginable that assessments regarding offspring fitness may be made by nonhumans, who do not experience the conscience and morality that seem to be the hallmark of humanity, but questions arise when one considers the applicability of this model for human parenting. Is there evidence for differential parental investment in humans? Although many—if not the majority—of children who have disabilities are lucky to receive the highest quality of caregiving in warm, loving, and nurturing environments, there are alarming statistics regarding vulnerability to abuse and neglect in this population (see Fisher, Hodapp & Dykens, in press; see the following section for a discussion of the "naturalistic fallacy"). In fact, children with ID and other disabilities are up to ten times more likely to be physically abused than their nondisabled counterparts (Daly &Wilson, 1984; Sobsey, 2002). Low estimates place North American children with disabilities at 1.67 to 3.4 times more likely to experienced maltreatment than their nondisabled counterparts (Sobsey & Varnhagen, 1989; Sullivan & Knutson, 2000). European estimates of children and adolescents with disabilities place the relative risk at 7.7 (Verdugo, Bermajo, & Fuertes, 1995). One study of an entire population of children with disabilities receiving school services in Omaha, Nebraska, found that one-quarter of children with ID and/or health impairments had experienced abuse (Sullivan & Knutson, 2000). Types of abuse encountered included physical abuse, neglect, sexual abuse, and emotional abuse. These outcomes may not be represented in the current literature on families of children with disabilities in that caregivers who may show abusive behaviors may be less likely to volunteer their time to become involved in research projects. Thus, much of the empirical literature on families of children with disabilities is likely a "best-case scenario" for family outcomes, because each of the families involved has the time, resources, and motivation necessary to volunteer for research of this sort.

Few bio-anthropological accounts have taken on the topic of parental investment and children with disabilities. A small number of cross-cultural studies demonstrate that patterns of abuse in children with disabilities exist in preindustrialized cultures (Daly & Wilson, 1984). Ethnographic studies using the Human Relation Area File have found that, in 21 of 35 societies studied, infanticide was attributed to the presence of an infant who was "deformed or very ill." In some cases, justification for infanticide is observed in stories about defeating supernatural forces (Daly & Wilson, 1984; Scrimshaw, 1984). Scrimshaw (1984) describes these instances of infanticide as the most extreme manifestation of a termination of parental investment, a process that can be either deliberate or unconscious.

A distinction should be made between parenting behavior that is evolutionarily adaptive and fixed patterns of parenting behavior. Gardiner and Bjorklund (2007) note that parenting adaptations are not specifically hardwired into human adults who become parents. Instead, they are best "thought of as developed strategies that will vary as a function of early experiences and general ecological conditions" (p. 338). Because of the great degree of variability in the environments in which humans live, behavioral flexibility in parenting was likely selected for over the selection of a hardwired species-specific set of parenting behaviors (Gardiner & Bjorklund, 2007). The notion of when certain parenting strategies are recruited, and under which conditions, is of primary interest in this discussion.

Child Characteristics and Parental "Preparedness"

Within parental investment theory lays the notion that human parenting behaviors likely evolved in close connection to certain child eliciting characteristics. Throughout human evolutionary history, certain physical and behavioral features came to signal a typical healthy, viable, immature member of a species—a good investment—and other features came to signal poor health and a greater investment risk for parents. These features can be described in terms of what parents are "prepared" to see in their offspring, thus contributing to the construct of *parental preparedness*. Mann (1992) describes this phenomenon in terms of a "template" or "prototype for normal, healthy infants" that involves expectancies regarding physical and behavioral features in a newborn that may be refined through direct and indirect experiences (p. 373). In his discussion of the critical role of the healthy human infant's predisposition to exhibiting behaviors that promote social relationships, Trevarthen (2001) notes that, "[y]oung humans are adapted to elicit sympathetic action by caregivers who know more and have greater powers of effective action in obtaining benefits and giving protection" (p. 113). But he continues with the point that a great deal of the evolutionary adaptation "is on the parent's side" (p. 113). In other words, child characteristics can only evoke responses when a parenting partner is prepared to recognize those characteristics as salient and is likely to respond to those characteristics in nurturing ways.

Across different mammalian species, there is much evidence that certain prepared parental responses are elicited by specific child characteristics and behaviors, in what Stern (1997) calls "offspring induced nurturance." Maternal responsiveness across species can be impaired by inappropriate, insufficient, or nonreciprocal interactions with her offspring. In rats, for example, tactile and other forms of stimulation from pups impels specific maternal caregiving behaviors (Stern, 1997). If the appropriate tactile, olfactory, and other somatosensory stimuli from pups are not received or sensed by mother, maternal behavioral sequences are truncated. This provides a clear cross-species delineation of the child effects model. If an offspring is not presenting a parent with appropriate types or amounts of certain behaviors or other characteristics, then they may not elicit certain types of parental responses that are typically seen in most parent–child dyads in a given species.

This may be important for researchers interested in studying parent behavior toward children with disabilities, who may deviate from normative child behaviors, physical features, and other characteristics. Consider a 6-month-old human infant. There are certain behavioral features that one expects from that infant, including crying, cooing, babbling, and selective social smiling. There are also certain physical features one expects to observe in that infant, including certain craniofacial proportions, musculature, and size. Deviations from those expectations, for example when a child is born with craniofacial anomalies like cleft lip and palate, may lead to a different set of elicited responses in the parent. In fact, observable differences in parenting behaviors has been reported in parents of children with craniofacial anomalies, including less face-to-face interaction than in parents of children without craniofacial anomalies (Wasserman & Allen, 1985).

Parental Preparedness and Disabilities

But is there evidence that human parents respond differentially to child eliciting characteristics? Findings in the disability literature are scarce, but there is some evidence that certain child characteristics elicit and set into motion parenting behaviors in typically developing children that are not elicited in atypical groups. In a study of 3- to 5-month-old preterm and typical babies and their mothers, Lester, Hoffman, and Brazelton (1985) showed synchrony in behavior cycles between full-term infants and their mothers, with full-term babies showing high levels of dominance in initiating interactions. In contrast, preterm babies had difficulty with self-regulation, and thus showed less coordinated cycles of affect and attention with their mothers. As a result, mothers of preterm infants in this study reported that their infants were "hard to read," and that they could not respond easily to their infants' behavior. In another study, the maternal responses to prematurely born twins were analyzed (Mann, 1992).

In each twin pair, one infant was identified as showing poorer health status than the other. When maternal responses to each twin were analyzed at 8 months, each mother in the study was found to direct more positive nurturing behaviors (holding, soothing, stimulating, giving affection, and vocalizing) toward the infant that was initially designated as healthier (Mann, 1992), a finding reported in another study of low-birth-weight twins as well (Minde, Perrotta, & Corter, 1982). These studies highlight the crucial role of the infant in bringing a coherent repertoire of behaviors to the parent–child relationship, and the differential parenting response based on the absence or presence of those behaviors.

Child eliciting effects can also be observed in retrospective video taped studies of children who are later diagnosed with autism. Trevarthen and Daniel (2005) describe that important intersubjective milestones, such as "a seeking for 'protoconversational' play" at 3–4 months and the development of "cooperative understanding of intentions, interests, and feelings" after 9 months, are reached by typically developing infants throughout the first 2 years of life. They argue that this developmental progression is critical for healthy social, emotional, and cognitive development in typically developing infants. A disruption in the achievement of these intersubjective milestones can have a profound impact not only on a child's development, but on the parenting behaviors and the parent–child dyad.

In one study, video tapes of 11-month-old monozygotic twin sisters were retrospectively coded for parent–child interaction patterns (Trevarthen & Daniel, 2005). One of the twins was later diagnosed with autism, whereas the second continued to show typical development throughout her childhood. When compared with the normative dyadic pattern of the parent and the typically developing infant— which included cycles of attention, anticipation, changes in emotional expression, and shared enjoyment— the dyadic pattern with the infant who was later diagnosed with autism was markedly different. This infant showed attenuated eye contact, no shared attention, no anticipation of the parent's behavior, and no affect sharing (Trevarthen & Daniel, 2005). The authors describe that, with the infant who was later diagnosed with autism, the parent received:

No reinforcement for the interpersonal elements of his behavior, as he does consistently from the developmentally normal twin. The absence of these normal, regulated social rewards affects the father's style of interaction. With the autistic twin, he misses the stages of shared tension and emotional build-up.

He resorts to repeatedly stimulating the infant in an attempt to engage her (S30).

Although this evidence comes from a case study involving only one set of twins, the in-depth analysis reported is suggestive of an important set of child-eliciting effects in infants and young children who are later diagnosed with autism or similar pervasive developmental disorders (or at least those who do not show developmental regression in the second year of life). Trevarthen and Daniel (2005) suggest that the dyadic pattern that is set in motion may be unhelpful for the infant who is later diagnosed with autism and that a different "platform of parental support" should be established to support a healthier development of intersubjective skills in vulnerable infants.

Given these findings, it is therefore not surprising that child eliciting characteristics have been shown to influence a parent's self-esteem and sense of self-competence. In a study of 80 full-term and preterm infants and their mothers, McGrath, Boudykis, and Lester (1993) used the Maternal Self-Report Inventory and found that maternal self-esteem was correlated with infant health status, as well as with infant autonomic stability, self-regulation, and non-fussiness. In children with poor health status as operationalized by these qualities, such as preterm infants, mothers showed lower levels of self-esteem. The authors concluded that the delivery of a healthy, typically functioning infant has an important influence on maternal self-concept, and ultimately on her adjustment and attitude toward her child.

Specific Cues

There is evidence, then, that overall atypical patterns of child behavior and development may elicit specific responses in parents that involve changed parenting behavior and sense of self-competence. But, in addition to studying general atypical patterns of child behavior, a parallel line of research has taken a narrower approach to characterize the impact of specific child behavioral or appearance cues on parenting.

For example, crying behavior is clearly a communicative signal that elicits responses from parents in almost any parent–child dyad. But there is evidence that the acoustic features of crying can be related to infant risk status, and thus, may serve as a direct indicator of health in a young infant. Premature infants, low-birth-weight infants, infants prenatally exposed to illicit drugs, and infants with intrauterine growth retardation have all been shown to demonstrate atypical crying patterns (see Boukydis & Lester, 1998, for a review). Changes in mean fundamental frequency, variability in mean fundamental frequency, shorter cry bursts, and greater frequency of pauses between cry bursts, are among the features that have been demonstrated in these populations (see Boukydis & Lester, 1998, for a review). The impact of these features on parent perception and response may be an example of a specific child cue that elicits parental responses in atypically developing populations. In one study, the acoustics of an infant's cry were strongly related to maternal ratings of infant temperament and emotional reactivity (Huffman et al., 1994). In another study, mothers of colicky infants gave higher perceived sadness ratings than did control mothers at the sound of their infant's cry, and they also rated their colicky infant's cry as more grating to hear (Lester, Boukydis, Garcia-Coll, Hole, & Peuker, 1992). These findings demonstrate that crying behavior can elicit perceptions and responses in parents that may affect their behavior. But there is even evidence for a wider impact of crying behavior on families. In one study, some acoustic features of preterm and full-term infants' crying behaviors were shown to be associated with help-seeking behavior and the elicitation of social support by parents (Boukydis & Lester, 1998).

Maternal responses to constitutional characteristics of their infants can also be found in studies of infant physical appearance. Infants differ in the degree to which they possess certain "attractive" infant-like facial features: fatter cheeks, larger eyes, larger foreheads, or rounder heads. Adults prefer to look at pictures of babies who have these facial characteristics; they also look at them longer, and can reliably rank infants in terms of their attractiveness (Maier, Holmes, Slaymaker, & Reich, 1984). Maier et al. (1984) showed that when compared to preterm infants (who do not usually possess these attractive features due to incomplete gestation), full-term infants are rated as more likable, normal, cute, and attractive. Raters in this study also predicted that attractive full-term babies would eat well, would be fun to be with, would make them happy, and that they would like to take care of and baby-sit the full-term babies more than preterm babies.

Other evidence for child eliciting characteristics and parental preparedness comes from a series of studies performed by Fidler and colleagues examining the effects of the craniofacial appearance of children with DS (Fidler & Hodapp, 1999; Fidler, 2003). Children with DS are known to have a unique craniofacial appearance that shares features commonly associated with infant-like facial dimensions (see Zebrowitz, 1997, for a review), including a lower nasal bridge and lower placement of features on the face. In one study, naïve observers were more likely to rate pictures of children with DS in line with perceptions of youthfulness and immaturity when compared with pictures of typically developing children and children with another genetic disorder (Fidler & Hodapp, 1999). Furthermore, pictures of more physically "baby-faced" children with DS were rated more strongly in accordance with this stereotype, as well (Fidler & Hodapp, 1999). In a follow-up study, Fidler (2003) found that parents of children with DS were more likely to make infant-directed speech voice prosody adjustments in their speech to their children than were parents of other children with developmental disabilities. These two studies suggest that parents and naïve observers may be responding to specific cues that a child with disabilities generates as a result of their disabling condition. It is likely that neither group of participants—neither parents nor naïve observers—had any awareness of these influences, yet the findings support the presence of such patterns of unconscious perceptions and adjustments.

An important caveat must be noted. From an evolutionary perspective, many of the specific cues that were discussed in this section may be reliable indicators of health status and one's likelihood to reproduce, but some may not be. For example, the presence of cleft lip and/or palate may be an observable atypical cue in a child at birth, but such a condition likely has no bearing on overall health and/or reproductive outcomes in adulthood. Thus, it is important to note that not all child factors that elicit parenting behavior do so in ways that maximize parental investment based on child reproductive fitness. In contrast, cues such as the craniofacial appearance in DS may also be similarly misleading, as some individuals with DS are not able to reproduce, but their craniofacial appearance elicits increased parental adjustments in the direction of caregiving for a younger child.

Naturalistic Fallacy

This discussion regarding parenting children with disabilities has aimed to bring into focus the ways in which children with disabilities elicit various responses from parents, which may in turn impact the environment in which they develop and ultimately, their developmental outcomes. However, it is worth noting that discussing these issues from a bio-anthropological or evolutionary perspective has the potential to offend our sense of right and wrong from a moral perspective, especially for those who are interested in improving the lives of children with disabilities. It is important to clarify, then, that this discussion aims only to characterize patterns of parent–child relationship behaviors and identify when they are likely to appear. As Salmon and Shackelford (2007) note, "[m]aking a claim or giving evidence that a behavior has evolved . . . says nothing about how such a behavior should be viewed from a moral stance. In fact, using what *is* to justify what *ought to be* is referred to as the naturalistic fallacy" (p. 3, emphasis added). The preceding discussion, then, is meant to shed greater light on patterns of parenting behavior, but not to recommend that such patterns ought to exist from a moral perspective. Rather, examining parenting behaviors more closely may inform decisions that are made from a moral perspective regarding how to support and provide services for parents of children with disabilities during their most vulnerable periods of time.

Future Directions

The findings presented in this section offer preliminary support for the notion that parenting behavior in families of children with disabilities is shaped by the construct of parental preparedness and child eliciting characteristics. The behavioral and physical cues observed in human infants can signal typicality or atypicality to parents in the earliest stages of development, which may then impact the parent–child relationship in a transactional manner over time. Although the evidence presented in this section is limited to physical and behavioral characteristics in infancy for the most part, it is possible that such features remain at play throughout development, as demonstrated in the studies described involving the craniofacial appearance in DS.

It is also likely that a more rigorous investigation of specific child factors, such as specific primary intersubjective behaviors that emerge between 3 and 6 months in typically developing children, will shed even greater light on the notion of child eliciting characteristics (Trevarthen & Aitken, 2001). The absence or attenuation of emotional signaling and emotional responsivity in infants who are later diagnosed with autism—if these findings hold—may have profound transactional implications on the developing relationship between a caregiver and infant (Trevarthen & Aitken, 2001), and will likely be the subject of greater research attention in prospective studies of early development in autism.

Other behavioral cues, such as the atypical development of eye contact in young children with FXS may also elicit parenting perceptions and responses that signal atypicality as well, and may have critical implications for the quality of parent–child interactions in this population (Lachiewicz, Spiridigliozzi, Gullion, Ransford, & Rao, 1994; Murphy, Abbeduto, Schroeder, & Serlin, 2007).

In addition, when examining the child effects of specific disorders on parenting perceptions and behavior, it may also be important to consider changes in the manifestation of these disorders over time. There is evidence that the expression of behavioral phenotypes is not static across development, and thus, syndrome outcomes may not influence families in monolithic ways throughout the child's entire developmental period (Paterson, Brown, Gsodl, Johson, & Karmiloff-Smith, 1999). As we come to understand how outcomes emerge and change during childhood in specific syndromes, we may be able to identify unique trajectories of stress associated with specific syndromes (Most et al., 2006). In one study, families of young children with DS were found to show lower stress levels at 15 months than were families of children with other developmental disabilities, yet, by 45 months, these families were shown to have equivalent levels of stress (Most, et al., 2006). These changes in stress were found to be closely linked to changes in behavioral functioning in young children with DS in the areas of cognition, language, and maladaptive behavior. Thus, the nature of child eliciting factors may be strongly linked to child chronological age, and therefore, may impact family outcomes differentially as changes in phenotypic expression emerge over time.

Conclusion

As a part of a larger movement toward understanding outcomes in families of children with disabilities, the study of child effects on parents offers a potentially critical contribution to characterizing the complex dynamic that develops between children with disabilities and their caregivers. With continued research into the nature of child eliciting effects, it may be possible to adopt even more sophisticated approaches to studying families of children with ID, including examination of how different syndromes elicit different family responses, and examining how clusters of behavioral strengths and weaknesses tap into the set of parental preparedness responses from a bio-anthropological perspective. These proximal and distal frameworks presented in this chapter have the potential to facilitate new clinical interpretations that deepen our understanding of parenting behaviors and responses beyond our current stress and coping models. Moving forward with these frameworks, we can develop more sophisticated approaches to supporting and improving outcomes for families of children with ID, and ultimately reduce the degree of vulnerability observed in this population.

References

American Academy of Pediatrics Newborn Screening Task Force (2000). Newborn Screening: A blueprint for the future. *Pediatrics, 106 Supplement*, 389–427.

Bailey, D. B., Skinner, D., & Sparkman, K. L. (2003). Discovering fragile X syndrome: Family experiences and perceptions. *Pediatrics, 111*, 407–416.

Bailey, D. B., Skinner, D., Hatton, D., & Roberts, J. (2000). Family experiences and factors associated with the diagnosis of fragile X syndrome. *Journal of Developmental and Behavioral Pediatrics, 21*, 315–321.

Baker, B., Blacher, J., Crnic, K. A., & Edelbrock, C. (2002). Behavior problems and parenting stress in families of three-year-old children with and without developmental delays. *American Journal on Mental Retardation, 107*, 433–444.

Bell, R. Q. (1968). A reinterpretation of the direction of effects in studies of socialization. *Psychological Review, 75*, 81–95.

Belsky, J. (1984). The determinants of parenting: A process model. *Child Development, 55*, 83–96.

Birenbaum, A. (1970). On managing a courtesy stigma. *Journal of Health and Social Behavior, 11*, 196–206.

Bjorklund, D.F. & Pellegrini, A.D. (2002). *The origins of human nature: Evolutionary developmental psychology.* Washington DC: American Psychological Association.

Bjorklund, D. F., Yunger, J. L. & Pellegrini, A. D. (2002). The evolution of parenting and evolutionary approaches to child-drearing. In M. H. Bornstein (Ed.), *Handbook of parenting:* Vol. 2. *Biology and Ecology of Parenting* (pp. 3–30). Mahwah, NJ: Erlbaum.

Blacher, J. (1984). Sequential stages of parental adjustment to the birth of the child with handicaps: Fact or artifact? *Mental Retardation, 22*, 55–68.

Blurton Jones, N. (1972). *Ethological studies of child behavior.* Oxford, UK: Cambridge University Press.

Boukydis, C. F. Z, & Lester, B. M. (1998). Infant crying, risk status and social support in families of preterm and term infants. *Early Development and Parenting, 7*, 31–39.

Bowlby, J. (1969). *Attachment and loss: Attachment.* New York: Basic.

Bristol, M. M., Gallagher, J. J., & Schopler, E. (1988). Mothers and fathers of young developmentally disabled and nondisabled boys: Adaptation and spousal support. *Developmental Psychology, 24*, 441–451.

Cahill, B. M., & Glidden, L. M. (1996). Influence of child diagnosis on family and parental functioning: Down syndrome versus other disabilities. *American Journal on Mental Retardation, 101*, 149–160.

Carmichael, B., Pembrey, M., Turner, G., & Barnicoat, A. (1999). Diagnosis of fragile X syndrome: The experiences of parents. *Journal of Intellectual Disability Research, 43*, 47–53.

Cummings, S. T. (1976). The impact of the child's deficiency on the father: A study of fathers of mentally retarded and of chronically ill children. *American Journal of Orthopsychiatry, 46,* 246–255.

Cummings, S. T., Bayley, H. C. & Rie, H. E. (1966). Effects of the child's deficiency on the mother: A study of mothers of mentally retarded, chronically ill and neurotic children. *American Journal of Orthopsychiatry, 36,* 595–608.

Daly, M., & Wilson, M. I. (1984). A sociobiological analysis of human infanticide. In G. Hausfater, & S. B. Hrdy (Eds.), *Infanticide: Comparative and evolutionary perspectives* (pp. 487–502). New York: Aldine Press.

Donovan, A. M. (1988). Family stress and ways of coping with adolescents who have handicaps: Maternal perceptions. *American Journal on Mental Retardation, 92,* 502–509.

Drotar, D., Baskiewicz, A., Irvin, N., Kennell, J., & Klaus, M. (1975). The adaptation of parents to the birth of an infant with a congenital malformation: A hypothetical model. *Pediatrics, 56,* 710–717.

Dumas, J., Wolf, L. C., Fisman, S. N., & Culligan, A. (1991). Parenting stress, child behavior problems, and dysphoria in parents of children with autism, Down syndrome, behavior disorders, and normal development. *Exceptionality, 2,* 97–110.

Dykens, E. M., Hodapp, R. M., & Finucane, B. M. (2000). *Genetics and mental retardation syndromes: A new look at behavior and interventions.* Baltimore: Paul H. Brookes Publishing.

Dykens, E. M. (1995). Measuring behavioral phenotypes: Provocations from the "New Genetics." *American Journal on Mental Retardation, 99,* 522–532.

Dyson, L. L. (1993). Response to the presence of a child with disabilities: Parental stress and family functioning over time. *American Journal on Mental Retardation, 98,* 207–218.

Emerson, E. (2003). Mothers of children and adolescents with intellectual disability: Social and economic situation, mental health status, and the self-assesses social and psychological impact of the child's difficulties. *Journal of Intellectual Disability Research, 47,* 385–399.

Farber, B., & Kirk, S. A. (1959). Effects of a severely mentally retarded child on family integration. *Monographs of the Society for Research in Child Development, 24,* 1–112.

Fidler, D. J. (2003). Parental vocalization patterns and perceived immaturity in Down syndrome. *American Journal on Mental Retardation, 108,* 425–434.

Fidler, D. J., Hodapp, R. M., & Dykens, E. M. (2000). Stress in families of young children with Down syndrome, Williams syndrome, and Smith-Magenis syndrome. *Early Education and Development, 11,* 395–406.

Fidler, D. J. & Hodapp, R. M. (1999). Craniofacial maturity and perceived personality in Down syndrome. *American Journal of Mental Retardation, 104,* 410–421.

Fisher, M. H., Hodapp, R. M., & Dykens, E. M. (2008). Child abuse among children with disabilities: What we know and what we need to know. *International Review of Research in Mental Retardation, 35,* 251–289.

Floyd, F. J., & Gallagher, E. M. (1997). Parental stress, care demands, and use of support services for school age children with disabilities and behavior problems. *Family Relations, 46,* 359–371.

Frey, K. S., Fewell, R. R., & Vadasy, P. F. (1989). Parental adjustment and changes in child outcome among families of young handicapped children. *Topics in Early Childhood Special Education, 8,* 38–57.

Frey, K.S., Greenberg, M.T., & Frewell, R.R. (1989). Stress and coping among parents of handicapped children: A multidimensional approach. *American Journal on Mental Retardation, 94,* 240–249.

Gardiner, A., & Bjorklund, D. F. (2007). All in the family: An evolutionary developmental perspective. In C. Salmon, & T. K. Shakelford (Eds.), *Family relationships: An evolutionary perspective* (pp. 337–358). New York: Oxford University Press.

Geary, D. C., & Bjorklund, D. F. (2000). Evolutionary developmental psychology. *Child Development, 71,* 57–65.

Geary, D. C., & Flinn, M. V. (2001). Evolution of human parental behavior and the human family. *Parenting: Science and Practice, 1,* 5–61.

Glidden, L. M. (2002). Parenting children with developmental disabilities: A ladder of influence. In J. G. Borkowski, & S. L. Ramey (Eds.), *Parenting and the child's world: Influences on academic, intellectual, and social-emotional development* (pp. 329–233). Mahwah, NJ: Lawrence Erlbaum Associates, Inc.

Gowen, J. W., Johnson-Martin, N., Goldman, B. D., & Appelbaum, M. (1989). Feelings of depression and parenting competence of mothers of handicapped and nonhandicapped infants: A longitudinal study. *American Journal on Mental Retardation, 94,* 259–271.

Grant, G., Ramcharan, P., McGrath, M., Nolan, M., & Keady, J. (1998). Rewards and gratifications among family caregivers: Towards a refined model of caring and coping. *Journal of Intellectual Disability Research, 42,* 58–71.

Haldy, M. B., & Hanzlik, J. R. (1990). A comparison of perceived competence in child-rearing between mothers of children with Down syndrome and mothers of children without delays. *Education and Training in Mental Retardation, 25,* 333–343.

Hall, S. S., Burns, D. D., & Reiss, A. L. (2007). Modeling family dynamics in children with fragile X syndrome. *Journal of Abnormal Psychology, 35,* 29–42.

Hanson, M. J., & Hanline, M. F. (1990). Parenting a child with a disability: A longitudinal study of parental stress and adaptation. *Journal of Early Intervention, 14,* 234–248.

Harper, L. V. (1975). The scope of offspring effects: From caregiver to culture. *Psychological Bulletin, 82,* 784–801.

Harris, V. S., & McHale, S. M. (1989). Family life problems, daily caregiving activities, and the psychological well-being of mothers of mentally retarded children. *American Journal on Mental Retardation, 94,* 231–239.

Hastings, R. P., & Taunt, H. M. (2002). Positive perceptions in families of children with developmental disabilities. *American Journal on Mental Retardation, 107,* 116–127.

Hayden, M. F., & Goldman, J. (1996). Families of adults with mental retardation: Stress levels and need for services. *Social Work, 41,* 657–667.

Hinde, R. A. (1987). *Individuals, relationships, and culture: Links between ethology and the social sciences.* New York: Cambridge University Press.

Hodapp, R. M. (1997). Direct and indirect behavioral effects of different genetic disorders of mental retardation. *American Journal on Mental Retardation, 102,* 67–79.

Hodapp, R. M., Dykens, E. M. & Masino, L. L. (1997). Families of children with Prader-Willi syndrome: Stress-support and relations to child characteristics. *Journal of Autism and Developmental Disorders, 27,* 11–24.

Hodapp, R. M., Fidler, D. J., & Smith, A. C. M. (1998). Stress and coping in families of children with Smith-Magenis syndrome. *Journal of Intellectual Disability Research, 42,* 331–340.

Hodapp, R. M., Ricci, L. A., Ly, T. M., & Fidler, D. J. (2003). The effects of the child with Down syndrome on maternal stress. *British Journal of Developmental Psychology, 21*, 137–151.

Hodapp, R. M., Wijma, C. A., & Masino, L. L. (1997). Families of children with 5- (cri du chat) syndrome: Familial stress and sibling reaction. *Developmental Medicine and Child Neurology, 39*, 757–761.

Holroyd, J., & McArthur, D. (1976). Mental retardation and stress on the parents: A contrast between Down's syndrome and childhood autism. *American Journal on Mental Deficiency, 80*, 431–436.

Holroyd, J., & McArthur, D. (1976). Mental retardation and stress on the parents: A contrast between Down's syndrome and childhood autism. *American Journal on Mental Deficiency, 80*, 431–436.

Hoppes, K., & Harris, S. L. (1990). Perceptions of child attachment and maternal gratification in mothers of children with autism and Down syndrome. *Journal of Clinical Child Psychology, 19*, 365–371.

Huang, L., Sadler, L., O'Riordan, M., & Robin, N. H. (2002). Delay of diagnosis in Williams syndrome. *Clinical Pediatrics, 41*, 257–261.

Huffman, L. C., Bryan, Y. E., Pedersen, F. A., Lester, B. M., Newman, J. D., & Del Carmen, R. (1994). Infant cry acoustics and maternal ratings of temperament. *Infant Behavior and Development, 17*, 45–53.

Kay, E., & Kingston, H. (2002). Feelings associated with being a carrier and characteristics of reproductive decision making in women known to be carriers of X-linked conditions. *Journal of Health Psychology, 7*, 169–181.

Kazak, A. E., & Clark, M. W. (1986). Stress in families of children with myelomeningocele. *Developmental Medicine and Child Neurology, 28*, 220–228.

Koch, R. K. (1999). Issues in newborn screening for phenylketonuria. *American Family Physician, 60*, 1462–1466.

Lachiewicz, A. M., Spiridigliozzi, G. A., Gullion, C.M., Ransford, S. N., & Rao, K. (1994). Aberrant behaviors of young boys with fragile X syndrome. *American Journal on Mental Retardation, 98*, 567–579.

Lester, B. M., Boukydis, C. F. Z, Garcia-Coll, C. T., Hole, W., & Peuker, M. (1992). Infantile colic: Acoustic cry characteristics, maternal perception of cry, and temperament. *Infant Behavior and Development, 15*, 15–26.

Lester, B. M., Hoffman, J., & Brazelton, T. B. (1985). The rhythmic structure of mother-infant interaction in term and preterm infants. *Child Development, 56*, 15–27.

Lewis, P., Abbeduto, L., Murphy, M., Richmond, E., Giles, N., Bruno, L., et al. (2007). Psychological well-being of mothers of youth with fragile X syndrome: Syndrome specificity and within-syndrome variability. *Journal of Intellectual Disability Research, 50*, 894–904.

Maier, R. A., Holmes, D. L., Slaymaker, F. L., & Reich, J. N. (1984). The perceived attractiveness of preterm infants. *Infant Behavior and Development, 7*, 403–414.

Malone, F. D., Canick, J. A., Ball, R. H., Nyberg, D. A., Comstock, C. H., Bukowski, R., et al. (2005). First and second-trimester screening, or both, for Down's syndrome. *New England Journal of Medicine, 353*, 2001–2011.

Mann, J. (1992). Nurturance or negligence: Maternal psychology and behavioral preference among preterm twins. In J. H. Barkow, L. Cosmides, & J. Tooby (Eds.), *The adapted mind: Evolutionary psychology and the generation of culture* (pp. 367–390). New York: Oxford University Press.

McGrath, M., Boudykis, C. F. Z., & Lester, B. M. (1993). Determinants of maternal self-esteem in the neonatal period. *Infant Mental Health Journal, 14*, 35–48.

McKinney, B., & Peterson, R. A. (1987). Predictors of stress in parents of developmentally disabled children. *Journal of Pediatric Psychology, 12*, 133–150.

Mickelson, K. D., Wroble, M., & Helgeson, V. S. (1999). "Why my child?" Parental attributions for children's special needs. *Journal of Applied Social Psychology, 29*, 1263–1291.

Minde, K. K., Perrotta, M., & Corter, C. (1982). The effects of neonatal complications in same-sexed premature twins on their mothers' preference. *Journal of the American Academy of Child and Adolescent Psychiatry, 21*, 446–452.

Mink, I. T., Meyers, C. E., & Nihira, K. (1984). Taxonomy of family lifestyle: II. Homes with slow learning children. *American Journal of Mental Deficiency, 89*, 111–123.

Most, D. E., Fidler, D. J., Booth-LaForce, C., & Kelly, J. (2006). Stress trajectories in mothers of young children with Down syndrome. *Journal of Intellectual Disability Research, 50*, 501–514.

Murphy, M. M., Abbeduto, L., Schroeder, S., & Serlin, R. (2007). Contribution of social and information-processing factors to eye-gaze avoidance in fragile X syndrome. *American Journal on Mental Retardation, 112*, 349–360.

Noh, S., Dumas, J. E., Wolf, L. C., & Fisman, S. N. (1989). Delineating sources of stress in parents of exceptional children. *Family Relations: Journal of Applied Family and Child Studies, 38*, 456–461.

Paterson, S. J., Brown, J. H., Gsodl, M. K., Johson, M. H. & Karmiloff-Smith, A. (1999). Cognitive modularity and genetic disorders. *Science, 286*, 2283–2284.

Poehlmann, J., Clements, M., Abbeduto, L., & Farsad, V. (2005). Family experiences associated with a child's diagnosis of fragile X syndrome or Down syndrome: Evidence for disruption and resilience. *Mental Retardation, 43*, 255–267.

Price, G. R. (1970). Selection and covariance. *Nature, 227*, 520–521.

Roach, M. A. Orsmond, G. I., & Barratt, M. S. (1999). Mothers and fathers of children with Down syndrome: Parental stress and involvement in childcare. *American Journal on Mental Retardation, 104*, 422–436.

Salmon, C., & Shackelford, T. (2007). *Family relationships: An evolutionary perspective.* New York: Oxford University Press.

Sameroff, A., & Chandler, M. (1975). Reproductive risk and the continuum of caretaking casualty. In F.D. Horowitz (Ed), *Child development research* Vol. 4. Chicago: University of Chicago Press.

Sander, J. L., & Morgan, S. B. (1997). Family stress and adjustment as perceived by parents of children with autism or Down syndrome: Implications for intervention. *Child and Family Behavior Therapy, 19*, 15–32.

Sarimski, K. (1997). Behavioural phenotypes and family stress in three mental retardation syndromes. *European Child & Adolescent Psychiatry, 6*, 26–31.

Scott, B. S., Atkinson, L., Minton, H. L., & Bowman, T. (1997). Psychological distress of parents of infants with Down syndrome. *American Journal on Mental Retardation, 102*, 161–171.

Scrimshaw, S. C. M. (1984). Infanticide in human populations: Societal and individual concerns. In S. B. Hrdy, & G. Hausfater (Eds.), *Comparative and evolutionary perspectives on infanticide: Introduction and overview.* New York: Aldine.

Seltzer, M. M., Abbeduto, L., Krauss, M. W., Greenberg, J., & Swe, A. (2004). Comparison groups in autism family research: Down syndrome, fragile X syndrome, and schizophrenia. *Journal of Autism and Developmental Disorders, 34*, 41–48.

Seltzer, M. M., Krauss, M. W., & Tsunematsu, N. (1993). Adults with Down syndrome and their aging mothers: Diagnostic group differences. *American Journal on Mental Retardation, 97*, 496–508.

Sobsey, D. (2002). Exceptionality, education, and maltreatment. *Exceptionality, 10*, 29–46.

Sobsey, D., & Varnhagen, C. (1989). Sexual abuse of people with disabilities. In M. Csapo, & L. Gougen (Eds.), *Special education across canada: Challenges for the 90s* (pp. 199–218). Vancouver: Centre for Human Development & Research.

Solnit, A., & Stark, M. (1961). Mourning and the birth of a defective child. *The Psychoanalytic Study of the Child, 16*, 523–537.

Stern, J. M. (1997). Offspring-induced nurturance: Animal-human parallels. *Developmental Psychobiology, 31*, 19–37.

Stoneman, Z. (2007). Examining the Down syndrome advantage: Mothers and fathers of young children with disabilities. *Journal of Intellectual Disability Research, 51*, 1006–1017.

Stores, R., Stores, G., Fellows., B., & Buckley, S. (1998). Daytime behaviour problems and maternal stress in children with Down's syndrome, their siblings, and other intellectual disabled peers. *Journal of Intellectual Disability Research, 42*, 228–238.

Sullivan, P. M., & Knutson, J. (2000). Maltreatment and disabilities: A population-based epidemiological study. *Child Abuse & Neglect, 24*, 1257–1273.

Trevarthen, C., & Aitken, K. J. (2001). Infant intersubjectivity: Research, theory, and clinical applications. *Journal of Child Psychology and Psychiatry, 42*, 3–48.

Trevarthen, C., & Daniel, S. (2005). Disorganized rhythm and synchrony: Early signs of autism and Rett syndrome. *Brain and Development, 27*, S25–S34.

Trivers, R. (1972). Parental investment and sexual selection. In B. Campbell (Ed.), *Sexual selection and the descent of man* (pp. 136–179). London: Heinemann.

Trute, B. (1990). Child and parent predictors of family adjustment in households containing young developmentally disabled children. *Family Relations, 39*, 292–297.

Van den Borne, H. W., van Hooren, R. H., van Gestel, M., Reinmeijer, P., Fryns, J. P., & Curfs, L. M. G. (1999). Psychosocial problems, coping strategies, and the need for information of parents of children with Prader-Willi syndrome and Angelman syndrome. *Parent Education and Counseling, 38*, 205–216.

Van Riper, M. (1999). Maternal perceptions of family-provider relationships and well-being in families of children with Down syndrome. *Research in Nursing and Health, 22*, 357–368.

Van Riper, M., Ryff C., & Pridham, K. (1992). Parental and family well-being in families of children with Down syndrome: A comparative study. *Research in Nursing and Health, 15*, 227–235.

Verdugo, M. A., Bermejo, B. G., & Fuertes, J. (1995). The maltreatment of intellectually handicapped children and adolescents. *Child Abuse & Neglect, 19*, 205–215.

von Gontard, A., Backes, M., Lausfersweiler-Plass, C., Wendland, C., Lehmkul, G., Zerres, K., & Rudnik-Schoneborn, S. (2002). Psychopathology and familial stress—Comparison of boys with fragile X syndrome and spinal muscular atrophy. *Journal of Child Psychology and Psychiatry, 43*, 949–957.

Wapner, R., Thom, E., Simpson, J. L., Pergament, E., Silver, R., Filkins, K., et al. (2003). First-trimester screening for trisomies 21 and 18. *New England Journal of Medicine, 349*, 1405–1413.

Ward, K. (2005). Microarray technology in obstetrics and gynecology: A guide for clinicians. *American Journal of Obstetrics and Gynecology, 195*, 364–372.

Wasserman, G., & Allen, R. (1985). Maternal withdrawal from handicapped toddlers. *Journal of Child Psychology and Psychology, 26*, 381–387.

Wikler, L., Wasow, M., & Hatfield, E. (1983). Chronic sorrow revisited: Parent vs. professional depiction of the adjustment of parents of mentally retarded children. *American Journal of Orthopsychiatry, 51*, 63–70.

Yau, M. K., & Li-Tsang, C. W. P. (1999). Adjustment and adaptation in parents of children with developmental disability in two-parent families: A review of the characteristics and attributes. *British Journal of Developmental Disabilities, 45*, 38–51.

Zebrowitz, L. A. (1997). *Reading faces: Window to the soul?* Boulder, CO: Westview Press.

Life Course Perspectives in Intellectual Disability Research: The Case of Family Caregiving

Anna J. Esbensen, Marsha Mailick Seltzer, *and* Marty Wyngaarden Krauss

Abstract

This chapter examines how a life course perspective contributes to research on families of persons with intellectual disability (ID), highlighting the contribution to research on families of persons with specific genetic syndromes or defined disorders. It considers the applicability of general theories of family development to families of persons with ID. It discusses salient and enduring differences in family development based on having a member with ID. It then presents specific applications of a life course perspective, with a focus on family development when the child has a specific genetic syndrome or defined disorder. The chapter concludes with suggestions for future research.

Keywords: Life course perspective, intellectual disability, families, caregiving

In this chapter, we examine how a life course perspective contributes to research on families of persons with intellectual disability (ID), highlighting the contribution to research on families of persons with specific genetic syndromes or defined disorders. The study of the life course is focused on patterns of individual development, with an emphasis on the effect of specific contextual phenomena on life outcomes. One of the central tenets of this perspective is that no single period of life dominates the continuous process of human development (Lerner & Ryff, 1978). Further, historical time and individual characteristics, including genetic syndromes or defined disorders, are salient influences in understanding the trajectories of experience and events that constitute the lifespan of an individual (Elder & Liker, 1982).

This perspective casts a wide lens on the antecedents and consequences of development across the life course. Consequently, it challenges researchers to conceptualize the importance of the past, present, and future developmental status of an individual with ID and his or her family. In this chapter, our goal is to use the life course perspective to interpret findings of ID family research. To this end,

we focus on the example of life-long care provided by families to their members with ID for two reasons. First, because the care provided by parents for a child with an ID often spans five or six decades (Krauss & Seltzer, 1993), it is equally important to focus research in this field on adults as on children, and on families at later stages of the life course as on families with young children. Unfortunately, far more is known about the initial adaptations and accommodations of such families than about the influence of early experiences on the subsequent experiences of affected families (Ferguson, 2002; Gallimore, Coots, Weisner, Garnier, & Guthrie, 1996). Similarly, most family research on specific genetic syndromes or defined disorders is focused primarily on children rather than adolescents or adults (for exceptions, see Abbeduto et al., 2004; Seltzer, Krauss, Orsmond, & Vestal, 2001b; Seltzer, Shattuck, Abbeduto, & Greenberg, 2004b) and little is known about how the adaptations and accommodations made by families of individuals with specific genetic syndromes or defined disorders shift as these individuals become adults, or what impact these changes have on the development of the individuals themselves (Esbensen,

Seltzer, & Abbeduto, 2007). Within the life course perspective, although adult development is firmly rooted in childhood and adolescence, change as well as continuity is characteristic of the transition from one stage to the next (Hetherington, Lerner, & Perlmutter, 1988).

Similar to individual development, family well-being evolves over time. Early stages of family life influence family functioning in later stages (Parke, 1988). Parenting is an enduring commitment that continues even after the child has become an adult (Lancaster, Altmann, Rossi, & Sherrod, 1987). This durable role may assume the attributes of a "career"—namely, the acquisition of specialized skills, the development of competence and particularized knowledge, and an ability to contextualize routine and acute events within a larger time frame (Aneshensel, Pearlin, Mullin, Zarit, & Whitlatch, 1995; Pearlin, 1992). Therefore, research on parental caregiving can be informed by knowledge about patterns established early on, by expectations of the years to come, and by the impact of genetic syndromes, defined disorders, or a diagnosis of ID on these patterns and expectations. Some research has been conducted on intrafamilial change and development over the full life course for families with a child with ID (Krauss & Seltzer, 1999; Seltzer, Greenberg, Floyd, Pettee, & Hong, 2001; Seltzer & Ryff, 1994), but less is known about how the family life course unfolds differentially for families with children with specific genetic syndromes or defined disorders. Thus, the focus of research must continue to extend throughout the adulthood of the son or daughter with ID, specific genetic syndromes, or defined disorders and into the old age of the parents.

Second, this chapter's focus is on the family unit because although the diagnosis of ID is an "event" that affects one member of the family, such events have ripple effects on all family members (Pruchno, Peters, & Burant, 1996). These effects are manifested on the levels of both family functioning and individual well-being, and differ between mothers and fathers (Essex, 2002; Essex, Seltzer, & Krauss, 1999; Krauss, 1993; Noh, Dumas, Wolf, & Fisman, 1989) and among siblings (Krauss, Seltzer, Gordon, & Friedman, 1996; Orsmond & Seltzer, 2000, 2007a,b; Seltzer, Begun, Seltzer, & Krauss, 1991; Stoneman & Berman, 1993). The focus of a life course perspective is on the developmental trajectories of each family member and of the family unit collectively. Having a family member with ID has a dynamic influence on family and individual development, with a mix of negative and positive impacts over time (Esbensen, Seltzer, & Greenberg, 2006; Lounds, Seltzer, Greenberg, & Shattuck, 2007; Seltzer et al., 2001b; Seltzer & Ryff, 1994). Further, having a family member with a specific genetic syndrome or defined disorder can have differential influences on the family and individual development, as a result of degree of heritability, supports, information available, and behavioral characteristics of the disorder (Abbeduto et al., 2004; Esbensen et al., 2007).

Thus, in this chapter, we examine the applicability of general theories of family development to families of persons with ID. We discuss salient and enduring differences in family development based on having a member with ID. We then present specific applications of a life course perspective, with a focus on family development in which the child has a specific genetic syndrome or defined disorder. The chapter concludes with suggestions for future research.

Overview of Our Research

A primary focus of the Lifespan Family Research Project is on the impacts of later life coresidence on parent caregivers and on their adolescent or adult son or daughters with developmental disabilities. It has particularly been focused on the antecedents and consequences of transitions in caregiving during the later stages of the parents' life course. The Lifespan Family Research Project has included three studies. In one, 461 families were studied in which the mother was between the age of 55 and 85 and a son or daughter with ID lived at home with her. In this study, 169 of these sons or daughters also had a diagnosis of Down syndrome (DS). In the second study, 406 families were studied in which the son or daughter had a confirmed diagnosis of an autism spectrum disorder (ASD) and was age 10–52 at the beginning of the study. The third study involves 115 families of adolescents (age 12 or older) and adults with fragile X syndrome (FXS). The designs of these studies involve multiple visits or phone contact with each family every 18 months, during which both quantitative and qualitative data are collected about characteristics of the son or daughter with the disability, the services he or she receives and needs, family characteristics, and maternal physical, social, and psychological well-being (for a description of the research, see Krauss & Seltzer, 1999; Seltzer et al., 2003). In our analyses, the primary focus is on the mothers. This selection is not arbitrary.

Consistent with most families, the mothers in our samples provide the bulk of the daily care needed and received by their adult child with developmental disabilities (Essex, Seltzer, & Krauss, 2002). However, data are also collected from fathers, nondisabled siblings, and when possible, with the individual with the disability (for summary of research findings on other family members, see Lounds & Seltzer, 2007).

In the first study, which included families of adults with ID, eight waves of data were collected from 1988 to 2000. At the beginning of the study, the average age of the son (54%) or daughter with ID was 34, and over a third (37%) had DS. Most of the sample members had mild (38%) or moderate (41%) ID, although 21% had severe/profound ID. The average age of the mothers at the start of the study was 66. Mothers were mostly married (66%) and had other children in addition to the son or daughter with ID (93%).

In our ongoing study of families of adolescents and adults with autism, five waves of data have thus far been collected since 1999, with two additional rounds of data collected specific to the individual with ASD and to the measurement of stress. At the start of the study, the average age of the son (73%) or daughter with autism was 22, and nearly two-thirds of the sample lived at home with their parents. More than half (60%) of the sample had been given a diagnosis of ID at some point in their life, according to parental report. The average age of the mothers at the start of the study was 52, and most mothers were married (78%).

The study of families of adolescents and adults with FXS is currently recruiting sample members.

Intellectual Disability Family Research and the Family Life Course

Scholars of the family articulate a "family life cycle" that explores the "expansion, contraction, and realignment of the relationship system to support the entry, exit, and development of family members" (Carter & McGoldrick, 1989, p. 13; Duvall, 1962). In general, six basic stages in the family life cycle are enumerated: leaving home as single young adults, the joining of families through marriage and the new couple, families with young children, families of adolescents, launching children and moving on, and families in later life (Carter & McGoldrick, 2005).

One focus of our research (Krauss & Seltzer, 1999) has been on the launching stage, which is considered the most problematic for families in general, and for families with a child with a disability in particular. This stage begins with the departure of the first child from the home and ends with the exit of the last child. It is the stage with the largest number of exits (i.e., launching, death, divorce) and entries (i.e., spouses, grandchildren) of family members. Consequently, realignments of previously stable roles and relationships, familial conflict, and renegotiation of relationships are primary problems to be overcome during this period (Nydegger & Mitteness, 1996; Silverberg, 1996). An additional factor influencing the launching stage among families with a child with ID is that the onset of the launching stage may occur prematurely (i.e., placement of the child with the disability prior to adulthood), on time (i.e., around the time of majority), or may be postponed (i.e., delayed until well into the child's adult years or not accomplished during the parents' lifetime).

Premature and Postponed Launching

With respect to the incidence of premature launching, rates are dropping in recent years among children with ID. Of all individuals served in out-of-home placements, 36.8% were under the age of 21 in 1977, 18.2% were under the age of 21 in 1987, 7.6% were under the age of 21 in 1997, and 6.2% were under the age of 21 in 2005 (Lakin, Anderson, & Prouty, 1998; Prouty, Lakin, Coucouvanis, & Anderson, 2005). Postponed launching for individuals with ID is more common, with many adults living with their aging parents until the death of the parents (Krauss & Seltzer, 1999). However, the prevalence of out-of-home placement for persons with ID (mainly adults) has risen in the last 20 years. In the 1980s, between 15% and 20% of persons with ID lived outside of the parental home (Lakin, 1985). In the 1990s and 2000s, the prevalence of out-of-home placement for persons with ID had risen to about 40% (Fujiura, 1998; Rizzolo, Hemp, Braddock, & Promeranz-Essley, 2004).

Although the incidence of premature launching is low, it constitutes a major alteration of the family life course. The most dramatic consequence of premature launching is the transfer of parenting roles from the family of origin to professionals before the time the child reaches adulthood (Blacher, 1994). Research on premature launching is quite dated, due to the declining likelihood of this transition, but such research remains important. A small number of factors have been found in such research to predict premature launching: more severe ID, presence of behavioral and physical problems, and the inability of the parents to meet the daily needs of the child (Blacher, Hanneman, & Rousey, 1992; Seltzer & Krauss, 1984). However, levels of stress among parents of *young children* with ID have not been found to differ if the child lives at home or in an out-of-home placement, whereas stress is reportedly lower for parents of *adult children* with ID who live outside the home as compared to those who coreside (Hayden & Heller, 1997). Also, families of young children with ID who have been placed report more stress and caregiving burden than do families of adults who have been placed (Baker & Blacher, 2002). Thus, premature launching does not appear to lessen the stress experienced by parents of young children with ID. Longitudinal studies are needed to sort out the direction of effects of stress and caregiving burden. It may be that a high level of caregiving stress during childhood leads to premature out-of-home placement, leaving a residual group of families who do not find coresidence to be stressful and for whom long-term coresidence is preferred.

Impact of Launching on Families of Persons with Intellectual Disability

An examination of the literature on premature and postponed launching from a life course perspective helps to identify associated factors that may be associated with the higher stress associated with premature launching. Heller and Factor (1994) noted that placement is more likely when the child has more severe ID and more serious maladaptive behaviors, when the parents are older and in worse health, when the family is larger, and when there are few informal and formal community supports. Although these trends are strong predictors of placement, they may be mediated by the stage of life of the family. Tausig (1985) examined differences in the factors associated with premature launching and launching during adulthood. He examined placement requests from families whose child was under age 21 in contrast to those whose child was 21 years or over. For families of children under the age of 21, placement requests were associated with the child's poor social behavior rather than with characteristics of the family. For children over the age of 21, placement requests were associated with disruptions of family relations rather than with characteristics of the child. Suelzle and Keenan (1981) examined age-related placement patterns and found that the risk of out-of-home placement is highest when the child is around 6 years of age, and again between 19 and 21 years of age. These periods are marked by the child's entry or exit from school systems and may therefore prompt higher levels of stress typically associated with transition points in the child's and family's life. However, the results of these two studies (Suelzle & Keenan, 1981; Tausig, 1985) are over 20 years old and need to be interpreted within their historical context. The reasons and timing of premature placement in the 1970s and 1980s may not be the same today, given the changes in services and supports available to families of individuals with ID.

In relation to the increasing rates of postponed launching, we examined the effects of postponed launching on the family as a unit, the parents as individuals, the siblings, other immediate family members, and the person with ID (Abbeduto et al., 2004; Esbensen et al., 2006; Essex, 2002; Hong, Seltzer, & Krauss, 2001; Kim, Greenberg, Seltzer, & Krauss, 2003; Orsmond & Seltzer, 2000; Seltzer, Krauss, Hong, & Orsmond, 2001a). The prevalence of life-long family care raises questions about why some families postpone launching or never plan to have their child live away from family. In contrast to the normative family life course, families of children with ID, specific genetic syndromes, or defined disorders may "know" from early on that their life course will be altered and may therefore forestall launching until after the child has reached chronologically based adulthood. The adaptation within such families may indeed be affected by *when* and *why* parents make decisions about the probability of launching their child.

Continued coresidence (or postponed launching) of an adult with ID with his or her parents may occur for many reasons. Krauss (1990) noted five commonly expressed motivations for life-long family-based care: family responsibility willingly accepted, misgivings about the alternatives, recognition of the child's need for stability, mutual benefits at this stage of life, and resignation to one's fate. These five motivations only hint at the complexity involved in parental decision-making of placing their child. Continued coresidence may also result from parental concerns associated with the transition to adulthood that include the personal welfare of the child, worries about the capacity of the adult service system to meet the child's needs, and the realization that parenting responsibilities extend beyond the time anticipated among families of typically developing children (Krauss et al., 2005).

Although launching may be postponed in many families of adults with ID, placement becomes more likely with advancing parental age

(Meyers, Borthwick, & Eyman, 1985). Placement during adulthood is predicted by parental health problems, parental feelings of burden, high levels of dependent and maladaptive behaviors in the adults with ID, and already being on a placement waiting list (Essex, Seltzer, & Krauss, 1997; Heller & Factor, 1994; Pruchno & Patrick, 1999; Seltzer, Greenberg, Krauss, & Hong, 1997). In addition, greater use of formal services is associated with an increased probability that caregivers will request residential placement (Blacher & Hanneman, 1993). This may be because use of services may decrease family apprehensiveness toward the community residential service system and may thus be a first step toward placement.

Although rates of postponed launching are increasing, long-term coresidence is still the preferred plan for the majority of families of individuals with ID (Freedman, Krauss, & Seltzer, 1997). Families preferring continued coresidence tend to have more positive well-being as compared to the families planning for a residential placement. This does not imply that families planning for a residential placement are disadvantaged. Families seeking residential placement not in times of family crisis tend to be highly involved in the relocation process, and continue to maintain contact with the adult with ID, similar to what is observed in premature or on-time launching of children with ID (Blacher, Baker, & Feinfeld, 1999; Eisenberg, Baker, & Blacher, 1998; Seltzer et al., 2001a). Further, we have found that maternal worries about the son or daughter's future care that may have prompted the residential placement significantly abate after a planned residential relocation, and are lower in comparison to the worries reported by mothers who chose to not place their adult son or daughter (Seltzer et al., 2001a).

Impact of Launching on Families of Persons with Genetic Syndromes and Defined Disorders

Only a limited amount of research has been conducted on the impact and pattern of postponed launching on families of adults with specific disorders (e.g., autism) or genetic syndromes (e.g., DS, FXS). There is a need to better understand what role genetic syndromes have on placement patterns and predictors thereof in order to provide syndrome-specific support to these families during the launching period. The differing behavioral phenotype of specific disabilities or genetic syndromes may contribute to differing age-related patterns of launching.

We also need to better understand how the behavioral phenotype of specific disorders and genetic syndromes contributes to the differing impact of launching on families. For example, mothers of adults with autism exhibit a high level of contact and maternal involvement with their son or daughter after launching (Krauss et al., 2005), similar to patterns evident for other types of disabilities. However, for individuals with autism, maternal worries about the future of their son or daughter with autism are reported to be even greater after a residential relocation outside the home (Krauss et al., 2005), whereas mothers of adults with other types of disabilities tend to have reduced levels of worries after their son or daughter is placed (Seltzer et al., 2001a). The need for sameness in the environment exhibited by many individuals with autism may constrain the successful transition of the individual to a new residential placement, and in turn affect the mother's level of worries.

Coresidence of aging parents and their adult child with ID, autism, or specific genetic syndromes can easily be cast into a pathological framework. Having an adult child living at home can be construed as a violation of the life course expectation of independent functioning for adult children and freedom from parenting tasks in old age. However, Aquilino (1990) notes that having an adult child live at home is increasingly common in the general population. Specifically, nearly half (45%) of parents in the United States between 45 to 54 years of age have adult children at home. This trend challenges traditional expectations about the launching of adult children from the family home and represents an alteration of the stages posited by family development theory.

The Aquilino study illustrates variations in the family life course in the general population that offer new interpretations to findings from research on families with a member with ID. Postponed launching has been shown to be increasingly normative and generally positively experienced. In this regard, the experience of families of coresident adults with ID, including those with autism or specific genetic syndromes, may be more similar to than different from those of other families without this special status.

The Impact of Life Course Family Caregiving in the Context of Different Diagnostic Groups

In examining the impact of family-based care, two hypotheses have been proposed. According to the *wear-and-tear hypothesis*, caregiving takes an increasing toll on the health and psychological well-being of caregiving parents, leading to higher rates and earlier timing of out-of-home placement (Townsend, Noelker, Deimling, & Bass, 1989). Alternatively, according to the *adaptational hypothesis*, over time, caregivers adapt by incorporating their specialized roles within their daily routines (Townsend et al., 1989). Our research of life-long family-based care of adults with ID revealed that this type of caregiving brings both psychological and emotional rewards, as well as stresses and burdens, to parents and siblings of persons with ID (Krauss et al., 1996; Seltzer & Krauss, 1994). Conversely, we found that families of adolescents and adults with autism appear to experience elevated levels of stress and caregiving demands as compared to parents of adolescents and adults with other types of disabilities (Abbeduto et al., 2004; Greenberg, Seltzer, Krauss, Chou, & Hong, 2004; Seltzer, Shattuck, Abbeduto, & Greenberg, 2004b). Thus, for families of individuals with ID, we found support for the adaptational hypothesis of the impact of family-based care. In contrast, for families of individuals with autism, the wear-and-tear hypothesis of the impact of family-based care may be more applicable.

Down Syndrome

A comparative advantage in adaptation is found in families of children with DS in contrast to families of children with autism or those whose ID is caused by other factors (Fidler, Hodapp, & Dykens, 2000; Fisman, Wolf, & Noh, 1989; Hauser-Cram, Warfield, Shonkoff, & Krauss, 2001; Holroyd & McArthur, 1976; Kasari & Sigman, 1997; Marcovitch, Goldberg, MacGregor, & Lojkasek, 1986; Shonkoff, Hauser-Cram, Krauss, & Upshur, 1992). And when compared to mothers of children with other genetic syndromes, mothers of children with DS are less pessimistic about their child's future and report fewer family problems (Fidler et al., 2000). The extent to which such early differences in family experiences are durable over the life course is a pivotal question that only recently has begun to be examined.

In our research, we have found that this comparative advantage indeed extends from childhood to adolescence, with families of adolescents with DS continuing to fare better than families of adolescents with autism or other types of IDs (Abbeduto et al., 2004; also, see Burack, Hodapp, Iarocci & Zigler, 2011, this volume). Mothers of adolescents and young adults with DS display better psychological well-being, less pessimism about their child's future, and more reciprocated feelings of closeness than do mothers of adolescents and young adults with autism or FXS (Abbeduto et al., 2004). Mothers of adolescents with DS also report more closeness in the relationship with their child and less depressive symptoms than do mothers of adolescents and young adults with autism (Abbeduto et al., 2004).

This advantage continues well into adulthood (Seltzer, Krauss, & Tsunematsu, 1993). In comparison to mothers of adults with ID of unknown etiology, mothers of adults with DS report less conflicted family environments, less stress and burden, and more satisfaction with their social supports (Seltzer et al., 1993). Social support networks are also reported to be larger for mothers of adult children with DS compared to mothers of adult children with other types of ID (Seltzer & Krauss, 1998). These findings suggest that there is a life course pattern of continuity in positive profiles of adaptation in mothers with a son or daughter with DS. There is also an increase in positive well-being afforded to mothers of adults with DS as their children get older. These mothers report a sense of optimism and acceptance of their adult child's disability and have developed an appreciation for their child's strengths (Krauss & Seltzer, 1995, 1999; Seltzer et al., 1993). This does not imply that mothers of adults with DS do not experience frustrations and stresses; however, these mothers typically report more gratifications than frustrations with raising their adult child (Krauss & Seltzer, 1995).

Autism

Although families of individuals with autism tend to be "disadvantaged" in childhood and adolescence, there is data to suggest that this disadvantage may lessen with age. Although when compared to mothers of adults with DS, mothers of adults with autism show poorer well-being on some outcomes, including having a more distant relationship with their son or daughter and more pessimism about their child's future (Greenberg et al., 2004; Seltzer et al., 2001b), many areas of physical and psychological similarity also exist (Greenberg et al., 2004; Lounds et al., 2007). For example, similar patterns have been found between mothers of adults with autism and DS on measures of depressive symptoms, optimism, positive psychological well-being, and physical health (Greenberg et al., 2004). This increasing similarity in adulthood may reflect improvements in symptoms of autism that are evident among adolescents and adults with autism (Seltzer et al., 2004b;

Shattuck et al., 2007), which in turn have been associated with improving maternal well-being (Lounds et al., 2007).

Fragile X Syndrome
Mothers of children with FXS are at a disadvantage in their well-being as compared to mothers of children with DS (Poehlmann, Clements, Abbeduto, & Farsad, 2005), but are advantaged in their well-being when compared to mothers of children with Prader-Willi syndrome, Williams syndrome, or ID of unknown etiology (Perry, Harris, & Minnes, 2004; Sarimski, 1997; van Lieshout, de Meyer, Curfs, & Fryns, 1998). They are less stressed, less depressed, have less marital conflict, less anger, and a lower need for control. And their disadvantage with respect to DS may also abate with age. In a comparative study, mothers of adolescents and young adults with FXS were contrasted with mothers of adolescents and young adults with DS or autism (Abbeduto et al., 2004). After controlling for contextual variables, no differences between mothers of individuals with FXS and DS were observed on measures of depressive symptoms, maternal ratings of perceived closeness with her child, or coping style. These findings suggest that, by the time their children reach adolescence, mothers of children with FXS may cope more comparably to mothers of children with DS than during childhood.

The different patterns from earlier to later stages of the family life course in DS, FXS, and autism underscore the importance of a life course perspective in understanding the experiences and adaptation of these families. We need to better understand what characteristics of genetic syndromes or of the individual child, such as behavioral characteristics and time since diagnosis, contribute to these differing life-long patterns in well-being. Further, the variable pattern from earlier to later stages of the family life course in these comparison studies highlights the importance of comparative life course analyses across different genetic syndromes and diagnostic groups.

The Influence of Support on Families Across the Life Course: Stress and Coping
Normative and Non-normative Sources of Stress
Mothers of persons with autism, genetic syndromes, or other types of ID are at risk for two particular types of stress. They face non-normative stress associated with the special challenges in rearing their son or daughter with the disability, and normative stress ordinarily experienced during the later years of adulthood. It is important to focus on both of these sources of stress. If families are viewed exclusively through the lens of the adult child with a disability (or what is non-normative), only one aspect of family life is cast in relief, whereas there is much that is normative or typical about these families' lives. Most families also have nondisabled children and experience a variety of the "expected" stressors that occur in later years. Our examination provides insights into parental reactions to these expected sources of stress during the later years of parenting.

Expected sources of stress, such as negative life events, are a relatively common feature of mid-life and old age. Persons who experience such life events are at increased risk for psychological distress (Cohen & Wills, 1985; Pearlin, 1989). In our sample of coresiding mothers of adults with ID, during an 18-month period, nearly half the mothers (45%) experienced at least one of the following stressful life events: widowhood, divorce, retirement, retirement of husband, moving from one home to another, declining health, or declining health in the child with ID (Seltzer et al., 1996). Although mothers who experienced stressful life events had higher levels of depressive symptoms than did mothers who experienced no negative life events in the past 18 months, these mothers were not significantly different in their depressive symptoms from a comparison group of mothers with children without disabilities who also experienced stress (Seltzer et al., 1996). In other words, mothers of adult children with ID respond to stressful life events *similarly* to their age peers who have had a normative parenting history. Mothers of adults with ID have adapted well to the role of parenting a child with special needs and, at this stage of life, they are not uniquely vulnerable to stressful life events. When limiting our sample of mothers of adults with autism to those who coreside with their adult child, over half of the mothers of adults with autism (60%) experienced similar stressful live events as those experienced by mothers of adults with ID. Studies are needed to explore what stressors are experienced by mothers of adults with genetic syndromes and how they cope with these stressors. Such studies are needed to determine if the particular behavioral phenotype of the disorder or genetic syndrome contribute to adapting to normative and non-normative stressors.

Daily stressors experienced by parents of adolescents and adults also provide insights into the lives of families. Mothers of adolescents and adults with ASD are much more likely to experience a day with at least one stressor, and to experience days with multiple stressors, than are mothers of individuals without disabilities (Smith, Hong, Seltzer, Greenberg, Almeida, & Bishop, 2009). Consistent with prior research, the mothers of adolescents and adults with ASD also reported higher levels of negative affect and lower levels of positive affect than the comparison group. The increased experience of daily stress likely contributes to the poorer outcomes in well-being observed in mothers of individuals with ASD as compared to mothers of individuals with no disabilities. Thus, the normative experience of daily stressors is magnified in families of individuals with disability and likely accumulates over years of caregiving, potentially taking a cumulative toll on the well-being of mothers of individuals with disability.

Coping with Psychological Distress

In adapting to their non-normative life course, mothers of adult children with ID develop and use effective coping mechanisms to reduce their risk for psychological distress. Mothers of adults with ID often use problem-focused coping strategies, which are particularly effective in reducing psychological distress under high caregiving demands, such as caring for an adult child with ID and either severe functional limitations or frequent behavior problems (Essex et al., 1999). Use of problem-focused coping, in place of emotion-focused coping, has been associated with a reduction in subjective burden associated with caregiving (Essex et al., 1999; Kim et al., 2003) and fewer depressive symptoms (Seltzer, Greenberg & Krauss, 1995).

Other research has examined how mothers of individuals with autism use coping techniques to alleviate their psychological distress (Abbeduto et al., 2004; Smith, Seltzer, Greenberg, Tager-Flusberg, & Carter, 2008). Mothers of adolescents with autism use problem- and emotion-focused coping in the same way as do mothers of adolescents with DS or FXS (Abbeduto et al., 2004). For mothers of adolescents with autism, use of problem-focused coping strategies buffers maternal distress, particularly when the son or daughter exhibits more severe autism symptoms (Smith et al., 2008). More research is needed regarding how coping techniques are employed by mothers of adults with autism and by mothers of adults with other disorders to manage the stress associated with non-normative parenting.

Other Factors Related to Psychological Distress

In addition to using coping techniques, having adequate social supports has also been found to reduce the risk of psychological distress. However, the effect of social support may vary over the life course for mothers of adults with ID (Greenberg, Seltzer, Krauss, & Kim, 1997). Mothers caring for adults with ID who have larger social support networks report lower levels of depressive symptoms 18 months later. However, being a member of a support group did not mitigate depressive symptoms when the mother was also faced with a stressful event (Greenberg et al., 1997). This finding may be due to the age of the maternal caregivers in the Greenberg et al. (1997) study. Mothers of adults with ID may have been involved in support groups earlier in life, at a time closer to their child's diagnosis, which may have impacted their well-being. But during mid-life and old age, participation in such groups may have less of an impact on well-being. We also found age-related differences in the effect of emotional support. For mothers over the age of 65 who had of adult children with ID, increases in the amount of emotional support received from social network members enhances positive well-being, but this was not the case for mothers aged 55–65 (Hong et al., 2001).

Conclusion

In this chapter, we brought a life course perspective to the study of family caregiving, particularly among families with an adult child with ID. Because the family environment is one of the most durable influences on the development and quality of life for persons with ID, it is important for researchers, policy makers, and service providers to attend carefully to the general and specific life course patterns of those families.

Interventions in the lives of persons with ID and their families require a more sophisticated understanding of *how* families change over time, their *motivations* to provide family-based care, and their *expectations* for themselves as a family unit and for each individual member. A life course perspective underscores the need for a more robust and active program of research on families. Most families achieve positive adaptations to the challenge of having a child with ID (Hastings, Allen, McDermott, & Still, 2002; Turnbull, Summers, & Brotherson, 1986) and, to a lesser extent, to having a child with autism (Greenberg et al., 2004). However, although some of the mechanisms that account for the adaptability and well-being of families of children with ID across the life course have been identified and tested empirically, the same needs to be accomplished for families of children with specific genetic syndromes. Identifying the most powerful mechanisms over time, and determining the extent to which these vary from syndrome to syndrome, represent important challenges for current and future research.

The study of family caregiving over the life course has come of age. There is an interest in the extent to which family development is characterized by discontinuities or by persistence of patterns established in the early, formative years of family life. We need to better understand the impact of getting off to a "rough start" within a family versus the impact of having a supportive and caring environment that is responsive to the early stresses families typically experience. Many of the early patterns of family adaptation persist over several decades, including the observation that families of persons with DS experience a more favorable level of parental well-being than do families of persons with other causes of ID. Similarly, the impact of coping as a personal resource appears to persist across the life course. Other early patterns of family adaptation change with time. Families of persons with autism experience less favorable levels of parental well-being to those whose children have DS when the children are younger, but become somewhat more comparable in parental well-being when the children are older.

The methodological challenges of conducting research over the life course warrant comment. Many technical issues remain unresolved, such as comparability of measures from childhood to adolescence to adulthood, disentangling developmental trends from cohort effects, and sampling issues (Seltzer, Floyd, & Hindes, 2004a). However, a life course approach reflects a set of tenets about the nature of human development, rather than a specific methodology applied to developmental research. A long lens from which to view the patterns of continuities and discontinuities in human development helps social and behavioral scientists from a variety of disciplines to provide answers to enduring questions about how parents who must cope with the daunting challenge of caring for a child with a disability overcome their sources of stress and display life-long patterns of adaptation.

Acknowledgments

This chapter was prepared with support from the National Institute on Child Health and Human Development (P30 HD03352, T32 HD07489), the National Institute on Aging (R01 AG08768), and the Autism Society of South Eastern Wisconsin.

References

Abbeduto, L., Seltzer, M. M., Shattuck, P., Krauss, M. W., Orsmond, G., & Murphy, M. M. (2004). Psychological well-being and coping in mothers of youths with autism, Down syndrome, or fragile X syndrome. *American Journal on Mental Retardation, 109,* 237–254.

Aneshensel, C., Pearlin, L., Mullin, J., Zarit, S., & Whitlatch, C. (1995). *Profiles in caregiving: The unexpected career.* New York: Academic Press.

Aquilino, W. S. (1990). The likelihood of parent-adult child coresidence: Effects on family structure and parental characteristics. *Journal of Marriage and the Family, 52,* 405–419.

Baker, B. L., & Blacher, J. (2002). For better or worse? Impact of residential placement on families. *Mental Retardation, 40,* 1–13.

Blacher, J. (1994). *When there's no place like home: Options for children living apart from their natural families.* Baltimore: Brookes.

Blacher, J., Baker, B., & Feinfeld, K. A. (1999). Leaving or launching? Continuing family involvement with children and adolescents in placement. *American Journal on Mental Retardation, 104,* 452–465.

Blacher, J., & Hanneman, R. (1993). Out-of-home placement of children and adolescents with severe handicaps: Behavioral intentions and behavior. *Research in Developmental Disabilities, 14,* 145–160.

Blacher, J., Hanneman, R. A., & Rousey, A. B. (1992). Out-of-home placement of children with severe handicaps: A comparison of approaches. *American Journal of Mental Retardation, 96,* 607–616.

Burack, J. A., Hodapp, R. M., Iarocci, G., & Zigler, E. (2011). On knowing more: Future issues for developmental approaches to understanding persons with intellectual disabilities. In J. A. Burack, R. M. Hodapp, G. Iarocci, & E. Zigler (Eds.), *The Oxford Handbook of Intellectual Disability and Development.* (pp. 395–402). New York, NY: Oxford University Press.

Carter, B., & McGoldrick, M. (1989). *The changing family life cycle: A framework for family therapy* (2nd ed.). Boston: Allyn & Bacon.

Carter, B., & McGoldrick, M. (2005). *The expanded family life cycle: Individual, family and social perspectives* (3rd ed.). Needham Heights, MA: Allyn & Bacon.

Cohen, S., & Wills, T. A. (1985). Stress, social support and the buffering hypothesis. *Psychological Bulletin, 98,* 310–357.

Duvall, E. (1962). *Family development.* Philadelphia: Lippincott.

Eisenberg, L., Baker, B., & Blacher, J. (1998). Siblings of children with mental retardation living at home or in residential placement. *Journal of Child Psychology and Psychiatry, 39,* 355–363.

Elder, G. H., & Liker, J. K. (1982). Hard times in women's lives: Historical influences across forty years. *American Journal of Sociology, 88,* 241–269.

Esbensen, A. J., Seltzer, M. M., & Abbeduto, L. (2007). Family well-being in Down syndrome and fragile X syndrome. In J. E. Roberts, R. Chapman, & S. Warren (Eds.), *Speech and language development and intervention in Down syndrome and Fragile X syndrome* (pp. 275–295). Baltimore: Brookes.

Esbensen, A. J., Seltzer, M. M., & Greenberg, J. S. (2006). Depressive symptoms of adults with mild to moderate intellectual disability and their relation to maternal well-being. *Journal of Policy and Practice in Intellectual Disabilities, 3*, 229–237.

Essex, E. L. (2002). Mothers and fathers of adults with mental retardation: Feelings of intergenerational closeness. *Family Relations, 51*, 156–165.

Essex, E. L., Seltzer, M. M., & Krauss, M. W. (2002). Fathers as caregivers for adult children with mental retardation. In B. J. Kramer, & E. Thompson (Eds.), *Men as caregivers: Theory, research and service implications.* New York: Springer.

Essex, E. L., Seltzer, M. M., & Krauss, M. W. (1997). Residential transitions of adults with mental retardation: Predictors of waiting list use and placement. *American Journal on Mental Retardation, 101*, 613–629.

Essex, E. L., Seltzer, M. M., & Krauss, M. W. (1999). Differences in coping effectiveness and well-being among aging mothers and fathers of adults with mental retardation. *American Journal on Mental Retardation, 104*, 545–563.

Ferguson, P. M. (2002). A place in the family: A historical interpretation of research on parental reactions to having a child with a disability. *The Journal of Special Education, 36*, 124–130, 147.

Fidler, D. J., Hodapp, R. M., & Dykens, E. M. (2000). Stress in families of young children with Down syndrome, Williams syndrome, and Smith-Magenis syndrome. *Early Education and Development, 11*, 395–406.

Fisman, S., Wolf, N., & Noh, S. (1989). Marital intimacy in parents of exceptional children. *Canadian Journal of Psychiatry, 34*, 519–525.

Freedman, R. I., Krauss, M. K., & Seltzer, M. M. (1997). Aging parents' residential plans for adult children with mental retardation. *Mental Retardation, 35*, 114–123.

Fujiura, G. T. (1998). Demography of family households. *American Journal on Mental Retardation, 103*, 225–235.

Gallimore, R., Coots, J., Weisner, T., Garnier, H., & Guthrie, D. (1996). Family responses to children with early developmental delays II: Accommodation intensity and activity in early and middle childhood. *American Journal on Mental Retardation, 101*, 215–232.

Greenberg, J. S., Seltzer, M. M., Krauss, M. W., Chou, R. J., & Hong, J. (2004). The effect of quality of the relationship between mothers and adult children with schizophrenia, autism or Down syndrome on maternal well-being: The mediating role of optimism. *American Journal of Orthopsychiatry, 74*, 14–25.

Greenberg, J. S., Seltzer, M. M., Krauss, M. W., & Kim, H. (1997). The differential effects of social support on the psychological well-being of aging mothers of adults with mental illness or mental retardation. *Family Relations, 46*, 383–394.

Hastings, R. P., Allen, R., McDermott, K., & Still, D. (2002). Factors related to positive perceptions in mothers of children with intellectual disabilities. *Journal of Applied Research in Intellectual Disabilities, 15*, 269–275.

Hauser-Cram, P., Warfield, M. E., Shonkoff, J. P., & Krauss, M. W. (2001). Children with disabilities: A longitudinal study of child development and parent well-being. *Monographs of the Society for Research in Child Development, 66*, 3.

Hayden, M. F., & Heller, T. (1997). Support, problem-solving/coping ability, and personal burden of younger and older caregivers of adults with mental retardation. *Mental Retardation, 35*, 364–372.

Heller, T., & Factor, A. (1994). Facilitating future planning and transitions out of the home. In M. M. Seltzer, M. W. Krauss, & M. P. Janicki (Eds.), *Life course perspectives on adulthood and old age.* Washington, DC: American Association on Mental Retardation.

Heller, T., Hsieh, K., & Rowitz, L. (1997). Maternal and paternal caregiving of persons with mental retardation across the lifespan. *Family Relations, 46*, 407–415.

Hetherington, E. M., Lerner, R. M., & Perlmutter, M. (Eds.). (1988). *Child development in life-span perspective.* Hillsdale, NJ: Erlbaum.

Holroyd, J., & McArthur, D. (1976). Mental retardation and stress on the parents: A contrast between Down's syndrome and childhood autism. *American Journal of Mental Deficiency, 80*, 431–436.

Hong, J., Seltzer, M. M., & Krauss, M. W. (2001). Change in social support and psychological well-being: A longitudinal study of aging mothers of adults with mental retardation. *Family Relations, 50*, 154–163.

Kasari, C., & Sigman, M. (1997). Linking parental perceptions to interactions in young children with autism. *Journal of Autism and Developmental Disorders, 27*, 39–57.

Kim. H. W., Greenberg, J. S., Seltzer, M. M., & Krauss, M. W. (2003). The role of coping in maintaining the psychological well-being of mothers of adults with intellectual disability and mental illness. *Journal of Intellectual Disability Research, 47*, 313–327.

Krauss, M. W. (1990). *Later life placements: Precipitating factors and family profiles.* Paper presented at the 114th Annual Meeting of the American Association on Mental Retardation, Atlanta, GA.

Krauss, M. W. (1993). Child-related and parenting stress: Similarities and differences between mothers and fathers of children with disabilities. *American Journal on Mental Retardation, 97*, 393–404.

Krauss, M. W., & Seltzer, M. M. (1993). Current well-being and future plans of older caregiving mothers. *Irish Journal of Psychology, 14*, 47–64.

Krauss, M. W., & Seltzer, M. M. (1995). Long-term caring: Family experiences over the life course. In L. Nadel, & D. Rosenthal (Eds.), *Down syndrome: Living and learning in the community* (pp. 91–98). New York: Wiley-Liss.

Krauss, M. W., & Seltzer, M. M. (1999). An unanticipated life: The impact of lifelong caregiving. In H. Bersani (Ed.), *Responding to the challenge: International trends and current issues in developmental disabilities.* Brookline, MA: Brookline Books.

Krauss, M. W., Seltzer, M. M., Gordon, R., & Friedman, D. H. (1996). Binding ties: The roles of adult siblings of persons with mental retardation. *Mental Retardation, 34*, 83–93.

Krauss, M. W., Seltzer, M. M., & Jacobson, H. T. (2005). Adults with autism living at home or in non-family settings: Positive and negative aspects of residential status. *Journal of Intellectual Disability Research, 49*, 111–124.

Lakin, K. C., Anderson, L., & Prouty, R. (1998). Decreases continue in out-of-home residential placements of children and youth with mental retardation. *Mental Retardation, 36*, 165–167.

Lakin, K. C. (1985). *Demographic studies of residential families for mentally retarded people: A historical overview of methodologies and findings.* Minneapolis: University of Minneapolis, Department of Educational Psychology.

Lancaster, J. B., Altmann, J., Rossi, A. S., & Sherrod, L. T. (Eds.). (1987). *Parenting across the life span: Biosocial dimensions.* New York: Aldine de Gruyter.

Lerner, R. M., & Ryff, C. D. (1978). Implementation of the life-span view of human development: The sample case of attachment. In P. B. Baltes (Ed.), *Life-span development and behavior* (pp. 2–45). New York: Academic Press.

Lounds, J. J., & Seltzer, M. M. (2007). Family impact in adulthood. In S. L. Odom, R. H. Horner, M. Snell, & J. Blancher (Eds.), *Handbook on developmental disabilities* (pp. 552–569). New York: Guilford Press.

Lounds, J. J., Seltzer, M. M., Greenberg, J. S., & Shattuck, P. (2007). Transition and change in adolescents and young adults with autism: Longitudinal effects on maternal well-being. *American Journal on Mental Retardation, 112*, 401–417.

Marcovitch, S., Goldberg, S., MacGregor, D., & Lojkasek, M. (1986). Patterns of temperament in three groups of developmentally delayed preschool children: Mother and father ratings. *Developmental and Behavioral Pediatrics, 7*, 247–252.

Meyers, C. D., Borthwick, S. A., & Eyman, R. (1985). Place of residence by age, ethnicity, and level of retardation of the mentally retarded/developmentally disabled population in California. *American Journal of Mental Deficiency, 90*, 266–270.

Noh, S., Dumas, J. E., Wolf, L. C., & Fisman, S. N. (1989). Delineating sources of stress in parents of exceptional children. *Family Relations, 38*, 456–461.

Nydegger, C. N., & Mitteness, L. S. (1996). Midlife: The prime of fathers. In C. Ryff, & M. Seltzer (Eds.), *The parental experience at midlife*. Chicago: University of Chicago Press.

Orsmond, G. I., & Seltzer, M. M. (2000). Brothers and sisters of adults with mental retardation: The gendered nature of the sibling relationship. *American Journal on Mental Retardation, 105*, 486–508.

Orsmond, G. I., & Seltzer, M. M. (2007a). Siblings of individuals with autism or Down syndrome: Effects on adult lives. *Journal of Intellectual Disability Research, 51*, 682–696.

Orsmond, G. I., & Seltzer, M. M. (2007b). Siblings of individuals with autism spectrum disorders across the life course. *Mental Retardation and Developmental Disabilities Research Reviews, 13*, 313–320.

Orsmond, G. I., Seltzer, M. M., Krauss, M. W., & Hong, J. (2003). Behavior problems in adults with mental retardation and maternal well-being: Examination of the direction of effects. *American Journal on Mental Retardation, 108*, 257–271.

Orsmond, G. I., Seltzer, M. M., Greenberg, J. S., & Krauss, M. W. (2006). Mother-child relationship quality among adolescents and adults with autism. *American Journal on Mental Retardation, 111*, 121–137.

Parke, R. D. (1988). Families in life-span perspective: A multilevel developmental approach. In E. M. Hetherington, R. M. Lerner, & M. Perlmutter (Eds.), *Child development in life-span perspective*. Hillsdale, NJ: Erlbaum.

Pearlin, L. I. (1989). The sociological study of stress. *Journal of Health and Social Behavior, 30*, 241–256.

Pearlin, L. I. (1992). The careers of caregivers. *The Gerontologist, 32*, 647.

Perry, A., Harris, K., & Minnes, P. (2004). Family environments and family harmony: An exploration across severity, age, and type of DD. *Journal on Developmental Disabilities, 11*, 17–29.

Poehlmann, J., Clements, M., Abbeduto, L., & Farsad, V. (2005). Family experiences associated with a child's diagnosis of fragile X or Down syndrome: Evidence for disruption and resilience. *Mental Retardation, 43*, 255–267.

Prouty, R., Lakin, K. C., Coucouvanis, K., & Anderson, L. (2005). Progress toward a national objective of Healthy People 2010: "Reduce to zero the number of children 17 years and younger living in congregate care." *Mental Retardation, 43*, 456–460.

Pruchno, R. A., & Patrick, J. H. (1999). Effects of formal and familial residential plans for adults with mental retardation on the aging mothers. *American Journal on Mental Retardation, 104*, 38–52.

Pruchno, R. A., Peters, N. P. & Burant, C. J. (1996). Child life events, parent child disagreements, and parent well-being: Model development and testing. In C. Ryff, & M. Seltzer (Eds.), *The parental experience at midlife*. Chicago: University of Chicago Press.

Rizzolo, M. C., Hemp, R., Braddock, D. & Pomeranz-Essley, A. (2004). *The state of the states in developmental disabilities*. Washington, DC: American Association on Mental Retardation.

Sarimski, K. (1997). Behavioural phenotypes and family stress in three mental retardation syndromes. *European Child and Adolescent Psychiatry, 6*, 26–31.

Seltzer, G. B., Begun, A., Seltzer, M. M., & Krauss, M. W. (1991). Adults with mental retardation and their aging mothers: Impacts of siblings. *Family Relations, 40*, 310–317.

Seltzer, M. M., Floyd, F. J., & Hindes, A. R. (2004a). Research methods in intellectual disabilities: The family context. In E. Emerson, C. Hatton, T. Thompson & T. R. Parmenter (Eds.), *The international handbook of applied research in intellectual disabilities*. Hoboken, NJ: Wiley.

Seltzer, M. M., Greenberg, J. S., Floyd, F. J., Pettee, Y., & Hong, J. (2001). Life course impacts of parenting a child with a disability. *American Journal on Mental Retardation, 106*, 265–286.

Seltzer, M. M., Greenberg, J. S., & Krauss, M. W. (1995). A comparison of coping strategies of aging mothers of adults with mental illness or mental retardation. *Psychology and Aging, 10*, 64–75.

Seltzer, M. M., Greenberg, J. S., Krauss, M. W., & Hong, J. (1997). Predictors of outcomes of the end of co-resident caregiving in aging families of adults with mental retardation or mental illness. *Family Relations, 46*, 13–22.

Seltzer, M. M., & Krauss, M. W. (1984). Placement alternatives for mentally retarded children and their families. In J. Blacher (Ed.), *Severely handicapped children and their families: Research in review* (pp. 143–175). New York: Academic Press.

Seltzer, M. M., & Krauss, M. W. (1994). Aging parents with co-resident adult children: The impact of lifelong caregiving. In M. M. Seltzer, M. W. Krauss, & M. P. Janicki (Eds.), *Life course perspectives on adulthood and old age* (pp. 105–114). Washington, DC: American Association on Mental Retardation.

Seltzer, M. M., & Krauss, M. W. (1998). Families of adults with Down syndrome. In J. F. Miller, L. A. Leavitt, & M. Leddy (Eds.), *Communication development in young children with Down syndrome*. Baltimore: Brookes.

Seltzer, M. M., Krauss, M. W., Hong, J., & Orsmond, G. I. (2001a). Continuity or discontinuity of family involvement following residential transitions of adults who have mental retardation. *Mental Retardation, 39*, 181–194.

Seltzer, M. M., Krauss, M. W., Orsmond, G. I., & Vestal, C. (2001b). Families of adolescents and adults with autism: Uncharted territory. In L. M. Glidden (Ed.), *International review of research on mental retardation* Vol. 23 (pp. 267–294). San Diego: Academic Press.

Seltzer, M. M., Krauss, M. W., Shattuck, P. T., Orsmond, G., Swe, A., & Lord, C. (2003). The symptoms of autism spectrum disorders in adolescence and adulthood. *Journal of Autism and Developmental Disorders, 33*, 565–581.

Seltzer, M. M., Krauss, M. W., & Tsunematsu, N. (1993). Adults with Down syndrome and their aging mothers: Diagnostic group differences. *American Journal on Mental Retardation, 97,* 464–508.

Seltzer, M. M., & Ryff, C. (1994). Parenting across the lifespan: The normative and nonnormative cases. In D. L. Fetherman, R. Lerner, & M. Perlmutter (Eds.), *Life-span development and behavior* Vol. 12 (pp. 1–40). Hillsdale, NJ: Erlbaum.

Seltzer, M. M., Shattuck, P., Abbeduto, L., & Greenberg, J. (2004b). The trajectory of development in adolescents and adults with autism. *Mental Retardation and Developmental Disabilities Research Reviews, 10,* 234–247.

Shattuck, P. T., Seltzer, M. M., Greenberg, J. S., Orsmond, G. I., Bolt, D., Kring, S., et al. (2007). Change in autism symptoms and maladaptive behaviors in adolescents and adults with an autism spectrum disorder. *Journal of Autism and Developmental Disorders, 37,* 1735–1747.

Shonkoff, J. P., Hauser-Cram, P., Krauss, M. W., & Upshur, C. (1992). Development of infants with disabilities and their families: Implications for theory and service delivery. *Monographs of the Society for Research in Child Development (57, Serial No. 6).* Chicago, IL: University of Chicago Press.

Silverberg, S. B. (1996). Parent well-being at their children's transition to adolescence. In C. Ryff, & M. Seltzer (Eds.), *The parental experience at midlife.* Chicago: University of Chicago Press.

Smith, L. E., Hong, J., Seltzer, M. M., Greenberg, J. S., Almeida, D. M., & Bishop, S. L. (2009). *Daily experiences among mothers of adolescents and adults with autism spectrum disorder, 40,* 167–178.

Smith, L. E., Seltzer, M. M., Greenberg, J. S., Tager-Flusberg, H., & Carter, A. S. (2008). A comparative analysis of well-being and coping among mothers of toddlers and mothers of adolescents with ASD. *Journal of Autism and Developmental Disorders, 38,* 876–889.

Stoneman, Z., & Berman, P. W. (Eds.). (1993). *The effects of mental retardation, disability, and illness on sibling relationships.* Baltimore: Brookes.

Suelzle, M., & Keenan, V. (1981). Changes in family support networks over the life cycle of mentally retarded persons. *American Journal of Mental Deficiency, 86,* 267–274.

Tausig, M. (1985). Factors in family decision-making about placement for developmentally disabled individuals. *American Journal of Mental Deficiency, 89,* 352–361.

Townsend, A., Noelker, L., Deimling, G., & Bass, D. (1989). Longitudinal impact of interhousehold caregiving on adult children's mental health. *Psychology and Aging, 4,* 393–401.

Turnbull, A. P., Summers, J. A., & Brotherson, M. J. (1986). Family life cycle: Theoretical and empirical implications and future directions for families with mentally retarded members. In J. J. Gallagher, & P. M. Vietze (Eds.), *Families of handicapped persons: Research, programs, and policy issues.* Baltimore: Brookes.

van Lieshout, C. F. M., de Meyer, R. E., Curfs, L. M. G., & Fryns, J. P. (1998). Family contexts, parental behaviour, and personality profiles of children and adolescents with Prader-Willi, Fragile-X, or Williams syndrome. *Journal of Child Psychology and Psychiatry, 39,* 699–710.

PART 7

Conclusions and Future Directions

On Knowing More: Future Issues for Developmental Approaches to Understanding Persons with Intellectual Disability

Jacob A. Burack, Robert M. Hodapp, Grace Iarocci, *and* Edward Zigler

Abstract

In this chapter, we summarize the contributions to this volume and to the evolving field of developmental research on intellectual disability (ID). The developmental theory and methodology reviewed in this volume reflect a level of precision and sophistication that could not have been imagined in our previous volumes from 1990 and 1998. These advances have led to an increasingly nuanced understanding of syndrome-specific cognitive and social developmental pathways, gene-brain-behavior relations, and transactions of individuals with their families and environments.

Keywords: Intellectual disability, developmental disability, genetics, etiology

In the opening chapter of this volume, we offered the adage that "the more you know the less you know." The book's many excellent contributions highlight this state of affairs, documenting both considerable advances and vast gaps in our understanding of the development of persons with ID. By encouraging authors to provide the framework for their own chapters, we hoped to provide greater insight into the ways in which the development of persons with ID is conceptualized, studied, and discussed.

Partly as a result, the contributions are organized in different ways, with a range of emphases and implications. Some chapters primarily concern single topical areas, which are examined across different syndromes. Others are focused on a single syndrome and provide insight into the etiology-related profiles or development of that specific group. In some cases, the emphasis is on what can be learned about the development of one or more syndromes; in others the lesson concerns development more generally. In some chapters, the focus is on the person's own development, while in others the effects on others in that person's life are highlighted.

Such cross-chapter diversity represents significant progress in studying ID from a developmental perspective. Consider the history of our several volumes on this topic. The title of our volume from two decades ago, *Issues in the Developmental Approach to Mental Retardation* (Hodapp, Burack, & Zigler, 1990b) implied a single developmental framework for understanding ID. That volume included the work of the small group of developmental researchers concerned with ID. Although the theory espoused was not entirely uniform, much discussion was based on the initial conceptualization of the developmental approach by Zigler (1967, 1969) and colleagues (Zigler & Balla, 1982; Zigler & Hodapp, 1986). Several chapters were focused on individuals with familial IDs (then called *familial mental retardation*), those whose ID is not due to any specific organic insult but who simply fall at the low end of the IQ curve (see Hodapp, Burack, & Zigler, 1990a; Zigler, 1967, 1969)). With the emphasis on persons with familial ID, developmental conceptualizations mostly concerned Piagetian-type cognitive sequences (Hodapp, 1990; Weisz & Zigler, 1979) and structures (Weiss, Weisz, & Bromfield, 1986; Weisz & Yeates, 1981). In this framework, development among persons with ID was generally considered to be typical, albeit at a slower rate and with a lower eventual asymptote (see Weisz, 1990; Weisz, Yeates, & Zigler, 1982; for a slightly differing perspective, see Mundy & Kasari, 1990).

In contrast to his developmental formulations about persons with familial ID, Zigler (1967, 1969) had long contended that "all bets were off" with regard to the uniformity of development among persons with clear physiological or neurological damage. He noted that, "if the etiology of the phenotypic intelligence (as measured by an IQ) of the two groups differs, it is far from logical to assert that the course of development is the same, or even that similar contents in their behaviors are mediated by exactly the same processes. . . ." (Zigler, 1969, p. 533).

Even in that earlier volume, however, attempts were made to extend the so-called developmental approach to individuals with different genetic etiologies. Although articulated when the Zeitgeist was to study persons with ID as a single population with a common defect, Zigler's perspective was more prophetic than he realized. In particular, many syndromes are now associated with specific developmental profiles, with relative strengths in some domains of functioning and relative weaknesses in others (Burack, 1990; Burack, Hodapp, & Zigler, 1988; Dykens, Hodapp, & Finucane, 2000). In parallel with the wider field of developmental psychology, researchers of persons with ID began calling into question the universality of Piagetian developmental structures, or relations across areas, even if Piagetian sequences might in many cases remain tenable.

Within this context, the developmental approach found a champion in Cicchetti, who, along with colleagues, argued for a liberal, or expanded, developmental approach. As articulated by Cicchetti (1990) in our original volume, meaningful organization across developmental structures might be found even among persons with specific syndromes, including those with Down syndrome (DS; Cicchetti, 1990; Cicchetti & Pogge-Hesse, 1982). Rather than use the difference in the development of children with DS as a reason for abandoning traditional developmental theory, Cicchetti and Pogge-Hesse (1982) used it as an opportunity to expand developmental theory and to provide lessons about development more generally (see also Hodapp & Burack, 1990). The second chapter on a specific syndrome, by Dykens and Leckman (1990), concerned

fragile X syndrome (FXS). That chapter reflected research on a little understood syndrome and highlighted the nature of potential etiology-related patterns and trajectories of development.

The need to differentiate by etiology was clearly articulated throughout our second edited volume, the *Handbook of Mental Retardation and Development* (Burack, Hodapp, & Zigler, 1998). With overview chapters on genetics (Simonoff, Bolton, & Rutter, 1998) and neuropsychology (Pennington & Bennetto, 1998), essential differences in behavior were highlighted across various etiological groups. Such profiles of relative strengths and weaknesses in different etiological group were considered in sensorimotor processing (Dunst, 1998), early communication (Mundy, 1998), language (Fowler, 1998; Tager-Flusberg & Sullivan 1998), symbolic play (Beeghly, 1998), attention (Iarocci & Burack, 1998), and metacognitive processing (Bebko & Luhaorg, 1998). Granted, at this time, more fine-tuned analyses revealed similarities among some syndromes on certain developmental domains (Hodapp & Dykens, 1994; Hodapp, 1997) and that the behavioral effects of etiologies were probabilistic (Dykens, 1995; Rondal, 1995)—rarely does every person with a syndrome show every characteristic, nor is every characteristic found in every person with the syndrome. Still, etiology-related behavioral characteristics vary greatly from one syndrome to another, and most individuals with a specific syndrome show many of their syndrome's behavioral characteristics.

Beyond the emphasis of etiology per se, Zigler's original developmental approach was also expanded in other ways in our earlier volumes. One, in line with his focus on the noncognitive lives of persons with ID, Zigler (1970) had emphasized that social-personality-motivational processes were identical for those with and without ID, but that the behavior of persons with ID is influenced by their life experiences, which often included some combination of institutionalization, social and educational exclusion, and histories of failure. For example, to avoid inevitable failure, these persons are more likely to use outer-directed, rather than self-chosen strategies, and to choose small-but-safe rewards rather than bigger but less certain rewards (Hodapp & Zigler, 1986; Zigler, 1970; Zigler & Balla, 1982). By including social and emotional domains within the purview of the developmental approach, the researchers highlighted the humanity—the "whole person"—of persons with ID.

But a whole-person approach would only be complete when persons with ID were also considered within their actual environments, and within the context of how they are influenced by and influence these environments. By our first volume in 1990, the environment had already been extensively addressed in two ways. One was the centuries-old discussion of the influence of the environment on IQ, now reframed within developmental ideas of risk and resilience (e.g., Sameroff, 1990). The second was the work by Zigler and colleagues on how different social-educational environments influenced the personality-motivational characteristics of persons with ID (e.g., Merighi, Edison, & Zigler, 1990).

Although both areas imply bidirectional person–environment interactions, neither highlighted the continuing, ongoing transactions between persons with ID and the world around them. Again influenced by advances in the broader field of developmental psychology (Bronfenbrenner, 1979, 1986), researchers began to consider persons with ID within the contexts of many different aspects of the environment (also see Sameroff, 1990). By our second volume in 1998 (Burack, Hodapp, & Zigler, 1998), one of those environments—the family—had begun to receive extended attention. In addition to a chapter on the broader environment (Greenbaum & Auerbach, 1998), that second volume featured individual chapters on mothers (Marfo, Dedrik, & Barbour, 1998; Shapiro, Blacher, & Lopez, 1998), siblings (Stoneman, 1998), and the larger family (Stoneman, 1998). This broader theoretical perspective on the systems of influences on the developing child was needed in order to consider the potential variability in development that may be associated with unique experiences and environmental conditions. The understanding of the genetic constraints on development are now balanced with a more nuanced understanding of the way choices in parenting styles, siblings, and family relations may be powerful determinants of variability in development. There is now a clearer commitment to the importance of considering the impact of the disability on both the individuals and on meaningful others in their lives. The path was open for fuller, more elaborated developmental approaches to children and adults with disabilities.

Summing Up: "The More We Know . . ."

If the prior two decades are seen as a prelude to the current volume, advances are evident on a number of levels. Most important, the research reviewed in these chapters is characterized by a level of precision and diversity that could not have been imagined in 1990 or in 1998. Beyond advances in clinical or behavioral genetics, electroencephalograms, or magnetic resonance imaging, the sophistication in understanding the domains and even the subdomains of development for specific etiological groups is apparent. For example, researchers can no longer simply note that children with DS have a relative weakness in language, but rather must juxtapose areas and subareas of grammar, vocabulary, and pragmatics. On topics in which we once only had questions and theories, we now have concrete evidence, and our subsequent questions and theories have become increasingly sophisticated. The cycle continues as increasing precision leads to new findings, questions, and theories, which in turn lead to new studies and evidence, leading to even further questions and theories.

In a similar way, virtually every chapter in this volume is characterized by links of etiology to subdomains within the general field of developmental psychology. More fine-tuned relations between genetics and particular areas of cognitive functioning are presented with regard to specific etiological groups, as are more detailed understandings of neuropsychological processes and brain–behavior relations. Such precision led to better understandings of specific syndromes, but also to advances in the relevant scientific subfields. Increasingly, we have fine-tuned profiles of relative strengths and weaknesses across many different subareas of cognition for increasing numbers of etiological groups.

At this point, a few general conclusions seem justified. For example, researchers and practitioners must now abandon their earlier notions of some universal deficit as underlying behavioral functioning for all persons with ID. There is no single "core" deficit that accounts for behavioral functioning for all persons with IDs. Similarly, individuals with specific etiologies often are prone to etiology-related maladaptive behavior and psychopathology, such as the extremely high prevalence rates of hyperphagia in Prader-Willi syndrome (Dykens & Cassidy, 1999), increased rates of fears and anxieties in Williams syndrome (Dykens, 2003), and social avoidance and autistic symptoms (and ASD itself) in high percentages of children with FXS (Philofsky et al., 2004; Scambler et al., 2007).

Even the relations with and impact on the family are increasingly studied within the context of etiology. Accordingly, we see a movement to determine whether—and why—families of children with DS seem to cope better than families of children with other ID conditions (Hodapp, 2007).

Do certain child characteristics "elicit" reactions from others (e.g., Fidler, 2011, Chapter 23, this volume), or might characteristics of the mother, father, or family overall most influence parent–family functioning? How does the child's cognitive-linguistic profile, behavior problems, or other characteristics predispose reactions from mothers, fathers, siblings, or the family as a whole (Hodapp, 2004)? Such questions are actively being studied by today's developmentally-oriented researchers.

Going Forward: "The More We Will Know . . ."

We end this chapter by discussing three issues for future work. In various ways, all are foreshadowed in many of this volume's chapters.

Greater Understanding of Etiology-related Trajectories and Profiles

As researchers increasingly examine development in children with different genetic etiologies, they appreciate how an individual child's developmental rate can change. Some changes seemingly relate to changes in the children themselves—for example, changes related to puberty or brain maturation—whereas others may relate to task difficulties. Young children with DS, who often show relatively high IQs in the infant and toddler years, may slow in their development as they experience difficulties in mastering their language's earliest grammatical relations. This issue of "age-related" versus "task-related" slowing, earlier discussed in relation to children with DS (Hodapp & Zigler, 1990), is now examined in terms of children with Williams syndrome, autism, and other conditions. The workings of such age- and task-related changes—both the "when" and the "why"—will increasingly be examined in future years.

Increased attention will also undoubtedly be devoted to the development of etiology-specific profiles. For example, in many cases of the early cognitive-linguistic development of children with different genetic disorders, very slight advantages and disadvantages at earlier ages may, over time, grow into the etiology-specific profiles that are evident among older children. This is seen in the recent work on the growing connection between cognitive-linguistic weaknesses and sociability among infants and toddlers with DS. For example, in examining mother–child interactions, Fidler, Philofsky, Hepburn, and Rogers (2005) found that infants with DS show particular difficulties in means–ends thinking, or tasks that involve the idea that objects

(e.g., stick, stool) can be used as a means for obtaining desired other objects. Such deficits seemingly then relate to increased amounts of looking to others for solutions to difficult problems among these children. Eventually, "the coupling of poor strategic [i.e., means–ends] thinking and strengths in social relatedness is hypothesized to lead to the less persistent and overly social personality-motivational orientation observed in this population" (Fidler, 2006, p. 147). Although much remains to be studied, such early developments—and their effects on emerging cognitive-linguistic profiles and personality-motivational characteristics—may hold the key to understanding many etiology-related behaviors among persons with DS and other genetic etiologies of ID.

Understanding Better the Role of Genetics

A second future area of increased work involves genetics. Three aspects of upcoming genetic studies seem noteworthy. One area is how particular genetic anomalies eventually predispose children to certain behavioral outcomes. For example, what is it about having a third chromosome 21 (i.e., DS) that ultimately leads to specific behavioral profiles, trajectories, or personality styles? What is it about having a missing part of the long arm of chromosome 15 (deletion form of Prader-Willi syndrome) that predisposes individuals to show extreme, sometimes even life-threatening, hyperphagia (i.e., overeating)? Why is FXS so tied to gaze aversion and other symptoms of ASD? Such questions are increasingly studied, and ideas of critical genetic regions and pathways from gene to brain to behavior are increasingly raised.

Two, "background genetics" play an essential role, as the genetic contribution to most behavioral characteristics does not solely involve trisomy, deletion, or other genetic anomaly. As shown by behavior geneticists for typically developing children, a person's personality, general intelligence, specific intellectual abilities (the various "s" factors in intelligence), and other behavioral characteristics are partially attributable to their genetic inheritance. Over the next few years, researchers will likely examine heredibility for components of intelligence, language, personality, and maladaptive behavior/psychopathology (e.g., depression, anxiety) among children with different etiological conditions. Similarly, we do not yet know whether one of behavior genetics' most intriguing findings—that for many behavioral traits heritability rates rise (instead of decline) as children get older (Plomin & Spinath,

2006)—will replicate for children with any or all of the different genetic etiologies.

A final genetic issue concerns interactions between genes and environment, or so-called G × E interactions. G × E interactions concern the ways in which specific environments do not affect everyone equally, but instead most affect those who already show certain genetic susceptibilities. One potential example for IDs involves the connections between child abuse and subsequent antisocial behavior. As Caspi et al. (2002) demonstrated, only those children who experienced child abuse *and* had a particular variant of the *MAOA* gene were at high risk of becoming antisocial; neither child abuse nor the presence of the *MAOA* variant, by itself, was usually enough for antisocial behavior to develop. These types of relationships among factors may be particularly essential to outcome as children with IDs are four to ten times more likely to be abused as compared to nondisabled children (Fisher, Hodapp, & Dykens, 2007).

Beyond child abuse per se, the general concept of G × E interactions should prove helpful to developmentally oriented research on ID. Especially for children with particular genetic syndromes, almost all outcomes are probabilistic, with not every individual showing any expected outcome. Some variability in outcome may be associated with polymorphisms that alter the expression or function of genes, and these may interact with poor or stressful environments that lead to less-than-optimal developmental outcomes. In this regard, the impact of poverty on the outcomes of children and adults with specific etiologies and their families would be especially informative as children with disabilities more often reside in single-parent, poorer, and minority families (Emerson, 2007; Fujiura & Yamaki, 1997)

Connecting Person–Environmental Reactions to Etiology-related Characteristics

A third focus of future research is how certain child characteristics elicit reactions from others in their environment (see Fidler, 2011, Chapter 23, this volume). This listing of potential elicitors is fairly long, with many elicitors appearing more often among persons with certain genetic conditions (Hodapp & Dykens, 2009). For example, compared to other children (with or without IDs), children with DS are more likely to have immature faces, with large and round faces, large eyes, and lower-set facial features. Among children and adults without disabilities, such "baby faces" elicit warm, caring,

and caretaking responses from others (Zebrowitz, 1997). So, too, do such caregiving responses appear to occur in reaction to faces of children with DS, at least as compared to same-aged children without disabilities and to those with other, more angular and adult-like faces (Fidler & Hodapp, 1999). In the same way, children with particular conditions are also more likely to display other eliciting characteristics (Hodapp & Dykens, 2009). Certain of these characteristics relate to personality; others relate to the presence, type, timing, or severity of psychopathology-maladaptive behaviors; health problems; motor or physical problems or other caregiving challenges; or even the onset of specific problems (e.g., onset of schizophrenia in adolescence-young adulthood; Seltzer et al., 2004). Although few potential elicitors have yet received sustained research attention, each likely influences family members and others in the child's environment.

Conversely, certain conditions show what might be termed "associated characteristics" (Hodapp, 1999). For example, infants with DS continue to be born to mothers who are on average older, more educated, more likely to be married, and of higher family socioeconomic status (Grosse, 2010). As compared to parents of children without disabilities, the parents of children with DS are slightly less likely to divorce (Urbano & Hodapp, 2007). Are these differences due to characteristics of the child (e.g., most children with DS display a more sociable personality), to characteristics of their parents or families (older, more educated parents), to the child's having a more well-known syndrome, or to some combination of the above? Such advantages and disadvantages may even change over the child's development. In a recent comparison of families of children with autism versus families of children without disability, Hartley et al. (2010) found that divorce rates were comparable for the two groups early on, but were higher among the families with children with autism as the children got older. In future studies, many of these elicitation factors, as well as how they operate as the child develops, should be discussed.

Conclusion: Up the Spiral Staircase?

We began this concluding chapter, as well as the book itself, with the idea that the more one knows, the less one knows. In some ways, this idea seems depressing. Why study anything, after all, if one ends up further behind than one started?

Ultimately, however, we feel that science progresses, and that even as we end with more questions than which we started, a general upward progression can be cited. This issue, long discussed in the philosophy of science (e.g., Kuhn, 1970), also applies to studies of individuals with ID when examined with developmental approaches. Do we know more today than we did when Zigler (1967) formally began developmental approaches over 40 years ago? Do we know more today compared to the information reviewed in our own volumes in 1990 and 1998?

To us, the answer seems obvious. We know much more today about development in specific etiological conditions, in specific areas and subareas of development, in connections among these subareas themselves, and in how different behavioral subareas connect to underlying brain structures. Similarly, concerning the environment, we know much more about mothers, fathers, siblings, and families as a whole, about schools, communities, and the workings of environments and gene–environment and environment–person interactions more generally. Some of this knowledge even links diverse levels of environment together, whereas some concerns the lifespan development of the person with specific etiologies or changing interpersonal (mostly familial) environments in which they live.

Ultimately, then, we may indeed be left with more questions over time, but our questions become more specific, more interesting, and (we hope) more relevant to the lives of these individuals. In some sense, we are becoming more "differentiated" and, to some extent, also more "hierarchically integrated." And, as we have been repeatedly instructed by Werner (1948) and other developmental thinkers, increasing differentiation and hierarchic integration constitute the hallmarks of higher levels of development, of any living organism (or living field of study).

References

Bebko, J. M., & Luhaorg, H. (1998). The development of strategy use and metacognitive processing in mental retardation: Some sources of difficulty. In J. A. Burack, R. M. Hodapp, & E. Zigler (Eds.), *Handbook of mental retardation and development* (pp. 382–408). New York: Cambridge University Press.

Beeghly, M. (1998). Emergence of symbolic play: Perspectives from typical and atypical development. In J. A. Burack, R. M. Hodapp, & E. Zigler (Eds.), *Handbook of mental retardation and development* (pp. 242–279). New York: Cambridge University Press.

Bronfenbrenner, U. (1979). *The ecology of human development: Experiments by design and nature.* Cambridge, MA: Harvard University Press.

Bronfenbrenner, U. (1986). Ecology of the family as a context of human development: Research perspectives. *Developmental Psychology, 22,* 723–742. doi: 10.1037/0012-1649.22.6.723.

Burack, J. A., Hodapp, R. M., & Zigler, E. (Eds.) (1998). *Handbook of mental retardation and development.* New York: Cambridge University Press.

Burack, J. A. (1990). Differentiating mental retardation: The two-group approach and beyond. In R. M. Hodapp, J. A. Burack, & E. Zigler (Eds.), *Issues in the developmental approach to mental retardation* (pp. 27–48). New York: Cambridge University Press.

Caspi, A., McClay, J., Moffitt, T.E., Mill, J., Martin, J., Craig, I.W., et al. (2002). Role of genotype in the cycle of violence in maltreated children. *Science, 297,* 851–854. doi: 10.1126/science.1072290.

Cicchetti, D. (1990). The organization and coherence of socioemotional, cognitive, and representational development: Illustrations through a developmental psychopathology perspective on Down syndrome and child maltreatment. In R. Thompson (Ed.), *Nebraska symposium on motivation:* Vol. 36. *Socioemotional development* (pp. 266–375). Lincoln: University of Nebraska Press.

Cicchetti, D., & Pogge-Hesse, P. (1982). Possible contributions of the study of organically retarded persons to developmental theory. In E. Zigler, & D. Balla (Eds.), *Mental retardation: the developmental difference controversy.* Hillsdale, NJ: Erlbaum.

Dunst, C. J. (1998). Sensorimotor development and developmental disabilities. In J. A. Burack, R. M. Hodapp, & E. Zigler (Eds.), *Handbook of mental retardation and development* (pp. 135–182). New York: Cambridge University Press.

Dykens, E. M. (1995). Measuring behavioral phenotypes: Provocations from the "new genetics." *American Journal on Mental Retardation, 99,* 522–532.

Dykens, E. M. (2003). Anxiety, fears, and phobias in persons with Williams syndrome. *Developmental Neuropsychology, 23,* 291–316. doi: 10.1207/S15326942DN231&2_13.

Dykens, E., Hodapp, R., & Finucane, B. (2000). *Genetics and mental retardation syndromes: A new look at behavior and interventions.* Baltimore: Paul Brookes.

Dykens, E. M., & Cassidy, S. B. (1999). Prader-Willi syndrome. In S. Goldstein, & C. Reynolds (Eds.), *Neurodevelopmental and genetic disorders in children* (pp. 525–545). New York, NY: Guilford Press.

Dykens, E. M., & Leckman, J. F. (1990). Developmental issues in fragile X syndrome. In R. M. Hodapp, J. A. Burack & E. Zigler (Eds.), *Issues in the developmental approach to mental retardation* (pp. 226–245). New York: Cambridge University Press.

Emerson, E. (2007). Poverty and people with intellectual disabilities. *Mental Retardation and Developmental Disabilities Research Reviews, 13,* 107–113. doi: 10.1002/mrdd.20144.

Fidler, D. J. (2006). The emergence of a syndrome-specific personality profile in young children with Down syndrome. In J. A. Rondal, & J. Perera (Eds.), *Down syndrome: Neurobehavioural specificity* (pp. 139–152). London: Wiley.

Fidler, D. J. (2011). Child eliciting effects in families of children with intellectual disability: Proximal and distal perspectives. In J. A. Burack, R. M. Hodapp, G. Iarocci, & E. Zigler (Eds.), *The Oxford handbook of intellectual disability and development,* 2nd ed. New York: Oxford University Press.

Fidler, D. J., & Hodapp, R. M. (1999). Craniofacial maturity and perceived personality in children with Down syndrome. *American Journal on Mental Retardation, 104,* 410–421.

Fidler, D. J., Philofsky, A., Hepburn, S. L., & Rogers, S. J. (2005). Nonverbal requesting and problem-solving by toddlers with Down syndrome. *American Journal on Mental Retardation, 110,* 312–322.

Fisher, M. H., Hodapp, R. M., & Dykens, E. M. (2007). Child abuse among children with disabilities: What we know and what we need to know. *International Review of Research in Mental Retardation, 35,* 251–289. doi: 10.1016/S0074–7750(07)35007–6.

Fujiura, G. T., & Yamaki, K. (1997). Analysis of ethnic variations in developmental disability prevalence and household economic status. *Mental Retardation, 35,* 286–294.

Greenbaum, C. W., & Auerbach, J. D. (1998). The environment of the child with mental retardation: Risk, vulnerability and resilience. In J. A. Burack, R. M. Hodapp, & E. Zigler (Eds.), *Handbook of mental retardation and development* (pp. 583–605). New York: Cambridge University Press.

Grosse, S. D. (2010). Sociodemographic characteristics of families of children with Down syndrome and the economic impacts of child disability on families. *International Review of Research in Mental Retardation, 39,* 257–294.

Hartley, S. L., Barker, E. T., Seltzer, M. M., Floyd, F., Greenberg, J., Orsmond, G., & Bolt, D. (2010). The relative risk and timing of divorce in families of children with an autism spectrum disorder. *Journal of Family Psychology, 24,* 449–457.

Hodapp, R. M. (1990). One road or many? Issues in the similar-sequence hypothesis. In R. M. Hodapp, J. A. Burack, & E. Zigler (Eds.), *Issues in the developmental approach to mental retardation.* New York: Cambridge University Press.

Hodapp, R. M. (1997). Direct and indirect effects of different genetic disorders of mental retardation. *American Journal on Mental Retardation, 102,* 67–79.

Hodapp, R. M. (1999). Indirect effects of genetic mental retardation disorders: Theoretical and methodological issues. *International Review of Research in Mental Retardation, 22,* 27–50. doi: 10.1016/S0074–7750(08)60130–5.

Hodapp, R. M. (2004). Studying interactions, reactions, and perceptions: Can genetic disorders serve as behavioral proxies? *Journal of Autism and Developmental Disorders, 34,* 29–34. doi: 10.1023/B:JADD.0000018071.02942.00.

Hodapp, R. M. (2007). Families of persons with Down syndrome: New perspectives, findings and research and service needs. *Mental Retardation and Developmental Disabilities Research Reviews, 13,* 279–287. doi: 10.1002/mrdd.20160.

Hodapp, R. M., & Burack, J. A. (1990). What mental retardation teaches us about typical development: The examples of sequences, rates, and cross-domain relations. *Development and Psychopathology, 2,* 213–225. doi:10.1017/S0954579400000730.

Hodapp, R. M., Burack, J. A., & Zigler, E. (1990a). The developmental perspective in the field of mental retardation. In R. M. Hodapp, J. A. Burack, & E. Zigler (Eds.), *Issues in the developmental approach to mental retardation* (pp. 3–26). New York: Cambridge University Press.

Hodapp, R. M., Burack, J. A., & Zigler, E. (1990b). Summing up and going forward: New directions in the developmental approach to mental retardation. In R. M. Hodapp, J. A. Burack, & E. Zigler (Eds.), *Issues in the developmental approach to mental retardation* (pp. 294–312). New York: Cambridge University Press.

Hodapp, R. M., Burack, J. A., & Zigler, E. (1998). Developmental approaches to mental retardation: A short introduction. In J. A. Burack, R. M. Hodapp, & E. Zigler (Eds.), *Handbook of mental retardation and development* (pp. 3–19). New York: Cambridge University Press.

Hodapp, R. M., & Dykens, E. M. (2009). Intellectual disabilities and child psychiatry: Looking to the future. *Journal of Child Psychology and Psychiatry, 50,* 99–107. doi: 10.1111/j.1469–7610.2008.02038.x.

Hodapp, R. M., & Zigler, E. (1986). Definition and classification of mental-retardation–Comments. *American Journal of Mental Deficiency, 91,* 117–119.

Hodapp, R. M., & Zigler, E. (1990). Applying the developmental perspective to individuals with Down Syndrome. In D. Cicchetti, & M. Beeghly (Eds.) *Children with Down syndrome: A developmental perspective* (pp. 1–28). New York: Cambridge University Press.

Iarocci, G., & Burack, J. A. (1998). Understanding the development of attention in persons with mental retardation: Challenging the myths. *Handbook of mental retardation and development.* New York: Cambridge University Press.

Kuhn, T. S. (1970). *The structure of scientific revolutions* (2nd ed.). Chicago: University of Chicago Press.

Marfo, K., Dedrick, C. F., & Barbour, N., 1998 Mother-child interactions and the development of children with mental retardation. *Handbook of mental retardation and development.* New York: Cambridge University Press.

Merighi J., Edison M., & Zigler E. (1990). The role of motivational factors in the functioning of mentally retarded individuals. In R. M. Hodapp, J. A. Burack, & E. Zigler (Eds.), *Issues in the developmental approach to mental retardation* (pp. 114–134). New York: Cambridge University Press.

Mundy, P., & Kasari, C. (1990). The similar-structure hypothesis and differential rate of development in mental retardation. In R. M. Hodapp, J. A. Burack, & E. Zigler (Eds.), *Issues in the developmental approach to mental retardation* (pp. 71–92). New York: Cambridge University Press.

Pennington, B. F., & Bennetto, L. (1998). Toward a neuropsychology of mental retardation. In J. A. Burack, R. M. Hodapp, & E. Zigler (Eds.), *Handbook of mental retardation and development* (pp 80–114). New York: Cambridge University Press.

Philofsky, A., Hepburn, S. L., Hayes, A., Hagerman, R. J., & Rogers, S. J. (2004). Linguistic and cognitive functioning and autism symptoms in children with fragile X syndrome. *American Journal on Mental Retardation, 109,* 208–218.

Plomin, R., & Spinath, F. M. (2006). Intelligence: Genetics, genes, and genomics. *Journal of Personality and Social Psychology, 86,* 112–129. doi: 10.1037/0022–3514.86.1.112.

Rondal, J. A. (1995). *Exceptional language development in Down syndrome: Implications for the cognition-language relationship.* Cambridge, UK: Cambridge University Press.

Sameroff, A. J. (1990). Neo-environmental perspectives on developmental theory. In R. M. Hodapp, J. A. Burack, & E. Zigler (Eds.), *Issues in the developmental approach to mental retardation* (pp. 93–113). Cambridge, UK: Cambridge University Press.

Scambler, D. J., Hepburn, S. L., Hagerman, R. J., & Rogers, S. J. (2007). A preliminary study of screening for risk of autism in children with fragile X syndrome: Testing two risk cut-offs for the Checklist for Autism in Toddlers. *Journal of Intellectual Disability Research, 51,* 269–276. doi: 10.1111/j.1365–2788.2006.00874.x.

Seltzer, M. M., Abbeduto, L., Krauss, M. W., Greenberg, J., & Swe, A. (2004). Comparison groups in autism family research: Down syndrome, fragile X syndrome, and schizophrenia. *Journal of Autism and Developmental Disorders, 34,* 41–48. doi: 10.1023/B:JADD.0000018073.92982.64.

Shapiro, J., Blacher, J., & Lopez, S. R. (1998). Maternal reactions to children with mental retardation. In J. A. Burack, R. M. Hodapp, & E. Zigler (Eds.), *Handbook of mental retardation and development* (pp. 606–636). New York: Cambridge University Press.

Simonoff, E., Bolton, P., & Rutter, M. (1998). Genetic perception on mental retardation. In J. A. Burack, R. M. Hodapp, & E. Zigler (Eds.), *Handbook of mental retardation and development* (pp. 41–79). New York: Cambridge University Press.

Stoneman, Z. (1998). Research on siblings of children with mental retardation: Contributions of developmental theory and etiology. In J. A. Burack, R. M. Hodapp, & E. Zigler (Eds.), *Handbook of mental retardation and development* (pp. 669–692). New York: Cambridge University Press.

Tager-Flusberg, H., & Sullivan, K. (1998). Early language development in children with mental retardation. In J. A. Burack, R. M. Hodapp, & E. Zigler (Eds.), *Handbook of mental retardation and development* (pp. 208–239). New York: Cambridge University Press.

Urbano, R. C., & Hodapp, R. M. (2007). Divorce in families of children with Down syndrome: A population-based study. *American Journal on Mental Retardation, 112,* 261–274.

Weisz, J. R. (1990). Cultural-familial mental retardation: A developmental perspective on cognitive performance and "helpless" behavior. In R. M. Hodapp, J. A. Burack, & E. Zigler (Eds.), *Issues in the developmental approach to mental retardation* (pp. 137–168). New York: Cambridge University Press.

Weisz, B., Weisz, J. R., & Bromfield, R. (1986). Performance of retarded and nonretarded persons on information-processing tasks: Further tests of the similar structure hypothesis. *Psychological Bulletin, 100,* 157–175. doi:10.1037/0033-2909.100.2.157.

Weisz, J. R., & Yeates, K. O. (1981). Cognitive development in retarded and nonretarded persons: Piagetian tests of the similar structure hypothesis. *Psychological Bulletin, 90,* 153–178.

Weisz, J. R., Yeates, K. O., & Zigler, E. (1982). Piagetian evidence and the developmental-difference controversy. In E. Zigler, & D. A. Balla (Eds.), *Mental retardation, the developmental-difference controversy* (pp. 213–269). Hillsdale, New Jersey: Lawrence Erlbaum Associates Inc.

Weisz, J. R., & Zigler, E. (1979). Cognitive development in retarded and nonretarded persons: Piagetian tests of the similar sequence hypothesis. *Psychological Bulletin, 86,* 831–851. doi:10.1037/0033-2909.86.4.831.

Werner, H. (1948). *Comparative psychology of mental development* (2nd ed.). Chicago: Follett.

Zebrowitz, L. A. (1997). *Reading faces: Window to the soul?* Boulder, CO: Westview Press.

Zigler, E. (1967). Familial mental retardation: A continuing dilemma. *Science, 155,* 292–298. doi:10.1126/science.155.3760.292.

Zigler, E. (1969). Developmental versus difference theories of mental retardation and the problem of motivation. *American Journal of Mental Deficiency, 73,* 536–556.

Zigler, E. (1970). The environmental mystique: Training the intellect versus development of the child. *Childhood Education, 46,* 402–412.

Zigler, E., & Balla, D. (1982). Selecting outcome variables in evaluation of early childhood special education programs. *Topics in Early Childhood Special Education, 1,* 1–22. doi:10.1177/027112148200100406.

Zigler, E., & Hodapp, R. (1986). *Understanding Mental Retardation.* New York: Cambridge University Press.

INDEX

Note: Page numbers followed by "*f*" and "*t*" denote figures and tables, respectively.

ERPs. *See* event-related potentials
etiology, 25
etiology-related trajectories and
      profiles, 398
event-related potentials (ERPs), 37, 45,
      47–48, 94, 149
   DS and, 151–53
   FXS and, 158
   PWS and, 154
   WS and, 155–57
evolutionary developmental psychology,
      371, 375
executive function (EF), 8
   cognitive-behavioral interventions and,
      248
   defining, 125
   in DS, 128, 129–32
   experimental tracking of development
      of, 127–28
   in FXS, 128, 132–33
   in ID, 128–29
   organization of, 126
   PFC and, 126–27
   in PKU, 128, 133–34
   in PWS, 128, 134
   in typically developing children,
      126–28
   WCST and, 125, 127–28
   working memory and, 117–19
explicit memory, 98
   verbal, 99–100
   visual-spatial, 100–101
exploration, 90, 90*f*
   visual, 91
expressive language development
   auditory-verbal working memory
      deficits and, 176
   DS and, 168, 170–73, 191–92
   joint attention and, 320
   literacy development and, 191–92
   studies of, 168, 170–73
   WS and, 328
expressive pragmatics, 171–73
expressive syntax, DS and acquisition of,
      171
expressive vocabulary
   in DS, 168, 170
   in WS, 223
Expressive Vocabulary Test (EVT),
      223, 228
externalizing behavior, in DS, 256
eye gaze
   aversion of, 259, 267, 398
   in DS, 255
   in typically developing children, 255
   WS and long, 327

F

face inversion effect, 70, 71
facial processing, emotion recognition
      and, 240
facial recognition, WS and, 326–28
familial intellectual disabilities, 395–96

familial mental retardation, 14–17, 16*t*,
      23, 395
   polygenic inheritance of, 20–22
families
   child characteristic-related stress in, 368
   child psychopathology and stress
      in, 369
   direct and indirect effects of, 9
   ID and functioning of, 366–67
   impact of launching on, 383–84
   life course perspective on, 380–81
   life cycle stages of, 382
   uncertain diagnosis and stress in, 370
family-centered support programs, 361
family-focused programs, 360
family pedigree, 25
family quality of life, 309
family studies, 25
family unit, 309
F-COPES, 313, 368
fetal alcohol syndrome, 102
5p syndrome, 369
FMR1. *See* fragile X mental retardation
      1 gene
fMRI. *See* functional magnetic resonance
      imaging
FMRP. *See* fragile X mental retardation
      protein
fragile X mental retardation 1 gene
      (FMR1), 46–48, 158–59, 207
   language development and, 210
fragile X mental retardation protein
      (FMRP), 43–44, 46–48, 132, 207
   cognition and level of, 49–50
   language development variations and
      levels of, 210
fragile X syndrome (FXS), 7, 8, 9, 25,
      35, 257
   ADHD and, 50–51
   ASD and, 50–52, 209–10, 258, 267,
      275, 277–78, 277*t*, 290, 397
   attention and, 37, 89–90, 92*t*, 93–94
   behavioral phenotype of, 212
   behavioral problems in, 50–52
   brain development and
      psychophysiology in, 258–59
   brain level, 47–48
   CdLS *vs.*, 279–80
   cognitive level, 48–49
   cross-cultural differences and, 52
   cross-syndrome comparisons with,
      52–53
   dendritic spine abnormalities in, 44, 47
   depression in, 211
   DS *vs.*, 52–53, 240
   EF in, 128, 132–33
   emotional development in, 258
   emotional expression in, 244
   emotion recognition and understanding
      and, 240, 242
   emotion regulation in, 246–47
   environmental contributions in,
      210–11

ERP studies of, 158
family stress and, 368, 369
future research avenues for, 52–53
gaze aversion in, 259, 267, 398
genetic and cellular level, 46–47
genetic disruption in, 43–44
HPA in, 259
hyperarousal in, 258, 259, 267
inhibition in, 132
language development and, 200, 210
language learning and use in, 202
life course family caregiving and, 386
linguistic phenotype of
   gender differences in, 207–9
   morphosyntax, 203–5, 212
   pragmatics, 205–7
   transition into language, 202
   vocabulary, 202–3
   within-syndrome variation in,
      207–10
mental retardation in, 48
MLU in, 204
MRI studies of, 158–59
musical ability and, 138, 143
neuroconstructivist approach and, 44
parent-child interactions in, 212
pragmatics and, 45, 205–9
receptive language and, 203
set-shifting in, 132–33
shyness in, 255, 258, 397
social and behavioral development in,
      258
speech fluency and, 45
temperament in, 258
theory of mind and, 278
uncertainty period for diagnosis of, 370
vocabulary and, 202–3
WS *vs.*, 52
fragile X tremor and ataxia syndrome
      (FXTAS), 49–50
Friedrich Questionnaire on Resources and
      Stress, 307
functional dissociations, 98
functional magnetic resonance imaging
      (fMRI), 46–49, 81, 93–94,
      139, 151
   comparison group issues for, 159–60
   DS and, 153
   FXS and, 159
   social cognition and, 157
   WS and, 157
FXS. *See* fragile X syndrome
FXTAS. *See* fragile X tremor and ataxia
      syndrome

G

Gage, Phineas, 125
gamete, 25
GARS. *See* Gilliam Autism Rating Scale
gaze aversion, 259, 267, 398
GCE. *See* group common environment
generalized attention deficit, 89
genetic modularity, 32